Skin Stress Response Pathways

Georg T. Wondrak
Editor

Skin Stress Response Pathways

Environmental Factors and Molecular Opportunities

Springer

Editor
Georg T. Wondrak
Department of Pharmacology
and Toxicology
College of Pharmacy & The University
of Arizona Cancer Center
University of Arizona
Tucson, AZ
USA

ISBN 978-3-319-43155-0 ISBN 978-3-319-43157-4 (eBook)
DOI 10.1007/978-3-319-43157-4

Library of Congress Control Number: 2016946320

Printed on acid-free paper

This Springer imprint is published by Springer Nature
The registered company is Springer International Publishing AG Switzerland

Preface

If the skin were parchment and the blows you gave were ink,
Your own handwriting would tell you what I think.

(William Shakespeare, *The Comedy of Errors*)

It is now understood that the interplay between environmental exposure and cellular stress response pathways plays a critical role in skin structure and function, and a refined mechanistic understanding of this phenomenon at the molecular level promises to open novel avenues for targeted therapeutic strategies that may benefit skin health of patients in the near future. The comprehensive coverage of cutaneous cell stress response pathways as presented for the first time in this book is intended to provide a state-of-the-art perspective that is of interest to both basic researchers focusing on fundamental skin biology in the context of environmental exposure as well as translational biomedical health care professionals.

With the completion of this project, I would like to express my gratitude to those who were instrumental in its creation. First and foremost, I would like to thank my co-authors from four continents who have graciously contributed their talent and time to assemble this first in a kind perspective on skin stress response pathways. Second, I am indebted to my department head Walt Klimecki for allowing me to pursue this project. Moreover, I am grateful for this outstanding opportunity and the expert support provided by Melania Ruiz and Ilse Hensen-Kooijman at Springer Science+Business Media B.V.

Finally, I would like to thank my family, Claudia, Gil, Philip, and Annie, for letting me divert precious time and energy from them in pursuit of this book project.

Tucson
June 2016

Georg T. Wondrak

Contents

Chapter 1
The Skin Lipidome Under Environmental Stress—Technological Platforms, Molecular Pathways and Translational Opportunities

Florian Gruber

Abstract The skin is an organ with a high level of lipid metabolism and is divided into regions with very differing lipid composition. Skin lipids determine the barrier function of the skin but are also important signaling mediators. Environmental stressors can modify lipid composition, reactivity and distribution and thereby influence skin biology. In the last decade the technology to investigate the lipids made explosive progress, allowing now for in-depth investigation of the role of lipids in skin biology. In this chapter the current developments in lipidomic analysis of environmental skin stress and the translational opportunities of this technology are discussed.

Keywords Oxidized lipids · Lipidomic · Mass spectrometry · Redox · Stress · Eicosanoids · Reactive oxygen species · Ultraviolet · Skin · Keratinocyte · Fibroblast · Phospholipids

1.1 Introduction

Redox biologists, (bio-) chemists, skin researchers, physicians—we are all usually not trained to deal with the *big data* from the inflationary—*omics* approaches that pour in over us. As soon as we have accepted that such projects are interdisciplinary, require adequate statistics, that they often are exploratory and hypothesis generating—then the benefits of such approaches become accessible. We learn to use the huge potential of lipidomic/metabolomic—*postgenomic*—data formats that

F. Gruber (✉)
Department of Dermatology, Division for Biology and Pathobiology of the Skin and Christian Doppler Laboratory for the Biotechnology of Skin Aging, Medical University of Vienna, Währinger Gürtel 18-20, 1090 Vienna, Austria
e-mail: florian.gruber@meduniwien.ac.at

G.T. Wondrak (ed.), *Skin Stress Response Pathways*,
DOI 10.1007/978-3-319-43157-4_1

do not adhere to the familiar linear information format provided under the central dogma of molecular biology (DNA-RNAs-protein).

The ultimate aim of lipidomic analyses of the skin, its cells or the subcellular structures like membrane subdomains is to identify those compounds, networks, pathways, physical forces, and interactions that keep the skin functioning in a hostile, changing milieu. In this chapter I will review, from the viewpoint of a molecular biologist of the skin, what has been learned by lipidomic approaches about how environmental stress affect the skin's lipids in their function as signaling mediators or structural molecules, and what translational potential such technology may yield.

1.1.1 *Lipids of the Skin—Distribution of Stress Accessible Lipid Classes*

The skin displays an active and diverse lipid metabolism, and lipids are essential for the barrier—and signaling functions of this organ (Feingold and Elias 2014; van Smeden et al. 2014b; Kendall et al. 2015). Any disturbance of lipid homeostasis by environmental stressors thus may result in impairment of these functions, and may cause disease or accelerated aging. The most common stressor the skin is exposed to and affects the lipids is sunlight, with very distinct effects on skin biology that are governed by wavelength and penetration depth. But also physical, chemical or biological stress can affect the cutaneous biology by changing lipid composition or structure (Fig. 1.1).

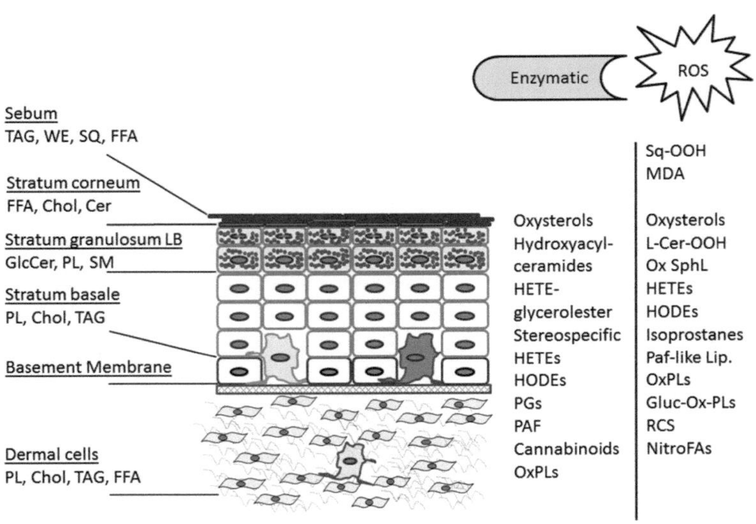

Fig. 1.1 Lipids of the skin

Environmental stressors affect lipids of the skin from its surface down to the dermis, which houses fibroblasts, epithelial structures of the hair follicle, nerve cells, microvasculature, dermal resident cells of the immune system and—depending on stimulation—infiltrating immune cells. The cells but also the dermal matrix gives evidence on stress related changes to lipids, as reactive carbonyls that originate from lipid peroxidation are detectable throughout the epidermis and can crosslink collagen and elastic fibers in the dermis (Larroque-Cardoso et al. 2015; Williams et al. 2014).

The lipid composition of the cells residing in the dermis (excluding the hair follicle and sebaceous gland) is very rich (75 %) in phosphatidylcholine (PC) and phosphatidylethanolamine (PE) phospholipids (PL), with low amounts of triglycerides, cholesterol, free fatty acids (FFA) and the other classes. The basement membrane separates the dermis from the epidermis, made up mostly of keratinocytes (KC) in various grades of terminal differentiation, and epidermal lipid preparations will mostly reflect KC lipids.

The lipid composition within the differentiating epidermis changes in a highly dynamic process, as on the one hand KC in the basal layer take up lipids (most polyunsaturated fatty acids) from the circulation and the microenvironment. On the other hand lipids inside vesicles and as part of vesicle membranes are transferred intracellularly for major metabolic conversion, and finally relocate to the extracellular lipid matrix or to the lipid envelope of terminally differentiated keratinocytes (corneocytes). Lipid content of keratinocytes in the basal layer of the epidermis (and in cultured cells) is made up mostly of phospholipids (70 %), cholesterol (13 %), triacylglycerides (11 %) (Ponec et al. 1988). Upon terminal differentiation there are drastic changes to the lipid composition. In the lamellar bodies (LB) of the granular layer KC glucosylceramides (GlcCERs), phospholipids and sphingomyelin are stored. These are substrates for the enzymes that catalyze the final stratum corneum lipids. The LB content is released by exocytose together with these enzymes beyond the SG and forms the low permeable and flexible connection (lipid matrix) between the rigid corneocytes which are themselves surrounded by the "lipid envelope" of hydroxylated ceramides that are esterified to involucrin by transglutaminase. The composition of stratum corneum lipids is dominated by FFA (40 %), cholesterol and ceramides (both 30 %) (Thakoersing et al. 2012). The FFA are mostly saturated in the SC, and are rather long-chained with C18, C24 and C26 being the dominant ones. The composition was determined first by GC-MS and could recently be confirmed with novel methodology that also detects other lipid species at the same time (see below, van Smeden et al. 2014a).

The lipids at the skin's surface have however a second major source, the sebaceous glands. The lipids synthesized in these glands consist mainly of triglycerides (45 %, TAG), wax esters, (25 %, WE), squalene (12 %), and FFA (10 %). How much sebum contributes to the total surface lipids depends on the body site, the abundance and activity of the sebaceous glands.

1.2 Lipidomic Methods to Analyze One or More Lipid Classes

Recently, a broad consensus was found by the lipid researchers organized in the lipid MAPS community, on a common systematic nomenclature of lipids, grouping them into eight categories (fatty acyls, glycerolipids, glycerophospholipids, sphingolipids, sterol lipids, prenol lipids, saccharolipids, and polyketides) based on their chemical properties (Fahy et al. 2005). Due to the differences in hydrophobicity, polarity, molecule size, quantitative isolation procedures and other aspects, it is technically difficult, and until recently regarded too complex to analyze in depth with lipidomics several lipid classes at one time. However, in the last decade the field made remarkable progress regarding sensitivity, accuracy and in data processing. The classical thin layer chromatography analysis is still a useful standard to identify major changes in lipid classes, but the selectivity of mass spectrometry (MS), and the possibility to couple it with numerous separation methods makes MS todays gold standard for identification and quantification of lipids, also in skin research.

MS analysis requires ionization of the analytes, which is usually achieved by electrospray ionization (ESI), matrix-assisted laser desorption ionization (MALDI) or atmospheric pressure chemical ionization (APCI). The sample can be injected without or with prior separation, and the unseparated direct infusion approach, usually termed "shotgun lipidomics" usually utilizes a triple quadrupole analyzer to scan precursor ions and neutral loss. The data generated this way usually base on lipid class specific fragments (e.g. Phosphocholine) but do not permit interpretation of the individual FA composition but rather the sum of fatty acyl carbons. However, quantification of analytes can be more robust as direct infusion is not subject to quantitative bias brought in by chromatographic separation.

Chromatographic separation prior to MS makes the analysis of some complex lipid classes possible because it adds retention time as a parameter that boosts the method's specificity. After the separation and ionization, several detection modes are applicable. For fingerprinting the intact molecular adduct ions can be scanned (single ion monitoring—MS), the advent of triple quadrupole devices then allowed to use one of the quadrupoles to be used as a collision cell between two mass resolving quadrupole units. After passing the first quadrupole (Q1), the precursor ions are collided in the second quadrupole with an inert gas and there noncovalent bonds dissociate (neutral loss, NL) or at higher collision energy the precursors are fragmented. The fragmented product ions are then detected with the third quadrupole (Q3) as mass analyzer at high frequency, in either of various modes: Product ion scan, where for a given precursor in Q1 the fragments are scanned in Q3, or the reverse, precursor ion scan, where for a specific fragment the precursors are scanned, or in multiple reaction monitoring (MRM) mode, where a number of preselected *m/z* pairs (targeted approach) are detected by the quadrupoles.

The sensitivity and mass resolution of MS/MS was multiplied by several technologies that emerged in the last decade. First, hybrid mass spectrometers that combine a quadrupole mass analyzer with a time of flight (TOF) device, which allow a higher scan rate and mass accuracy. The latest generation detectors are equipped with orbitrap or linear ion trap devices combined to TOF or Fourier transform ion cyclotron resonance—MS. These, together with novel separation techniques like ultra-performance HPLC, and hydrophilic interaction liquid chromatography (HILIC), and ion mobility detection, provide the accuracy needed for the structural identification in some approaches described below. MALDI-TOF, which cannot be coupled to chromatography, is not nearly as frequently used for (skin) lipidomics, but combining it with TLC may be very useful. For in-depth reviews on the technological platforms, application fields, biological settings and data processing for lipidomic research and identification strategies the reader is referred to Murphy and Gaskell (2011), Brügger (2014), Cajka and Fiehn (2014), Köfeler et al. (2012), Lam and Shui (2013), Serhan et al. (2007)—a list without claim to completeness.

The various variants of liquid chromatography coupled to MS, followed by direct infusion MS are the overwhelmingly dominant methods for lipidomic analysis in life sciences over the last years (Cajka and Fiehn 2014), and below I provide a collection of state of the art technical approaches that have been undertaken in the skin lipidomic field or at least would be applicable to study stress related changes in the skin lipidome.

1.2.1 Fatty Acyls (Fatty Acids, Eicosanoids, Endocannabinoids)

An early lipidomic study of eicosanoids in mouse skin utilized GC/MS of eicosanoid derivatives to identify and quantify the major lipoxygenase products of arachidonic and linoleic acid in mouse epidermis (Lehmann et al. 1992). Also more recent studies show that with high-temperature gas chromatography coupled to electron impact or chemical ionization MS large numbers of compounds including fatty acids, eicosanoids but also other skin surface lipids can be identified in one analytical run (Michael-Jubeli et al. 2011). Most of the recent analyses of fatty acyls, including eicosanoids are performed by ESI-MS/MS coupled to high or ultra-performance HPLC (rev. in Astarita et al. 2015). For the detection of potentially beneficial resolvins and other DHA derived mediators Hong et al. applied LC–ultraviolet spectrometer–tandem MS; the UV absorption data added information about conjugated di-ene arrangement in the species (Hong et al. 2005). A method to identify positional isomers in FA by Yang et al. used charge switching derivatization and MS/MS (Yang et al. 2013). A current standard method to analyze endocannabinoids inserts a lipid fractionation step on silica gel before RP-LC coupled to ESI-MS (Astarita and Piomelli 2009). Chlorinated fatty acids were analyzed in detail by TLC combined with ESI-MS (Schroter et al. 2015) and nitrated and nitro-oxidized fatty acids with a targeted high resolution LC-MS/MS method (Milic et al. 2015). The lipidomic analyses of PUFA derived bioactive lipids were reviewed by Massey and Nicolaou (2011).

1.2.2 Glycerolipids (Tri- and, Di-Acylglycerols)

Canine skin glycerolipids and ceramides were analyzed with HP-TLC, and partially bands (could be identified via a TLC-MS interface (Angelbeck-Schulze et al. 2014). A more comprehensive method to identify and quantify TAG and DAG of murine skin was recently presented by King et al. (2015) where an ESI-MS/MS—neutral loss (NL) scan approach was successful in identifying and quantifying most relevant acylglycerol species, and found that dietary restriction and exercise reduces skin TG species containing 18:1 fatty acid chains.

1.2.3 Glycerophospholipids (PC, PE, PI, PS, PG, PA, Cardiolipin)

On the lipidomic analysis of the phospholipid species several excellent reviews have been recently published (Spickett and Pitt 2015; O'Donnell 2011), which reflect that as broad standard HPLC-ESI-MS/MS is used for identification and quantification of phospholipid (PL) species, native or oxidized. The high end laboratories introduced high resolution equipment including q-TOF, spin trapping, orbitrap and FT-IR-MS in combination with high performance columns for PL analysis (Sala et al. 2015), also very recently for nitrated PL (Melo et al. 2016) and for glycated and glycoxidized PLs (Simoes et al. 2012). The generated big data are used for smart scanning approaches that facilitate lipid identification (Simons et al. 2012). Chlorinated phospholipids have been detected by also by MALDI-TOF approaches (Panasenko et al. 2007) and TLC-ESI-MS (Schroter et al. 2015). Cardiolipin analysis with HILIC-MC/MS together with phosphatidylglycerol (PG) and phosphatidic acid (PA) species is described by Scherer et al. (2010), and a recent review on the topic by Tyurina et al. (2014) is recommended.

1.2.4 Sphingolipids (Sphingomyelin, Sulfatides, Sphingosine, Ceramides, Gangliosides)

Ceramides (Cer) and sphingomyelin (SM) species have been profiled in mouse epidermis at various prenatal developmental stages with HPLC-MS/MS using a triple-quadrupole mass spectrometer operated in positive mode and ultrahigh-pressure LC coupled with hybrid quadrupole TOF mass spectrometer by

Wang et al. (2013). For structural identification of non-hydroxyacyl epidermal ceramides Shin et al. applied chip-based direct infusion nanoelectrospray-ion trap mass spectrometry, generating characteristic fragmentation patterns of acyl and sphingoid units that allow identification of numerous compounds (Shin et al. 2014). A more complex approach by van Smeden et al. that utilized LC/MS/MS with an ion trap (IT) system, a Fourier transform-ion cyclotron resonance system, and a triple quadrupole system, which did not only detect all 11 known subclasses of ceramides but identified the presence of other lipid subclasses using a 3D multi mass chromatogram [12]. More than 300 Cer species in 11 known and one unknown class were detected with a NPLC-ESI-MS/MS method (Masukawa et al. 2009). With reversed-phase LC coupled to high-resolution quadrupole time-of-flight MS operated in both positive and negative ESI mode T'Kindt et al. detected that Cer species display skeletal isomers due to varying length of the sphingoid and FA components (t'Kindt et al. 2012). The effect of sphingoid bases on the sphingolipidome of differentiating KC was investigated using HPLC ESI-MS/MS (Sigruener et al. 2013). To specifically investigate phosphorylated ceramides very recently a method including phosphate tagging and MALDI-MS was introduced for skin and other tissues (Yamashita et al. 2016). Gangliosides were quantified in skin fibroblasts from gangliosidosis patients with RP-LC-ESI-MS/MS in MRM mode (Fuller et al. 2014).

1.2.5 Sterol Lipids

Cholesterol hydroperoxides were quantified and identified with TLC coupled to GC-MS(SIM) in mouse fibroblasts (Nakamura et al. 2013), and cholesterol esters (CE) from epidermis of fetal, adult and keloid skin were investigated with silica gel purification followed by chemical ionization and MS (Tachi and Iwamori 2008).

1.2.6 Prenol Lipids

Today's standard method to quantify squalene in biological samples is GC-MS (Hall et al. 2016), also applicable for squalene analysis in hair (Wu et al. 2016). The in vitro non-volatile ozonolysis products of squalene were analyzed by ESI-high resolution MS (Fooshee et al. 2015).

As there is yet no literature available to the author on the lipidomic study of saccharolipids and polyketides as metabolites deriving from skin itself, these classes will not be dealt with in this chapter.

1.2.7 Methods for Several Lipid Classes

High resolution and mass accuracy detectors allow to cover wide ranges of lipid classes in single experiments: UPLC-ESI-MS (+ and- mode) analysis of 11 of the major lipid subclasses [FA, cholesterolsulfates, PA, PE, PS, PC, phosphatidyl glycerols (PG), Cers, SM, diacylglycerols (DG), triacylglycerols (TG)] was performed. A combination of TOF and triple quadrupole MS following LC was applied to comprehensively study non-invasively sampled sebaceous lipids (Camera et al. 2010). Using a non-targeted approach that first creates a data base with retention time (tR) values, equivalent of carbon numbers (ECN) for each lipid class, and then a MS/MS fragmentation pattern, Lanzini and colleagues could perform structure assignments within each analyzed subclass of skin lipids. For that they utilized LIPID MAPS and METLIN data with high mass accuracy (5 ppm tolerance), a lipid class specific relation between equivalent number of carbon (ECN) and retention time, and MS/MS fragmentation patterns. By that they could identify over 100 lipids of different classes (Lanzini et al. 2015). van Smeden et al. describe a dual injection method with RPLC–negative ion mode APCI-MS (for detection of FFA) and NPLC-Positive ion mode APCI-MS (to detect Cer and Chol) which was also very useful for analysis of a broader range of SC lipids in one step (van Smeden et al. 2014a).

1.2.8 Lipid Organization

Organization of lipids in the lamellae between the corneocytes (lateral organization) can be analyzed by Fourier transform infrared spectroscopy (FTIR), electron diffraction and wide- and small angle X-ray diffraction (WAXD/SAXD). The localization of ceramides, cholesterol and fatty acids in the lipid matrix was also studied with neutron diffraction analysis (Mojumdar et al. 2015). Barrier function impairment can also be caused by changes in the lateral lipid organization (van Smeden et al. 2014b). A recent review summarizes the methodologies to study lipid organization in stratum corneum function (Wertz 2013).

1.2.9 Lipid Imaging

Using the specificity of MS together with an imaging technique for tissues or even cells to determine the distribution of lipids is another technical breakthrough with potential. The ionization methods applied for that approach include positively charged fullerenes (C60) with secondary ion MS (SIMS) (Kurczy et al. 2010), and MALDI which was successfully used to impressively image lipids in total skin

(Hart et al. 2011) or cholesterol sulphate (Enthaler et al. 2013) and phospholipids (Patterson et al. 2014) in sections.

1.3 How Stressors Affect the Lipidome

Extracellular stress can affect the cutaneous lipid composition (and—ordering) directly or indirectly. The most prominent stressor—ultraviolet light—can directly generate reactive oxygen species (ROS) within the tissue down to the dermal compartment, which are capable of modifying lipids, as is contact to topical reactive chemicals. At the same time, stressors may induce rapid intracellular lipid modifying cascades, as the enzymatic production of lipid mediators from stored precursors, or de novo synthesis of variant lipid species, or they set free intracellular reactive oxygen—or nitrogen—species that again act non-enzymatically on lipids. In the longer run, as reaction to stress, cells of the immune system can be directed to the skin, and secrete novel lipid mediator classes or oxidize lipids in their microenvironment by releasing ROS, as in the respiratory burst. And on an even larger time scale, cells of the skin can photo age or become senescent after chemotherapy, both resulting in changed cellular redox state, damaged mitochondria and resulting in changes to intracellular and secreted lipids. Last, when stress leads to cell death, the dying cell may expose special modified lipid moieties from its membrane that act as danger signals to the immune system and neighboring cells.

1.3.1 Stress Induced Enzymatic Pathways that Affect the Lipidome

Most of the research on ultraviolet induced bioactive lipid generation via enzymatic pathways was done on eicosanoid synthesis by the actions of phospholipases, cyclooxygenases and lipoxygenases, and a review by Nicolaou and colleagues systematically deals with synthesis and action of these and other enzymatically generated mediators (Nicolaou et al. 2011). Below listed are the most prominent lipid metabolizing enzymes that are UV-regulated.

1.3.1.1 Phospholipase A2 (PLA2) and Other Phospholipases

Phospholipase A2 (PLA2) hydrolyzes fatty acids from the *sn*-2 position of phospholipids. Phospholipase activity in mammalian epidermis after UV was first described by Black and Anglin (1971) and later studies detected phospholipase activation after UVB (DeLeo et al. 1988) and UVA (Hanson and DeLeo 1990) exposure of keratinocytes. Pentlands group identified that cytosolic PLA2 (cPLA2,

PLA2G4A) induced by secondary oxidative stress after UVB was responsible for the immediate increase in E type prostaglandins (Gresham et al. 1996; Chen et al. 1996). In epidermis cPLA2 and the secreted sPLA2 are the main enzymes for eicosanoid production in homeostasis and to maintain barrier function. These enzymes are regulated in inflammation but also by UV, reviewed in Dan et al. (2012), Ilic et al. (2014). Lipidomic analyses upon selective PLA2 inhibition identified novel substrates and metabolites (Duvernay et al. 2015), which has yet to be done for epidermal PLAs. In addition to PLA2, also PLC and PLD, both generating 1,2 diacylglycerols (DAG) out of phospholipids, were activated by UVR (broadband) in mouse transformed melanocytes and fibroblasts and human keratinocytes and melanocytes, where these lipids may contribute to pigment production (Carsberg et al. 1995).

1.3.1.2 Cyclooxygenases and Prostaglandin Synthases

The free fatty acids (e.g. those set free by UV induced PLA2) can be metabolized to further bioactive products by enzymes of which several are also stress regulated. In keratinocytes, Cyclooxygenase-2 (COX-2, PTGS2) induction by UV was observed in first in guinea pig (KC differentiation dependent), where it induced five prostaglandin species (Karmali and Safai 1984). COX-2 is also induced by H_2O_2 and by PMA in mouse skin (Nakamura et al. 2003). COX-2 catalyzes the oxidation of PGH2 out of AA, but also utilizes other unsaturated fatty acids as substrates. Further, COX-2 can oxygenate endocannabinoids like anandamide to prostamides (PG-EAs). Using PGH2 as substrate, UV induced prostaglandin synthases form PGD and PGEs which were quantified with lipidomics (Black et al. 2008). Prostaglandin E synthase is induced in human skin after UV and heat stress (Weinkauf et al. 2012).

1.3.1.3 Lipoxygenases

Lipoxygenases synthesize oxygenated products from unsaturated fatty acids but also from complex lipids, and give rise to many important signaling mediators (HETEs and HODEs) but also structural lipid species of the skin (hydroxyacyl ceramides of the cornified lipid envelope), reviewed in Krieg and Furstenberger (2014). In HaCaT keratinocytes a UV mediated switch in the lipoxygenase activities from 12-LOX to 15-LOX. 15-LOX1 metabolizes LA to 13-HODE, whereas 15-Lox2 AA to 15-HETE. 12-LOX was decreased by UVB 100–300 and UVA 10–30. The UV-induced switch in LOX activity was enhanced by 15-LOX metabolites which inhibited 12-LOX expression when added to the medium (Yoo et al. 2008). 12-LOX can produce 12-Hete Glycerol Ester (GE) from the endocannabinoid anandamide (Kozak et al. 2002).

1.3.1.4 Peroxiredoxins

Peroxiredoxins (PRDX1) is UV inducible and have documented photo-protective activity, and PRDX6 has PLA2 and PL-OOH reductase-, and newly described also lysophosphocholine acyltransferase (LPCAT) (Fisher et al. 2016; Fisher 2011) activities that affect OxPL levels and is important in skin chemical stress response, carcinogenesis and wound healing (Rolfs et al. 2013).

1.3.1.5 PAF Acetyltransferase and PAF Hydrolase

PAF and PAF like lipids are inflammatory mediators important in skin inflammation associated with UV and oxidative stress (Barber et al. 1998; Travers 1999). Whereas PAF can be generated in keratinocytes nonenzymatically upon UV (see below), PAF can be formed also by PAF acetyltransferase metabolizing the LysoPC generated by PLA2. PAF acetylhydrolase, the enzyme degrading PAF translocates to the cell membrane after UVB irradiation (Marques et al. 2002).

1.3.1.6 Other UV/Chemical Stress Regulated Lipid Metabolizing Enzymes

Cytochrome oxidases can produce eicosanoids from PUFA and endocannabinoids, and Cyp1B1 (Villard et al. 2002), CYP4A11 (Villard et al. 2002) are inducible by UVB. P450 family enzymes can also induce oxysterol generation from cholesterol (Jusakul et al. 2011). Keratinocyte ATP binding casette transporters important for epidermal lipid transport were differentially regulated by UVB (Marko et al. 2012). UV inducible glutathione peroxidases (GPx) detoxify lipid hydroperoxides (Girotti and Kriska 2004). Leukotriene A4 hydrolase, together with COX-2, mPGES-2, PGDS, 5-LOX are regulated by sulphur mustard (Black et al. 2010). UVB reduces ceramidase activity, but also a ceramide mediated pro apoptotic effect was observed after high doses of UVB (Uchida et al. 2010).

1.3.2 Non-enzymatic Pathways that Affect the Skin Lipidome

Free radicals (molecules with a single unpaired electron) are produced in normal cell metabolism. When mitochondria are damaged and the electron transport into the respiratory chain is impaired, superoxide anion is formed (and not further processed) by one-electron reduction of oxygen. O_2^- is also physiologically produced by, e.g. NADPH oxidases to load the phagocytic vacuole.

Superoxide anion can promote LDL (and phospholipid-) oxidation in various cell types including skin fibroblasts (Steinbrecher 1988). Superoxide is rapidly converted to H_2O_2 and O_2 by abundant superoxide dismutases.

Hydrogen peroxide is not a free radical and quite stable, but rapidly destroyed by antioxidants like catalase or glutathione peroxidase. It can react with thiols and reduced transition metals and can influence activity of metal containing enzymes. Low concentrations of H_2O_2 activate cyclooxygenases and lipoxygenases (Forman 2010), catalyzing lipid modifications. Catalase reduces H_2O_2 to O_2 and H_2O, when H_2O_2 levels are high, Glutathione peroxidase (GPx) is more important to detoxify H_2O_2 with reduced glutathione, which upon oxidation is reduced back using NADPH. However, H_2O_2 can be cleaved hemolytically by UV radiation to give rise to hydroxyl radicals ($^{\cdot}OH$), and in the presence of redox metal ions it gives rise to hydroxyl radicals in the Fenton reaction.

Hydroxyl radical is the most reactive species and reacts almost unselectively with most compounds. Lipid peroxidation chain reaction starts most effectively with hydrogen abstraction by hydroxyl radical. Lipid peroxidation generates lipid peroxy radicals ($LOO^{\cdot}$) which abstract hydrogen from another lipid molecule generating LOOH and another carbon centered lipid radical, and this continues unless chain terminated by e.g. phenolic antioxidants. Recently a role for hydroxyl radical in sphingolipid modification was demonstrated using lipidomics (Couto et al. 2015).

Molecular Oxygen O_2 is not a free radical but reacts rapidly with radicals. A non-radical ROS is the long wave UV (UVA) photo-excited singlet oxygen $^1O_2$ which has two paired electrons in the same orbital, leaving an empty orbital for reactivity. It reacts rapidly with histidine and cysteinyls in proteins, with lipids (PUFA phospholipids, cholesterol and others) and nucleic acids. Interestingly $^1O_2$ is also formed during the UVA irradiation of polyunsaturated fatty acids in free and esterified form (Baier et al. 2008).

NO radical and superoxide anion can form peroxynitrite ($ONOO^-$) and the much more reactive protonated peroxinitrous acid can oxidize unsaturated fatty acids in biological membranes to form nitrated fatty acids that have biological activity and damages DNA (8OHdG, 8 nitroguanine). Also $^{\cdot}NO_2$ can react with unsaturated lipids yielding e.g. nitrohydroxy derivatives (Rubbo et al. 2009; Trostchansky et al. 2011). ONOOH can be reduced by GPx and PRDX.

Hypochlorous acid (HOCl, bleach) is formed by myeloperoxidase/H_2O_2 dependent oxidation of Cl^- anion. HOCl can form chlorohydrin derivatives of lipids but obviously also more complex modifications (Schroter et al. 2015).

Chemotherapy using Doxorubicin, *cis*-platin or bleomycin, quinones and the use of photosensitizers result in generation of ROS which then may affect skin lipid oxidation. The more unsaturated the free or esterified fatty acids is, the more prone to oxidation they are, but also the head groups of e.g. phosphatidylethanolamines are subject to ROS mediated modification.

1.4 Stress Generated Lipid Modifications and Bioactive Lipid Mediators

1.4.1 Fatty Acyls Derived Bioactive Lipids

1.4.1.1 EICOSANOIDS

In a study combining several analytic approaches, the GC-TOF-MS analysis of mouse liver lipids revealed significantly increased un-oxidized linoleic and palmitic—but decreased elaidic acid 6 weeks after UVB irradiation (Park et al. 2014). Black et al. studied UVB induced changes in prostaglandin levels of mouse keratinocytes with HPLC of derivatized PGs using a UV detector, and found increased PGE(2) and PGJ (2) levels, while PGD(2) decreased after 24 h (Black et al. 2008). Using microdialysis to isolate dermal interstitial fluid Grundmann et al. identified eicosanoids generated in the first 5 h and 24 h post UVB irradiation with GC-MS (Grundmann et al. 2004) and found several hydroxyeicosatetraeonic acids (HETEs), 8-isoPGF2a and other prostanoid lipid species increased, several of them non-enzymatically generated lipid mediators. Rhodes, et al. studied the eicosanoid profiles during the sunburn response of human skin in detail using LC-ESI MS/MS (Rhodes et al. 2009) and show that early erythema was accompanied by vasodilatory PGE2, PGF2a, and PGE3, immediate appearance of 11-, 12-, 8-HETE and a late increase of pro-resolving 15-HETE. Lipidomic analysis of eicosanoids (HPLC-ESI MS/MS negative mode) in chemically (DMBA/phorbolester) induced papillomas identified PGE2 and PGF2a as the most promising candidates and the COX-2 pathway as important factor for tumor progression (Jiao et al. 2014).

The bioactivity of hydroperoxyoctadecadienoic acids, (HODEs; linoleate oxidation products) was investigated with respect to the mechanism of generation by Akazawa-Ogawa et al., and they differentiated singlet oxygen derived, peroxidation products and enzymatic products on their ability to induce Nrf2 (Akazawa-Ogawa et al. 2015). Interestingly, two $^1O_2$ specific HODE isomers (10-HODE and 12-HODE), that had earlier been identified by lipidomic analysis in UVA exposed mouse skin using GC/MS/SIM (single ion monitoring) of trimethylsilyl HODE derivatives(Bando et al. 2004), turned out to be very efficient inducers of Nrf2. 9-HODE which is also formed by radical oxidation and 13-ZE-HODE, a 15-lipoxygenase product, both are peroxisome proliferator activated receptor γ (PPARγ) agonists (Itoh et al. 2008). These lipids were no efficient Nrf2 inducers, nicely showing stereo specificity of HODEs and the importance of how they were generated (Akazawa-Ogawa et al. 2015). The balance between 12-LOX and 15-LOX activity is disturbed in psoriatic keratinocytes (FADS1 and 15-LOX-2 are downregulated, increased 12-HETE leads to hyperproliferation). UV-induced 15-LOX metabolites (Yoo et al. 2008) detected by lipidomics ameliorate the inflammation.

1.4.1.2 Endocannabinoids

N-acylethanolamines (NAE) are strongly increased in necrosis and in ischemic stress, but may function as a cyto-protective response that stabilizes membranes, especially in preventing the mitochondrial permeability transition (Epps et al. 1982) Among the NAE are however also agonists for the endocannabinoid receptors like anandamide, therefore Berdyshev et al. studied generation of NAEs and their precursor N-acyl phosphatidylethanolamines by GC-MS, and found that 18:1 n-9 N-acyl PE and NAE in general were increased after UVB, but levels recovered over time, especially when serum containing media was supplemented (Berdyshev et al. 2000).

1.4.2 Glycerolipids (Tri-, Di-Acylglycerols)

Epidermal samples from UVB irradiated volunteers were analyzed for triacylglycerols TAG (and FFA), and decrease of both observed at 48 and 72 h post irradiation, however no further identification was performed (Kim et al. 2010). In a study combining several analytic approaches, the LTQ-MS analysis of mouse liver lipids revealed significantly decreased triglycerides (56:4) 6 weeks after UVB irradiation (Park et al. 2014).

1.4.3 Glycerophospholipids Derived Bioactive Mediators

1.4.3.1 Phosphatidylethanolamines

In an elegant study Melo et al. identified many UV induced oxidation and glycoxidation products of phosphatidylethanolamine PLs (Melo et al. 2013). The chemical reactivity of glycated PEs was additionally investigated with a spin trapping approach (Simoes et al. 2012) and immuno-modulating activity on monocyte derived cells was subsequently identified for selected glycoxidized compounds (Simoes et al. 2013).

1.4.3.2 Phosphatidylcholines

Our group investigated with HPLC MS/MS in cell culture the generation of oxidation specific lipid species immediately after exposure to physiologic fluences of UVA-1 in fibroblasts. We could identify roughly two hundred fluence dependent induced lipid species (Gruber et al. 2012). One product tentatively identified as epoxy isoprostanoid modification of the arachidonoyl residue by us and others was a strong Nrf2 activator in dermal FB (Gruber et al. 2007). The method was applied to study PL oxidation in autophagy deficient versus wildtype keratinocytes (Zhao et al. 2013) and melanocytes (Zhang et al. 2015), and we found that autophagy deficiency seems to result in impaired OxPL degradation. We detected in murine dendritic cells deficient in 15-lipoxygenase a decrease in PL hydroperoxides (Bluml et al. 2005), which caused excessive DC maturation. Also in vivo, in the epidermis of peroxiredoxin reductase 6 (PRDX6) deficient or transgenic mice (Rolfs et al. 2013) changes in oxPL species could be quantified that suggested a role for PRDX6 in the degradation of oxidized lipids. Some of the lipids we detected as UV-inducible are cytotoxic to melanoma cells (Ramprecht et al. 2015). In a study combining several analytic approaches, the UPLC-Q-TOF-MS analysis mouse hepatic lipids revealed significantly decreased PUFA lysophosphocholines 6 weeks after UVB irradiation (Park et al. 2014). For more advanced, high resolution methods to detect oxidized PC and PE species a recent review by O'Donnell (2011) is highly recommended.

1.4.3.3 PAF-Like Lipids

The Travers group found that UVB induces formation of PAF receptor agonists and PPARγ agonists that derive from 1-alkyl-GPC, and the first PPARγ ligand they could identify with HPLC—tandem MS was 1-hexaydecyl-2-AzPC (Zhang et al. 2005) and C4 PAF analogs with butanoyl and butenoyl moieties esterified to the sn-2 position (Marathe et al. 2005), subsequently they characterized with HPLC-ESI-tandem MS in MRM mode several 1-alkyl but also 1-acyl PAFr agonists (Yao et al. 2012). UVB generated PAF-agonists mediate systemic immunosuppression in a PAF-R and IL10 dependent way, thereby inhibiting antitumor immunity (Sahu et al. 2012)—an important finding based on initial lipidomic study of stressed skin cells. Cigarette smoke exposure is associated with a redox imbalance in keratinocytes, and causes increased formation of carbonyl adducts but also the regulation of keratinocyte lipid scavenger receptors (Sticozzi et al. 2012), but also less reactive lipid mediators are produced, as PAF-like lipids that are immunosuppressive (Sahu et al. 2013). A recent study has highlighted that chemotherapy could limit its own efficacy by generation of PAF-agonistic lipids that reduce antitumor immunity, but that could be inhibited by COX-2 inhibition (Sahu et al. 2014). Similarly, photodynamic therapy, where a photosensitizer is taken up by (pre) malignant cells and makes them susceptible to directed photo toxicity can lead to production of immunosuppressive PAF agonists (Ferracini et al. 2015). Aluminium (for US: aluminum) cytotoxicity in skin fibroblasts caused lipid peroxidation, that was however studied by TBARS only (Anane and Creppy 2001).

1.4.4 *Sphingolipid Changes*

1.4.4.1 Ceramides

Early lipidomic studies found ceramide III and cholesterol sulphate in stratum corneum lipid models to be inert to oxidative stress (Trommer et al. 2003), however a major ceramide transport protein CERT is UV regulated, changing the intracellular ceramide distribution and sphingomyelin production after UVB (Charruyer et al. 2008).

1.4.4.2 Glycosphingolipids

In vitro photo-oxidation of glycosphingolipids was studied with ESI-MS (QTOF) and LC-MS/MS, which allowed in combination to identify novel hydroperoxyl derivatives of galactosyl- and lactosyl ceramides (Santinha et al. 2014). These modifications (if detectable in vivo) likely affect organization and signaling in lipid rafts and sphingolipid signaling under redox stress, as observed Parkinson's disease.

1.4.5 *Bioactive Sterol Lipids*

Yamazaki found UV to induce oxidation of Cholesterol in human skin (Yamazaki et al. 1999), and later study with lipidomic methods has identified three significantly increased ChOOH isomers after 2 h and their ability to induce MMP9 activity was confirmed (Nakamura et al. 2013). Oxysterols can act as pro-inflammatory signaling mediators and are linked to carcinogenesis also as some types are highly reactive, other oxysterols can signal via liver-X-receptor (Jusakul et al. 2011).

1.4.6 *Bioactive Prenol Lipids*

Squalene as a quantitatively prominent skin surface lipid is long known to be UV oxidized, and also found increased after cigarette smoke exposure but a recently developed lipidomic method (QTRAP MS/MS) allowed analyzing the positional isomers of SQ-OOHs on skin after 3 h of sunlight exposure. As Sq-OOH is so prominent can further oxidize to carbonylic malondialdehyde, it is believed to play a role in UV induced lipid peroxidation damage in skin (Nakagawa et al. 2007).

1.5 Translational Applications and Therapeutic Opportunities of Lipidomics

In the last paragraph I will discuss novel ongoing, developing and feasible applications of skin lipidomic technology.

1.5.1 Drug Development Opportunities

COX-2 induction and the metabolites are not only implicated in UV induced inflammation but also in photo carcinogenesis (Elmets et al. 2014) and chemically induced skin cancer (Jiao et al. 2014), so it is feasible that lipidomic analysis may identify carcinogenic metabolites as pharmacological targets for prevention. In a recent review by Lamaziere et al. discuss how lipidomic analysis could be best used to screen chemical libraries for substances that inhibit lipogenesis and have thus potential as anticancer drugs (Lamaziere et al. 2014). Restoration of the 12-HETE to 15-HETE balance in psoriasis may be a treatment option to develop out of lipidomic analysis of psoriasis and UV therapy, which identified lipid mediators that are affected by disease and therapy (Yoo et al. 2008). Novel lipid based approaches to ameliorate diseases with epidermal barrier defects are being initiated recently and would be impossible without the knowledge gained by- and surveillance performed with lipidomic analysis (Elias 2014).

1.5.2 Mechanistic Insights into Disease from Lipidomics

Melanoma—Lipidomics revealed that melanoma cells take up palmitic acid, probably from adjacent adipocytes, ant that may promote melanoma cell growth (Kwan et al. 2014) and autophagy (Jia et al. 2016).

Alopecia—The Foxn1 gene, responsible for the nude phenotype of mice, is another example where lipidomic analysis complemented and widened the classical phenotypical investigations. The alopecia and the epidermal changes (irregular corneocytes, abnormal differentiation, barrier defect) observed in nude mice made can be explained in part by major changes in lipids classes. Cholesterol sulfate is synthesized in the stratum granulosum by cholesterol sulfotransferase and hydrolyzed to cholesterol in the SC by steroid sulfatase. This process is necessary for desquamation, and thus changes in CS levels affect proper corneocyte shedding but also influence expression of differentiation associated proteins, signaling function via RORa- and CS may affect the Nude phenotype of the Foxn1 deficient mouse (Lanzini et al. 2015).

Xeroderma pigmentosum A (XPA)—PAF agonistic lipids identified by lipidomics account for the increased photosensitivity observed in XPA (Yao et al. 2012).

Epidermal Barrier and Defects—In a study investigating the effect of transcription factor Ctip2 in developing mouse epidermis, a lipidomic study found less short chain unsaturated (16:1) ceramides but more short chain saturated sphingomyelin (16:0) and more long chain unsaturated sphingomyelins, identifying this TF as a target for controlling epidermal lipid metabolism (Wang et al. 2013). Lipidomic study of defects in epidermal TAG catabolism contributed to characterization of one form of ichthyosis, reviewed in Radner and Fischer (2014). Recessive X-linked ichthyosis is caused by excessive sulfatation of cholesterol which is then not available in its free form, and the molecular species of CS were identified in Sanchez-Guijo et al. (2015).

Psoriasis—In Psoriasis, increased 12-HETE, PGE(2), PGF(2a) have been detected long ago (Hammarstrom et al. 1975), thus influencing eicosanoid levels with dietary intervention and performing lipid analyses for surveillance may help in disease management. Lipidomics identified effects of ALOX12 and ALOX15 polymorphisms on urinary excretion of 12-HETE but not on severity of disease (Setkowicz et al. 2015).

Atopic Dermatitis—The EOS ceramides, which are esterified by transglutaminase to involucrin to form the lipid envelope of the corneocytes, are strongly reduced in AD (Imokawa et al. 1991). Lipidomic analyses with LC/MSD found an association between increased very short chain ceramides (C34) in the [NS] class and permeability barrier function impairment (Ishikawa et al. 2010) in AD, a finding that was repeated by others who also confirmed that at the same time reduced FFA chain length and reduced lipid organization (van Smeden et al. 2014c). Not epidermal, but serum lipids of childhood AD patients were investigated and eicosanoids could be correlated to IgE levels (Huang et al. 2014).

Airway/skin irritants—In vitro ozone mediated oxidation of squalene yielded peroxyl, hydroxyl and ether modifications, and such compounds may have relevance as skin scale derived indoor dust that may be an irritant by its reactivity (Fooshee et al. 2015).

Influenza—Protectin D1, a 12/15 lipoxygenase metabolite inhibits influenza virus replication—epithelial stimulation of protect in synthesis is thus a promising concept to counteract influenza.

Diabetes—The Domingues group investigated oxidation and glycoxidation of phosphatidylethanol-amine PLs, identifying potential mediators in diabetes and redox stress diseases (Melo et al. 2013).

1.5.3 Cosmetic Applications

A major application of all "oxidized lipidomics" of the skin is to test for the ability of active compounds to prevent stress induced oxidative damage to the skin and thus to unsaturated lipids as excellent endogenous oxidation sensors. A method applicable to study nutriceutical manipulation of ceramide content and thereby skin moisturization utilized GC-combustion isotope ratio mass spectrometry to identify carbon labeled ceramide species in skin (Haraguchi et al. 2014), and LC/MS-MS was used to determine how surfactant alkyl chain length influences their penetration into a epidermal model system (Yamaguchi et al. 2014). Elaborate models to study compound-skin interactions could include investigation of lipid organization in addition to lipid composition (Groen et al. 2014). Oxidation of sebum lipids by UV or chemical stressors has been implicated to affect premature skin ageing and acne (Oyewole and Birch-Machin 2015). An example of lipid organization analysis is a study on the impact of volatile organic compounds on lipid assembly by X-ray diffraction in an artificial matrix resembling the SC lipid matrix, presenting an objective alternative to studies in ex vivo human epidermis (Groen et al. 2014).

1.5.4 Lipidomics for Biomarker Discovery

Epidermal and skin surface lipids have the highest potential as biomarkers because the sample can be acquired in a non- or minimally invasive way. Disorders where lipid metabolism is affected or correlated to disease manifestation are most promising, as disease specific metabolites can reach the epidermis via the vasculature but also could affect keratinocyte metabolism or sebum synthesis. Skin sensitization—With various lipidomic methods Santhina et al. have identified oxidized PC and PS species isolated from cultured Keratinocytes that might allow discriminating between irritant and immunogenic topical compounds tested on these in vitro (Santinha et al. 2013). Alzheimer's disease—the first promising results on peripheral (skin) lipid biomarkers for Alzheimer's disease, which is obviously correlated with lipid oxidation not only in plaque areas, is discussed in Khan and Alkon (2015). Leprosy—A MS method that identifies diagnostic lipids from pathogenic mycobacteria within superficial skin lipids was developed (Lima et al. 2015). Skin ulcers—Proteomic and lipidomic analysis revealed potential lipid biomarkers for impaired wound healing in pressure ulcers (Taverna et al. 2011). Environmental pollution—Oxidization of squalene measured by lipidomics may yield new biomarkers of environmental pollution (Pham et al. 2015). Forensics—Forensic use of lipidomics is reported by Girod and Weyermann, who detected 104 lipids from different classes (mostly wax esters) in fingermark residues with GC-EI-MS (Girod and Weyermann 2014).

References

Akazawa-Ogawa Y, Shichiri M, Nishio K, Yoshida Y, Niki E, Hagihara Y (2015) Singlet-oxygen-derived products from linoleate activate Nrf2 signaling in skin cells. Free Radic Biol Med 79:164–175

Anane R, Creppy EE (2001) Lipid peroxidation as pathway of aluminium cytotoxicity in human skin fibroblast cultures: prevention by superoxide dismutase+ catalase and vitamins E and C. Hum Exp Toxicol 20:477–481

Angelbeck-Schulze M, Mischke R, Rohn K, Hewicker-Trautwein M, Naim HY, Baumer W (2014) Canine epidermal lipid sampling by skin scrub revealed variations between different body sites and normal and atopic dogs. BMC Vet Res 10:152

Astarita G, Piomelli D (2009) Lipidomic analysis of endocannabinoid metabolism in biological samples. J Chromatogr B Anal Technol Biomed Life Sci 877:2755–2767

Astarita G, Kendall AC, Dennis EA, Nicolaou A (2015) Targeted lipidomic strategies for oxygenated metabolites of polyunsaturated fatty acids. Biochim Biophys Acta 1851:456–468

Baier J, Maisch T, Regensburger J, Pollmann C, Baumler W (2008) Optical detection of singlet oxygen produced by fatty acids and phospholipids under ultraviolet A irradiation. J Biomed Opt 13:044029

Bando N, Hayashi H, Wakamatsu S, Inakuma T, Miyoshi M, Nagao A, Yamauchi R, Terao J (2004) Participation of singlet oxygen in ultraviolet-a-induced lipid peroxidation in mouse skin and its inhibition by dietary beta-carotene: an ex vivo study. Free Radic Biol Med 37:1854–1863

Barber LA, Spandau DF, Rathman SC, Murphy RC, Johnson CA, Kelley SW, Hurwitz SA, Travers JB (1998) Expression of the platelet-activating factor receptor results in enhanced ultraviolet B radiation-induced apoptosis in a human epidermal cell line. J Biol Chem 273:18891–18897

Berdyshev EV, Schmid PC, Dong Z, Schmid HH (2000) Stress-induced generation of N-acylethanolamines in mouse epidermal JB6 P+ cells. Biochem J 346(2):369–374

Black O Jr, Anglin JH Jr (1971) Release of a guinea pig epidermal cellular component by ultraviolet light. J Invest Dermatol 57:87–93

Black AT, Gray JP, Shakarjian MP, Mishin V, Laskin DL, Heck DE, Laskin JD (2008) UVB light upregulates prostaglandin synthases and prostaglandin receptors in mouse keratinocytes. Toxicol Appl Pharmacol 232:14–24

Black AT, Joseph LB, Casillas RP, Heck DE, Gerecke DR, Sinko PJ, Laskin DL, Laskin JD (2010) Role of MAP kinases in regulating expression of antioxidants and inflammatory mediators in mouse keratinocytes following exposure to the half mustard, 2-chloroethyl ethyl sulfide. Toxicol Appl Pharmacol 245:352–360

Bluml S, Kirchberger S, Bochkov VN, Kronke G, Stuhlmeier K, Majdic O, Zlabinger GJ, Knapp W, Binder BR, Stockl J, Leitinger N (2005) Oxidized phospholipids negatively regulate dendritic cell maturation induced by TLRs and CD40. J Immunol 175:501–508

Brugger B (2014) Lipidomics: analysis of the lipid composition of cells and subcellular organelles by electrospray ionization mass spectrometry. Annu Rev Biochem 83:79–98

Cajka T, Fiehn O (2014) Comprehensive analysis of lipids in biological systems by liquid chromatography-mass spectrometry. Trends Anal Chem 61:192–206

Camera E, Ludovici M, Galante M, Sinagra JL, Picardo M (2010) Comprehensive analysis of the major lipid classes in sebum by rapid resolution high-performance liquid chromatography and electrospray mass spectrometry. J Lipid Res 51:3377–3388

Carsberg CJ, Ohanian J, Friedmann PS (1995) Ultraviolet radiation stimulates a biphasic pattern of 1,2-diacylglycerol formation in cultured human melanocytes and keratinocytes by activation of phospholipases C and D. Biochem J 305(2):471–477

Charruyer A, Bell SM, Kawano M, Douangpanya S, Yen TY, Macher BA, Kumagai K, Hanada K, Holleran WM, Uchida Y (2008) Decreased ceramide transport protein (CERT) function alters sphingomyelin production following UVB irradiation. J Biol Chem 283:16682–16692

Chen X, Gresham A, Morrison A, Pentland AP (1996) Oxidative stress mediates synthesis of cytosolic phospholipase A2 after UVB injury. Biochim Biophys Acta 1299:23–33

Couto D, Santinha D, Melo T, Ferreira-Fernandes E, Videira RA, Campos A, Fardilha M, Domingues P, Domingues MR (2015) Glycosphingolipids and oxidative stress: evaluation of hydroxyl radical oxidation of galactosyl and lactosylceramides using mass spectrometry. Chem Phys Lipids 191:106–114

Dan P, Rosenblat G, Yedgar S (2012) Phospholipase A(2) activities in skin physiology and pathology. Eur J Pharmacol 691:1–8

DeLeo V, Scheide S, Meshulam J, Hanson D, Cardullo A (1988) Ultraviolet radiation alters choline phospholipid metabolism in human keratinocytes. J Invest Dermatol 91:303–308

Duvernay MT, Matafonov A, Lindsley CW, Hamm HE (2015) Platelet lipidomic profiling: novel insight into cytosolic phospholipase A2α activity and its role in human platelet activation. Biochemistry 54:5578–5588

Elias PM (2014) Lipid abnormalities and lipid-based repair strategies in atopic dermatitis. Biochim Biophys Acta 1841:323–330

Elmets CA, Ledet JJ, Athar M (2014) Cyclooxygenases: mediators of UV-induced skin cancer and potential targets for prevention. J Invest Dermatol 134:2497–2502

Enthaler B, Trusch M, Fischer M, Rapp C, Pruns JK, Vietzke JP (2013) MALDI imaging in human skin tissue sections: focus on various matrices and enzymes. Anal Bioanal Chem 405:1159–1170

Epps DE, Palmer JW, Schmid HH, Pfeiffer DR (1982) Inhibition of permeability-dependent $Ca2^{+}$ release from mitochondria by N-acylethanolamines, a class of lipids synthesized in ischemic heart tissue. J Biol Chem 257:1383–1391

Fahy E, Subramaniam S, Brown HA, Glass CK, Merrill AH Jr, Murphy RC, Raetz CR, Russell DW, Seyama Y, Shaw W, Shimizu T, Spener F, van Meer G, VanNieuwenhze MS, White SH, Witztum JL, Dennis EA (2005) A comprehensive classification system for lipids. J Lipid Res 46:839–861

Feingold KR, Elias PM (2014) Role of lipids in the formation and maintenance of the cutaneous permeability barrier. Biochim Biophys Acta 1841:280–294

Ferracini M, Sahu RP, Harrison KA, Waeiss RA, Murphy RC, Jancar S, Konger RL, Travers JB (2015) Topical photodynamic therapy induces systemic immunosuppression via generation of platelet-activating factor receptor ligands. J Invest Dermatol 135:321–323

Fisher AB (2011) Peroxiredoxin 6: a bifunctional enzyme with glutathione peroxidase and phospholipase A(2) activities. Antioxid Redox Signal 15:831–844

Fisher AB, Dodia C, Sorokina EM, Li H, Zhou S, Raabe T, Feinstein SI (2016) A novel lysophosphatidylcholine acyl transferase activity is expressed by peroxiredoxin 6. J Lipid Res 57:587–596

Fooshee DR, Aiona PK, Laskin A, Laskin J, Nizkorodov SA, Baldi PF (2015) Atmospheric oxidation of squalene: molecular study using COBRA modeling and high-resolution mass spectrometry. Environ Sci Technol 49:13304–13313

Forman HJ (2010) Reactive oxygen species and alpha, beta-unsaturated aldehydes as second messengers in signal transduction. Ann NY Acad Sci 1203:35–44

Fuller M, Duplock S, Hein LK, Rigat BA, Mahuran DJ (2014) Liquid chromatography/electrospray ionisation-tandem mass spectrometry quantification of GM2 gangliosides in human peripheral cells and plasma. Anal Biochem 458:20–26

Girod A, Weyermann C (2014) Lipid composition of fingermark residue and donor classification using GC/MS. Forensic Sci Int 238:68–82

Girotti AW, Kriska T (2004) Role of lipid hydroperoxides in photo-oxidative stress signaling. Antioxid Redox Signal 6:301–310

Gresham A, Masferrer J, Chen X, Leal-Khouri S, Pentland AP (1996) Increased synthesis of high-molecular-weight cPLA2 mediates early UV-induced PGE2 in human skin. Am J Physiol 270:C1037–C1050

Groen D, Berthaud F, Bouwstra JA, Chapuis C, Gooris GS, Boncheva M (2014) In vitro model systems for studying the impact of organic chemicals on the skin barrier lipids. Biochim Biophys Acta 1838:310–318

Gruber F, Oskolkova O, Leitner A, Mildner M, Mlitz V, Lengauer B, Kadl A, Mrass P, Kronke G, Binder BR, Bochkov VN, Leitinger N, Tschachler E (2007) Photooxidation generates biologically active phospholipids that induce heme oxygenase-1 in skin cells. J Biol Chem 282:16934–16941

Gruber F, Bicker W, Oskolkova OV, Tschachler E, Bochkov VN (2012) A simplified procedure for semi-targeted lipidomic analysis of oxidized phosphatidylcholines induced by UVA irradiation. J Lipid Res 53:1232–1242

Grundmann JU, Wiswedel I, Hirsch D, Gollnick HP (2004) Detection of monohydroxyeicosatetraenoic acids and F2-isoprostanes in microdialysis samples of human UV-irradiated skin by gas chromatography-mass spectrometry. Skin Pharmacol Physiol 17:37–41

Hall DW, Marshall SN, Gordon KC, Killeen DP (2016) Rapid quantitative determination of squalene in shark liver oils by Raman and IR spectroscopy. Lipids 51:139–147

Hammarstrom S, Hamberg M, Samuelsson B, Duell EA, Stawiski M, Voorhees JJ (1975) Increased concentrations of nonesterified arachidonic acid, 12L-hydroxy-5,8,10,14-eicosatetraenoic acid, prostaglandin E2, and prostaglandin F2alpha in epidermis of psoriasis. Proc Natl Acad Sci USA 72:5130–5134

Hanson D, DeLeo V (1990) Long-wave ultraviolet light induces phospholipase activation in cultured human epidermal keratinocytes. J Invest Dermatol 95:158–163

Haraguchi H, Yamada K, Miyashita R, Aida K, Ohnishi M, Gilbert A, Yoshida N (2014) Determination of carbon isotopic measurement conditions for ceramide in skin using gas chromatography-combustion-isotope ratio mass spectrometry. J Oleo Sci 63:1283–1291

Hart PJ, Francese S, Claude E, Woodroofe MN, Clench MR (2011) MALDI-MS imaging of lipids in ex vivo human skin. Anal Bioanal Chem 401:115–125

Hong S, Tjonahen E, Morgan EL, Lu Y, Serhan CN, Rowley AF (2005) Rainbow trout (Oncorhynchus mykiss) brain cells biosynthesize novel docosahexaenoic acid-derived resolvins and protectins-mediator lipidomic analysis. Prostaglandins Other Lipid Mediat 78:107–116

Huang Y, Chen G, Liu X, Shao Y, Gao P, Xin C, Cui Z, Zhao X, Xu G (2014) Serum metabolomics study and eicosanoid analysis of childhood atopic dermatitis based on liquid chromatography-mass spectrometry. J Proteome Res 13:5715–5723

Ilic D, Bollinger JM, Gelb M, Mauro TM (2014) sPLA2 and the epidermal barrier. Biochim Biophys Acta 1841:416–421

Imokawa G, Abe A, Jin K, Higaki Y, Kawashima M, Hidano A (1991) Decreased level of ceramides in stratum corneum of atopic dermatitis: an etiologic factor in atopic dry skin? J Invest Dermatol 96:523–526

Ishikawa J, Narita H, Kondo N, Hotta M, Takagi Y, Masukawa Y, Kitahara T, Takema Y, Koyano S, Yamazaki S, Hatamochi A (2010) Changes in the ceramide profile of atopic dermatitis patients. J Invest Dermatol 130:2511–2514

Itoh T, Fairall L, Amin K, Inaba Y, Szanto A, Balint BL, Nagy L, Yamamoto K, Schwabe JW (2008) Structural basis for the activation of PPARγ by oxidized fatty acids. Nat Struct Mol Biol 15:924–931

Jia SN, Lin C, Chen DF, Li AQ, Dai L, Zhang L, Zhao LL, Yang JS, Yang F, Yang WJ (2016) The transcription factor p 8 regulates autophagy in response to palmitic acid stress via a mammalian target of rapamycin (mTOR)-independent signaling pathway. J Biol Chem 291:4462–4472

Jiao J, Ishikawa TO, Dumlao DS, Norris PC, Magyar CE, Mikulec C, Catapang A, Dennis EA, Fischer SM, Herschman HR (2014) Targeted deletion and lipidomic analysis identify epithelial cell COX-2 as a major driver of chemically induced skin cancer. Mol Cancer Res 12: 1677–1688

Jusakul A, Yongvanit P, Loilome W, Namwat N, Kuver R (2011) Mechanisms of oxysterol-induced carcinogenesis. Lipids Health Dis 10:44

Karmali RA, Safai B (1984) Ultraviolet-evoked prostaglandin biosynthesis in varying stages of keratinocyte differentiation in guinea pig skin. Prostaglandins Leukot Med 15:277–286

Kendall AC, Pilkington SM, Massey KA, Sassano G, Rhodes LE, Nicolaou A (2015) Distribution of bioactive lipid mediators in human skin. J Invest Dermatol 135:1510–1520

Khan TK, Alkon DL (2015) Peripheral biomarkers of Alzheimer's disease. J Alzheimers Dis 44:729–744

Kim EJ, Jin XJ, Kim YK, Oh IK, Kim JE, Park CH, Chung JH (2010) UV decreases the synthesis of free fatty acids and triglycerides in the epidermis of human skin in vivo, contributing to development of skin photoaging. J Dermatol Sci 57:19–26

King BS, Lu L, Yu M, Jiang Y, Standard J, Su X, Zhao Z, Wang W (2015) Lipidomic profiling of di- and tri-acylglycerol species in weight-controlled mice. PLoS ONE 10:e0116398

Kofeler HC, Fauland A, Rechberger GN, Trotzmuller M (2012) Mass spectrometry based lipidomics: an overview of technological platforms. Metabolites 2:19–38

Kozak KR, Crews BC, Morrow JD, Wang LH, Ma YH, Weinander R, Jakobsson PJ, Marnett LJ (2002) Metabolism of the endocannabinoids, 2-arachidonylglycerol and anandamide, into prostaglandin, thromboxane, and prostacyclin glycerol esters and ethanolamides. J Biol Chem 277:44877–44885

Krieg P, Furstenberger G (2014) The role of lipoxygenases in epidermis. Biochim Biophys Acta 1841:390–400

Kurczy ME, Piehowsky PD, Willingham D, Molyneaux KA, Heien ML, Winograd N, Ewing AG (2010) Nanotome cluster bombardment to recover spatial chemistry after preparation of biological samples for SIMS imaging. J Am Soc Mass Spectrom 21:833–836

Kwan HY, Fu X, Liu B, Chao X, Chan CL, Cao H, Su T, Tse AK, Fong WF, Yu ZL (2014) Subcutaneous adipocytes promote melanoma cell growth by activating the Akt signaling pathway: role of palmitic acid. J Biol Chem 289:30525–30537

Lam SM, Shui G (2013) Lipidomics as a principal tool for advancing biomedical research. J Genet Genomics 40:375–390

Lamaziere A, Wolf C, Quinn PJ (2014) How lipidomics provides new insight into drug discovery. Expert Opin Drug Discov 9:819–836

Lanzini J, Dargere D, Regazzetti A Tebani A, Laprevote O, Auzeil N (2015) Changing in lipid profile induced by the mutation of Foxn1 gene: a lipidomic analysis of Nude mice skin. Biochimie 118:234–243

Larroque-Cardoso P, Camare C, Nadal-Wollbold F, Grazide MH, Pucelle M, Garoby-Salom S, Bogdanowicz P, Josse G, Schmitt AM, Uchida K, Zarkovic K, Salvayre R, Negre-Salvayre A (2015) Elastin modification by 4-hydroxynonenal in hairless mice exposed to UV-A. role in photoaging and actinic elastosis J Invest Dermatol 135:1873–1881

Lehmann WD, Stephan M, Furstenberger G (1992) Profiling assay for lipoxygenase products of linoleic and arachidonic acid by gas chromatography-mass spectrometry. Anal Biochem 204:158–170

Lima EO, de Macedo CS, Esteves CZ, de Oliveira DN, Pessolani MC, Nery JA, Sarno EN, Catharino RR (2015) Skin imprinting in silica plates: a potential diagnostic methodology for leprosy using high-resolution mass spectrometry. Anal Chem 87:3585–3592

Marathe GK, Johnson C, Billings SD, Southall MD, Pei Y, Spandau D, Murphy RC, Zimmerman GA, McIntyre TM, Travers JB (2005) Ultraviolet B radiation generates platelet-activating factor-like phospholipids underlying cutaneous damage. J Biol Chem 280:35448–35457

Marko L, Paragh G, Ugocsai P, Boettcher A, Vogt T, Schling P, Balogh A, Tarabin V, Orso E, Wikonkal N, Mandl J, Remenyik E, Schmitz G (2012) Keratinocyte ATP binding cassette transporter expression is regulated by ultraviolet light. J Photochem Photobiol, B 116:79–88

Marques SA, Dy LC, Southall MD, Yi Q, Smietana E, Kapur R, Marques M, Travers JB, Spandau DF (2002) The platelet-activating factor receptor activates the extracellular signal-regulated kinase mitogen-activated protein kinase and induces proliferation of epidermal cells through an epidermal growth factor-receptor-dependent pathway. J Pharmacol Exp Ther 300:1026–1035

Massey KA, Nicolaou A (2011) Lipidomics of polyunsaturated-fatty-acid-derived oxygenated metabolites. Biochem Soc Trans 39:1240–1246

Masukawa Y, Narita H, Sato H, Naoe A, Kondo N, Sugai Y, Oba T, Homma R, Ishikawa J, Takagi Y, Kitahara T (2009) Comprehensive quantification of ceramide species in human stratum corneum. J Lipid Res 50:1708–1719

Melo T, Silva EM, Simoes C, Domingues P, Domingues MR (2013) Photooxidation of glycated and non-glycated phosphatidylethanolamines monitored by mass spectrometry. J Mass Spectrom 48:68–78

Melo T, Domingues P, Ferreira R, Milic I, Fedorova M, Santos SM, Segundo MA, Domingues MR (2016) Recent advances on mass spectrometry analysis of nitrated phospholipids. Anal Chem 88:2622–2629

Michael-Jubeli R, Bleton J, Baillet-Guffroy A (2011) High-temperature gas chromatography-mass spectrometry for skin surface lipids profiling. J Lipid Res 52:143–151

Milic I, Griesser E, Vemula V, Ieda N, Nakagawa H, Miyata N, Galano JM, Oger C, Durand T, Fedorova M (2015) Profiling and relative quantification of multiply nitrated and oxidized fatty acids. Anal Bioanal Chem 407:5587–5602

Mojumdar EH, Gooris GS, Barlow DJ, Lawrence MJ, Deme B, Bouwstra JA (2015) Skin lipids: localization of ceramide and fatty acid in the unit cell of the long periodicity phase. Biophys J 108:2670–2679

Murphy RC, Gaskell SJ (2011) New applications of mass spectrometry in lipid analysis. J Biol Chem 286:25427–25433

Nakagawa K, Ibusuki D, Suzuki Y, Yamashita S, Higuchi O, Oikawa S, Miyazawa T (2007) Ion-trap tandem mass spectrometric analysis of squalene monohydroperoxide isomers in sunlight-exposed human skin. J Lipid Res 48:2779–2787

Nakamura Y, Kozuka M, Naniwa K, Takabayashi S, Torikai K, Hayashi R, Sato T, Ohigashi H, Osawa T (2003) Arachidonic acid cascade inhibitors modulate phorbol ester-induced oxidative stress in female ICR mouse skin: differential roles of 5-lipoxygenase and cyclooxygenase-2 in leukocyte infiltration and activation. Free Radic Biol Med 35:997–1007

Nakamura T, Noma A, Shimada S, Ishii N, Bando N, Kawai Y, Terao J (2013) Non-selective distribution of isomeric cholesterol hydroperoxides to microdomains in cell membranes and activation of matrix metalloproteinase activity in a model of dermal cells. Chem Phys Lipids 174:17–23

Nicolaou A, Pilkington SM, Rhodes LE (2011) Ultraviolet-radiation induced skin inflammation: dissecting the role of bioactive lipids. Chem Phys Lipids 164:535–543

O'Donnell VB (2011) Mass spectrometry analysis of oxidized phosphatidylcholine and phosphatidylethanolamine. Biochim Biophys Acta 1811:818–826

Oyewole AO, Birch-Machin MA (2015) Sebum, inflammasomes and the skin: current concepts and future perspective. Exp Dermatol 24:651–654

Panasenko OM, Vakhrusheva T, Tretyakov V, Spalteholz H, Arnhold J (2007) Influence of chloride on modification of unsaturated phosphatidylcholines by the myeloperoxidase/hydrogen peroxide/bromide system. Chem Phys Lipids 149:40–51

Park HM, Shon JC, Lee MY, Liu KH, Kim JK, Lee SJ, Lee CH (2014) Mass spectrometry-based metabolite profiling in the mouse liver following exposure to ultraviolet B radiation. PLoS ONE 9:e109479

Patterson NH, Thomas A, Chaurand P (2014) Monitoring time-dependent degradation of phospholipids in sectioned tissues by MALDI imaging mass spectrometry. J Mass Spectrom 49:622–627

Pham DM, Boussouira B, Moyal D, Nguyen QL (2015) Oxidization of squalene, a human skin lipid: a new and reliable marker of environmental pollution studies. Int J Cosmet Sci 37: 357–365

Ponec M, Weerheim A, Kempenaar J, Mommaas AM, Nugteren DH (1988) Lipid composition of cultured human keratinocytes in relation to their differentiation. J Lipid Res 29:949–961

Radner FP, Fischer J (2014) The important role of epidermal triacylglycerol metabolism for maintenance of the skin permeability barrier function. Biochim Biophys Acta 1841:409–415

Ramprecht C, Jaritz H, Streith I, Zenzmaier E, Kofeler H, Hofmann-Wellenhof R, Schaider H, Hermetter A (2015) Toxicity of oxidized phosphatidylcholines in cultured human melanoma cells. Chem Phys Lipids 189:39–47

Rhodes LE, Gledhill K, Masoodi M, Haylett AK, Brownrigg M, Thody AJ, Tobin DJ, Nicolaou A (2009) The sunburn response in human skin is characterized by sequential eicosanoid profiles that may mediate its early and late phases. FASEB J 23:3947–3956

Rolfs F, Huber M, Gruber F, Bohm F, Pfister HJ, Bochkov VN, Tschachler E, Dummer R, Hohl D, Schafer M, Werner S (2013) Dual role of the antioxidant enzyme peroxiredoxin 6 in skin carcinogenesis. Cancer Res 73:3460–3469

Rubbo H, Trostchansky A, O'Donnell VB (2009) Peroxynitrite-mediated lipid oxidation and nitration: mechanisms and consequences. Arch Biochem Biophys 484:167–172

Sahu RP, Turner MJ, Dasilva SC, Rashid BM, Ocana JA, Perkins SM, Konger RL, Touloukian CE, Kaplan MH, Travers JB (2012) The environmental stressor ultraviolet B radiation inhibits murine antitumor immunity through its ability to generate platelet-activating factor agonists. Carcinogenesis

Sahu RP, Petrache I, Van Demark MJ, Rashid BM, Ocana JA, Tang Y, Yi Q, Turner MJ, Konger RL, Travers JB (2013) Cigarette smoke exposure inhibits contact hypersensitivity via the generation of platelet-activating factor agonists. J Immunol 190:2447–2454

Sahu RP, Ocana JA, Harrison KA, Ferracini M, Touloukian CE, Al-Hassani M, Sun L, Loesch M, Murphy RC, Althouse SK, Perkins SM, Speicher PJ, Tyler DS, Konger RL, Travers JB (2014) Chemotherapeutic agents subvert tumor immunity by generating agonists of platelet-activating factor. Cancer Res 74:7069–7078

Sala P, Potz S, Brunner M, Trotzmuller M, Fauland A, Triebl A, Hartler J, Lankmayr E, Kofeler HC (2015) Determination of oxidized phosphatidylcholines by hydrophilic interaction liquid chromatography coupled to Fourier transform mass spectrometry. Int J Mol Sci 16:8351–8363

Sanchez-Guijo A, Oji V, Hartmann MF, Schuppe HC, Traupe H, Wudy SA (2015) High levels of oxysterol sulfates in serum of patients with steroid sulfatase deficiency. J Lipid Res 56: 403–412

Santinha DR, Doria ML, Neves BM, Maciel EA, Martins J, Helguero L, Domingues P, Cruz MT, Domingues MR (2013) Prospective phospholipid markers for skin sensitization prediction in keratinocytes: a phospholipidomic approach. Arch Biochem Biophys 533:33–41

Santinha D, Ferreira-Fernandes E, Melo T, Silva EM, Maciel E, Fardilha M, Domingues P, Domingues MR (2014) Evaluation of the photooxidation of galactosyl- and lactosylceramide by electrospray ionization mass spectrometry. Rapid Commun Mass Spectrom 28:2275–2284

Scherer M, Schmitz G, Liebisch G (2010) Simultaneous quantification of cardiolipin, bis (monoacylglycero) phosphate and their precursors by hydrophilic interaction LC-MS/MS including correction of isotopic overlap. Anal Chem 82:8794–8799

Schroter J, Griesinger H, Reuss E, Schulz M, Riemer T, Suss R, Schiller J, Fuchs B (2015) Unexpected products of the hypochlorous acid-induced oxidation of oleic acid: a study using high performance thin-layer chromatography-electrospray ionization mass spectrometry. J Chromatogr A 1439:89–96

Serhan CN, Lu Y, Hong S, Yang R (2007) Mediator lipidomics: search algorithms for eicosanoids, resolvins, and protectins. Methods Enzymol 432:275–317

Setkowicz M, Mastalerz L, Gielicz A, Wojas-Pelc A, Sanak M (2015) Lack of association of ALOX12 and ALOX15B polymorphisms with psoriasis despite altered urinary excretion of 12 (S)-hydroxyeicosatetraenoic acid. Br J Dermatol 172:337–344

Shin JH, Shon JC, Lee K, Kim S, Park CS, Choi EH, Lee CH, Lee HS, Liu KH (2014) A lipidomic platform establishment for structural identification of skin ceramides with non-hydroxyacyl chains. Anal Bioanal Chem 406:1917–1932

Sigruener A, Tarabin V, Paragh G, Liebisch G, Koehler T, Farwick M, Schmitz G (2013) Effects of sphingoid bases on the sphingolipidome in early keratinocyte differentiation. Exp Dermatol 22:677–679

Simoes C, Domingues P, Domingues MR (2012) Identification of free radicals in oxidized and glycoxidized phosphatidylethanolamines by spin trapping combined with tandem mass spectrometry. Rapid Commun Mass Spectrom 26:931–939
Simoes C, Silva AC, Domingues P, Laranjeira P, Paiva A, Domingues MR (2013) Phosphatidylethanolamines glycation, oxidation, and glycoxidation: effects on monocyte and dendritic cell stimulation. Cell Biochem Biophys 66:477–487
Simons B, Kauhanen D, Sylvanne T, Tarasov K, Duchoslav E, Ekroos K (2012) Shotgun lipidomics by sequential precursor ion fragmentation on a hybrid quadrupole time-of-flight mass spectrometer. Metabolites 2:195–213
Spickett CM, Pitt AR (2015) Oxidiative lipidomics coming of age: advances in analysis of oxidized phospholipids in physiology and pathology. Antioxid Redox Signal 22:1646–1666
Steinbrecher UP (1988) Role of superoxide in endothelial-cell modification of low-density lipoproteins. Biochim Biophys Acta 959:20–30
Sticozzi C, Belmonte G, Pecorelli A, Arezzini B, Gardi C, Maioli E, Miracco C, Toscano M, Forman HJ, Valacchi G (2012) Cigarette smoke affects keratinocytes SRB1 expression and localization via H2O2 production and HNE protein adducts formation. PLoS ONE 7:e33592
Tachi M, Iwamori M (2008) Mass spectrometric characterization of cholesterol esters and wax esters in epidermis of fetal, adult and keloidal human skin. Exp Dermatol 17:318–323
Taverna D, Nanney LB, Pollins AC, Sindona G, Caprioli R (2011) Multiplexed molecular descriptors of pressure ulcers defined by imaging mass spectrometry. Wound Repair Regen 19:734–744
Thakoersing VS, Gooris GS, Mulder A, Rietveld M, El GA, Bouwstra JA (2012) Unraveling barrier properties of three different in-house human skin equivalents. Tissue Eng Part C Methods 18:1–11
t'Kindt R, Jorge L, Dumont E, Couturon P, David F, Sandra P, Sandra K (2012) Profiling and characterizing skin ceramides using reversed-phase liquid chromatography-quadrupole time-of-flight mass spectrometry. Anal Chem 84:403–411
Travers JB (1999) Oxidative stress can activate the epidermal platelet-activating factor receptor. J Invest Dermatol 112:279–283
Trommer H, Platzer M, Wolf R, Neubert RH (2003) Mass spectrometric examinations of stratum corneum lipid models exposed to ultraviolet irradiation. Skin Pharmacol Appl Skin Physiol 16:291–304
Trostchansky A, Bonilla L, Thomas CP, O'Donnell VB, Marnett LJ, Radi R, Rubbo H (2011) Nitroarachidonic acid, a novel peroxidase inhibitor of prostaglandin endoperoxide H synthases 1 and 2. J Biol Chem 286:12891–12900
Tyurina YY, Domingues RM, Tyurin VA, Maciel E, Domingues P, Amoscato AA, Bayir H, Kagan VE (2014) Characterization of cardiolipins and their oxidation products by LC-MS analysis. Chem Phys Lipids 179:3–10
Uchida Y, Houben E, Park K, Douangpanya S, Lee YM, Wu BX, Hannun YA, Radin NS, Elias PM, Holleran WM (2010) Hydrolytic pathway protects against ceramide-induced apoptosis in keratinocytes exposed to UVB. J Invest Dermatol 130:2472–2480
van Smeden J, Boiten WA, Hankemeier T, Rissmann R, Bouwstra JA, Vreeken RJ (2014a) Combined LC/MS-platform for analysis of all major stratum corneum lipids, and the profiling of skin substitutes. Biochim Biophys Acta 1841:70–79
van Smeden J, Janssens M, Gooris GS, Bouwstra JA (2014b) The important role of stratum corneum lipids for the cutaneous barrier function. Biochim Biophys Acta 1841:295–313
van Smeden J, Janssens M, Kaye EC, Caspers PJ, Lavrijsen AP, Vreeken RJ, Bouwstra JA (2014c) The importance of free fatty acid chain length for the skin barrier function in atopic eczema patients. Exp Dermatol 23:45–52
Villard PH, Sampol E, Elkaim JL, Puyoou F, Casanova D, Seree E, Durand A, Lacarelle B (2002) Increase of CYP1B1 transcription in human keratinocytes and HaCaT cells after UV-B exposure. Toxicol Appl Pharmacol 178:137–143
Wang Z, Kirkwood JS, Taylor AW, Stevens JF, Leid M, Ganguli-Indra G, Indra AK (2013) Transcription factor Ctip2 controls epidermal lipid metabolism and regulates expression of

genes involved in sphingolipid biosynthesis during skin development. J Invest Dermatol 133:668–676

Weinkauf B, Rukwied R, Quiding H, Dahllund L, Johansson P, Schmelz M (2012) Local gene expression changes after UV-irradiation of human skin. PLoS ONE 7:e39411

Wertz PW (2013) Current understanding of skin biology pertinent to skin penetration: skin biochemistry. Skin Pharmacol Physiol 26:217–226

Williams JD, Bermudez Y, Park SL, Stratton SP, Uchida K, Hurst CA, Wondrak GT (2014) Malondialdehyde-derived epitopes in human skin result from acute exposure to solar UV and occur in nonmelanoma skin cancer tissue. J Photochem Photobiol, B 132:56–65

Wu Y, Chen G, Ji C, Hoptroff M, Jones A, Collins LZ, Janssen HG (2016) Gas chromatography-mass spectrometry and Raman imaging measurement of squalene content and distribution in human hair. Anal Bioanal Chem 408:2357–2362

Yamaguchi F, Watanabe S, Harada F, Miyake M, Yoshida M, Okano T (2014) In vitro analysis of the effect of alkyl-chain length of anionic surfactants on the skin by using a reconstructed human epidermal model. J Oleo Sci 63:995–1004

Yamashita R, Tabata Y, Iga E, Nakao M, Sano S, Kogure K, Tokumura A, Tanaka T (2016) Analysis of molecular species profiles of ceramide-1-phosphate and sphingomyelin using MALDI-TOF mass spectrometry. Lipids 51:263–270

Yamazaki S, Ozawa N, Hiratsuka A, Watabe T (1999) Increases in cholesterol 7-hydroperoxides in lipids of human skin by sunlight exposure. Free Radic Biol Med 26:1126–1133

Yang K, Dilthey BG, Gross RW (2013) Identification and quantitation of fatty acid double bond positional isomers: a shotgun lipidomics approach using charge-switch derivatization. Anal Chem 85:9742–9750

Yao Y, Harrison KA, Al-Hassani M, Murphy RC, Rezania S, Konger RL, Travers JB (2012) Platelet-activating factor receptor agonists mediate xeroderma pigmentosum A photosensitivity. J Biol Chem 287:9311–9321

Yoo H, Jeon B, Jeon MS, Lee H, Kim TY (2008) Reciprocal regulation of 12- and 15-lipoxygenases by UV-irradiation in human keratinocytes. FEBS Lett 582:3249–3253

Zhang Q, Southall MD, Mezsick SM, Johnson C, Murphy RC, Konger RL, Travers JB (2005) Epidermal peroxisome proliferator-activated receptor gamma as a target for ultraviolet B radiation. J Biol Chem 280:73–79

Zhang CF, Gruber F, Ni C, Mildner M, Koenig U, Karner S, Barresi C, Rossiter H, Narzt MS, Nagelreiter IM, Larue L, Tobin DJ, Eckhart L, Tschachler E (2015) Suppression of autophagy dysregulates the antioxidant response and causes premature senescence of melanocytes. J Invest Dermatol 135:1348–1357

Zhao Y, Zhang CF, Rossiter H, Eckhart L, Konig U, Karner S, Mildner M, Bochkov VN, Tschachler E, Gruber F (2013) Autophagy is induced by UVA and promotes removal of oxidized phospholipids and protein aggregates in epidermal keratinocytes. J Invest Dermatol 133:1629–1637

Chapter 2
Squalene and Skin Barrier Function: From Molecular Target to Biomarker of Environmental Exposure

Boudiaf Boussouira and Dang Man Pham

Abstract The human skin naturally faces an aerial oxidative environment. The environment presents however a variable oxidative potential since enhanced by solar rays (UV, Visible) possibly combined to aerial-borne pollutants that most often act as catalysts in the different oxidative pathways. The poly-unsaturated human sebum highly present on the upper parts of the body (face, torso) is therefore a natural "receptor" of these oxidative actions. Comprised at 10–20 % within sebum, Squalene ($C_{30}H_{50}$) is not only specific to human sebum but its 6 double bonds make it a highly sensitive molecule towards various forms of Reactive Oxygen Species, singlet oxygen included, leading to different per-oxidized by-products. The latter thus appear as natural bio-markers of most oxidative actions upon the cutaneous tissue. Some mechanisms can easily be modelled in vitro, thereby demonstrating the influences of UVA rays, cigarette smoke, particulate matters or some porphyrins that are synthesized by the resident skin flora. These models allow the structures of various forms of squalene peroxides to being determined and to quantify the quenching properties of some known anti-oxidants (Carotenoids, Vitamin E). These chains of events were logically traced in vivo, by comparing the contents of Squalene and Vitamin E in the sebum of subjects living in differently polluted but close geographical locations. The oxidized state of Squalene then represents a reliable biomarker of most oxidative events induced by various environmental factors. Their possible biological impacts upon the skin physiology, which greatly remain to being documented, are discussed.

Keywords Squalene · Skin lipids · Oxidation · Barrier function

B. Boussouira (✉) · D.M. Pham
L'Oréal Research and Innovation, 188, rue Paul Hochart,
94152 Chevilly Larue, France
e-mail: bboussouira@rd.loreal.com

D.M. Pham
e-mail: dmpham@rd.loreal.com

G.T. Wondrak (ed.), *Skin Stress Response Pathways*,
DOI 10.1007/978-3-319-43157-4_2

2.1 Introduction: The Human Skin, a Constantly Adaptive Organ

The adaptation of skin to environmental changes is as old as humanity. Ethnological findings (Tishkoff and Verelli 2003; Jablonski 2004; Lucock et al. 2014) indicate that some of our far ancestors migrated from Eastern Africa 60,000 to 30,000 years ago towards Northern regions. Such moves necessarily implied drastic environmental changes to which successive genetic and phenotypic adaptations responded to various Darwinian *imperata*. Long periods of time, different sun irradiance, food/vitamins supply led numerous genetic mutations to be selected, among which those concerning skin pigmentation-related genes are rather well documented (Jablonski 2011; Basu Mallick et al. 2013; Jablonski and Chaplin 2013; Wilde et al. 2014).

With a 1.5–2 m^2 developed surface (in adults), the human skin offers a rather large exchange capacity with its close environment (Hadgraft 2001), being exogenous (sun, wind, cold, heat) or man-made (soap, water, cosmetic products, frictions). With regard to skin, the term "environment" can hardly be restricted to the sole physico-chemical conditions of the surrounding world. It includes many other factors to which skin (and body) may be exposed, all being now covered by the generic term "exposome" (Patel and Manrai 2015). This generic term comprises all factors that, over time, possibly influence the skin physiology such as food, psychological stress, medications, fatigue, smoking, alcohol consumption, etc. The notion of exposome, with regard to skin, may be even extended to the assembly (the so-called microbiome) of a resident and transient microflora (the so-called microbiome) that is permanently found on the skin surface and within the depth of the hair follicle canal (Grice and Segre 2011).

Hence, the effects of this microbiome upon the skin and, vice versa, those from the host tissue towards these micro-organisms represent constant mutual relationships.

2.1.1 Age-Related Changes

In utero, during the first two months needed for its full constitution, the human skin exposes to an aquatic and sterile medium, free from any stress. It then sets up a natural barrier to this environment, produced by already active sebaceous glands (stimulated by maternal hormones), thus delivering an important lipid-rich hydrophobic "film" (5–15 g all along the whole infant's body), called the Vernix Caseosa (Mikova et al. 2014; Visscher et al. 2015). The latter is in fact a very early sebum that nurses wipe off at the very first minutes post delivery, using sterile cotton pads.

At birth, all conditions drastically change. The skin now faces a totally different environment: dry, of a high oxygen tension (≈20 %) and non-sterile. Skin is almost immediately colonized by a resident microflora that will permanently thrive on the skin surface all along life span (Marples et al. 1974; Baviera et al. 2014). Later, skin will be progressively exposed to sunlight (UV, Visible and Infra-red ranges). These four major elements represent its early exposome.

Progressively, age-related physiological changes make skin more prone to adapted responses to various assaults. Melanocytes have become fully operational by inducing a protecting pigmentation in the fairer skin tones (Phototypes II–III) (Fitzpatrick 1988; Chardon et al. 1991). The epidermal physiology has then set up an efficiently regulated anti-oxidant network including various enzymes (Super Oxide Dismutase, Glutathione Peroxidase) and molecules (Vitamin E, Selenium, Vitamin C) (Thiele et al. 2001). Possible contacts with exogenous allergens are normally fought by an efficient immune response, most ensured initially by the epidermal Langerhans cells (Haniffa et al. 2015).

2.1.2 Environment Exposure Changes

Since the 19th century, our aerial environment has been strongly modified with regard to growing industrialization, transporting systems, agricultural changes etc. Nowadays, pollutants of various natures and origins are, in additional to natural sources (soil erosion, volcanic eruptions, forest fires), clearly linked to human activities. These cover the increases in emitted volatiles such as CO_2, CO, NO, NO_2, O_3 (ozone), Polycyclic Aromatic Hydrocarbons (PAH's) and Particulate Matters (PM) covering a wide range in size (0.1–100 μm) and nature (Ning et al. 2006; Ding et al. 2006; Zheng et al. 2002). Combined with solar rays (UV's, Visible, Infra-Red), most of these human-related pollutants are now shown as efficient catalytic agents in many oxidizing processes (Colin et al. 1994; Tai-Long et al. 2015a, b).

2.2 Specificities of the Stratum Corneum

The present chapter mostly focuses on the various effects of an oxidative environment upon the facial skin surface. The latter is indeed a privileged skin site for assessing the impacts of some environmental assaults for the following reasons:

- It is usually (in common with hands) the most constantly exposed skin region to the external environment.
- It is a skin site that gathers highly functional appendages (apocrine and eccrine Sweat glands, Sebaceous glands). Hence, many epidermal by-products (horny cells, sebum, epidermal lipids, peptides and amino acids, salts, organic acids, urea, water, etc.) are daily found at its surface, exposed to environment.

2.2.1 A Cornified Protecting Barrier Covered by Sebum

The Stratum Corneum (SC) comprises stacked flat dead cells (corneocytes) of usually 15–20 μm in thickness, embedded in a lipid-rich medium within intercellular spaces (the so-called brick and mortar organization), as shown by Fig. 2.1.

The SC is a powerful and vital barrier that ensures a wide array of defensive functions (Elias 2005). It is constantly produced by the epidermal cells (keratinocytes) renewal and their progressive keratinization process that ends up with natural desquamation, as single cells. A normal epidermis shows in fact a rather low mitotic index (about 10 %), i.e. the ratio of dividing cells at a given moment. In other words, epidermis possesses a high potential in speeding up the renewal of keratinocytes. The latter then allows the SC thickness (number of cell layers) to being adapted by an increase in cell layers according to needs (cut, wound, burn, frictions).

The Stratum Corneum, through both multilayer corneocytes and inter-cellular lipid medium, ensures a dual barrier function. Internally, it controls the Trans Epidermal Water Loss (TEWL, 5–10 g m^{-2} h^{-1}). The latter parameter is a precious marker of SC cohesion and thickness, since rapidly elevated in the case of a loose, damaged or thinned SC (Rawlings and Matts 2005; Rawlings and Leyden 2009). Externally, SC controls the flux of exogenous substances, acts as a thermo-insulating tissue and is an efficient shield against UV rays.

As a mantle exposed to various environments, the SC surface is daily covered by sebum (and traces of sweat according to the thermo-regulation function). Depending on the skin sites, the density of sebaceous glands (and eccrine glands) and consequently the amount of sebum (and sweat) presents some local variations.

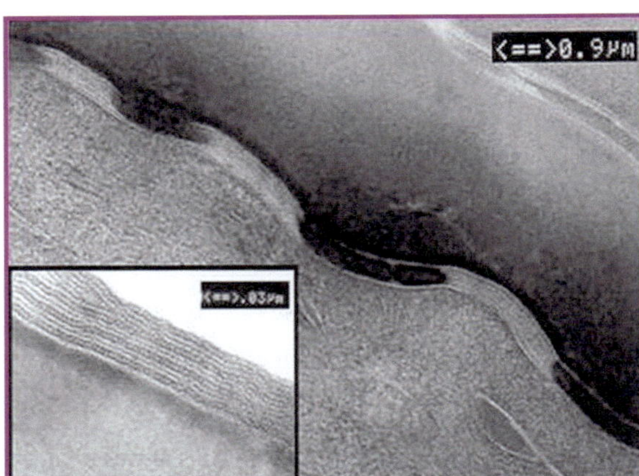

Fig. 2.1 Transversal section of the Stratum Corneum showing its organization in multi layered corneocytes, separated by an inter-cellular lipid medium (*zoomed section*). The corneodesmosomes (in *black*) ensure the attachments between corneocytes. The progressive degradation of corneodesmosomes drives the desquamation process that further delivers corneocytes as single cells in normal conditions (Courtesy of A. Potter, A.M. Minondo, F. Fiat. Life Sciences, L'Oréal Research and Innovation)

2.2.2 *The Human Sebum*

2.2.2.1 Quantitative Aspects

This complex lipid mixture is constantly produced by the Sebaceous Glands (Bernard and Saint-Léger 2000) and delivered within the follicular canal under the disintegration (holocrine process) of their cells (sebocytes). Excreted to the skin surface from the follicular ostia (about 250 per cm^2), at a rate ranging 0.4–2.5 μg cm^{-2} min^{-1} according to gender, age, ethnics, circadian rhythms. Sebum further spreads over the skin surface to reach an equilibrium level (the so-called casual level) of some 50–300 μg cm^{-2} which could be reached within a few hours post cleaning (Saint-Leger et al. 1982). The human face (surface $\approx$ 500 cm^2) appears then daily covered by 25–150 mg of sebum, in addition to admixed lipids of epidermal origin (Cholesterol, Ceramides, Triglycerides). On face, the ratio of Sebum to Epidermal lipids is about 97/3 (Wilkinson 1969). Such a lipid mantle then represents a "film" of a theoretical thickness of 3–10 μm, hence greatly facilitating exchanges with the environment.

2.2.2.2 Qualitative Aspects

The human sebum is an oil, unlike that, waxy, of most animals. This fluid behavior mostly results from a high proportion of mono and poly unsaturated lipid chains that, by nature, are highly sensitive to oxidization process. At a native state (within the sebaceous glands), sebum initially comprises a mixture of 3 lipid classes: Triglycerides (TG) 60 %, Wax esters 25 % and Squalene 15 %. Later, excreted sebum will transform. TG's are hydrolyzed by lipases emitted by the resident and

Table 2.1 Description of the major classes (approximate figures) and properties of lipids within sebum daily present on face

Lipid class	Number of C atoms	Unsaturated chains (iso and ante-iso methyl branched)	Relative concentrations present at the skin surface	Linked to
Triglycerides (TG)	30–60	66 % (2/3)	0–60 %	Sebaceous glands
Free fatty acids (FFA)	10–20	66 % (2/3)	60–0 %	Lipases/microflora, S.C hydrolases
Wax esters (WE)	20–60	50 % (1/2)	25 %, stable, untransformed	Sebaceous glands
Squalene (SQ)	30	100 %	10–20 %	Sebaceous glands and oxidization processes

The ratio TG/FFA is a precious reflection of the metabolic activity of the skin microflora and may greatly vary between individuals and regimen (e.g. intake)

lipophilic microflora, yielding Free Fatty Acids of 10–20 carbon chain lengths at the skin surface (Nicolaides 1974). Table 2.1 summarizes the major events of the sebum transformation steps and their major effectors or origins.

2.3 Squalene (SQ), a Key Element

2.3.1 A Biological Human Curiosity

Squalene is a specific marker of human sebum since absent in the sebum of almost all mammalian species (Lindholm and Downing 1980). As a readily precursor of Cholesterol and since rapidly transformed, it is present in almost all cells at minute amount. The major exception remains the case of the liver of the Squalidea family (its derived name) where large amount of SQ are found. The human sebaceous glands do not achieve a complete synthesis of Cholesterol and thus liberate pure squalene. The human sebaceous glands therefore clearly diverge from those of all animals where sebum is almost uniquely Cholesterol or Sterol-based, (e.g. Lanolin in sheep).

2.3.2 Structure/Properties of SQ

Squalene is a triterpene of the general formula $C_{30}H_{50}$ (see Fig. 2.2) that comprises 6 non-conjugated double bonds, making this compound one of the most unsaturated lipids.

It is a transparent oil, of a specific gravity of 0.855, fluid under normal conditions (Fusion T° = −20 °C). As most lipids, it is readily soluble in organic solvents and totally insoluble in water.

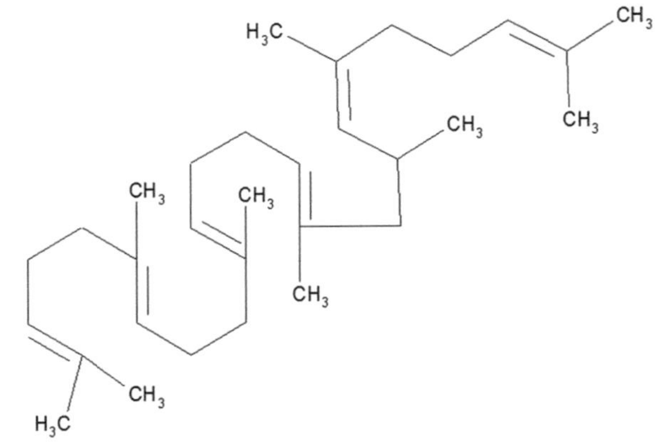

Fig. 2.2 Simplified chemical structure of squalene. Such representation illustrates how, when cyclized, squalene generates the future sterol ring

2.3.3 Squalene, a Strong Acceptor of All Forms of Oxygen

Such a richly unsaturated level naturally makes squalene highly prone to oxidization processes. The latter phenomenon was early described (Chapman 1923) showing that, when completely oxidized, squalene can absorb oxygen up to ¼ of its weight. However, squalene is highly sensitive to singlet oxygen ($^1O_2$), a very reactive oxidative species, that could be generated by various ionizing sources. This Singlet Oxygen rapidly reacts with the double bonds of squalene (Leong et al. 1976; Miquel et al. 1989; Petrick and Dubowski 2009). Yielding families of squalene peroxydes (SQOOH) and, to a lesser extent, squalene hydroxides (SQOH) (Ekanayake Mudiyanselage 2003). A slower but progressive oxidization can however be obtained by simply exposing a thin film of pure squalene to an ambient air free from singlet oxygen. In days, regular increases of its oxidized forms concomitant to decreased values of pure squalene are observed. Chemically speaking, all these chain-reaction processes lead to the addition of "ene" types of mechanisms into which the 6 electron-rich carbon double bonds (C=C) play a central role. Such finding was later confirmed (Saint-Leger et al. 1986; Tochio et al. 2009).

Sebum extracted from forehead, analyzed by liquid chromatography with UV and Light Diffracted Detector shows the presence of squalene and also squalene peroxides (SQOOH) and squalene hydroxides (SQOH). Further works using LC/MS (Thiele et al. 2003) confirmed that levels of squalene monohydroperoxides were strongly increased under low doses of UV exposures.

An alternative analytical method to quantify SQ and SQOOH was early developed in our laboratories and currently used, allowing low amount of SQOOH forms to being detected. Post solvent extraction and filtration, squalene peroxides are quantified by ultra-performance liquid chromatography (UPLC), on reversed phase, coupled with atmospheric pressure chemical ionization (APCI) tandem mass spectrometry (MS/MS) on positive mode (UPLC-APCI-MS/MS). Residual squalene (i.e. non-oxidized) is quantified on the same run with PDA detection at 205 nm, using pure squalene as standard. Under such conditions, the Limit Of Detection (LOD) and Limit Of Quantification (LOQ) of squalene monohydroperoxides are 10 and 50 ng ml^{-1}, respectively, together with an acceptable reproducibility (coefficient of variation <10 %). LOD and LOQ for residual squalene are 0.1 µg and 1 µg ml^{-1}, respectively. These limits allow very low amount of SQOOH and squalene to be determined on a freshly collected sebum (basal values) since slightly (per)oxidized before its excretion over the skin surface.

2.3.4 Squalene and the Resident Oxidative Skin Microflora

Within the depth of the follicular canal, porphyrins are synthesized and excreted by *Propionibacteria* spp. (Cornelius and Ludwig 1967; Fuhrhop et al. 1980). These compounds strongly absorb in the 360–450 nm range (UVA and Visible),

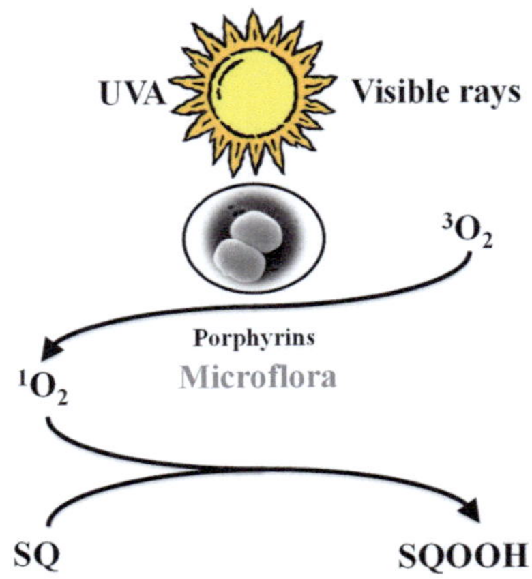

Fig. 2.3 Simplified scheme of the chain of reactions induced by photo-catalytic porphyrins, yielding singlet oxygen ($^1O_2$) that further reacts with squalene (SQ) to generate SQOOH forms

according to their structures, and generate Singlet Oxygen ($^1O_2$) from oxygen (Ekanayake Mudiyanselage 2003). This explains why squalene (per)oxides are naturally found within the sebum of most subjects.

This presence of porphyrins could also explain the reason why a high level of SQOOH is found within the comedones of acneic subjects (Motoyoshi 1983; Saint-Leger et al. 1986).

In brief, squalene, before facing additional external oxidative environments, is already- and partly-oxidized. The simplified scheme in Fig. 2.3 illustrates such chain of events.

This scheme allows a better understanding of the possible impact of Vitamin E (α tocopherol) since, supplied by food, it is eliminated through the sebaceous gland metabolism and further excreted within sebum (Thiele et al. 1999). A follicular canal enriched with Vitamin E is therefore likely more prone to inhibit such chain reactions, that can be quenched by well-known singlet oxygen scavengers such as Carotenoids, Vitamin E, Butyl Hydroxy Toluene (BHT) etc. as exposed later in this chapter.

The scheme also indicates how UVA sunscreens may efficiently slow down these oxidative pathways through controlling the penetration of UVA rays within the depth of the follicular canal, in agreement with previous findings (Fourtanier et al. 2006; Battie et al. 2014).

2.3.5 *Squalene Facing Singlet Oxygen Released by Porphyrins*

As previously mentioned, porphyrins are prone to generate singlet oxygen under UVA exposure. This can be easily demonstrated by simple preliminary assays. First, under UVA exposure, a methanolic solution of pure squalene (Sigma Aldrich, ref S3626) leads to a rather low SQOOH/SQ ratio whereas the methanolic extract of

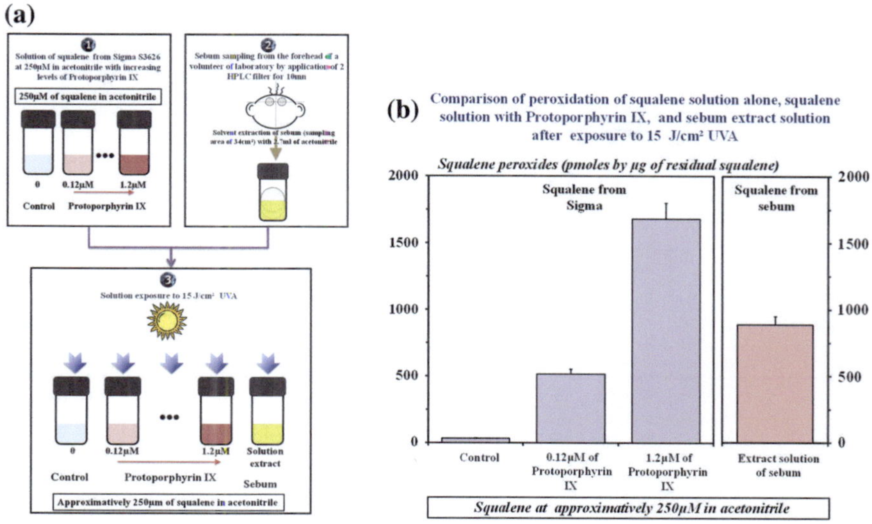

Fig. 2.4 **a** Examples of experimental protocols using either pure squalene and Protoporphyrin IX or squalene from sebum without addition of Protoporphyrin IX. All samples were exposed to 15 J/cm^2 UVA. **b** Ratios of SQOOH/SQ obtained under the two protocols exposed in (**a**)

a sebum collected from a human forehead (that contains traces of porphyrins) leads, in same conditions of UVA exposure, to a much higher SQOOH/SQ ratio, as shown by Fig. 2.4a, b.

Second, adding increased concentrations of a porphyrin, Protoporphyrin IX (Sigma Aldrich, ref P8293) to a methanolic solution of pure squalene shows a dose dependent increase in the generation of SQOOH forms under UVA exposure, as illustrated by Fig. 2.5a, b, at least within the studied concentrations of porphyrin IX.

Figure 2.5a, b illustrate the linear dependence of generated SQOOH with increasing amount of squalene and a fixed amount of Protoporphyrin IX or, at a constant concentration of squalene, with increasing amount of Protoporphyrin IX.

The latter assays indicate that the follow up of SQOOH forms is a precious indicator of an oxidative stress driven by singlet oxygen and obviously paves the road to in vitro testing of known or candidate molecular scavengers of this reactive form of oxygen (see next paragraph).

2.3.5.1 Effect of Some Anti-oxidants

With regard to the high sensitivity of the analytical technique, the in vitro tests exposed above can be applied for determine the amount of the decreased SQOOH forms induced by five common anti-oxidant molecules. Figure 2.6a, b illustrate the various amplitudes of their effects, outlining (and confirming) the very high potency

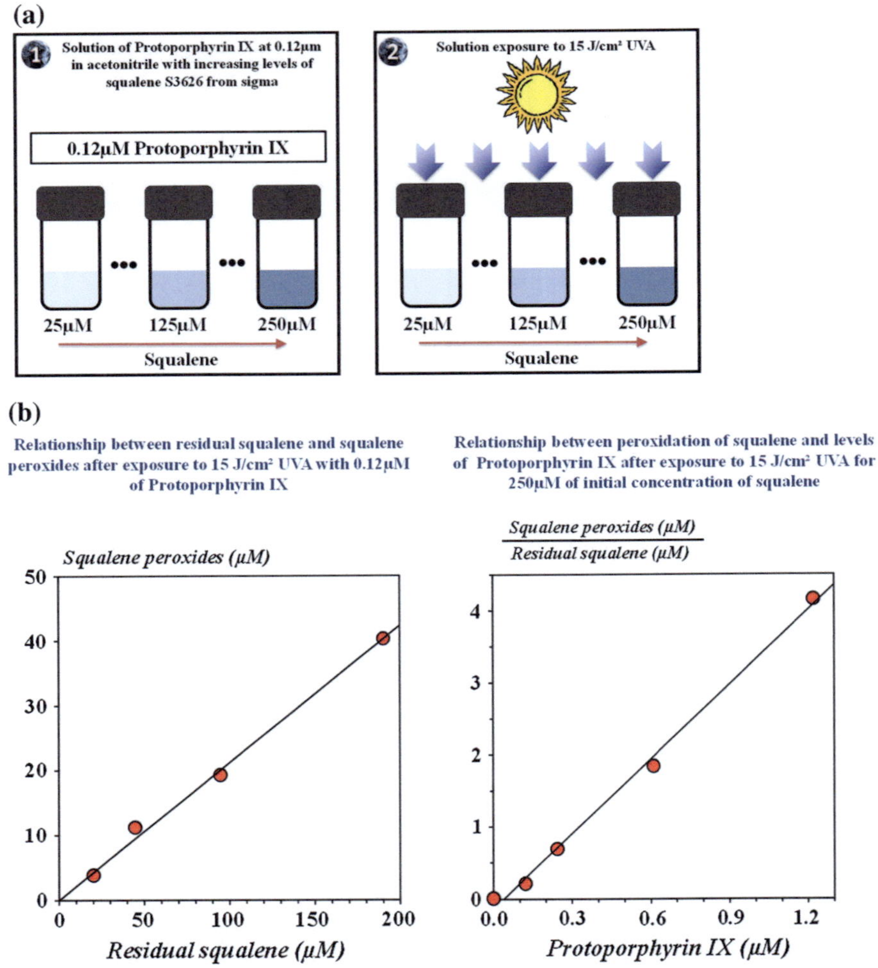

Fig. 2.5 **a** Global protocols used to precise the dose dependence of SQOOH forms with squalene and Protoporphyrin IX. **b** Dose responses of generated SQOOH forms with different amount of squalene and/or Protoporphyrin IX

of β Carotene to inhibit the peroxidization of squalene, as a potent scavenger of singlet oxygen, a property shared by most Carotenoids (Hosaka et al. 2005).

2.3.5.2 SQOOH Properties

The easiness in preparing, in vitro, oxidized forms of squalene, under the above methodologies given as examples, allows their major characteristics to be precised. It has to be kept in mind that other oxidizing methods can be used, such as exposing

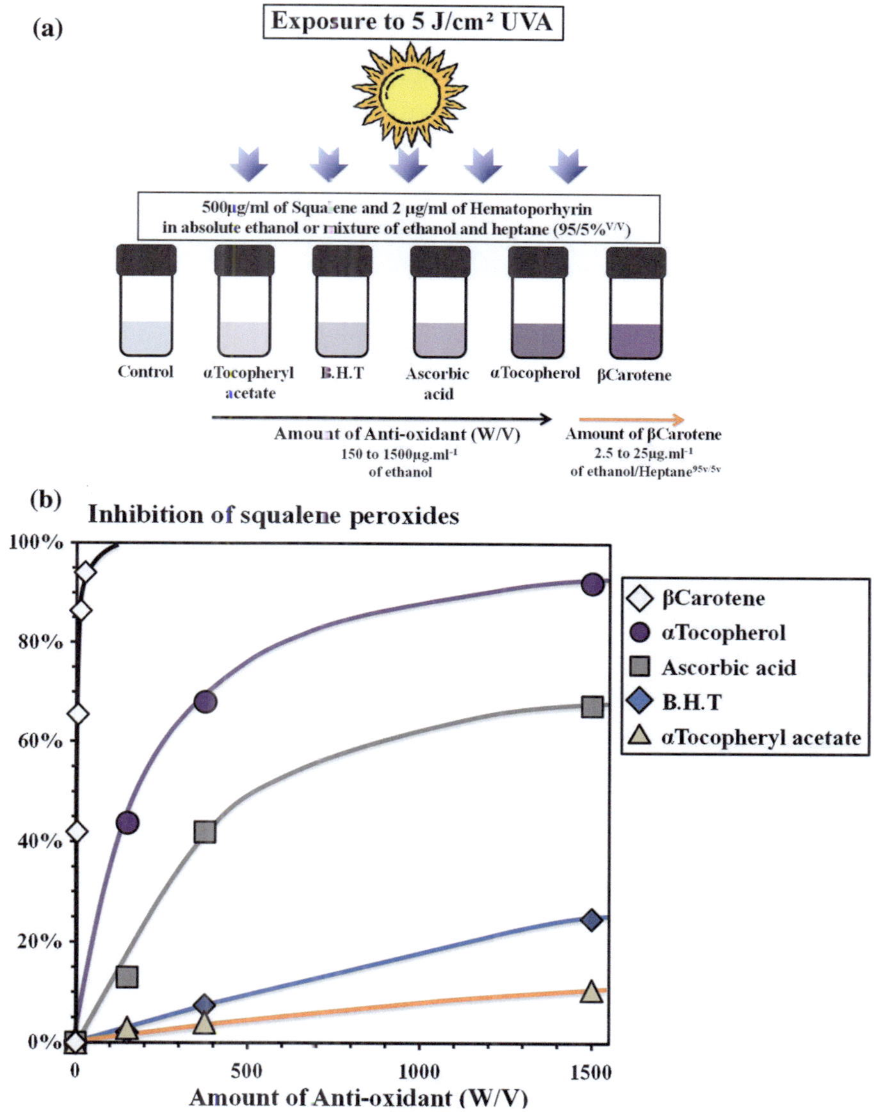

Fig. 2.6 **a** General protocol used for determining the efficacy of some common anti-oxidant molecules. **b** Effects of some anti-oxidant molecules upon the genesis of SQOOH from squalene in the presence of porphyrin and exposure to UVA. β-Carotene shows a high anti-oxidant activity whereas the acetate form of vitamin E brings the lower activity

squalene to Ozone (O_3), a marker of aerial pollution, according to a previously quoted work (Petrick and Dubowski 2009). Little is known, however, whether such a procedure leads to a similar chemical family of SQOOH forms.

- In our experimental conditions, the production of SQOOH's is UVA dose-dependent.
- The minimum UVA dose at which such SQOOH production starts being detected corresponds to a reasonable (not extreme) sun exposure of the skin at zenith time during a European summer climatic condition.
- Chemical instability is the hallmark of most peroxides. Despite, SQOOH forms appear relatively stable under the experimental conditions exposed above and can be kept at −20 °C under Nitrogen without significant losses. However, high UVA doses lead to their transformation/disappearance.
- Oxidizing different amounts of squalene by a same dose of UVA leads to similar SQOOH/SQ ratios.

These reasons are then crucial in the establishment of in vitro testing, in the need of adopting adequate and realistic conditions such as UV doses, initial SQ amount, respective ratio with a photocatalytic agent etc.

2.4 Squalene as a Reliable Bio-marker of an Oxidative Environment

Squalene then appears as a privileged molecule in studies dealing with oxidization-related processes for the following reasons:

- Easily oxidizable under mild conditions.
- Its oxidized by-products (SQOOH, SQOH) can be detected at very low amount.
- Apart from using pure squalene, human sebum as a source of squalene is an easy alternative model that better integrates or mimics the actual in vivo situation.

Indeed (i) it is of an easy collection (forehead), (ii) it is constantly renewed by the skin, and (iii) it comprises physiological components (porphyrins, unsaturated fatty acids).

A recent paper from our group (Pham et al. 2015) explored and illustrated some possible technical approaches for assessing the rate, amplitude and specificity of some factors (UVA, aerial pollutants) at enhancing the (per)oxidization of squalene, either in a pure form or present within human sebum. Their results, summarized below, suggest that the latter could be a reliable bio-marker of the impacts of aerial pollution upon human skin, of an easy collection, i.e. adapted to various protocols of in vivo studies.

2.4.1 In Real Life (In Vivo) Conditions

Two comparable in vivo studies were carried out by our group of research in 2000 and 2008 in Mexico city/Mexico and Shanghai/P.R. China regions, respectively (Nguyen et al. 2015a, b). In both cases, half of subjects under study (a total of 348

Table 2.2 Record of some pollution markers

Average of 8 h	O_3 ($\mu g\ m^{-3}\ h^{-1}$)	NOx ($\mu g\ m^{-3}\ h^{-1}$)	SO_2 ($\mu g\ m^{-3}\ h^{-1}$)	PM_{10} ($\mu g\ m^{-3}$)
Mexico city (2000)	170 ± 46	109 ± 26	N.A	N.A
Shanghai center (2007)	N.A	75 ± 25	100 ± 35	86 ± 30

N.A Not addressed

Table 2.3 Distribution of subjects under study in the 4 different Mexican and Chinese locations

Regions	Number of subjects	Women (average age)	Men (average age)
Mexico city	96	56 (32y ± 15)	40 (30y ± 12)
Cuernavaca	93	57 (34y ± 13)	36 (31y ± 15)
Shanghai/center	79	40 (33y ± 12)	39 (36y ± 10)
Chongming	80	40 (35y ± 10)	40 (35y ± 10)

women and men of comparable ages) were recruited as residing in city center whereas the other half were living in a close surrounding (<100 km, Cuernavaca in Mexico, Chongming in China) that is much less daily exposed to aerial pollution. The records of Air Pollution Indexes issued by local official bureaus confirm higher contents of pollution markers (NO, NO_x, SO_2, PM, O_3) in the atmosphere of both city centers (Table 2.2).

Table 2.3 summarizes the composition of the four cohorts of studied subjects.

Non-invasive samplings, using cotton pads imbibed with an ethanol water solution 70/30 v/v solution or adhesive D'Squame® stripping were performed on various sites of the faces of all subjects. Prior to samplings, some instrumental measurements were performed on the same facial locations (skin pH, Sebum Excretion Rate, Skin colour, Skin hydration) using standardized techniques. From cotton pads, following extraction by methanol, analytical assays of total lipids, squalene, Vitamin E, Cholesterol, lactic acid were carried out whereas the adhesive D'Squame® disks allowed collected proteins, ATP and interleukin (IL1α) residual content to be analyzed. All technical details can be found in the two previously quoted publications from Nguyen et al. For practical reasons (un-availability of equipment, methods still in development at these periods), the SQOOH forms could not unfortunately be analyzed.

Overall, most results of these two studies converge and showed significant differences in many parameters between a polluted environment and a less polluted one, in both countries and independent of gender. With regard to squalene and lipids, two major and significant ($p < 0.01$) findings were as follows:

– Squalene content (versus total lipids) much decreased (by approximately 50 %) in a polluted environment, suggesting that its (per)oxidized forms increased by a comparable extent.

- The ratio Vitamin E/Squalene strongly decreased in a polluted environment (by almost 90 %). In other words, a possible protective action towards (per)oxidization of squalene becomes abolished by an environmental pollution. Such decrease in Vitamin E (likely unrelated to differences in Vitamin E intakes by such close subjects) is in agreement with a previous work (Thiele et al. 1997) showing how ozone may deplete Vitamin E.

These results confirm an oxidative boosting impact of polluted environments.

2.4.2 *Possible Influences of Other Factors from a Polluted Aerial Environment*

On a practical basis, sampling skin surface lipids on the face is easily performed non-invasively and the regular sebum excretion affords a constant supply of a "fresh" sebum/squalene, as control of ulterior oxidative events. The latter may be driven by various factors present in an aerial polluted environment, susceptible (or not) to generate singlet oxygen from O_2 through UV irradiance. Some of these are listed in Table 2.4, showing that their implication of some airborne pollutants in the Squalene oxidization process largely remains to being explored.

In real life conditions, assessing the actual impact(s) of UVA and Visible rays, shown as important (direct or indirect via Porphyrins) inducers of oxidizing agents, is a rather difficult task since airborne particles, fumes of all kinds in a heavily polluted environment, shield (filter out) almost all sun rays. This paradoxical situation creates ambiguities when aiming at evaluating the relative contributions of solar rays and airborne pollutants in the oxidization processes of squalene. Whatsoever, from a protective aspect, applications of UVB-UVA sunscreens, intakes of natural anti-oxidants (Vitamin E in vegetable oils, Vitamin C in fruits) seem being logical measures. With regard to environment, it has to be kept in mind that indoor conditions more concentrate some volatile oxidizing compounds than an outdoor environment. This is particularly relevant to PAHs that are generated by cigarette smoke as previously mentioned, confirmed by our in vitro approach

Table 2.4 Summary of some major factors susceptible to enhance the (per)oxidization of squalene

Airborne compounds/aerial pollution	Pro-oxidant action/SQ
Ozone (O_3)	Yes. Depletes vitamin E and reacts with vitamin C to generate singlet oxygen
Particulate matters (PM)	Probable but still unexplored Influence of size and content (heavy metals)?
Volatile organic and non organic compounds (NO, SO_2, NO_2, CO, PAH's, aldehydes)	Probable but still unexplored, PAH's excepted
Metallic atoms (Ni, Cd, Pb, Fe)	Probable but still unexplored

exposed above. Apart from volatile elements, the biological consequences of possible contacts between skin and particulate matters still remain largely unknown. A recent work (Tai Long 2015a, b), using pig skin in vivo, indicates that such contacts induce changes in both structural elements and functions of the SC, thereby modifying the skin absorption of drugs.

2.4.3 *Mimicking, In Vitro and/or Ex Vivo, the Impact of Some Environmental Factors upon Squalene Oxidization*

There are many variants and applied purposes (effect of anti-oxidants) that appear versatile and sensitive enough for assessing the impact of UV exposure, aerial or solid compounds upon the oxidization of the oxygen-sensitive (and naturally present) squalene molecule.

Squalene samples:

Two complementary approaches can be used, as previously described (Pham et al. 2015).

(a) Using a squalene standard solution as a model for studying the effect of oxidative processes. This option obviously allows a full control of various in vitro testing, by adding possible effector molecules of a known structure.
(b) Sebum could be collected from skin (face or forehead are the most easily accessible skin sites) using non-invasive procedures (contacts of the skin surface with polytetrafluoroethylene (PTFE) disks or cotton pad wipes, for instance). Sebum collected could be used directly as a thin film (adsorbed in the PTFE disks) or as solution extracted from cotton pad. In this case, squalene is surrounded with other compounds present in sebum (unsaturated fatty acids, porphyrins). In all cases, the determination of basal SQOOH within the collected sebum is paramount since, as mentioned above, excreted sebum is already partially and weakly (per)oxidized. This point is fundamental when collecting, in vivo, a sebum that has been exposed to various conditions (UV, Pollutants).

Stress exposures and further analysis:

In a thin support like PTFE disks, samples of collected human sebum were placed into chamber with a quartz window to allow UVA exposures. To simulate different forms of aerial stress, cigarette smoke (2 puffs as example) or an aerosol mixture (gases or PM) can fill the volume of the quartz chambers.

Solvent extraction of sebum or pure squalene from the Teflon Disks is further carried out, using methanol as solvent. Following filtration, the extract is analyzed through the method exposed earlier. In brief, these technical approaches can offer in vitro, or ex vivo methods to evaluate oxidative effects upon skin lipids from various aerial environments.

2.5 Biological Consequences of Squalene (Per)oxides on the Skin

Many findings from previous works converge. As previously mentioned, the link between Sun exposure and comedogenesis (onset of acneic lesions) was early suggested and the pivotal role of squalene in such a process was further specified (Chiba et al. 2000; Ottaviani et al. 2006). Squalene (per)oxides were shown active mediators in the development of inflammatory acne (Picardo et al. 1991; Ottaviani et al. 2010). At the cellular level, squalene monohydroperoxide was shown depleting glutathione, an important compound within the natural anti-oxidant cellular system (Chiba et al. 2001). Topical applications of squalene monohydroperoxide onto the skin of hairless mice enhanced the skin roughness and induced a wrinkling process (Chiba et al. 1999, 2003). Little is known, however, whether same effects can occur on the human skin as a response. When applied onto the skin of guinea pigs, squalene peroxides led to a hyperpigmentation via the release of prostaglandin E_2 by keratinocytes (Ryu et al. 2009). In humans, oxidized surface lipids are viewed as potent inflammatory mediators in many skin afflictions such as pityriasis versicolor or seborrheic dermatitis (De Luca and Valacchi 2010). A very recent paper (Oyewole and Birch-Machin 2015) examines the mediating role of UVR-oxidized lipids as activators of NALP3 inflammasome (Nod Like Receptor Proteins).

2.6 Perspectives/Conclusion

The in vitro and in vivo data presented here indicate that squalene may be considered as a reliable biomarker of the impact of some pollution-related oxidative processes upon the human skin. Although other skin lipids (unsaturated fatty acids, cholesterol) might be used as markers of oxidative events, their oxidized forms may pose technical limits in detection, stability or specificity. The analytical determination of oxidized forms of squalene affords a reliable detection of very low signals of an oxidative environment, i.e. prone to record subtle impacts of oxygen-driven assaults upon the skin.

An external environment implies the combination of many different elements, gaseous and/or solid, at variable concentrations according to external, changing and often uncontrollable conditions (weather, air-ventilation, time of the day, geographical location). This aspect makes it hardly possible, in real life condition, to assess the precise contribution of each given element in the formation of (per) oxidized forms of squalene.

However, although squalene is particularly sensitive to singlet oxygen, it appears clear that the SQOOH/SQ index shall be viewed as a global signal since induced by various oxidative mechanisms (and agents).

On the one hand, as sebum is constantly renewed by the skin and easily collected from the skin surface, squalene and its oxidized forms could be used to record a short term and low external oxidative stress such as the one induced by low doses of UVA (2.5 J/cm^2). On the other hand, with regard to peroxides instability, our own experience on repeated exposures to oxidative environment, such as UV, has revealed that these do not lead to a progressive accumulation of SQOOH forms onto the skin surface. Longer exposures probably need to record other—and possibly secondary—oxidative radical side events (induced or not by SQOOH) such as carbonyl adducts on SC proteins, as example.

Such considerations call for the complementary and practical in routine uses of in vitro models where an aerial environment can be more easily controlled, by introducing a given gaseous element (Ozone, NO, SO_2) at realistic dosages. To such perspective, the use of reconstructed skin techniques (Marionnet et al. 2010, 2014; Duval et al. 2012) is possibly a valuable approach since also allowing contacts with PM or lipids, squalene included. These reconstructed tissues, that can be used for safety or efficacy purposes, offer structures and functions of much similarities with those of real skin, even allowing genes activated or shut-down by a given compound or electro-magnetic waves to being detected (Marionnet et al. 2012; Cottrez et al. 2015). These precious investigative tools have been proven reproducible and some are now introduced within the legal frame of U.E., as alternative testing methods to animals. In addition, they offer a wide pattern of applications since possibly composed by different cell types, i.e. extended to other tissues than skin alone. For instance, the impact of a given pollutant upon a reconstructed cornea (Skinethic, France) may help to decipher the mechanisms involved in ocular irritation, a frequent symptom that occurs during a period of heavy aerial pollution (Wieslander and Norbäck 2010; Novaes et al. 2010). The availability of in vitro techniques of hair growth (Thibaut et al. 2003; Collin et al. 2006) may well contribute to explore the possible and specific impacts of some pollutants upon the hair follicle physiology.

These available in vitro models seem much complementary to in vivo experiments such as those exposed above, by describing skin parameters that specifically reflect the impact of a given air pollutant. In addition, future in vivo experimental protocols should include, in the next future, non-invasive measurements offered by (bio)physical technics. Their possible contributions (e.g. Skin Imaging under UVA or IR rays, Photo-acoustics, Skin Fluorescence recorded by using Confocal laser Microscopy or Multi-photon microscopy etc.) should obviously be initially explored on the skin of subjects who are daily exposed to differently polluted indoor or outdoor environments. The combination of all possible non-invasive techniques is likely a pre-requisite for better evaluating the actual cumulative impacts of this complex aerosol upon the human skin and their related possible side effects. Meanwhile, from a skincare viewpoint, the use of UVB-UVA sunscreens, anti-oxidant enriched formulations, together with efficient and well-tolerated cleansing products offer practical preventive and corrective actions against undesired—and possibly deleterious—oxidative events that daily assault and challenge the cutaneous tissue.

Acknowledgments The authors wish to deeply thank Mr Q.L. Nguyen who initially paved their professional roads towards the mechanisms of lipid oxidization and to acknowledge the precious helps from Mrs D. Saint-Leger and B.A. Bernard in the preparation of this chapter.

References

Basu Mallick C et al (2013) The light skin allele of SCL24A5 in South Asians and Europeans shares identity by descent. PLoS Genet 9(11):e1003912

Battie C et al (2014) New insights in photoaging, UVA induced damage and skin types. Exp Dermatol 1:7–12

Baviera G et al (2014) Microbiota in healthy skin and in atopic eczema. Biomed Res Int. doi:10.1155/2014/436921

Bernard BA, Saint-Léger D (2000) Sécrétion sébacée. Encyclopédie Médico-chirurgicale, Cosmétologie et Dermatologie esthétique, 50-020-F-10, 1–6

Chapman AC (1923) Spinacene: its oxidation and decomposition. J Chem Soc 123, 769

Chardon A, Cretois I, Hourseau C (1991) Skin color typology and suntanning pathways. Int J Cosm Sci 13(4):191–208

Chiba K et al (1999) Skin roughness and wrinkle formation induced by repeated applications of squalene monohydroperoxide to the hairless mouse. Exp Dermatol 8(6):471–479

Chiba K et al (2000) Comedogenicity of squalene monohydroperoxide in the skin after topical application. J Toxicol Sci 25(2):77–83

Chiba K et al (2001) Changes in the levels of glutathione after cellular and cutaneous damage induced by squalene monohydroperoxide. J Biochem Mol Toxicol 15(3):150–158

Chiba K, Kawakami K, Sone T, Onoue M (2003) Characteristics of skin wrinkling and dermal changes induced by repeated applications of squalene monohydroperoxide to hairless mouse skin. Skin Pharmacol Appl Skin Physiol 16(4):242–251

Colin C, Boussouira B, Bernard D, Moyal D, Nguyen QL (1994) Non invasive methods of evaluation of oxidative stress induced by low doses of ultra violet in humans. 18th IFSCC Congress report, pp 51–72

Collin C et al (2006) Protective effects of taurine on human hair follicle grown in vitro. Int J Cosmet Sci 28(4):289–298

Cornelius CE, Ludwig GD (1967) Red fluorescence for comedones: production of porphyrins by corynebacterium acnes. J Invest Dermatol 49:368–370

Cottrez F et al (2015) Genes specifically modulated in sensitized skins allow the detection of sensitizers in a reconstructed human skin model. Development of the SENS-IS assay. Toxicol in Vitro 29(4):787–802

De Luca C, Valacchi G (2010) Surface lipids as multifunctional mediators of skin responses to environmental stimuli. Mediators Inflamm. doi:10.1155/2010/321494

Ding YS et al (2006) Determination of 14 polycyclic aromatic hydrocarbons in mainstream smoke from US brand and non-US brand cigarettes. Environ Sci Technol 40(4):1133–1138

Duval C et al (2012) Human skin model containing melanocytes: essential role of keratinocyte growth factor for constitutive pigmentation-functional response to α-melanocyte stimulating hormone and forskolin. Tissue Eng Part C Methods 18(12):947–957

Ekanayake Mudiyanselage S et al (2003) Ultraviolet A induces generation of squalene monohydroperoxide isomers in human sebum and skin surface lipids in vitro and in vivo. J Invest Dermatol 120(6):915–923

Elias PM (2005) Stratum corneum defensive functions: an integrated view. J Invest Dermatol 125:183–200

Fitzpatrick TB (1988) The validity and practicability of sun-reactive skin type I through VI. Arch Dermatol 124:869–871

Fourtanier A et al (2006) Protection of skin biological targets by different types of sunscreens. Photodermatol Photoimmunol Photomed 22(1):22–32

Fuhrhop JH et al (1980) Metalloporphyrin catalyzed oxidation 3. Epoxidation and aldehyde formation by carbon bond cleavage in squalene. J Mol Catal 7:257–266

Grice EA, Segre JA (2011) The skin microbiome. Nat Rev Microbiol 9(4):244–253

Hadgraft J (2001) Skin, the final frontier. Int J Pharm 224:1–18

Haniffa M et al (2015) Human skin dendritic cells in health and disease. J Dermatol Sci 77(2): 85–92

Hosaka S, Obuki M, Nakajima J et al (2005) Comparative study of antioxidants as quenchers or scavengers of reactive oxygen species based on the quenching of MCLA-dependent chemiluminescence. Luminescence 20(6):419–427

Jablonski NG (2004) The evolution of human skin and skin color. Annu Rev Anthropol 33: 585–623

Jablonski NG (2011) Why humans come in colors. Anthro Notes 32:7–10

Jablonski NG, Chaplin G (2013) Epidermal pigmentation in the human lineage is an adaptation to ultraviolet radiation. J Hum Evol 65(5):671–675

Leong W et al (1976) Polyene oxidation: the oxidation of squalene with singlet oxygen. J Rub Res Instit Malays 24:215–220

Lindholm JS, Downing DT (1980) Occurrence of squalene in skin surface lipids of the otter, the beaver and the kinkajou. Lipids 15(12):1062–1063

Lucock M et al (2014) Vitamin D, folate and potential early lifecycle environmental adult phenotypes. Evol Med Public Health 1:69–91

Marionnet C et al (2010) Different oxidative stress response in keratinocytes and fibroblasts of reconstructed skin exposed to non extreme daily-ultraviolet radiation. PLoS One, e12059. doi:10.1371/journal.pone.0012059

Marionnet C et al (2012) Modulations of gene expression induced by daily ultraviolet light can be prevented by a broad spectrum sunscreen. J Photochem Photobiol 116:37–47

Marionnet C et al (2014) Diversity of biological effects induced by long wave UVA rays (UVA1) in reconstructed skin. PLoS One, e105263. doi:10.1371/journal.pone.0105263

Marples RR et al (1974) The microflora of the face and acne lesions. J Invest Dermatol 62(3): 326–331

Mikova R et al (2014) Newborn boys and girls differ in the lipid composition of vernix caseosa. PLoS One. doi:10.1371/journal pone.0099173

Miquel J, Quintanilha AT, Webber H (1989) Chemical and biochemical aspects of activated oxygen: singlet oxygen, superoxide anion and related species. In: Handbook of free radicals and antioxidants in biomedicine, vol 1. CRC press, Boca Raton, FL, USA

Motoyoshi K (1983) Enhanced comedo formation in rabbit ear skin by squalene and oleic acid peroxides. Br J Dermatol 109:191–196

Nicolaides N (1974) Skin lipids: their biochemical uniqueness. Science 186(4158):19–26

Ning Z, Cheung CS, Fu J, Liu MA, Schnell MA (2006) Experimental study of environmental tobacco smoke particles under actual indoor environment. Sci Total Environ 367:822–830

Nguyen QL et al (2015a) Consequence of urban pollution upon skin status. A controlled study in Shanghai area. Int J Cosmet Sci. doi:10.1111/ijcs12270

Nguyen QL et al (2015b) Evaluation of the impact of urban pollution on the quality of skin: a multicentre study in Mexico. Int J Cosmet Sci 37(3):329–338

Novaes P et al (2010) The effects of chronic exposure to traffic derived air pollution on the ocular surface. Environ Res 110(4):372–374

Ottaviani M et al (2006) Peroxidated squalene induces the production of inflammatory mediators in Ha Cat keratinocytes: a possible role in acne vulgaris. J Invest Dermatol 126(11):2430–2437

Ottaviani M et al (2010) Lipid mediator in acne. Mediator of Inflammation, vol 2010. Hindawi Publishing Corporation, Article ID 858176
Oyewole AO, Birch-Machin AA (2015) Sebum, inflammasomes and the skin: current concepts and future perspective. Exp Dermatol 24:651–654
Patel CJ, Manrai AK (2015) Development of exposome correlation globes to map out environment-wide associations. Pac Symp Biocomput, 231–242, PMC4299925
Petrick L, Dubowski Y (2009) Hetergeneous oxidation of squalene film by ozone under various indoor conditions. Indoor Air 19(5):381–391
Pham DM et al (2015) Oxidation of squalene, a human skin lipid. A new and reliable marker of environmental pollution studies. Int J Cosmet Sci 37:357–365
Picardo MS et al (1991) Squalene peroxides may contribute to ultraviolet light-induced immunological effects. Photodermatol Photoimmunol Photomed 8(3):105–110
Rawlings AV, Leyden JJ (2009) Skin mosturization, 2nd edn. Informa Healthcare, New York, USA
Rawlings AV, Matts PJ (2005) Stratum corneum moisturization at the molecular level: an update in relation to the dry skin cycle. J Invest Dermatol 124:1099–1110
Ryu A et al (2009) Squalene as a target molecule in skin hyperpigmentation caused by singlet oxygen. Biol Pharm Bull 32(9):1504–1509
Saint-Leger D et al (1982) A comparative study of refatting kinetics on the scalp and forehead. Br J Dermatol 106:669–675
Saint-Leger D et al (1986) A possible role for squalene in the pathogenesis of acne. I. In vitro study of squalene oxidation. Br J Dermatol 114:535–542
Tai-Long P et al (2015a) The impact of urban particulate pollution on skin barrier function and the subsequent drug absorption. J Dermatol Sci 78:51–60
Tai-Long P, Pei Wen W, Aljuffali IA et al (2015b) The impact of urban pollution on skin barrier function and the subsequent drug absorption. J Dermatol Sci 78:51–60
Thibaut S et al (2003) Hair keratin pattern in human hair follicles grown in vitro. Exp Dermatol 12 (2):160–164
Thiele JJ et al (1997) Ozone depletes tocopherols and tocotrienols topically applied to murine skin. FEBS Lett 401:167–170
Thiele JJ et al (1999) Sebaceous gland secretion is a major physiological route of vitamin E delivery to skin. J Invest Dermatol 113:1006–1010
Thiele JJ, Schroeter C, Hsieh SN, Podda M, Packer L (2001) The antioxidant network of the stratum corneum. Curr Probl Dermatol 29:26–42
Thiele JJ et al (2003) Ultraviolet a induces generation of squalene monohydroperoxide isomers in human sebum and skin surface lipids in vitro and in vivo. J Invest Dermatol 120(6):915–922
Tishkoff SA, Verelli B (2003) Patterns of human genetic diversity: implications for human evolutionary and disease. Annu Rev Genomics Hum Genet 4:293–340
Tochio T et al (2009) Accumulation of lipid peroxide in the content of comedones may be involved in the progression of comedogenesis and inflammatory changes in comedones. J Cosmet Dermatol 8(2):152–158
Visscher MO et al (2015) Newborn infant skin: physiology, development and care. Clin Dermatol 33(3):271–280
Wieslander G, Norbäck D (2010) Ocular symptoms, tear film stability, nasal patency and biomarkers in nasal lavage in indoor painters in relation to emissions from water-based paint. Int Arch Occup Environ Health 83(7):733–741
Wilde S et al (2014) Direct evidence for positive selection of skin, hair and eye pigmentation in Europeans during the last 5,000 years. PNAS 111(13):4832–4837
Wilkinson DI (1969) Variability in composition of surface lipids. The problem of epidermal contribution. J Invest Dermatol 52(4):339–343
Zheng M, Cass GR, Schauer JJ, Edgerton ES (2002) Source apportionment of PM2.5 in the southeastern United States using solvent-extractable organic compounds as tracers. Environ Sci Technol 36(11):2361–2371

Chapter 3
Sunlight-Induced DNA Damage: Molecular Mechanisms and Photoprotection Strategies

Thierry Douki

Abstract Epidemiological and biological studies point DNA damage as a major event in the induction of skin cancers. It is thus important to determine the nature of these DNA lesions and their main biological features like repair and mutagenicity. Available data allowed to identify pyrimidine dimers as the main carcinogenic class of DNA damage, with oxidative stress also playing a role to a lesser extent. Such information is important in order to design and evaluate appropriate photoprotective strategies. The present chapter summarizes the main data available on the formation of DNA damage caused by solar UV radiation. The repair and mutagenic properties of the different lesions are then compared in order to determine the most carcinogenic photo-induced mechanisms. Based on these data, a critical review of the main photoprotection approaches is proposed.

Keywords Skin cancer · DNA damage · DNA repair · Mutations · Pyrimidine dimers · Oxidative stress · Photoprotection · Sunscreen · Antioxidants

3.1 Introduction

Skin cancer is one of the most deleterious effects of overexposure to solar UV radiation (Melnikova and Ananthaswamy 2005). Evidence is growing that artificial UV sources such as tanning equipment constitute another risk factor for skin cancer (El Ghissassi et al. 2009). Depending on the age and the pattern of exposure, three main types of skin cancers can be induced in photo-exposed sites of the body. The two most frequent types of skin tumors arise from epidermal keratinocytes and

T. Douki
University of Grenoble Alpes, INAC, LCIB, LAN, 38000 Grenoble, France

T. Douki (✉)
CEA, INAC, SCIB, LAN, 38000, Grenoble, France
e-mail: thierry.douki@cea.fr

G.T. Wondrak (ed.), *Skin Stress Response Pathways*,
DOI 10.1007/978-3-319-43157-4_3

include basal cell (BCCs) and squamous cell carcinomas (SCCs). Melanocytes give rise to the less frequent but more severe melanomas. The carcinogenic potency of UV radiation is mainly explained by its ability to cause DNA damage. However, UV is considered as a complete carcinogen since it also triggers promotion and progression in tumorogenesis. Identifying the different DNA photoproducts and determining their specific contribution to mutagenesis is thus important in order to understand the initiation step of skin cancer and to find relevant prevention strategies. In this context, an important issue is the respective contribution of the different ranges of radiation, namely UVB (280–320 nm), UVA (320–400 nm) and visible (400–700 nm). In addition to the photochemical events leading to DNA damage and their consequences in terms of mutations, solar radiation induces numerous other cellular responses also associated with the tumorigenesis process in skin. Apoptosis is one of these important protective pathways since it prevents cells with heavily damaged DNA from undergoing replication. The immune response against skin tumors is another important protection against carcinogenesis and the immunosuppressive effect of sunlight is therefore a major issue to be considered. Large amounts of information on these aspects have been gathered in the recent years but they will not be discussed in the present chapter. This review will rather provide a survey of the main steps leading from DNA damage to mutations and to discuss possible strategies aimed at limiting the genotoxic impact of exposure to sunlight.

3.2 DNA Damage Formation

The DNA damaging portion of the solar spectrum reaching Earth includes UVB, UVA and visible radiations. The photochemical reactions leading to DNA damage in cells differ from one wavelengths range to the other, although the final photoproducts may, to some extent, be the same. In addition, it is becoming clearer that combinations of wavelengths must be considered in order to explain the distribution of DNA damage observed in sun-exposed cells and skin. Photochemical processes leading to DNA damage can be rationalized into two series of pathways: those involving direct absorption of the incident photons by DNA and those involving photosensitizers. These photoreactions lead to the formation of dimeric pyrimidine photoproducts and oxidative lesions. The chemical structures of the final photoproducts are now well established and most of the present research on DNA photochemistry deals with the identification of the reaction pathways and the nature of the short-lived intermediates produced immediately after interaction of DNA with incident photons.

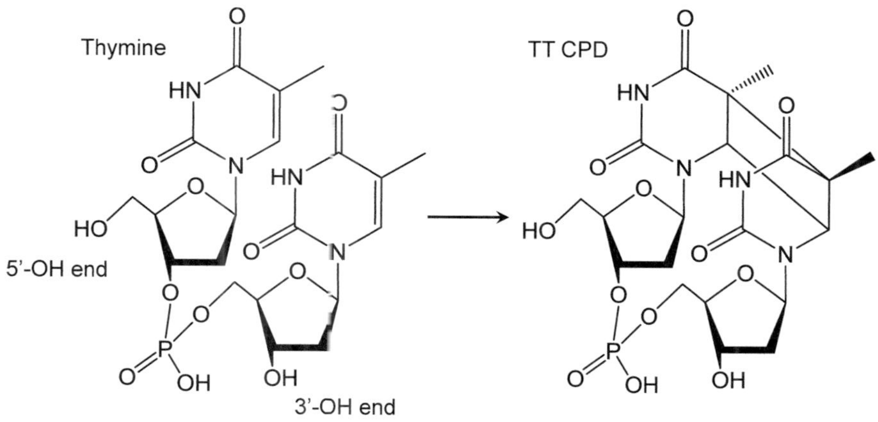

Fig. 3.1 Formation of CPD in a dinucleotide bearing two adjacent thymine bases. Several diastereoisomers can be produced but the CPDs found in double-stranded DNA all exhibit the illustrated *cis, syn* configuration

3.2.1 Cyclobutane Pyrimidine Dimers

Cyclobutane pyrimidine dimers (CPDs) represent the prototype of UV-induced DNA damage (Fig. 3.1). Since their first isolation and characterization at the end of the 1950s, numerous photochemical works and cellular studies have been devoted to the understanding of the parameters governing their formation. CPDs were actually found to be produced by several different photochemical processes as described below.

3.2.1.1 UVB Absorption

The maximal UV absorption of DNA occurs at around 260 nm, in the UVC range. However, DNA still efficiently absorbs UVB photons; the actual absorption at 280, 290 and 300 nm roughly represents 50, 20 and 4 % of that measured at 260 nm. The proportion of UVB in solar UV radiation is below 5 % but the corresponding photons are readily absorbed by DNA bases. In the recent years, numerous time-resolved studies have been carried out to understand the fate of the resulting excited states. In monomeric bases, the relaxation of the $^1\pi\pi^*$ excited states is very fast, on the picosecond time-scale (Middleton et al. 2009). The picture becomes much more complex in DNA. First, Frank-Codon excited states are partly delocalized over several bases (Emanuele et al. 2005). The absorbed energy may also transfer along stacked bases (Vaya et al. 2012). In addition, several types of excited states have been proposed, including $^1\pi\pi^*$, $^1n\pi^*$ and charge transfer states (Lange and Herbert 2009; Vaya et al. 2012). Formation of photoproducts is one pathway leading to the loss of the excess energy gathered by DNA. In particular, $^1\pi\pi^*$

excited states have been proposed by recent theoretical and spectroscopic studies to be at the origin of CPDs (Blancafort and Migani 2007; Schreier et al. 2009; McCullagh et al. 2010; Banyasz et al. 2012). The formation of this class of photoproducts involves a [2+2] cycloaddition between the C5–C6 double bonds of adjacent pyrimidine bases. The rate of reaction was found to be very high, in the ps time scale (Schreier et al. 2007). This observation strongly supports that singlet excited states are involved and that only adjacent bases in a proper orientation react with one another. The efficiency is yet limited, with a quantum yield of approximately 2 % (Garcès and Davila 1982). CPDs are formed at TT, TC, CT and CC sequences. However, the efficiency of the reaction is not the same for all these photoproducts. The ratio between the yields of the TT, TC, CT and CC CPDs were found to be 10/5/2/1 based on HPLC-mass spectrometry measurements (Douki and Cadet 2001). A larger contribution of CC CPD was recently determined by ligation-mediated PCR in several genes of UVC-irradiated fibroblasts (Bastien et al. 2013). Another important parameter is the presence in DNA of 5-methylcytosine, an epigenetic factor present mostly in CpG islands. Evidence has been provided that C5-methylation leads to a strong increase in the formation of CPDs upon exposure to UV radiation (Tommasi et al. 1997; You and Pfeifer 1999).

3.2.1.2 UVA-Induced CPDs

UVB is always mentioned as the source of CPDs in solar light. However, evidence has accumulated in the literature for the induction of CPDs also in cells exposed to UVA. A first report was made in 1973 in bacteria (Tyrrell 1973) and subsequently in cultured mammalian cells (Freeman and Ryan 1990; Kielbassa et al. 1997; Perdiz et al. 2000; Rochette et al. 2003; Besaratinia et al. 2005) and skin (Freeman et al. 1989; Young et al. 1998). These results have long been disregarded first because contamination of UVA sources by UVB was suspected and second because UVA was believed to mainly induce oxidative lesions. In addition, the yield of CPDs induced by UVA is two to three orders of magnitude lower than by UVB. The biological relevance of CPDs to UVA genotoxicity was first established by the fact that these photoproducts were produced in larger amounts than 8-oxo-7,8-dihydroguanine (8-oxoGua), the most frequent oxidative lesion (Douki et al. 2003; Courdavault et al. 2004; Mouret et al. 2006) and thus CPDs represent, at least quantitatively, the major photoproducts. In addition, precise determination of the distribution of UVA-induced photoproducts showed that the underlying photochemical processes were different from those involved with UVB. Indeed, no pyrimidine (6-4) pyrimidone photoproduct (64PP), the other main class of pyrimidine dimers, was produced. TT CPD was found to represent approximately 90 % of the CPDs in UVA-exposed cells while it is only 50 % with UVB. The presence of UVB radiation in the light sources could thus be ruled out. A possible explanation to the UVA-induction of CPDs could be the existence of a photosensitized mechanism involving endogenous cellular sensitizers. However, the observation that CPDs are also produced upon UVA irradiation of isolated DNA in yields similar to those observed in cells seems to rule out this pathway (Kuluncsics et al. 1999; Jiang et al. 2009). A direct photochemical process, resulting from the low but significant absorption of UVA photons by DNA seems involved (Mouret et al. 2010). Actually, spectroscopic studies on a model duplex oligonucleotide have shown that the proportion of excited states exhibiting a charge transfer character increases with increasing wavelength (Banyasz et al. 2011). This trend could explain why UVA and UVB, dominated by $^1\pi\pi^*$excited states, do not lead to the same distribution of dimeric photoproducts.

3.2.1.3 Triplet-Triplet Energy Transfer

In addition to the direct mechanisms involved with UVB and UVA, CPDs can be produced through a photosensitized pathway known as triplet-triplet energy transfer (TTET) (Cuquerella et al. 2011). This photoreaction may have an important impact in human health since several drugs such as anti-inflammatory compounds exhibiting an aromatic ketone motive (Cuquerella et al. 2012) or antibacterial agents of the fluoroquinolone family (Lhiaubet-Vallet et al. 2007) are potent TTET photosensitizers. TTET requires a chromophore that efficiently absorbs UVA and exhibits a large yield of intersystem crossing, a process converting singlet into triplet excited states. In addition, a high energy level of the triplet excited state of the sensitizer is necessary. Under these conditions, a triplet-triplet energy transfer process can take place between the excited sensitizer and nearby DNA bases. The excited triplet state of DNA is directly populated and gives specifically rise to CPDs. Thymine is the base exhibiting the lowest energy for its triplet excited state, slightly below 270 kJ/mol in double-stranded DNA (Bosca et al. 2006), and is thus expected to be the major target for TTET. Recent quantification of CPDs in DNA damaged by TTET suggests that a scheme where an isolated thymine base receives the whole triplet energy from the excited sensitizer may be too simplistic. Indeed, TT CPD represents 90 % or more of the CPDs depending on the sensitizer, while TC and CT CPDs account for less than 10 % (Douki et al. 2014). These proportions are far from those expected by a simple statistic distribution and strongly suggest that the nature of the base adjacent to the thymine strongly impacts the formation of CPDs. It may thus be proposed that the target for TTET spreads over two nucleotides. If a Dexter mechanism takes place, this could be a way to charge transfer excited states and could thus explain the similarity in photoproduct distribution upon pure UVA irradiation and TTET.

3.2.1.4 CPDS in the Dark in UVA-Irradiated Melanocytes

The formation of CPDs in cellular DNA in the absence of irradiation was recently reported (Premi et al. 2016). More precisely, CPDs were produced in UVA-irradiated human melanocytes in the minutes and hours following the end of the irradiation. This phenomenon was not observed in keratinocytes and in melanocytes from albino mice. These observations pointed to a role of melanin. It was actually shown in vitro that some monomeric precursors of melanin could be oxidized and CPDs were formed in DNA that was subsequently added. A likely explanation of this dark formation of CPDs could thus be the production of dioxetanes which are oxidation products undergoing decomposition into excited states and possibly leading to the formation of CPDs by energy transfer. It is worth mentioning that not only TT CPD but also the mutagenic TC CPD is produced by this pathway. These observations do not mean that melanin is not an efficient protective pigment in skin but point out the complexity of the interaction between UV and melanocytes. These results may provide an interesting insight into the molecular mechanisms leading to melanoma.

3.2.2 Pyrimidine (6-4) Photoproducts and Their Dewar Valence Isomers

Although TT CPD (often referred to as "thymine dimer") is the gold standard of UV-induced DNA damage, other photoproducts are induced upon UV irradiation. The second most frequent type of pyrimidine dimers are the pyrimidine (6-4) pyrimidine photoproducts (64PPs) which are also found in DNA in the form of their Dewar valence isomers (DEWs) (Fig. 3.2).

3.2.2.1 Formation of Pyrimidine (6-4) Pyrimidone Photoproducts

Formation of 64PPs is often explained in terms of a [2+2] Paterno-Büchi cycloaddition. This photoreaction involves the C5–C6 double bond of the 5′-end pyrimidine and either the C4 keto group of a 3′-end thymine or the C4 imino group of a 3′-end cytosine in a tautomeric form. An intermediate exhibiting an oxetane or an azetidine structure depending on whether the 3′-end base is T or C is produced. More recently, the same intermediates were proposed to arise from charge transfer excited state either through the triplet (Giussani et al. 2013) or more likely the

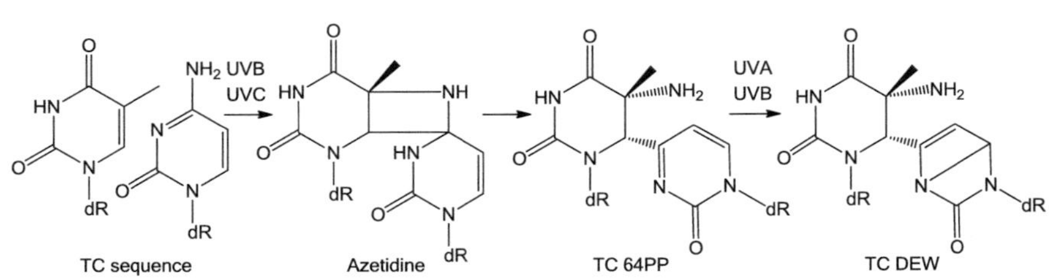

Fig. 3.2 Formation and structure of the TC 64PP and DEW (*dR* deoxyribose moieties in DNA)

singlet channel (Banyasz et al. 2012). In the latter case a large activation energy was calculated which could explain why 64PPs are produced by energetic UVB photons but not by UVA.

64PPs are produced in lower yields than CPDs in a ratio ranging between 1/2 and 1/8 depending on the detection methods (Mitchell et al. 1990; Perdiz et al. 2000; Douki and Cadet 2001). This proportion is yet very different from one bipyrimidine sequence to the other as shown by chromatographic assay (Douki and Cadet 2001). At TT sites, the ratio between CPDs and 64PPs is 10/1 while it is 5/4 at TC sites. CT 64PPs is hardly detected even in UVC irradiated isolated DNA while CC 64PP is produced in a 3-times lower yield than the corresponding CPD. Altogether, TC 64PP is the most frequent 64PP.

3.2.2.2 Photoisomerization into Dewar Valence Isomers

The pyrimidone ring exhibits absorption at 325 nm in TT and CT 64PPs, and at 315 nm in TC and CC 64PPs. The presence of this heterocyclic structure also provides fluorescence properties to 64PPs. In addition, a specific property of the pyrimidone rings is their ability to undergo 4π electrocyclization into their Dewar valence isomers (Taylor and Cohrs 1987; Haiser et al. 2012). Singlet excited states are the most likely intermediates in the photoreaction (Fingerhut et al. 2012). Time-resolved spectroscopic studies have shown that the reaction is quite slow, in the nanosecond time scale (Haiser et al. 2012). Photoisomerization of 64PPs exhibits a quantum yield of a few percent (Lemaire and Ruzsicska 1993; Haiser et al. 2012) and thus significantly contributes to UV-induced DNA damage. It should yet be emphasized that two photons are needed to produce a DEW, one to generate the initial 64PP and a second one to induce its photoisomerization.

Available data show that irradiation with a combination of UVB and UVA such as simulated solar radiation or sequential exposure to UVB and then to UVA is much more efficient at inducing DEWs in cells than pure UVB (Perdiz et al. 2000; Douki et al. 2003; Courdavault et al. 2005). This can be explained by the fact that UVB photons are absorbed by the normal bases present in large excess while UVA more efficiently reaches 64PPs. Because of the non-linear nature of the formation of DEWs, it is difficult to precisely determine their contribution to UV-induced DNA damage. The published data on the ratio between 64PPs and DEWs range from 10:1 to 1:4. This large variability reflects the overall UV dose and the emission spectra of the sources used in the different studies.

3.2.3 Oxidative Damage

Pyrimidine dimers are not the only DNA damage induced upon exposure to solar radiation. Other lesions arising from oxidation reactions are also produced. The

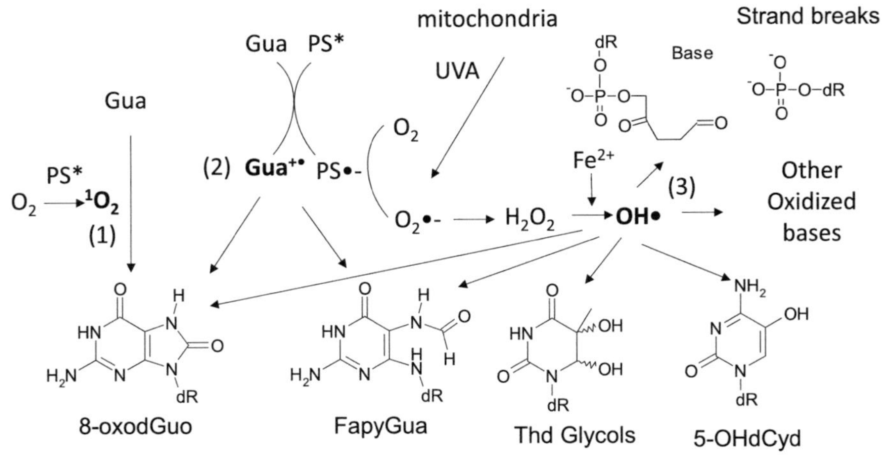

Fig. 3.3 The three oxidation pathways associated with exposure to UVA, (*1*) singlet oxygen production (*2*) electron abstraction and (*3*) production of hydroxyl radicals

underlying chemistry is quite complex since several pathways and different origins of reactive oxygen species (ROS) are involved (Fig. 3.3).

3.2.3.1 Photosensitized Formation

DNA is the main UVB chromophore in cells. In contrast, many other cellular components more efficiently absorb UVA and visible photons (Wondrak et al. 2006). Upon excitation, some of these endogenous chromophores may trigger photochemical processes leading to degradation of biomolecules including lipids, proteins and DNA. These photosensitization reactions mostly consist in oxidative pathways of various nature (Cadet et al. 2012). Because photosensitization requires biomolecular interactions, the reactive state of the photosensitizer is the long-lived triplet excited state rather than the singlet one. It should be stressed that exogenous compounds may also exhibit photosensitizing properties and enhance the photo-oxidative effect of solar radiation. Such properties are often associated with phototoxicity.

A first pathway involves transfer of the energy of the excited sensitizer to molecular oxygen. The latter is thus converted into its reactive singlet form (${}^1O_2$). In DNA, ${}^1O_2$ specifically reacts with guanine bases and leads almost exclusively to the formation of 8-oxoGua (Ravanat et al. 2001). Another photosensitization pathway involves electron abstraction from the substrate by the excited sensitizer. This reaction leads to the formation of a radical cation of the substrate and a radical anion of the sensitizer. In DNA, guanine is the main target because it exhibits the lowest oxidation potential among the DNA components. The guanine radical cation evolves into several final products. The major pathway is hydration into the

8-hydroxy-7,8-dihydroguanyl radical which may be either oxidized into 8-oxoGua or reduced into the ring opened 2,6-diamino-4-hydroxy-5-formamidopyrimidine (FapyGua) (Cadet et al. 2009). Addition of nucleophilic amino acid to the guanine radical cation is also an efficient reaction that may be one of the pathways leading to the formation of DNA-protein crosslinks observed in UVA-irradiated cells (Perrier et al. 2006).

A third oxidative pathway involves the highly reactive hydroxyl radical ($^{\cdot}OH$) (Cadet et al. 2012). The formation of $^{\cdot}OH$ involves the initial release of superoxide anion ($O_2^{\circ -}$) either by reaction of the photosensitizers' radical anions with oxygen or by release from mitochondria. $O_2^{\circ -}$ is poorly reactive with DNA. Yet it can dismutate into hydrogen peroxide H_2O_2, for instance through the action of cellular superoxide dismutase. The latter ROS is not reactive but is converted into $^{\cdot}OH$ by reaction with redox metal ions such as copper or iron. The fact that UVA leads to the release of iron from ferritin favors this deleterious pathway (Pourzand et al. 1999). In contrast to $^1O_2$ and electron abstraction, $^{\cdot}OH$ reacts in DNA without specificity. Not only guanine but all four bases are damaged into a wide variety of oxidation products. $^{\cdot}OH$ also damages deoxyribose moieties and thus leads to the induction of single strand breaks (SSBs). The formation of double strand breaks (DSBs) as a result of the photo-oxidative stress induced by UVA has been ruled out (Rizzo et al. 2010). This is expected since a DSB requires two simultaneous and closely located oxidation reactions. This is possible for instance along the track of ionizing radiations but is very unlikely to happen with UV radiation which spreads homogeneously over the exposed area. This does not preclude the formation of DSBs as a delayed response to UV exposure and especially by the collapse of replication forks at the site of photoproducts. The latter process explains why phosphorylation of the H2AX histone, a widely used marker of DSBs, is at its maximum several hours after exposure to UVB. In contrast, γ-H2AX is detected after a few minutes with ionizing radiations that cause DSB immediately after irradiation.

3.2.3.2 Secondary Oxidative DNA Damage

Oxidizing species are not only produced during the exposure period. They can be released in a subsequent phase as a response of skin cells to UV radiation. An important source of ROS and reactive nitrogen species is inflammation (Bickers and Athar 2006). This physiological mechanism, responsible among other of sunburns, is associated with the production of a series of oxidizing species including $O_2^{\circ -}$, H_2O_2, peroxynitrite and hypochlorous acid. UVB is also known to produce oxidizing species because of its interaction with several enzymes such as NADPH oxidase or cyclooxygenase (Beak et al. 2004; Wang and Kochevar 2005). The bulk of these processes lead to a delayed oxidative stress, well characterized in cultured keratinocytes (Rezvani et al. 2006).

Another indirect cause of DNA damage related to oxidative stress is the reaction of degradation products of other cellular components. It has been shown that the hydroperoxides present on oxidized proteins could generate oxidized bases in DNA (Furukawa et al. 2005). Photodegradation products of proteins have also been suggested to behave as secondary photosensitizers (Lamore et al. 2013). Another indirect genotoxic consequence of photo-oxidative stress could be the reaction of lipid peroxides breakdown products with DNA. UV radiation is indeed known to induce lipid peroxidation leading to the formation of reactive aldehydes (Winczura et al. 2012) such as malondialdehyde or 4-hydroxy-2,3-*trans*-nonenal. These compounds react with DNA bases, and in particular the exocyclic functions of adenine and guanine, to yield cyclic adducts. The formation of this class of DNA lesions has been well documented for other oxidative stress situations but remains poorly investigated in the case of UV exposure. Evidence that other biomolecules such as proteins react with lipid peroxidation by-products upon UV exposure (Larroque-Cardoso et al. 2015) strongly suggests that DNA could be another target.

3.2.3.3 Direct UV-Induced DNA Oxidation

Data are available that suggest the induction of oxidative lesions upon exposure of pure isolated DNA to UV radiations. A first evidence was the induction of strand breaks in the hyper sensitive plasmid relaxation assay by UVC, UVB and UVA (Boullard and Giacomoni 1988). It should be stressed that these experiments are difficult to perform because the DNA used must be free of any trace of contaminants which could behave as sensitizers. Yet, their results suggest that absorption of UV photons by DNA, both in the UVA and UVB range may lead to oxidative lesions. A first hypothesis based on the observation of the formation of 8-oxoGua was the production of singlet oxygen (Bishop et al. 1994; Mohammad and Morrison 1996). However, ionization cannot be ruled out (Marguet et al. 2006), although the energy provided by a single UV photon is below the ionization threshold of monomers. Further experiments are required to determine how the complexity of the fate of excited states in double stranded DNA could explain this result.

3.2.4 UV-Induced Photoproducts in Cells and Skin

Large amounts of information are available on the formation of DNA damage in cells exposed to UV radiation. Although some of these studies are not quantitative when non-calibrated immunoassays are used, other works made possible a comparison of the frequency of the different lesions following irradiation. Pure UVB causes an overwhelming formation of CPDs in mammalian cells compared to oxidized bases and strand breaks (Kielbassa et al. 1997; Douki et al. 2003), showing that the cellular context has only a limited impact on the overall photoreactivity of DNA. However, specificity in the formation of the pyrimidine dimers can be observed within the genome. For instance, quantification of CPDs at the nucleotide level in specific genes showed that the sequence context could enhance or inhibit the formation of photoproducts (Drouin and Therrien 1997; You et al. 2000). Data also show that the photoreactivity is modulated in telomeres (Rochette and Brash 2010). Interestingly, in vitro results suggest that inter-strand CPDs could be produced in quadruplex regions (Su et al. 2008). The yield of UVB-induced pyrimidine dimers is roughly the same in all types of cultured cells. In contrast, significant differences can be found between skins of different phototypes with less CPDs in dark than in light skin (Tadokoro et al. 2003). The same trend is observed for UVA-induced CPDs (Mouret et al. 2011b).

HPLC-mass spectrometry measurements allowed to compare the yield of formation of 8-oxoGua and TT CPDs in a series of cell types and in skin exposed to UVA. The ratio between the amounts of CPDs and 8-oxoGua is 9 (Mouret et al. 2006) in skin and approximately 6 in primary cultures of human keratinocytes and fibroblasts (Courdavault et al. 2004). Similar ratios were obtained by using biochemical assays in CHO cells (Kielbassa et al. 1997). CPDs are produced in a roughly 3 orders of magnitude lower yield in the UVA than in the UVB range. Interestingly, the ratio between the yields of CPDs and 8-oxoGua is only 1.4 in primary cultures of human melanocytes (Mouret et al. 2012). These in vitro results show that melanocytes are more sensitive to UVA-induced oxidative stress than other cell types (Wang et al. 2010; Mouret et al. 2012). These observations are in agreement with data obtained using either pigmented or albino mice and showing that melanoma is partly induced in the UVA range by oxidative stress mediated by melanin (Noonan et al. 2012). As far as the distribution of UVA-induced oxidative lesions is concerned, a series of studies using different cell types and quantification assays showed that oxidized purines (OxyPyr), and mostly 8-oxoGua, was the major oxidative lesion (Kielbassa et al. 1997; Pouget et al. 2000). SSBs are produced in 3-times and oxidized pyrimidines in 4-times lower yields. The formation of DNA-protein crosslinks (Peak and Peak 1991) represents roughly one tenth of that of 8-oxoGua.

Most of these data were obtained using pure UVB or UVA radiation. Some information is available on the distribution of pyrimidine dimers exposed to natural or simulated sunlight (SSL). CPDs are the main photoproducts in both cultured cells and skin. In addition, as expected from the experiments involving a combination of UVA and UVB, DEWs are produced in significant amounts at the expense of 64PPs in both cells and skin exposed to SSL (Rosenstein and Mitchell 1991; Clingen et al. 1995; Perdiz et al. 2000; Douki et al. 2003; Bacqueville et al. 2015) and sunlight (Clingen et al. 1995; Qin et al. 1996). It should be stressed that the proportion of DEWs was found to be dose dependent. In a recent study using human skin explants, the yield of isomerization of 64PPs ranged from 17 to 36 % between 1 and 3 minimal erythemal dose (Bacqueville et al. 2015). Using SSL, the yield of formation of oxidized bases is much lower than that of pyrimidine dimers (Douki et al. 2003). By combining all these pieces of information on the relative yields of the different UV-induced lesions and considering that the proportion of UVA in sunlight is higher than 95 %, it is possible to propose a semi-quantitative

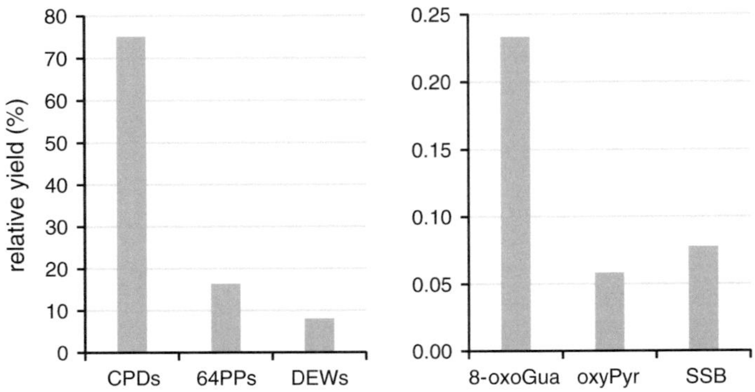

Fig. 3.4 Semi-quantitative distribution of the DNA damage induced by solar radiation. Results are expressed in percentage. Note that the scale of the *right* panel is different from that on the *left*. Calculation is based on a UVA to UVB ratio of 20. The yield of photoisomerization of 64PPs into DEWs is that observed after exposure to 3 MED in skin explants

distribution of DNA damage in skin cells exposed to solar radiation (Fig. 3.4). Pyrimidine dimers appear as the predominant lesions.

3.3 From Damage to Mutation

Determining the respective amounts of the different types of DNA damage is important in order to quantify the genotoxic effect of UV radiation. However, knowing the frequency of the different damage is not enough to predict the induction of mutations. Indeed, the differential repair efficiency and mutagenicity of the different DNA lesions must also be taken into account.

3.3.1 DNA Repair

DNA repair is a very complex machinery with several pathways handling the different types of damage. These pathways involve numerous proteins which are sometimes common to several mechanisms and are under the control of complex signaling cascades. The purpose here is not to summarize the enormous amounts of data gathered during the last years concerning the biochemical and cellular aspects of DNA repair. The paragraph will mostly consider the repair through the differential efficacy for the different lesions induced by UV radiation.

3.3.1.1 Nucleotide Excision Repair

Nucleotide excision repair (NER) removes lesions that significantly modify the tridimensional structure of DNA. Consequently, NER repairs all bulky lesions including UV-induced pyrimidine dimers. NER actually includes two distinct pathways depending on the DNA damage signaling step. The first one relies on arrest of RNA polymerases at the damaged site (transcription-coupled NER, TCR) (Fousteri and Mullenders 2008) with subsequent activation of CSB protein, while the other involves sensing proteins such as XPC that bind to photoproducts in the whole DNA (global genome NER, GGR) (Gillet and Scharer 2006). The last steps of the repair process are the same in both TCR and GGR, with recruitments of DNA unwinding proteins followed by cleavage of a short single-stranded portion of DNA containing the photoproduct. The resulting gap is filled by DNA polymerases and sealed by a DNA ligase. TCR is much faster than GGR and eliminates CPDs and 64PPs with a similar efficiency. TCR is yet limited to the lesions present in the transcribed strand of active genes. In contrast GGR handles lesions in the whole genome but with a lower efficiency. GGR removes 64PPs and DEWs faster than CPDs (Mitchell et al. 1985; Young et al. 1996; Courdavault et al. 2005). In cultured cells, 64PPs are typically removed within a few hours while CPDs can still be found three days after exposure. The rate of repair is even slower in skin. Interestingly, the four CPDs were found to be repaired at different rates. The half-life times were found to be in the following order in primary cultures of human skin cells and in skin explants: CT < CC < TC < TT (Mouret et al. 2008).

3.3.1.2 Base Excision Repair

Oxidative DNA lesions are handled by base excision repair (BER). This repair system is in charge of small DNA modifications such as oxidized or methylated bases. Key components of BER are DNA-*N*-glycosylases (Hegde et al. 2008; Zharkov 2008). These enzymes are substrate-specific and each recognizes a limited number of modified bases. For instance OGG1 is specific for 8-oxoGua while Nth-like DNA glycosylase 1 (NTHL1) and Nei-like DNA glycosylase 1 (NEIL1) removes oxidized pyrimidines. After binding to the modified bases, glycosylases cleave the *N*-glycosidic bond, leaving an abasic site in DNA. This abasic site is then cleaved by an endonuclease, in particular APE1, leaving a one-nucleotide gap with a 3′-end OH and a 5′-end ribosyl-phosphate. Some glycosylases are bifunctional and can cleave both the base-sugar bond and the abasic site. Depending on their catalytic mechanism, either a 3′-end phosphate/5′-end phosphate (β,δ-elimination) or a 3′-end sugar residue/5′-end phosphate (β-elimination) gap is obtained. APE-1 mediated nicks and 3′-end phospate/5′-end phosphate produced by β,δ-bifunctional enzymes are then converted into a gap with a 3′-OH end and a 5′-phosphate by action of polβ or PNK, respectively. A single nucleotide is incorporated using the complementary strand and the intact strand is obtained by action of a ligase. This BER pathway is known as short patch repair. In the case of the more complex products of β-bifunctional enzymes, polδ or ε synthesize a short piece of DNA by strand displacement from the site of the gap. The resulting 5′-flap segment is cleaved by FEN1 and the strand is sealed by a ligase. In BER, strand breaks are produced as intermediates in the mechanism. Consequently, BER is also the repair system handling SSBs from oxidative origin. BER is a rapid system compared to NER. The half-life time of SSBs is less than one hour after exposure to UVA and that of 8-oxoGua a few hours (Surjana et al. 2013). It may be added that repair of the latter lesion is completed by hMYH which removes adenine opposite 8-oxoGua and NUDT1 that cleaves 8-oxodGTP from the nucleotide pool in order to prevent the incorporation of the oxidized base.

3.3.1.3 Impact of UVA-Induced Oxidative Stress on Repair

When cells and skin are exposed to doses of UVA or UVB leading to the same level of CPDs in DNA, the rate of repair is slower with UVA than with UVB (Courdavault et al. 2005; Mouret et al. 2006). This observation is rather unexpected since the CPDs are the same whatever the mechanism they arise from. Furthermore, UVB induces 64PPs in addition to CPDs. Therefore, the amount of DNA damage which the cell has to deal with for a same level of CPDs is larger with UVB than with UVA and repair could be thought to be less efficient. Another unexpected result was that cells exposed to a low dose of UVA removed CPDs and 64PPs less efficiently after UVB irradiation than cells that did not receive the preliminary UVA treatment (Courdavault et al. 2005). This set of information strongly suggests that UVA interferes with the repair of pyrimidine dimers. Evidence has been provided that oxidation of repair proteins is at least one of the mechanisms involved. Indeed, it was shown that PCNA underwent oligomerization as the result of photo-oxidation in cells exposed to UVA both in the presence and the absence of photosensitizer (Montaner et al. 2007). More recently, oxidative photodegradation of RPA was also established (Guven et al. 2015). Decreased repair activity after exposure to UVA may also result from other mechanisms including modulation of signal transduction, but this remains to be explored.

3.3.2 *Mutagenic Properties of DNA Damage In Vitro*

The yield of formation and the repair efficiency determine the frequency of a specific lesion and its persistence within DNA. In order to assess its contribution to the overall mutagenesis, the mutagenic properties of all individual lesion must be taken into account. This kind of Information has been gathered in in vitro assays using synthetic DNA probes bearing specific lesions.

3.3.2.1 Pyrimidine Dimers

Numerous data on the mutagenic properties have been obtained using purified polymerases or the shuttle vector approach in yeasts and SOS-induced bacteria (Lawrence et al. 1993; Taylor 1994). TT CPD is a blocking lesion but when bypassed it induces mutations in less than 5 % of the times (Taylor and O'Day 1990). For other CPDs, an important aspect to consider is a secondary reaction involving cytosine moieties known as deamination. This spontaneous hydrolytic process converts the cytosine moiety of CPDs into uracil within a few hours (Frederico et al. 1990; Peng and Shaw 1996). The impact of deamination in mutagenesis is explained by the fact that uracil like thymine codes for adenine (Fig. 3.5). This is clearly illustrated by the observation that UU CPD, like TT CPD, leads to the incorporation of two adenines in 95 % of the bypass events (Gibbs and Lawrence 1993). Altogether, deamination is a key explanation to the induction of C → T transitions by C-containing CPDs as confirmed in biological assays (Jiang and Taylor 1993). The importance of deamination is also reinforced by the demonstration that non deaminated TC CPD is not mutagenic (Horsfall et al. 1997).

64PPs also exhibit mutational properties mostly resulting from the modulation of the hydrogen bonding capacities of the bases. Deamination is poorly involved because it takes place at the 5′-end C in the very minor CT and CC 64PPs but not in the abundant TC 64PP in which the exocyclic amino group of C is shifted to the C5

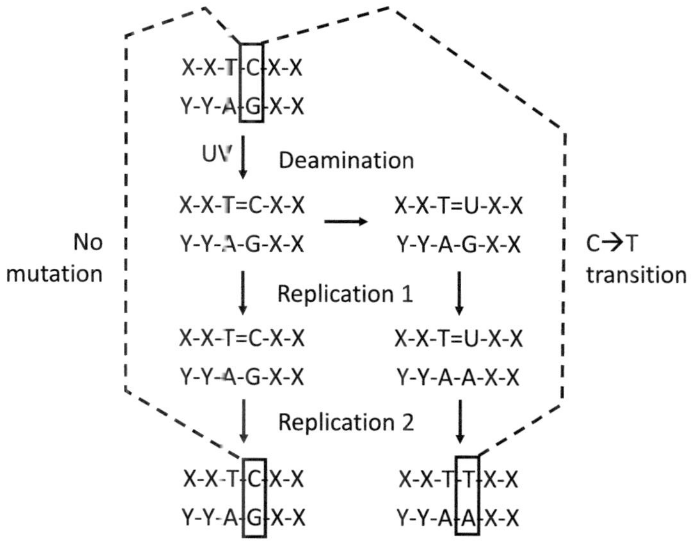

Fig. 3.5 Involvement of deamination in the mutagenesis of UV-induced photoproducts. The figure illustrates the case of TC CPD (T=C). Replication of the strand bearing the CPD leads to the respective incorporation of G and A opposite the cytosine and the uracil moieties depending whether the CPD is deaminated or not. During a second replication, the newly synthesized DNA strands lead to the formation of C:G and T:A base pairs, respectively

position of T. TT 64PP is highly mutagenic with mostly T → C mutations at the 3′-end (LeClerc et al. 1991). TT DEW is less mutagenic because the 3′-end ring is mostly non-coding and leads to the incorporation of adenine (Smith et al. 1996). The TC 64PP is poorly mutagenic but efficiently induces C → T transitions after conversion into its DEW (Horsfall and Lawrence 1993). This is explained by the fact that the 5′-end T codes for T in both 64PPs and DEWs while the 3′-end pyrimidone leads mostly to the incorporation of G with 64PPs and A with DEWs.

In terms of mutagenesis, an important finding in the recent years is the role played by a specific class of polymerases known as translesion synthesis (TLS) polymerases (Makridakis and Reichardt 2012). These enzymes replicate normal DNA with poor fidelity but process damaged sites with much more efficiency than normal replicative polymerases. Implication of TLS-polymerases can thus be considered as a tolerance mechanism. A drawback of such a pathway could be an increased risk for mutagenesis. Fortunately, TLS-polymerases are error-free for specific classes of DNA lesions. In response to UV radiation, polη plays a major role since it was shown to replicate TT, TC and CC CPDs with high fidelity (Yu et al. 2001; Yoon et al. 2009). Lack of polη like in XP-variant patients results in increased mutagenesis because replication of CPDs is performed by other polymerases in an error-prone way. An interesting point regarding polη is whether deaminated cytosine within CPDs code for A or G. Only the latter case would make the polymerase fully error-free for CPDs. The fact that TT CPDs are replicated by polη with high fidelity yet suggests that deamination may also lead to mutations due the coding of A by U with TLS-polymerases (Choi and Pfeifer 2005).

3.3.2.2 8-oxoGua

8-oxoGua has been shown to cause the incorporation of adenine and thereby inducing G → T transitions (Shibutani et al. 1991). This mutagenic action is governed by two properties: the hydrogen bonding properties of the base and the orientation of the *N*-glycosidic bond. When the purine ring of 8-oxoGua is in opposite orientation with respect to the deoxyribose ring, as in unmodified guanine, 8-oxoGua pairs with cytosine and thus does not induce mutations. However, the C8 oxo group of 8-oxoGua induces steric hindrance in the nucleotide and leads to a rotation along the N-glycosidic bond, placing the purine ring of 8-oxoGua above the sugar (Kouchakdjian et al. 1991; McAuley-Hecht et al. 1994). In this orientation, 8-oxoGua causes the incorporation of adenine instead to cytosine, with subsequent induction of G → T mutations. Like for CPDs, TLS-polymerases play an important role in the mutagenicity of 8-oxoGua. It is replicated with fidelity by polη but in an error-prone way by polι.

3.3.2.3 Other Oxidation Products

The mutagenicity of oxidized bases has also been investigated in vitro. 8-oxoadenine is an example of much less mutagenic lesions than 8-oxoGua (Tan et al. 1999). Information was also obtained on the Fapy derivatives showing that FapyGua induces G → T transversions while FapyAde is poorly mutagenic (Kalam et al. 2006). Thymine glycols are strongly blocking lesions but are poorly mutagenic. The latter property is also true for TLS-polymerases (Evans et al. 1993). 5-Formyluracil also leads to a low mutation frequency (Kamiya et al. 2002). In contrast to these thymine lesions, cytosine oxidation products are mutagenic, mostly under their deaminated form (Purmal et al. 1994; Kreutzer and Essigmann 1998).

3.3.3 Respective Contribution of the Photoproducts to Mutagenesis In Vivo

Large amounts of information have been gathered on the different mutations induced by UVB, mostly by sequencing UVB-irradiated plasmids replicated after transfection in bacteria or by sequencing specific genes in UVB-irradiated cells (Miller 1985; Romac et al. 1989). All these studies led to the same conclusion, namely that the most frequent mutations are C → T transition at TC sites and CC → TT tandem mutations. Interestingly, very few mutations occur at CT sites, likely reflecting the high repair efficiency of CT CPD. Experiments using cells (You et al. 2001) and mice (Jans et al. 2005) exhibiting increased repair of either 64PPs or CPDs have shown that the latter photoproducts were responsible for the majority of the mutations. This observation can be explained by the more efficient repair of 64PPs compared to CPDs. For the UVA range, early studies in rodent cells reported A:T → C:G transversions (Sage et al. 1996) as the most frequent events while more recent works, carried out in human cells, report mostly mutations at bipyrimidine sites (Kappes et al. 2006; Ikehata et al. 2008). Interestingly, the signature of 8-oxoGua, G → T, is never a predominant mutation although 8-oxoGua is the main oxidative lesion. This may again be explained by the very efficient repair system for 8-oxoGua. All these results provide information on the DNA damage leading to skin cancers. In tumors, the signature of CPDs is the predominant mutational event with C → T transition at TC sites and tandem CC → TT mutations accounting for more than 80 % of the mutations in targeted genes like p53 (Brash et al. 1991; Ziegler et al. 1993). Recent work using modern next generation sequencing showed that this UV mutation signature is found within the whole genome of melanoma (Pleasance et al. 2010). The overwhelming presence of mutations at bipyrimidine sites is obviously explained by the fact that pyrimidine dimers are by far the most frequent DNA lesions caused by exposure to solar radiation. Very few mutations corresponding to oxidative lesions like 8-oxoGua are detected except in tumors arising from the deepest layers of epidermis (Agar et al. 2004). The latter observation is in agreement with the idea that the ratio between UVB and UVA decreases with the penetration in skin. Chromosomal aberrations could be another minor type of mutational event caused by UV radiations. As discussed above, DSB can be indirectly produced by pyrimidine dimers or SSBs. This possible pathway remains though to be investigated.

3.4 Preventing UV-Induced DNA Damage

The data reported above unambiguously show that solar radiation is a very efficient DNA damaging and mutagenic agent. Natural tanning by induction of melanogenesis can be considered as a photoprotection but it requires significant exposure to UV radiation and the unavoidable induction of DNA damage. In addition, the protection afforded by tanning is limited (Sheehan et al. 1998). The most efficient photoprotection strategy is thus to avoid excessive exposure to sunlight, by seeking shade or using proper clothing, and to ban the use of artificial tanning equipments. Regrettably, such behavior is commonly not followed, either for occupational reasons or as the results of recreational habits. Alternative photoprotective approaches should thus be applied.

3.4.1 Sunscreens

As described above, mutations leading to skin tumors are mostly due to pyrimidine dimers. Because these lesions are produced by the direct absorption of UV by DNA bases, their formation can be prevented only by limiting the amount of photons reaching skin cells. Sunscreen is one of the best way to reach this goal. The efficiency of sunscreens at preventing the formation of CPDs and 64PPs has been shown both in vivo (Freeman et al. 1988; van Praag et al. 1993; Young et al. 2000) and ex vivo (Bissonauth et al. 2000; Rouabhia et al. 2002; Mouret et al. 2011a; Bacqueville et al. 2015). It should be stressed that sunscreens are characterized by their sun protection factor (SPF) which measures their ability at preventing sunburns. Although both formation of pyrimidine dimers and erythema induction depend on the applied UV dose, they drastically differ in terms of mechanism, one being a direct photoreaction and the other an inflammatory response. Moreover, sunburn is a threshold response while CPDs are detected even at sub-erythemal doses. It remains thus to be established whether SPF quantitatively reflects protection of DNA. The few available data are contradictory with some studies showing an identical efficiency (Freeman et al. 1988; Young et al. 2000) while others suggest that the DNA protection is slightly lower than the SPF (Bissonauth et al. 2000; Rouabhia et al. 2002; Mouret et al. 2011a; Bacqueville et al. 2015). However, it is unquestionable that sunscreens do protect skin against the formation of pyrimidine dimers.

A still pending question is why there are sometimes disappointing results of sunscreen-based photoprotection (Autier et al. 1998; Wachsmuth et al. 2005). Possibly, sunscreen users tend to increase their recreational exposure (Holman et al. 1986; Autier et al. 2007). Another likely explanation is that the amount of product used is too low. Sunscreens are tested at a dose of 2 mg/cm^2 which is much more than that the amount applied in general population (Reich et al. 2009). When the amount of sunscreen is better controlled and applied on a regular basis, studies do see a significant decrease of skin cancer in sunscreen users (Green et al. 1999, 2011). In addition to UV filters, modern sunscreens often contain antioxydants (Chen et al. 2012). Evidence that these compounds improve erythema, immunosuppression and carcinogenesis has been documented for instance for vitamin C (Darr et al. 1992; Nakamura et al. 1997), tocopherols (Gensler and Magdaleno 1991; Burke et al. 2000), and combination of both (Lin et al. 2003). Decreased formation of pyrimidine dimers (McVean and Liebler 1997, 1999) has been also reported, although the underlying mechanism remains unclear. Although these data are promising, use of antioxydants in complete sunscreens is disappointing because their formulation favors a local deposition on the upper layers of skin which prevents an efficient diffusion of antioxydants in the cells. The antioxydants effects of sunscreen may actually mostly result from the absorption of UVA radiation by the UV filters (Wang et al. 2008).

3.4.2 *Systemic Photoprotection*

Preventing absorption of UV photons by DNA and endogenous sensitizers is the most efficient way to protect skin against photocarcinogenesis. However, other physiological responses and systemic effects such as inflammation and immunosuppression play significant roles in tumor development. Preventive oral intake of active compounds modulating these effects was thus proposed as a way to provide additional photoprotection. In that respect, oxidative stress, that plays only a minor role in the initial insult to DNA but is an important mediator in other effects, is a key target. In contrast to sunscreens that provide immediate protection, the positive effects of systemic photoprotection are only seen after long term supplementation. A widely investigated class of compounds are retinoids (vitamin A) that were shown to protect against SCCs in a normal population (Moon et al. 1997) and in psoriasis patients (Nijsten and Stern 2003). Carotenoids also exhibit photoprotection against erythema (Stahl et al. 2006; Kopcke and Krutmann 2008) and photocarcinogenesis (Frieling et al. 2000). Nonsteroidal anti-inflammatory drugs are other potential photoprotective compounds, especially against SCCs (Kopcke and Krutmann 2008; Clouser et al. 2009). It should be stressed that little information is available on the mechanisms underlying the photoprotection afforded by these classes of compounds. DNA damage is rarely investigated in such studies and hypotheses are mostly related to inflammation and immunosuppression. More recently, a different strategy has been designed that involves supplementation with nicotinamide in order to favor ATP synthesis and maintain the energy level in irradiated cells. One of the major expected consequences is an increased DNA repair activity that strongly depends on ATP as observed in cells and skin explants (Surjana et al. 2013). Human supplementation studies showed that nicotinamide prevents actinic keratosis and suggest that it also prevents non-melanoma skin cancer (Moloney et al. 2010; Surjana et al. 2012). Finally, recent proposal is the use of melatonin as a factor against UV-induced skin damage (Goswami and Haldar 2015) mostly because it exhibits antioxidant properties. An additional interesting idea is that repair of DNA damage by NER and even induction of skin cancer in mice could be associated with circadian rhythms (Kang et al. 2010; Gaddameedhi et al. 2015).

3.4.3 Natural Products and Extracts

Most high SPF sunscreens include metal oxide nanoparticles and all contain a combination of different UV absorbing organic compounds. These ingredients have been questioned for their toxicity and their environmental impact. As a consequence, numerous studies have been devoted to the identification of natural compounds and extracts of various origin exhibiting photoprotective properties (Chen et al. 2013; Jansen et al. 2013; Saewan and Jimtaisong 2015). A well-documented example is green tea extracts that are rich in antioxidant polyphenols. Their topical application in animal models was found to protect against immunosuppression and photocarcinogenesis (Rutter et al. 2003; Yusuf et al. 2007). In addition, supplementation with polyphenols from green tea enhances DNA repair in skin (Meeran et al. 2009). In some in vitro studies, protection against DNA damage has been reported for instance for strawberry (Giampieri et al. 2012), pomegranate (Afaq et al. 2009) and alga extracts (Lyons and O'Brien 2002; Heo et al. 2009). In these studies, emphasis is often placed on oxidative damage reflecting the beneficial effects of antioxidants. Yet, the presence of UV absorbing molecules may also make them suitable for the production of natural sunscreens. In that respect, mycosporin isolated from lichens exhibit interesting photoprotective properties and was found to decrease the formation of pyrimidine dimers (Rancan et al. 2002; Russo et al. 2008). Similar photoprotection is provided by propolis extracts (Gregoris et al. 2011). Although the results obtained with natural products and extracts are encouraging, their large scale use in photoprotection still lacks validation in large human studies and a better understanding of the underlying mechanisms is necessary.

3.5 Concluding Remarks

Solar UV radiation is likely the mutagenic agent to which humans are the most frequently exposed. In terms of its tumorogenic actions, the very large amounts of information gathered in the last 50 years now allow us to describe the whole initiation phase from the induction of DNA damage to repair and mutagenesis. This chain of events unambiguously show the predominant role played by UVB-induced pyrimidine dimers. UVA can yet not be neglected since it clearly contributes although to a lesser extent to the load of DNA damage and interferes with major processes like repair and immune response. Formation of pyrimidine dimers by both UVB and UVA involve absorption by DNA and induction of oxidative stress in the UVA and visible ranges require absorption by endogenous chromophores. Therefore, the best way to protect skin from the deleterious effects of sunlight is obviously to prevent its interaction with incident photons. It is thus necessary to keep on communicating to the general public the importance of avoiding exposure at the time of day when the intensity of UV radiation and the proportion of UVB are maximal, and wearing hats and clothes under the sun. It should be also reminded that using tanning equipment represents an unnecessary exposure to a mutagenic agent and does not provide protection for subsequent exposure. When limitation of exposure is not possible or not wanted, other strategies can be applied. Sunscreen is then interesting but does not completely prevent the formation of DNA damage, especially when used in insufficient amounts as often. Supplementation with antioxidants and naturel products provide additional beneficial effects mostly related to reduced oxidative stress. However, they do not prevent the formation of the carcinogenic pyrimidine dimers.

References

Afaq F, Zaid MA, Khan N, Dreher M, Mukhtar H (2009) Protective effect of pomegranate-derived products on UVB-mediated damage in human reconstituted skin. Exp Dermatol 18:553–561

Agar NS, Halliday GM, Barnetson ESC, Ananthaswamy HN, Wheeler M, Jones AM (2004) The basal layer in human squamous tumors harbors more UVA than UVB fingerprints mutations: a role for UVA in human skin carcinogenesis. Proc Natl Acad Sci USA 101:4954–4959

Autier P, Dore JF, Cattaruzza MS, Renard F, Luther H, Gentiloni-Silverj F, Zantedeschi E, Mezzetti M, Monjaud I, Andry M et al (1998) Sunscreen use, wearing clothes, and number of nevi in 6- to 7-year-old European children. European Organization for Research and Treatment of Cancer Melanoma Cooperative Group. J Natl Cancer Inst 90:1873–1880

Autier P, Boniol M, Dore JF (2007) Sunscreen use and increased duration of intentional sun exposure: still a burning issue. Int J Cancer 121:1–5

Bacqueville D, Douki T, Duprat L, Rebelo-Moreira S, Guiraud B, Dromigny H, Perier V, Bessou-Touya S, Duplan H (2015) A new hair follicle-derived human epidermal model for the evaluation of sunscreen genoprotection. J Photochem Photobiol B Biol 151:31–38

Banyasz A, Vaya I, Changenet-Barret P, Gustavsson T, Douki T, Markovitsi D (2011) Base pairing enhances fluorescence and favors cyclobutane dimer formation induced upon absorption of UVA radiation by DNA. J Am Chem Soc 133:5163–5165

Banyasz A, Douki T, Improta R, Gustavsson T, Onidas D, Vaya I, Perron M, Markovitsi D (2012) Electronic excited states responsible for dimer formation upon UV absorption directly by thymine strands: joint experimental and theoretical study. J Am Chem Soc 134:14834–14845

Bastien N, Therrien JP, Drouin R (2013) Cytosine containing dipyrimidine sites can be hotspots of cyclobutane pyrimidine dimer formation after UVB exposure. Photochem Photobiol Sci 12:1544–1554

Beak SM, Lee YS, Kim JA (2004) NADPH oxidase and cyclooxygenase mediate the ultraviolet B-induced generation of reactive oxygen species and activation of nuclear factor-kappaB in HaCaT human keratinocytes. Biochimie 86:425–429

Besaratinia A, Synold TW, Chen H-H, Chang C, Xi B, Riggs A, Pfeifer GP (2005) DNA lesions induced by UV A1 and B radiation in human cells: comparative analyses in the overall genome and in the p53 tumor suppressor gene. Proc Natl Acad Sci USA 102:10058–10063

Bickers DR, Athar M (2006) Oxidative stress in the pathogenesis of skin disease. J Invest Dermatol 126:2565–2575

Bishop SM, Malone M, Phillips D, Parker AW, Symons CR (1994) Singlet oxygen sensitisation by excited state DNA. J Chem Soc Chem Comm, 871–872

Bissonauth V, Drouin R, Mitchell DL, Rhainds M, Claveau J, Rouabhia M (2000) The efficacy of a broad-spectrum sunscreen to protect engineered human skin from tissue and DNA damage induced by solar ultraviolet exposure. Clin Cancer Res 6:4128–4135

Blancafort L, Migani A (2007) Modeling thymine photodimerizations in DNA: mechanism and correlation diagrams. J Am Chem Soc 129:14540–14541

Bosca F, Lhiaubet-Vallet V, Cuquerella MC, Castell JV, Miranda MA (2006) The triplet energy of thymine in DNA. J Am Chem Soc 128:6318–6319

Boullard A, Giacomoni PU (1988) Effect of UV irradiation at defined wavelengths on the tertiary structure of double-stranded covalently closed circular DNA. J Photochem Photobiol B Biol 2:491–501

Brash DE, Rudolph JA, Simon JA, Lin A, McKenna GJ, Baden HP, Halperin AJ, Ponten J (1991) A role for sunlight in skin cancer: UV-induced p53 mutations in squamous cell carcinoma. Proc Natl Acad Sci USA 88:10124–10128

Burke KE, Clive J, Combs GF Jr, Commisso J, Keen CL, Nakamura RM (2000) Effects of topical and oral vitamin E on pigmentation and skin cancer induced by ultraviolet irradiation in Skh: 2 hairless mice. Nutr Cancer 38:87–97

Cadet J, Douki T, Ravanat JL, Di Mascio P (2009) Sensitized formation of oxidatively generated damage to cellular DNA by UVA radiation. Photochem Photobiol Sci 8:903–911

Cadet J, Mouret S, Ravanat JL, Douki T (2012) Photoinduced damage to cellular DNA: direct and photosensitized reactions. Photochem Photobiol 88:1048–1065

Chen L, Hu JY, Wang SQ (2012) The role of antioxidants in photoprotection: a critical review. J Am Acad Dermatol 67:1013–1024

Chen AC, Damian DL, Halliday GM (2013) Oral and systemic photoprotection. Photodermatol Photoimmunol Photomed 30:102–111

Choi JH, Pfeifer GP (2005) The role of DNA polymerase eta in UV mutational spectra. DNA Repair 4:211–220

Clingen PH, Arlett CF, Roza L, Mori T, Nikaido O, Green MHL (1995) Induction of cyclobutane pyrimidine dimers, pyrimidine(6-4)pyrimidone photoproducts, and Dewar valence isomers by natural sunlight in normal human mononuclear cells. Cancer Res 55:2245–2248

Clouser MC, Roe DJ, Foote JA, Harris RB (2009) Effect of non-steroidal anti-inflammatory drugs on non-melanoma skin cancer incidence in the SKICAP-AK trial. Pharmacoepidemiol Drug Saf 18:276–283

Courdavault S, Baudouin C, Charveron M, Favier A, Cadet J, Douki T (2004) Larger yield of cyclobutane dimers than 8 oxo-7,8-dihydroguanine in the DNA of UVA-irradiated human skin cells. Mutat Res 556:135–142

Courdavault S, Baudouin C, Charveron M, Canghilem B, Favier A, Cadet J, Douki T (2005) Repair of the three main types of bipyrimidine DNA photoproducts in human keratinocytes exposed to UVB and UVA radiations. DNA Repair 4:836–844

Cuquerella MC, Lhiaubet-Vallet V, Bosca F, Miranda MA (2011) Photosensitised pyrimidine dimerisation in DNA. Chem Sci 2:1219–1232

Cuquerella MC, Lhiaubet-Vallet V, Cadet J, Miranda MA (2012) Benzophenone photosensitized DNA damage. Account Chem Res 45:1558–1570

Darr D, Combs S, Dunston S, Manning T, Pinnell S (1992) Topical vitamin C protects porcine skin from ultraviolet radiation-induced damage. Br J Dermatol 127:247–253

Douki T, Cadet J (2001) Individual determination of the yield of the main-UV induced dimeric pyrimidine photoproducts in DNA suggests a high mutagenicity of CC photolesions. Biochemistry 40:2495–2501

Douki T, Reynaud-Angelin A, Cadet J, Sage E (2003) Bipyrimidine photoproducts rather than oxidative lesions are the main type of DNA damage involved in the genotoxic effect of solar UVA radiation. Biochemistry 42:9221–9226

Douki T, Berard I, Wack A, Andra S (2014) Contribution of cytosine-containing cyclobutane dimers to DNA damage produced by photosensitized triplet–triplet energy transfer. Chem Eur J 20:5787–5794

Drouin R, Therrien JP (1997) UVB-induced cyclobutane pyrimidine dimer frequency correlates with skin cancer mutational hotspots in p53. Photochem Photobiol 66:719–726

El Ghissassi F, Baan R, Straif K, Grosse Y, Secretan B, Bouvard V, Benbrahim-Tallaa L, Guha N, Freeman C, Galichet L et al (2009) A review of human carcinogens—part D: radiation. Lancet Oncol 10:751–752

Emanuele E, Zakrzewska K, Markovitsi D, Lavery R, Millie P (2005) Exciton states of dynamic DNA double helices: alternating dCdG sequences. J Phys Chem B 109:16109–16118

Evans J, Maccabee M, Hatahet Z, Courcelle J, Bockrath R, Ide H, Wallace S (1993) Thymine ring saturation and fragmentation products—lesion bypass, misinsertion and implications for mutagenesis. Mutat Res 299:147–156

Fingerhut BP, Herzog TT, Ryseck G, Haiser K, Graupner FF, Heil K, Gilch P, Schreier WJ, Carell T, de Vivie-Riedle R et al (2012) Dynamics of ultraviolet-induced DNA lesions: Dewar formation guided by pre-tension induced by the backbone. New J Phys 14

Fousteri M, Mullenders LH (2008) Transcription-coupled nucleotide excision repair in mammalian cells: molecular mechanisms and biological effects. Cell Res 18:73–84

Frederico LA, Kunkel TA, Shaw BR (1990) A sensitive genetic assay for the detection of cytosine deamination: determination of rate constants and the activation energy. Biochemistry 29:2532–2537

Freeman SE, Ryan SL (1990) Wavelength dependence for UV-induced pyrimidine dimer formation in DNA of human peripheral blood lymphocytes. Mutat Res 235:181–186

Freeman SE, Ley RD, Ley KD (1988) Sunscreen protection against UV-induced pyrimidine dimers in DNA of human skin in situ. Photodermatology 5:243–247

Freeman SE, Hacham H, Gange RW, Maytum DJ, Sutherland JC, Sutherland BM (1989) Wavelength dependence of pyrimidine dimer formation in DNA of human skin irradiated in situ with ultraviolet light. Proc Natl Acad Sci USA 86:5605–5609

Frieling UM, Schaumberg DA, Kupper TS, Muntwyler J, Hennekens CH (2000) A randomized, 12-year primary-prevention trial of beta carotene supplementation for nonmelanoma skin cancer in the physician's health study. Arch Dermatol 136:179–184

Furukawa A, Hiraku Y, Oikawa S, Luxford C, Davies MJ, Kawanishi S (2005) Guanine-specific DNA damage induced by gamma-irradiated histone. Biochem J 388:813–818

Gaddameedhi S, Selby CP, Kaufmann WK, Smart RC, Sancar A (2015) Control of skin cancer by the circadian rhythm. Proc Natl Acad Sci USA 108:18790–18795

Garcès F, Davila CA (1982) Alterations in DNA irradiated with ultraviolet radiation—I. The formation process of cyclobutylpyrimidine dimers: cross sections, action spectra and quantum yields. Photochem Photobiol 35:9–16

Gensler HL, Magdaleno M (1991) Topical vitamin E inhibition of immunosuppression and tumorigenesis induced by ultraviolet irradiation. Nutr Cancer 15:97–106

Giampieri F, Alvarez-Suarez JM, Tulipani S, Gonzales-Paramas AM, Santos-Buelga C, Bompadre S, Quiles JL, Mezzetti B, Battino M (2012) Photoprotective potential of strawberry

(Fragaria × ananassa) extract against UV-A irradiation damage on human fibroblasts. J Agric Food Chem 60:2322–2327
Gibbs PEM, Lawrence CW (1993) U-U and T-T cyclobutane dimers have different mutational properties. Nucleic Acids Res 21:4059–4065
Gillet LCJ, Scharer OD (2006) Molecular mechanisms of mammalian global genome nucleotide excision repair. Chem Rev 106:253–276
Giussani A, Serrano-Andres L, Merchan M, Roca-Sanjuan D, Garavelli M (2013) Photoinduced formation mechanism of the thymine-thymine (6-4) adduct. J Phys Chem B 117:1999–2004
Goswami S, Haldar C (2015) Melatonin as a possible antidote to UV radiation induced cutaneous damages and immune-suppression: an overview. J Photochem Photobiol B Biol 153:281–288
Green A, Williams G, Neale R, Hart V, Leslie D, Parsons P, Marks GC, Gaffney P, Battistutta D, Frost C et al (1999) Daily sunscreen application and betacarotene supplementation in prevention of basal-cell and squamous-cell carcinomas of the skin: a randomised controlled trial. Lancet 354:723–729
Green AC, Williams GM, Logan V, Strutton GM (2011) Reduced melanoma after regular sunscreen use: randomized trial follow-up. J Clin Oncol 29:257–263
Gregoris E, Fabris S, Bertelle M, Grassato L, Stevanato R (2011) Propolis as potential cosmeceutical sunscreen agent for its combined photoprotective and antioxidant properties. Int J Pharm 405:97–101
Guven M, Brem R, Macpherson P, Peacock M, Karran P (2015) Oxidative damage to RPA limits the nucleotide excision repair capacity of human cells. J Invest Dermatol 135:2834–2841
Haiser K, Fingerhut BP, Heil K, Glas A, Herzog TT, Pilles BM, Schreier WJ, Zinth W, de Vivie-Riedle R, Carell T (2012) Mechanism of UV-induced formation of Dewar lesions in DNA. Angew Chem Int Ed 51:408–411
Hegde ML, Hazra TK, Mitra S (2008) Early steps in the DNA base excision/single-strand interruption repair pathway in mammalian cells. Cell Res 18:27–47
Heo SJ, Ko SC, Cha SH, Kang DH, Park HS, Choi YU, Kim D, Jung WK, Jeon YJ (2009) Effect of phlorotannins isolated from Ecklonia cava on melanogenesis and their protective effect against photo-oxidative stress induced by UV-B radiation. Toxicol In Vitro 23:1123–1130
Holman CD, Armstrong BK, Heenan PJ (1986) Relationship of cutaneous malignant melanoma to individual sunlight-exposure habits. J Natl Cancer Inst 76:403–414
Horsfall MJ, Lawrence CW (1993) Accuracy of replication past the T-C (6-4) adduct. J Mol Biol 235:465–471
Horsfall MJ, Borden A, Lawrence CW (1997) Mutagenic properties of the T-C cyclobutane dimer. J Bacteriol 179:2835–2839
Ikehata H, Kawai K, Komura J, Sakatsume K, Wang LC, Imai M, Higashi S, Nikaido O, Yamamoto K, Hieda K et al (2008) UVA1 genotoxicity is mediated not by oxidative damage but by cyclobutane pyrimidine dimers in normal mouse skin. J Invest Dermatol 128:2289–2296
Jans J, Schul W, Sert YG, Rijksen Y, Rebel H, Eker AP, Nakajima S, van Steeg H, de Gruijl FR, Yasui A et al (2005) Powerful skin cancer protection by a CPD-photolyase transgene. Curr Biol 15:105–115
Jansen R, Wang SQ, Burnett M, Osterwalder U, Lim HW (2013) Photoprotection: part I. Photoprotection by naturally occurring, physical, and systemic agents. J Am Acad Dermatol 69:853 e851-812; quiz 865-856
Jiang N, Taylor J-S (1993) In vivo evidence that UV-induced C → T mutations at dipyrimidine sites could result from the replicative bypass of cis-syn cyclobutane dimers or their deamination products. Biochemistry 32:472–481
Jiang Y, Rabbi M, Kim M, Ke CH, Lee W, Clark RL, Mieczkowski PA, Marszalek PE (2009) UVA generates pyrimidine dimers in DNA directly. Biophys J 96:1151–1158
Kalam MA, Haraguchi K, Chandani S, Loechler EL, Moriya M, Greenberg MM, Basu AK (2006) Genetic effects of oxidative DNA damages: comparative mutagenesis of the imidazole ring-opened formamidopyrimidines (Fapy lesions) and 8-oxo-purines in simian kidney cells. Nucleic Acids Res 34:2305–2315

Kamiya H, Murata-Kamiya N, Karino N, Ueno Y, Matsuda A, Kasai H (2002) Induction of T → G and T → A transversions by 5-formyluracil in mammalian cells. Mutat Res 513:213–222

Kang T-H, Lindsey-Boltz LA, Reardon JT, Sancar A (2010) Circadian control of XPA and excision repair of cisplatin-DNA damage by cryptochrome and HERC2 ubiquitin ligase. Proc Natl Acad Sci USA 107:4890–4895

Kappes UP, Luo D, Potter M, Schulmeister K, Rünger TM (2006) Short- and long-wave light (UVB and UVA) induce similar mutations in human skin cells. J Invest Dermatol 126:667–675

Kielbassa C, Roza L, Epe B (1997) Wavelength dependence of oxidative DNA damage induced by UV and visible light. Carcinogenesis 18:811–816

Kopcke W, Krutmann J (2008) Protection from sunburn with beta-Carotene–a meta-analysis. Photochem Photobiol 84:284–288

Kouchakdjian M, Bodepudi V, Shibutani S, Eisenberg M, Johnson F, Grollman AP, Patel DJ (1991) NMR structural studies of the ionizing-radiation adduct 7-hydro-8-oxodeoxyguanosine (8-oxo-7h-dG) opposite deoxyadenosine in a DNA duplex—8-oxo-7h-dG(syn). dA(anti) alignment at lesion site. Biochemistry 30:1403–1412

Kreutzer DA, Essigmann JM (1998) Oxidized, deaminated cytosines are a source of C → T transitions in vivo. Proc Natl Acad Sci USA 95:3578–3582

Kuluncsics Z, Perdiz D, Brulay E, Muel B, Sage E (1999) Wavelength dependence of ultraviolet-induced DNA damage distribution: involvement of direct or indirect mechanisms and possible artefacts. J Photochem Photobiol B Biol 49:71–80

Lamore SD, Azimian S, Horn D, Anglin BL, Uchida K, Cabello CM, Wondrak GT (2013) The malondialdehyde-derived fluorophore DHP-lysine is a potent sensitizer of UVA-induced photooxidative stress in human skin cells. J Photochem Photobiol B Biol 101:251–264

Lange AW, Herbert JM (2009) Both intra- and interstrand charge-transfer excited states in aqueous B-DNA are present at energies comparable to, or just above, the (1)$\pi\pi^*$ excitonic bright states. J Am Chem Soc 131:3913–3922

Larroque-Cardoso P, Camare C, Nadal-Wollbold F, Grazide M-H, Pucelle M, Garoby-Salom S, Bogdanowicz P, Josse G, Schmitt A-M, Uchida K et al (2015) Elastin modification by 4-hydroxynonenal in hairless mice exposed to UV-A. Role in photoaging and actinic elastosis. J Invest Dermatol 135:1873–1881

Lawrence CW, Gibbs PEM, Borden A, Horsfall MJ, Kilbey BJ (1993) Mutagenesis induced by single UV photoproducts in *E. Coli* and yeast. Mutat Res 299:157–163

LeClerc JE, Borden A, Lawrence CW (1991) The thymine-thymine pyrimidine-pyrimidone (6-4) ultraviolet light photoproduct is highly mutagenic and specifically induces 3′ thymine-to-cytosine transitions in *Escherichia coli*. Proc Natl Acad Sci USA 88:9685–9689

Lemaire DGE, Ruzsicska BP (1993) Quantum yields and secondary photoreactions of the photoproducts of dTpdT, dTpdC and dTpdU. Photochem Photobiol 57:755–769

Lhiaubet-Vallet V, Cuquerella MC, Castell JV, Bosca F, Miranda MA (2007) Triplet excited fluoroquinolones as mediators for thymine cyclobutane dimer formation in DNA. J Phys Chem B 111:7409–7414

Lin JY, Selim MA, Shea CR, Grichnik JM, Omar MM, Monteiro-Riviere NA, Pinnell SR (2003) UV photoprotection by combination topical antioxidants vitamin C and vitamin E. J Am Acad Dermatol 48:866–874

Lyons NM, O'Brien NM (2002) Modulatory effects of an algal extract containing astaxanthin on UVA-irradiated cells in culture. J Dermatol Sci 30:73–84

Makridakis NM, Reichardt JK (2012) Translesion DNA polymerases and cancer. Front Genet 3:174

Marguet S, Markovitsi D, Talbot F (2006) One- and two-photon ionization of DNA single and double helices studied by laser flash photolysis at 266 nm. J Phys Chem B 110:11037–11039

McAuley-Hecht KE, Leonard GA, Gibson NJ, Thomson JB, Watson WP, Hunter WN, Brown T (1994) Crystal structure of a DNA duplex containing 8-hydroxydeoxyguanine-adenine base pairs. Biochemistry 33:10266–10270

McCullagh M, Hariharan M, Lewis FD, Markovitsi D, Douki T, Schatz GC (2010) Conformational control of TT dimerization in DNA conjugates. A molecular dynamics study. J Phys Chem B 114:5215–5221
McVean M, Liebler DC (1997) Inhibition of UVB induced DNA photodamage in mouse epidermis by topically applied alpha-tocopherol. Carcinogenesis 18:1617–1622
McVean M, Liebler DC (1999) Prevention of DNA photodamage by vitamin E compounds and sunscreens: roles of ultraviolet absorbance and cellular uptake. Mol Carcinog 24:169–176
Meeran SM, Akhtar S, Katiyar SK (2009) Inhibition of UVB-induced skin tumor development by drinking green tea polyphenols is mediated through DNA repair and subsequent inhibition of inflammation. J Invest Dermatol 129:1258–1270
Melnikova VO, Ananthaswamy HN (2005) Cellular and molecular events leading to the development of skin cancer. Mutat Res 571:91–106
Middleton CT, de La Harpe K, Su C, Law YK, Crespo-Hernandez CE, Kohler B (2009) DNA excited-state dynamics: from single bases to the double helix. Ann Rev Phys Chem 60:217–239
Miller JH (1985) Mutagenic specificity of ultraviolet-light. J Mol Biol 182:45–65
Mitchell DL, Haipek CA, Clarkson JM (1985) (6-4) Photoproducts are removed from the DNA of UV-irradiated mammalian cells more efficiently than cyclobutane pyrimidine dimers. Mutat Res 143:109–112
Mitchell DL, Allison JP, Nairn RS (1990) Immunoprecipitation of pyrimidine (6-4) pyrimidone photoproducts and cyclobutane pyrimidine dimers in UV-irradiated DNA. Radiat Res 123:299–303
Mohammad T, Morrison H (1996) Evidence for the photosensitized formation of singlet oxygen by UVB irradiation of 2′-deoxyguanosine 5′-monophosphate. J Am Chem Soc 118:1221–1222
Moloney F, Vestergaard M, Radojkovic B, Damian D (2010) Randomized, double-blinded, placebo controlled study to assess the effect of topical 1 % nicotinamide on actinic keratoses. Br J Dermatol 162:1138–1139
Montaner B, O'Donovan P, Reelfs O, Perrett CM, Zhang X, Xu YZ, Ren X, Macpherson P, Frith D, Karran P (2007) Reactive oxygen-mediated damage to a human DNA replication and repair protein. EMBO Rep 8:1074–1079
Moon TE, Levine N, Cartmel B, Bangert JL, Rodney S, Dong Q, Peng YM, Alberts DS (1997) Effect of retinol in preventing squamous cell skin cancer in moderate-risk subjects: a randomized, double-blind, controlled trial. Southwest Skin Cancer Prevention Study Group. Cancer Epidemiol Biomarkers Prev 6:949–956
Mouret S, Baudouin C, Charveron M, Favier A, Cadet J, Douki T (2006) Cyclobutane pyrimidine dimers are predominant DNA lesions in whole human skin exposed to UVA radiation. Proc Natl Acad Sci USA 103:13765–13770
Mouret S, Charveron M, Favier A, Cadet J, Douki T (2008) Differential repair of UVB-induced cyclobutane pyrimidine dimers in cultured human skin cells and whole human skin. DNA Repair 7:704–712
Mouret S, Philippe C, Gracia-Chantegrel J, Banyasz A, Karpati S, Markovitsi D, Douki T (2010) UVA-induced cyclobutane pyrimidine dimers in DNA: a direct photochemical mechanism? Org Biomolec Chem 8:1706 (in press)
Mouret S, Bogdanowicz P, Haure MJ, Castex-Rizzi N, Cadet J, Favier A, Douki T (2011a) Assessment of the photoprotection properties of sunscreens by chromatographic measurement of DNA damage in skin explants. Photochem Photobiol 87:109–116
Mouret S, Leccia MT, Bourrain JL, Douki T, Beani JC (2011b) Individual photosensitivity of human skin and UVA-induced pyrimidine dimers in DNA. J Invest Dermatol 131:1539–1546
Mouret S, Forestier A, Douki T (2012) The specificity of UVA-induced DNA damage in human melanocytes. Photochem Photobiol Sci 11:155–162
Nakamura T, Pinnell SR, Darr D, Kurimoto I, Itami S, Yoshikawa K, Streilein JW (1997) Vitamin C abrogates the deleterious effects of UVB radiation on cutaneous immunity by a mechanism that does not depend on TNF-alpha. J Invest Dermatol 109:20–24

Nijsten TE, Stern RS (2003) Oral retinoid use reduces cutaneous squamous cell carcinoma risk in patients with psoriasis treated with psoralen-UVA: a nested cohort study. J Am Acad Dermatol 49:644–650

Noonan FP, Zaidi MR, Wolnicka-Glubisz A, Anver MR, Bahn J, Wielgus A, Cadet J, Douki T, Mouret S, Tucker MA et al (2012) Melanoma induction by ultraviolet A but not ultraviolet B radiation requires melanin pigment. Nat Commun 3:884

Peak JG, Peak MJ (1991) Comparison of initial yields of DNA-to-protein crosslinks and single-strand breaks induced in cultured human cells by far- and near-ultraviolet light, blue light and X-rays. Mutat Res 246:187–191

Peng W, Shaw BR (1996) Accelerated deamination of cytosine residues in UV-induced cyclobutane dimers leads to CC-TT transitions. Biochemistry 35:10172–10181

Perdiz D, Grof P, Mezzina M, Nikaido O, Moustacchi E, Sage E (2000) Distribution and repair of bipyrimidine photoproducts in solar UV-irradiated mammalian cells. Possible role of Dewar photoproducts in solar mutagenesis. J Biol Chem 275:26732–26742

Perrier S, Hau J, Gasparutto D, Cadet J, Favier A, Ravanat J-L (2006) Characterization of lysine-guanine cross-links upon one-electron oxidation of a guanine-containing oligonucleotide in the presence of a trilysine peptide. J Am Chem Soc 128:5703–5710

Pleasance ED, Cheetham RK, Stephens PJ, McBride DJ, Humphray SJ, Greenman CD, Varela I, Lin ML, Ordonez GR, Bignell GR et al (2010) A comprehensive catalogue of somatic mutations from a human cancer genome. Nature 463:191–196

Pouget J-P, Douki T, Richard M-J, Cadet J (2000) DNA damage induced in cells by gamma and UVA radiations as measured by HPLC/GC-MS, HPLC-EC and comet assay. Chem Res Toxicol 13:541–549

Pourzand C, Watkin RD, Brown JE, Tyrrell RM (1999) Ultraviolet A radiation induces immediate release of iron in human primary skin fibroblasts: the role of ferritin. Proc Natl Acad Sci USA 96:6751–6756

Premi S, Wallisch S, Mano CM, Weiner AB, Bacchiocchi A, Wakamatsu K, Bechara EJ, Halaban R, Douki T, Brash DE (2016) Photochemistry. Chemiexcitation of melanin derivatives induces DNA photoproducts long after UV exposure. Science 347:842–847

Purmal AA, Kow YW, Wallace SS (1994) Major oxidative products of cytosine, 5-hydroxycytosine and 5-hydroxyuracil, exhibit sequence context-dependent mispairing in-vitro. Nucleic Acids Res 22 72–78

Qin XS, Zhang SM, Zarkovic M Nakatsuru Y, Shimizu S, Yamazaki Y, Oda H, Nikaido O, Ishikawa T (1996) Detection of ultraviolet photoproducts in mouse skin exposed to natural sunlight. Japan J Cancer Res 87:685–690

Rancan F, Rosan S, Boehm K, Fernandez E, Hidalgo ME, Quihot W, Rubio C, Boehm F, Piazena H, Oltmanns U (2002) Protection against UVB irradiation by natural filters extracted from lichens. J Photochem Photobiol B Biol 68:133–139

Ravanat J-L, Saint-Pierre C, Di Mascio P, Martinez GR, Medeiros MH, Cadet J (2001) Damage to isolated DNA mediated by singlet oxygen. Helvet Chim Acta 84:3702–3709

Reich A, Harupa M, Bury M, Chrzaszcz J, Starczewska A (2009) Application of sunscreen preparations: a need to change the regulations. Photodermatol Photoimmunol Photomed 25:242–244

Rezvani HR, Mazurier F, Cario-Andre M, Pain C, Ged C, Taieb A, de Verneuil H (2006) Protective effects of catalase overexpression on UVB-induced apoptosis in normal human keratinocytes. J Biol Chem 281:17999–18007

Rizzo JL, Dunn J, Rees A, Runger TM (2010) No formation of DNA double-strand breaks and no activation of recombination repair with UVA. J Invest Dermatol 131:1139–1148

Rochette PJ, Brash DE (2010) Human telomeres are hypersensitive to UV-induced DNA damage and refractory to repair. PLoS Genet 6:e1000926

Rochette PJ, Therrien J-P, Drouin R, Perdiz D, Bastien N, Drobetsky EA, Sage E (2003) UVA-induced cyclobutane pyrimidine dimers form predominantly at thymine-thymine dipyrimidines and correlate with the mutation spectrum in rodent cells. Nucleic Acids Res 31:2786–2794

Romac S, Leong P, Sockett H, Hutchinson F (1989) DNA-base sequence changes induced by ultraviolet-light mutagenesis of a gene on a chromosome in Chinese-hamster ovary cells. J Mol Biol 209:195–204

Rosenstein BS, Mitchell DL (1991) The repair of DNA damages induced in normal human skin fibroblasts exposed to simulated sunlight. Radiat Res 126:338–342

Rouabhia M, Mitchell DL, Rhainds M, Claveau J, Drouin R (2002) A physical sunscreen protects engineered human skin against artificial solar ultraviolet radiation-induced tissue and DNA damage. Photochem Photobiol Sci 1:471–477

Russo A, Piovano M, Lombardo L, Garbarino J, Cardile V (2008) Lichen metabolites prevent UV light and nitric oxide-mediated plasmid DNA damage and induce apoptosis in human melanoma cells. Life Sci 83:468–474

Rutter K, Sell DR, Fraser N, Obrenovich M, Zito M, Starke-Reed P, Monnier VM (2003) Green tea extract suppresses the age-related increase in collagen crosslinking and fluorescent products in C57BL/6 mice. Int J Vitam Nutr Res 73:453–460

Saewan N, Jimtaisong A (2015) Natural products as photoprotection. J Cosmet Dermatol 14:47–63

Sage E, Lamolet B, Brulay E, Moustacchi E, Chateauneuf A, Drobetsky EA (1996) Mutagenic specificity of solar UV light in nucleotide excision repair-deficient rodent cells. Proc Natl Acad Sci USA 93:176–180

Schreier WJ, Schrader TE, Koller FO, Gilch P, Crespo-Hernandez CE, Swaminathan VN, Carell T, Zinth W, Kohler B (2007) Thymine dimerization in DNA is an ultrafast photoreaction. Science 315:625–629

Schreier WJ, Kubon J, Regner N, Haiser K, Schrader TE, Zinth W, Clivio P, Gilch P (2009) Thymine dimerization in DNA model systems: cyclobutane photolesion is predominantly formed via the singlet channel. J Am Chem Soc 131:5038–5039

Sheehan JM, Potten CS, Young AR (1998) Tanning in human skin types II and III offers modest photoprotection against erythema. Photochem Photobiol 68:588–592

Shibutani S, Takeshita M, Grollman AP (1991) Insertion of specific bases during DNA synthesis past the oxidation-damaged base 8-oxodG. Nature 349:431–434

Smith CA, Wang M, Jiang N, Che L, Zhao XD, Taylor JS (1996) Mutation spectra of M13 vectors containing site-specific cis-syn, trans-syn-I, (6-4), and dewar pyrimidone photoproducts of thymidylyl-(3′ → 5′)-thymidine in *Escherichia coli* under SOS conditions. Biochemistry 35:4146–4154

Stahl W, Heinrich U, Aust O, Tronnier H, Sies H (2006) Lycopene-rich products and dietary photoprotection. Photochem Photobiol Sci 5:238–242

Su DG, Kao JL, Gross ML, Taylor JS (2008) Structure determination of an interstrand-type cis-anti cyclobutane thymine dimer produced in high yield by UVB light in an oligodeoxynucleotide at acidic pH. J Am Chem Soc 130:11328–11337

Surjana D, Halliday GM, Martin AJ, Moloney FJ, Damian DL (2012) Oral nicotinamide reduces actinic keratoses in phase II double-blinded randomized controlled trials. J Invest Dermatol 132:1497–1500

Surjana D, Halliday GM, Damian DL (2013) Nicotinamide enhances repair of ultraviolet radiation-induced DNA damage in human keratinocytes and ex vivo skin. Carcinogenesis 34:1144–1149

Tadokoro T, Kobayashi N, Zmudzka BZ, Ito S, Wakamatsu K, Yamaguchi Y, Korossy KS, Miller SA, Beer JZ, Hearing VJ (2003) UV-induced DNA damage and melanin content in human skin differing in racial/ethnic origin. FASEB J 17:1177–1179

Tan XZ, Grollman AP, Shibutani S (1999) Comparison of the mutagenic properties of 8-oxo-7,8-dihydro-2′-deoxyadenosine and 8-oxo-7,8-dihydro-2′-deoxyguanosine DNA lesions in mammalian cells. Carcinogenesis 20:2287–2292

Taylor J-S (1994) Unraveling the molecular pathway from sunlight to skin cancer. Account Chem Res 27:76–82

Taylor J-S, Cohrs MP (1987) DNA, light, and Dewar pyrimidones: the structure and biological significance of TpT3. J Am Chem Soc 109:2834–2835

Taylor J-S, O'Day CL (1990) Cis-syn thymine dimers are not absolute blocks to replication by DNA polymerase I of *Escherichia coli* in vitro. Biochemistry 29:1624–1632

Tommasi S, Denissenko MF, Pfeifer GP (1997) Sunlight induces pyrimidine dimers preferentially at 5-methylcytosine bases. Cancer Res 57:4727–4730

Tyrrell RM (1973) Induction of pyrimidine dimers in bacterial DNA by 365 nm radiation. Photochem Photobiol 17:69–73

van Praag MC, Roza L, Boom BW, Out-Luijting C, Henegouwen JB, Vermeer BJ, Mommaas AM (1993) Determination of the photoprotective efficacy of a topical sunscreen against UVB-induced DNA damage in human epidermis. J Photochem Photobiol B Biol 19:129–134

Vaya I, Gustavsson T, Douki T, Berlin Y, Markovitsi D (2012) Electronic excitation energy transfer between nucleobases of natural DNA. J Am Chem Soc 134:11366–11368

Wachsmuth RC, Turner F, Barrett JH, Gaut R, Randerson-Moor JA, Bishop DT, Bishop JA (2005) The effect of sun exposure in determining nevus density in UK adolescent twins. J Invest Dermatol 124:56–62

Wang H, Kochevar IE (2005) Involvement of UVB-induced reactive oxygen species in TGF-beta biosynthesis and activation in keratinocytes. Free Radic Biol Med 38:890–897

Wang SQ, Stanfield JW, Osterwalder U (2008) In vitro assessments of UVA protection by popular sunscreens available in the United States. J Am Acad Dermatol 59:934–942

Wang HT, Choi B, Tang MS (2010) Melanocytes are deficient in repair of oxidative DNA damage and UV-induced photoproducts. Proc Natl Acad Sci USA 107:12180–12185

Winczura A, Zdzalik D, Tudek B (2012) Damage of DNA and proteins by major lipid peroxidation products in genome stability. Free Radic Res 46:442–459

Wondrak GT, Jacobson MK, Jacobson EL (2006) Endogenous UVA-photosensitizers: mediators of skin photodamage and novel targets for skin photoprotection. Photochem Photobiol Sci 5:215–237

Yoon JH, Prakash L, Prakash S (2009) Highly error-free role of DNA polymerase eta in the replicative bypass of UV-induced pyrimidine dimers in mouse and human cells. Proc Natl Acad Sci USA 106:18219–18224

You Y-H, Pfeifer GP (1999) Involvement of 5-methylcytosine in sunlight-induced mutagenesis. J Mol Biol 293:493–503

You Y-H, Szabo PE, Pfeifer GP (2000) Cyclobutane pyrimidine dimers form preferentially at the major p53 mutational hotspot in UVB-induced mouse skin tumors. Carcinogenesis 21:2113–2117

You YH, Lee DH, Yoon JH, Nakajima S, Yasui A, Pfeifer GP (2001) Cyclobutane pyrimidine dimers are responsible for the vast majority of mutations induced by UVB irradiation in mammalian cells. J Biol Chem 276:44688–44694

Young AR, Chadwick CA, Harrison GI, Hawk JL, Nikaido O, Potten CS (1996) The in situ repair kinetics of epidermal thymine dimers and 6-4 photoproducts in human skin types I and II. J Invest Dermatol 106:1307–1313

Young AR, Potten CS, Nikaido O, Parsons PG, Boenders J, Ramsden JM, Chadmick CA (1998) Human melanocytes and keratinocytes exposed to UVB or UVA in vivo show comparable levels of thymine dimers. J Invest Dermatol 111:936–940

Young AR, Sheehan JM, Chadwick CA, Potten CS (2000) Protection by ultraviolet A and B sunscreens against in situ dipyrimidine photolesions in human epidermis is comparable to protection against sunburn. J Invest Dermatol 115:37–41

Yu SL, Johnson RE, Prakash S, Prakash L (2001) Requirement of DNA polymerase eta for error-free bypass of UV-induced CC and TC photoproducts. Mol Cell Biol 21:185–188

Yusuf N, Irby C, Katiyar SK, Elmets CA (2007) Photoprotective effects of green tea polyphenols. Photodermatol Photoimmunol Photomed 23:48–56

Zharkov DO (2008) Base excision DNA repair. Cell Mol Life Sci 65:1544–1565

Ziegler A, Leffel DJ, Kunala S, Sharma HW, Shapiro PE, Bale AE, Brash DE (1993) Mutation hotspots due to sunlight in the p53 gene of nonmelanoma skin cancers. Proc Natl Acad Sci USA 90:4216–4220

Chapter 4
Urocanic Acid and Skin Photodamage: New Light on an Old Chromophore

Leopold Eckhart

Abstract Urocanic acid (UCA) is one of the most efficient ultraviolet (UV) radiation-absorbing substances of the skin. UV irradiation leads to the interconversion of the two stereoisomers *trans*-UCA and *cis*-UCA, of which the latter is able to induce immunosuppression. Accordingly, the regulation of UCA biosynthesis, UV absorption by UCA in the cornified layer of the epidermis and the effects of UCA on the adaptive immune system are integral components of the cutaneous UV stress program. Here the evidence for the multiple roles of UCA in the skin and the associated open scientific questions are reviewed comprehensively.

Keywords Urocanic acid • Epidermis • Stratum corneum • Histidase • Ultraviolet radiation • Immunosuppression • Histidinemia • Atopic dermatitis • Filaggrin • Keratinocytes

4.1 Introduction: Urocanic Acid

4.1.1 Overview

Ultraviolet (UV) radiation is one of the most important environmental stressors of the skin and, for a long time, one of the main UV absorbing substances of the skin, urocanic acid (UCA), has been implicated in the protection of the tissue and in the initiation of cellular responses to UV exposure (Norval et al. 1995; Mohammad et al. 1999; Gibbs et al. 2008).

The history of UCA begins with its isolation from the urine of a dog, as reported by Jaffe in 1874 (Jaffe 1874). The structure of UCA was determined in 1912

L. Eckhart (✉)
Research Division of Biology and Pathobiology of the Skin, Department of Dermatology, Medical University of Vienna, Lazarettgasse 14, 1090 Vienna, Austria
e-mail: leopold.eckhart@meduniwien.ac.at

G.T. Wondrak (ed.), *Skin Stress Response Pathways*,
DOI 10.1007/978-3-319-43157-4_4

(Hunter 1912), and the link between UCA and the skin was established in the 1950s when UCA was isolated from the skin surface. Already at that time UCA was suggested to represent a major UV-absorbing compound of the epidermis (Zenisek and Kral 1953; Zenisek et al. 1955; Tabachnik 1957). Subsequently, UCA was added to cosmetics and sunscreens from the 1960s until the 1990s (Andersen 1995; Gibbs et al. 2008). Its use in sunscreens was discontinued because of evidence for immunosuppressive activity of UCA (Andersen 1995). Studies on the physiological functions and molecular mechanisms of action of UCA have continued and still promise new insights into the photobiology of the skin.

4.1.2 Chemical and Physical Properties of UCA

UCA, chemical formula $C_6H_6N_2O_2$, belongs to the class of imidazolyl carboxylic acids and has a molecular weight of 138.12 g/mol. It exists as either one of two isomers, *trans*-UCA and *cis*-UCA (Fig. 4.1). The presence of an imidazole ring and a carboxylic acid chain containing a double bond facilitate the high UV absorption capacity of UCA (Kurogochi et al. 1957).

UCA is a weak acid with an acid dissociation constant (pKa) 3.5 for the deprotonation of COOH and pKa 5.8 for the deprotonation of the first NH in the imidazole ring (Brookman et al. 2002). *trans*-UCA is relatively insoluble at its isoelectric point (pH 4.6) but well soluble at higher pH (Mehler and Tabor 1953). *cis*-UCA is more soluble than *trans*-UCA by an order of a magnitude (Mohammad et al. 1999).

Both isomers of UCA are hydrophilic (Joo et al. 2012) but both *trans*-UCA and *cis*-UCA also associate with liposomes whereby the association is higher at pH 7.4 than at pH 5.0. The liposome incorporation of *trans*-UCA is twice as efficient as that of *cis*-UCA (Campos et al. 2008). Pure UCA is not hygroscopic (Mehler and Tabor 1953).

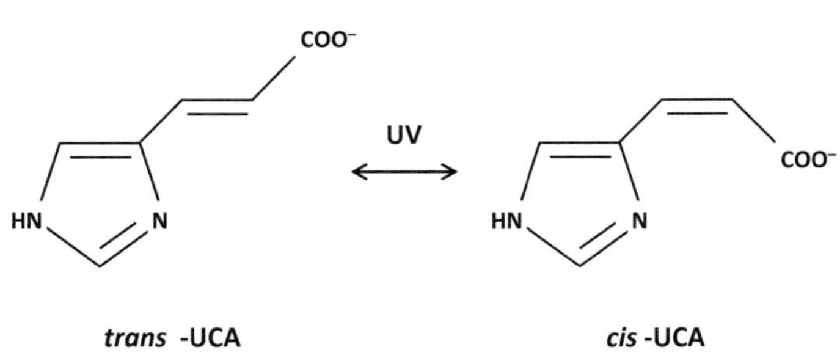

Fig. 4.1 *trans*-UCA and *cis*-UCA are isomers of UCA. UV irradiation converts *trans*-UCA to *cis*-UCA and *vice versa*

4.1.3 UV Absorption by UCA

UCA absorbs radiation mainly in the range of UVC (100–280 nm) and UVB (280–320 nm) but also significantly in the UVA range (320–380 nm) (Fig. 4.2). The absorption spectra of *trans*-UCA and *cis*-UCA are generally similar, with *cis*-UCA having approximately 25 % less molar absorptivity than *trans*-UCA. At pH 7, extinction coefficients (ε), also referred to as molar absorptivities, of $\varepsilon = 1.63 \times 10^4\ M^{-1}\ cm^{-1}$ at 280 nm and $\varepsilon = 1.19 \times 10^4\ M^{-1}\ cm^{-1}$ at 275 nm have been reported for the *trans*-UCA and *cis*-UCA, respectively (Brookman et al. 2002). These values compare to the maximal extinction coefficients (at 280 nm) of amino acids in proteins which are $\varepsilon = 0.57 \times 10^4\ M^{-1}\ cm^{-1}$ for tryptophan and $\varepsilon = 0.13 \times 10^4\ M^{-1}\ cm^{-1}$ for tyrosine, both at pH 6.5, and much smaller for all other amino acids including histidine (Gill and von Hippel 1989).

The absorption spectra of *trans*-UCA and *cis*-UCA are shifted to shorter wavelengths by reducing the pH in a physiologically relevant range between pH 5 and pH 7. *cis*-UCA has lower absorptivity than *trans*-UCA at all pH values (Brookman et al. 2002). As a consequence, a decrease in the pH in the upper layers of the stratum corneum is associated with a significant decrease of the effective UV extinction coefficient of UCA.

Most importantly, UV irradiation leads to the photoisomerization of UCA. *trans*-UCA is converted to *cis*-UCA and vice versa so that prolonged irradiation leads to an equilibrium of both isomers. Only *trans*-UCA is produced by keratinocytes in the absence of UV irradiation. Therefore, the amount of *cis*-UCA is a marker of previous UV exposure.

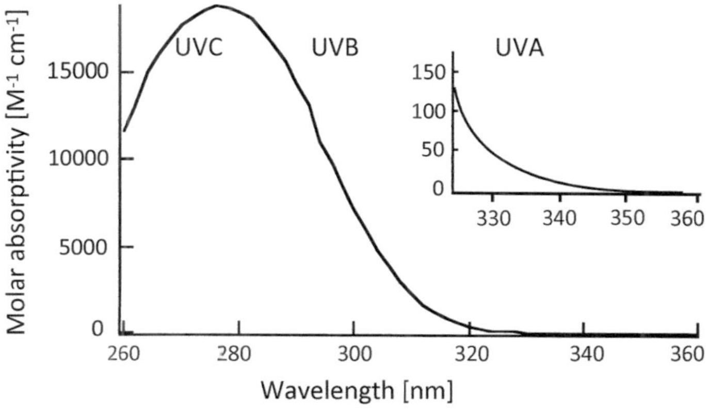

Fig. 4.2 UV absorption spectrum of *trans*-UCA. The molar absorptivity (extinction coefficient) is plotted over the wavelength in the range of UVC, UVB, and UVA radiation. This figure is modified from Hanson and Simon (1998) (with permission of the National Academy of Sciences of the United States of America (Copyright 1998))

4.2 Formation of Urocanic Acid in the Epidermis

4.2.1 Enzymatic Formation of UCA

The isomerization state and the removal of UCA in the epidermis are largely controlled by physical factors such as UV irradiation and elution from the skin surface. By contrast, the formation of UCA is controlled by biological factors active in epidermal keratinocytes. Hence this level of control is most amenable to stress response pathways of the skin. UCA is formed by the removal of the amino group (deamination) of histidine (Fig. 4.3). The reaction is catalyzed by the enzyme histidase, which is strictly stereospecific (Brand and Harper 1976). The substrate of the reaction is L-histidine, and the products are *trans*-UCA and ammonia. The reaction occurs only at approximately neutral pH so that all the involved substances carry charges, as indicated in Fig. 4.3.

4.2.2 Histidine Is the Precursor of UCA

The formation of UCA depends on the availability of the amino acid, histidine, the substrate of histidase. Histidine is synthesized in the liver and transported in the vasculature to the peripheral organs such as the skin. As the expression site of histidase in the epidermis, i.e. the granular layer, is not close to blood vessels, supply of free histidine is not effective. Therefore, formation of histidine by hydrolysis of proteins appears to be the limiting factor for the supply of histidine in keratinocytes capable of UCA formation.

In the epidermis, the "histidine-rich protein" filaggrin is expressed specifically in terminally differentiated keratinocytes. The *FLG* gene encodes profilaggrin, a large protein of more than 3000 amino acid residues, 10 % of which are histidine residues. Profilaggrin is proteolytically processed into filaggrin monomers in the granular layer by proteases such saspase and kallikreins. Filaggrin contributes to the aggregation of keratin intermediate filaments and subsequently is degraded further into peptides and ultimately free amino acids. The latter step involves caspase-14 and other proteases (Denecker et al. 2007).

Several lines of evidence suggest that filaggrin is the main source of histidine for UCA formation. The time course of breakdown of filaggrin fits to that of the appearance of free amino acids, including histidine, and the relative abundance of amino acids in filaggrin agrees well with the relative abundance of free amino acids in the stratum corneum (Scott et al. 1982). Knockout of filaggrin in the mouse results in a decrease in the stratum corneum concentrations of histidine and UCA (Kawasaki et al. 2012). The concentrations of histidine and UCA are also decreased in the stratum corneum of human individuals carrying heterozygous or homozygous mutations of FLG (Kezic et al. 2009). Knockdown of *FLG* expression reduces the level of UCA by 60 % in a human in vitro skin model (Mildner et al. 2010).

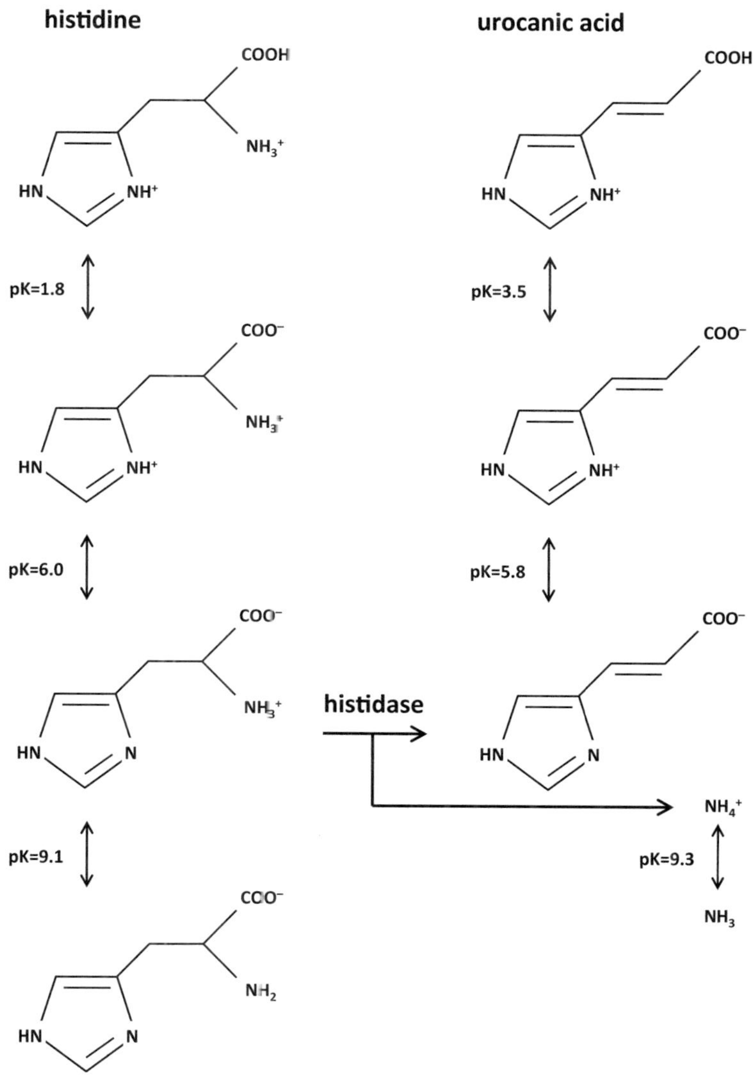

Fig. 4.3 Conversion of histidine to UCA in the context of the pH. Histidase catalyzes the conversion of histidine at neutral pH. The protonation status of the substrate and the products of this reaction are determined by their acid dissociation constants (pKa) and depend on the pH

The formation of UCA from histidine competes with the conjugation of histidine to its specific tRNA, which is catalyzed by histidyl-tRNA synthetase and represents the first step of histidine's incorporation into newly translated proteins. Moreover, histidine is the precursor of histamine. This conversion is catalyzed by L-histidine decarboxylase, an enzyme encoded by the *HDC* gene. The biosynthesis of histamine is active in keratinocytes at least under certain conditions (Shimizu et al.

2015). Thus, the deamination of histidine by histidase is integrated in the general metabolism of histidine in the epidermis.

4.2.3 Histidase Converts Histidine to UCA

The formation of epidermal UCA is catalyzed by histidase, also known as L-histidine ammonia lyase (HAL) (EC 4.3.1.3) (Zannoni and La Du 1963; Gibbs et al. 2008). Histidase belongs to the phylogenetically ancient aromatic amino acid lyase family which also includes the bacterial enzymes phenylalanine ammonia-lyase and tyrosine ammonia-lyase. In mammals, histidase is a cytosolic enzyme which catalyzes the nonoxidative deamination of L-histidine to *trans*-UCA in a highly selective manner. Determination of the crystal structure of bacterial histidase revealed a homotetramer and suggested a catalytic mechanism that depends on the autocatalytic cyclization and dehydration of 3 amino acid residues of histidase to form a reactive electrophile (4-methylidene-imidazole-5-one) (Schwede et al. 1999).

Human histidase has 657 amino acid residues. The aromatic amino acid lyase domain comprises residues 114–592 while the amino-terminus contains a Par-3 N-terminal domain (NTD)-like domain that has self-association capacity (Zhang et al. 2013). Isoforms of histidase are generated by alternative mRNA splicing, however, their physiological significance is unclear. Histidase is encoded by the *HAL* gene (localized on human chromosome 12q23.1) which is expressed in hepatocytes and epidermal keratinocytes (Taylor et al. 1990; Suchi et al. 1995; Eckhart et al. 2008). In the liver, the expression of *HAL* is upregulated by the availability of dietary protein (Torres et al. 1998). Similarly, addition of histidine and, paradoxically, also reduction of histidine in the diet result in increased epidermal UCA levels (De Fabo et al. 1997).

In proliferating keratinocytes of the basal layer of the epidermis the *HAL* gene is essentially not expressed but its transcription is induced during the last phase of keratinocyte differentiation in the epidermis (Eckhart et al. 2008). Expression can be induced in keratinocytes in vitro by maintaining cells in confluent culture or by triggering cell differentiation in a 3-dimensional skin model. The expression of *HAL* is suppressed by interleukin 1-α, tumor necrosis factor (TNF)-α and by treatment with retinoic acid (Eckhart et al. 2008). The latter effect indicates that a suppression of *HAL* expression and a consequent decrease in histidase-mediated formation of UCA might contribute to elevated UV sensitivity in response to retinoid treatment of human patients (Ferguson and Johnson 1986). However, expression levels of histidase in diseased and retinoid-treated human skin remain to be investigated.

In normal human skin as well as in mouse skin, histidase protein is confined to the granular and cornified layers of the epidermis (Barresi et al. 2011). This coincides with histidase activity (Scott 1981). Histidase is present in terminally differentiated keratinocytes and, after cornification, becomes a component of corneocytes. As the pH decreases, histidase activity is suppressed in corneocytes with the enzyme being almost inactive at pH values below 6 (Brand and Harper 1976; Scott 1981). The contribution of UCA to stratum corneum acidification has been suggested to establish a negative feedback on UCA production via suppression of histidase activity (Krien and Kermici 2000). Moreover, histidase may be inactivated by transglutamination, proteolytic processing by stratum corneum proteases and by the decreased water content of corneocytes. Interestingly, histidase has been reported to be less stable in human stratum corneum samples than in dried human nail samples where it retains enzymatic activity over more than 100 days (Fujitaka et al. 1993).

Histidase is inhibited by 8-methoxypsoralen and psoralen-oxidized photoproducts (Reilly et al. 2010). Increased histidase activity is present in psoriatic scales (Reaven and Cox 1965), and the epidermis of patients with psoriasis contains elevated amounts of UCA (Gilmour et al. 1993). Epidermal histidase activity is decreased by TPA treatment of mice (Colburn et al. 1975). Notably, the UCA content is significantly higher in the epidermis (from fingertips) of infants aged <3 months (70–110 μmol/g) than in adults (around 30 μmol/g) (Yokoya et al. 1983). Interestingly, skin histidase activity is also high in the first days of life of mice and declines later (Wright et al. 1982). The mechanism underlying these changes in histidase activity need further investigations but likely involve changes in gene expression.

4.2.4 *Histidinemia Is a Model for Reduced Histidase Activity*

Histidinemia (OMIM #235800) is associated with elevated concentrations of histidine in blood, urine, and cerebrospinal fluid, and with reduced concentrations of the UCA and the downstream metabolite formiminoglutamic acid in the blood. Histidinemia is considered a benign disorder (Lam et al. 1996; Baden et al. 1969a) after several studies have not supported the previous hypothesis of an association with mental retardation. Individuals with histidinemia have no or little UCA in the stratum corneum (Levy et al. 1969). Histidinemia was reported to be the most frequent inborn metabolic error in Japan with a prevalence (1:8400) (Suchi et al. 1995) while its prevalence is lower in Europe (Alm et al. 1981; Widhalm and Virmani 1994). Recently, rare loss-of-function alleles of *HAL* were found to be associated with increased serum histidine levels and decreased incidence of coronary heart disease (Yu et al. 2015). A potential pathomechanistic involvement of UCA has remained uninvestigated.

A single nucleotide mutation leading to the change of amino acid residue arginine 322 to glutamine has been identified in a mouse strain known as Peruvian mice (Kacser et al. 1973; Taylor et al. 1993). This mutation does not compromise histidase mRNA stability but strongly reduces the heat stability and the half life of the histidase protein (Wright et al. 1982; Taylor et al. 1993). Of note, the expression of the mutant protein in COS cells showed approximately 10 % of the normal enzymatic activity, and a specific activity of 60 % of the normal histidase was estimated (Taylor et al. 1993). Apparently due to histidase destabilization in vivo, the histidase enzymatic activity is essentially abolished in the liver of histidinemic mice (Bulfield and Kacser 1975; Wright et al. 1982; Taylor et al. 1993). Epidermal keratinocyte differentiation appears to be largely normal in these mice except for the lack of histidase immunoreactivity in the granular layer of the epidermis (Barresi et al. 2011). Accordingly, the concentration of UCA is strongly decreased in the stratum corneum of histidinemic mice, i.e. Peruvian mice backcrossed into a C57/BL6 background (Barresi et al. 2011).

Of note, defects in histidase lead to increased histamine concentrations in humans (Imamura et al. 1984) and mice (Kacser et al. 1973). Eczema-like dermatitis of the extremities or trunk were reported at increased incidence in histidinemic individuals (8/42 had mild eczema, 9/42 had severe eczema versus 0/10 in normal controls), and individuals with dermatitis had higher concentrations of histamine and N-methyl histamine (Imamura et al. 1984). Investigations of patients with histidinemia and atopic dermatitis patients without histidinemia suggested that hyperhistaminemia resulted primarily from increased decarboxylation of histidine present at higher levels in histidinemia (Tanabe and Sakura 1989). A low incidence of atopic dermatitis was detected in a European histidinemia patient cohort (Widhalm and Virmani 1994). Comparative studies of human individuals with and without loss-of-function mutations in histidase promise to yield important insights into the functions of UCA and other histidine metabolites in the skin.

4.2.5 UCA Is Removed by Various Processes

UCA is constantly generated in differentiated keratinocytes of the upper granular layer and/or the low cornified layer of the epidermis. The formation of UCA is balanced by loss of UCA from the epidermis. UCA is not catabolized by skin cells because the enzyme active on UCA, urocanase, is not expressed at appreciable amounts outside of the liver. Urocanase catabolizes UCA to 4,5-dihydro-4-oxo-5-imidazolepropanoate so that UCA concentrations are kept low in the liver and in body fluids. Rare mutations in the urocanase gene, *UROC1*, are associated with urocanic aciduria that is characterized by UCA levels above 150 mmol/mol creatinine, as compared to normal values below 10 (Espinós et al. 2009). Skin abnormalities are not present in patients with urocanic aciduria (Espinós et al. 2009), confirming that *UROC1* is not involved in normal skin homeostasis. Absence of urocanase from the skin implies that, during homeostasis, the removal and/or degradation of UCA is determined by other factors.

First, the majority of UCA leaves the skin into the environment. Corneocytes of the stratum corneum undergo desquamation and UCA present within corneocytes is thereby removed from the epidermis. The removal of UCA is enhanced by water which elutes UCA from the superficial layers of the stratum corneum. It is plausible that washing and bathing reduces the concentration of epidermal UCA and enhances the photosensitivity of normal skin (Gers-Balag et al. 1997). Likewise, sweat is able to extract UCA (Zenisek and Kral 1953; Brusilow and Ikai 1968). Interestingly, UCA has been identified as a chemoattractant for a skin-penetrating parasitic nematode (Safer et al. 2007).

Second, UCA can be metabolized by the microflora on the skin surface. Bacteria degrade UCA as a source of carbon and nitrogen (Hug et al. 1999). Interestingly, UCA is also utilized as a signaling molecule that allows bacteria to recognize eukaryotic hosts (Zhang et al. 2014). Miajlovic have suggested that filaggrin breakdown products such as UCA influence the growth of *Staphylococcus aureus* (Miajlovic et al. 2010).

Third, a fraction of UCA is chemically modified by hydroxyl radicals which are formed by cleavage of the O–O bond of H_2O_2 upon UV irradiation (Kammeyer et al. 1999, 2001). Photooxidation of UCA is induced by UVB but not by UVA. UCA yields imidazole-4-carboxaldehyde, imidazole-4-acetic acid and imidazole-4-carboxylic acid and probably other breakdown products upon UVB irradiation of the stratum corneum (Kammeyer et al. 2001). These substances may contribute to UCA-dependent UV-induced immunosuppression, but this hypothesis remains to be tested (Kammeyer et al. 2001).

Fourth, UCA diffuses from the stratum corneum into the deeper layers of the epidermis and also into the dermis where it can enter the circulation (Moodycliffe et al. 1993). Unlike *trans*-UCA, *cis*-UCA is not metabolized by urocanase in the liver but rather undergoes excretion in the urine (Sastry et al. 2005). However, a fraction of *cis*-UCA has been proposed to react with glutathione under the catalysis by glutathione S-transferase (Kinuta et al. 2003).

4.3 Absorption of UV Radiation by Endogenous UCA

4.3.1 UCA Absorbs UVB Radiation

As UCA has both high abundance in the epidermis and a high UVB absorption capacity, it has been hypothesized to act as a natural sunscreen of the skin (Zenisek et al. 1955; Tabachnik 1957). However, there were also reports that questioned the physiological significance of UCA's contribution to UVB absorption in the skin (de Fine Olivarius et al. 1996, 1998). In the latter study, the minimal erythema dose (MED) and the epidermal UCA concentration did not show a correlation in 22 children and 36 adults. Such a correlation might be obscured by the variation of human skin pigmentation which is certainly an important factor in determining photosensitivity, as measured by the MED approach. It is also important to notice that MED correlates only very loosely with the sensitivity to UV-induced DNA damage (Heenen et al. 2001).

A study in histidinemic mice provided strong evidence for significant UVB protection by endogenous UCA (Barresi et al. 2011). The stratum corneum of these mice contained only 10 % of the normal amounts of UCA and the UVB absorption capacity of the stratum corneum of histidinemic mice was reduced proportionally. This study also demonstrated that the UV absorption profile of stratum corneum from normal mice, but not of mutant mice, largely overlapped with that of UCA, supporting a major contribution of UCA to UV absorption in normal stratum corneum (Barresi et al. 2011). Of note, the quantification of UV absorption utilized the extracts from the stratum corneum whereas elution-resistant components of the stratum corneum were not analyzed.

To evaluate the effects of UV on the living cell layers of the epidermis, i.e. those beneath the stratum corneum, histidinemic mice were shaved, irradiated with UVB, and analyzed for the formation of DNA photoproducts as well as for the occurrence of cell death after irradiation. The results showed that the epidermis of histidinemic mice contained approximately 40 % more cyclobutane pyrimidine dimers (CPDs) than epidermis of normal mice. As a consequence of high levels of DNA damage, the cell death program of apoptosis was induced at significantly higher rate in epidermal cells of UV-irradiated histidinemic mice. The increased UVB-photosensitivity of histidinemic mice was reversed by topical application of UCA (Barresi et al. 2011).

The effect on *HAL* mutations on the UV absorption of the stratum corneum has not yet been studied in large numbers of human individuals. Irradiation of 2 patients of histidinemia showed an apparently above-normal UV sensitivity in one but not the other individual (Baden et al. 1969a). In another study, the comparison of 6 individuals with histidinemia and 6 skin phototype-matched control individuals revealed an approximately 40 % lower MED in histidinemics (Tye et al. 2008).

In contrast to the rare mutations of *HAL*, *FLG* mutations are relatively common and also known to decrease the epidermal UCA concentration (Kezic et al. 2009). Comparison of MED in 10 heterozygous carriers of *FLG* mutations versus 61 *FLG* wild-type subjects did not show significant differences (Forbes et al. 2016). In another study large cohorts of individuals with and without *FLG* mutations ($n > 80$ *FLG* heterozygous, $n > 1000$ *FLG* wild-type) were investigated for their vitamin D levels, which can be considered as a surrogate marker of UV penetration through the stratum corneum. UVB radiation of the skin drives the synthesis of vitamin D_3 which is converted to 25-hydroxy-vitamin D in the liver. Thyssen and colleagues showed that the serum concentration of 25-hydroxy-vitamin D was increased by approximately 10 % (confidence interval 6.7–13.6 %) in carriers of *FLG* mutations (Thyssen et al. 2012). These data suggest that UCA levels influence UV absorption and UVB-dependent processes such as vitamin D production in the skin.

The links between filaggrin, UCA and UV sensitivity were confirmed in vitro. Reduction of filaggrin by siRNA-mediated knockdown of *FLG* gene expression reduced the formation of UCA and elevated the sensitivity to UVB irradiation-induced DNA damage in a human skin equivalent model (Mildner et al. 2010).

The ability of UCA to absorb UVB under the conditions present in the outermost layer of the skin was confirmed by topical application of UCA onto human skin, which led to an increase in photoprotection (Baden and Pathak 1967). For several years, UCA was used as a component of commercial sunscreens until reports on the immunosuppressive properties of *cis*-UCA prompted UCA-containing sunscreens to be withdrawn from the market (De Fabo and Noonan 1983; Andersen 1995). A sun protection factor (as defined by the change in the MED) of 1.58 was reported for exogenous UCA on human skin (de Fine Olivarius et al. 1996). Topical UCA decreased UVB-induced DNA damage by a factor of 1.44 in wild-type versus histidinemic mouse skin (Barresi et al. 2011). For comparison, endogenous UCA reduced UVB-induced DNA damage in wild-type mouse epidermis by a factor of 1.52 relative to histidinemic mice (Barresi et al. 2011). Notably, the amounts of UCA per area of skin were different in the various studies.

Besides the mentioned negative effects of UV irradiation, also the positive effects of UVB, such as enhanced formation of vitamin D in the epidermis, are suppressed by UCA (Thyssen et al. 2012). Intriguingly, the reduced level of UCA and, as a consequence, increased UV-driven vitamin D synthesis have been hypothesized to act as evolutionary drivers of high prevalences of *FLG* mutations in northern Europeans (Thyssen et al. 2014). This hypothesis implies that the UV-protective effects of epidermal UCA outweigh the disadvantages of reduced vitamin D synthesis in human populations exposed to high doses of UV but not in populations exposed to low doses of UV.

This hypothesis leads to the question as to whether the sunscreening effect of UCA was the critical driver for the origin of epidermal UCA formation during human evolution. Epidermal UCA is present not only in humans but also in fury animals which do not require UV protection by absorption in the stratum corneum. This notion holds true for most mammals including the main biomedical model species, the mouse. All amphibians, reptiles and birds investigated so far have been reported to lack epidermal UCA (Baden et al. 1969b; Ley et al. 2000). This species distribution indicates that the UCA forming capability of the epidermis has evolved in "early" mammals. Notably, this event likely coincided with the origin of the *FLG* gene (Mlitz et al. 2014) which supported the production of histidine in the stratum corneum. This evolutionary pattern indicates an important role of epidermal UCA in mammals but argues against a primary role in UV protection. Thus, the photoprotective effect of UCA in humans and the immuno-suppressive effects of UV-induced *cis*-UCA, as discussed below, are likely to have secondarily gained physiological relevance only in humans and few other mammals that have lost a UV-protective pelage.

4.3.2 Interaction of UCA with Radicals and Possible Role in Photoaging

Besides directly absorbing UVB radiation, UCA also protects the epidermis by scavenging hydroxyl radicals that are generated by UVB irradiation (Kammeyer et al. 1999, 2001). Importantly, the UV absorption goes beyond the UVB range, although absorption of UVA is weaker than that of UVB by two orders of magnitude (Fig. 4.2). UVA irradiation of *trans*-UCA induces the formation of $^1O_2$ with an action spectrum that is highly similar to that of UVA-induced sagging of mouse skin (Hanson and Simon 1998). Consequently, it was proposed that UVA excitation of *trans*-UCA acid causes skin photo-aging via incompletely defined chemical processes. Later, theoretical calculations have supported the hypothesis that UCA contributes to photosensitization by generating various reactive oxygen species such as $^1O_2$ and O_2^- (Shen and Ji 2008). Other reports have suggested that *trans*-UCA acts as a strong triplet quencher. The physiological relevance of UCA in UVA photosensitization will need further studies (Wondrak et al. 2006).

4.4 Effects of UCA on Skin Cells and Immune Responses

4.4.1 Direct and Indirect Effects of UCA

UCA affects the physicochemical milieu and the UV exposure of skin cells, which will here be referred to as indirect effects, and it exerts direct effects by entering cells and/or binding to receptor protein(s) on cells (Fig. 4.4). The relative contributions of direct and indirect effects and the intercellular signaling (secondary effects) triggered by UCA are only incompletely understood. However, many studies (reviewed by Noonan and De Fabo 1992; Norval 2006) have provided evidence for an important role of the *cis* isomer of UCA in controlling immune responses. Therefore, the UCA effects on cells represent a promising area of skin research.

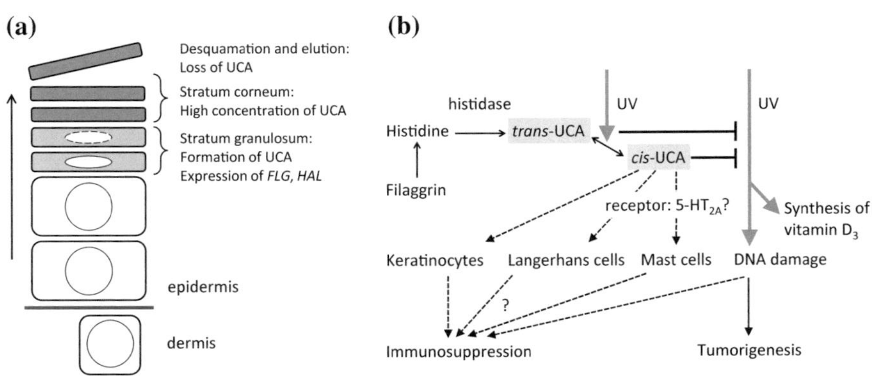

Fig. 4.4 Roles of UCA in UV-stressed skin. The localization of UCA formation in the epidermis **a** and the metabolism, UV absorption and signaling functions of UCA **b** are shown schematically. The *arrow* in panel **a** indicates the direction of keratinocyte differentiation. *Question marks* in panel **b** indicate major open questions concerning the signaling mechanism and the target cells of *cis*-UCA

The main indirect effect of UCA on skin cells is the absorption of UVB radiation in the stratum corneum, which reduces the UV doses on cells of deeper skin layers. As UVB radiation damages DNA, proteins and lipids and supports the synthesis of vitamin D, the UCA-mediated reduction of the UV reaching keratinocytes, melanocytes, Langerhans cells and other skin cells is physiologically important.

UCA has also been implicated in the control of the pH in the stratum corneum. The pH within the stratum corneum influences the proteolytic system that drives the desquamation of superficial corneocytes and controls the resident microflora. The analysis of proton donors extractable from the human skin surface showed that the pK of the proton donors matched that of UCA and the amount of UCA in the stratum corneum could explain the acidic pH on different individuals (Krien and Kermici 2000). Other studies have provided evidence against a critical role of UCA in skin surface pH control (Fluhr et al. 2010). Further experimental studies are necessary to determine whether UCA formation actively alters the stratum corneum pH or whether UCA contributes significantly to the buffering against changes of the pH.

4.4.2 Effects of UCA Via Receptors

UCA interacts with several cell components in a relatively unspecific manner whereas a specific binding to a cellular receptor has been postulated as the first step of the physiologically important immunosuppressive activity of *cis*-UCA (see below). It was suggested that UCA binds to DNA (Yarosh et al. 1992), however, other data argue against this interaction in vivo (Ijland et al. 1998). UCA associates with lipid membranes in a pH-sensitive manner (Campos et al. 2008), but the physiological role of this process remains to be tested. More significantly, UCA interacts with epidermal proteins leading to a red shift by 10 nm of the photoisomerization action spectrum of UCA in the stratum corneum relative to that in vitro (Jones et al. 1996). *trans*-UCA and *cis*-UCA interact with BSA, with *cis*-UCA binding more strongly than *trans*-UCA (Campos et al. 2008). Binding to the aforementioned tissue components is not believed to evoke a biological response to UCA.

By contrast, specific binding of UCA to cellular receptor(s) has been hypothesized to initiate signaling and important responses (reviewed by Gibbs et al. 2008). Most notably, 5-hydroxytryptamine (serotonin) receptor 2A (5-HT_{2A}) has been identified as a high-affinity receptor (Kd = 4.6 nM) for *cis*-UCA whereas *trans*-UCA does not bind to 5-HT_{2A} (Walterscheid et al. 2006). Binding of *cis*-UCA to 5-HT2A was competitively inhibited by the main ligand of the receptor, i.e. serotonin (5-hydroxytryptamine, 5-HT), a neurotransmitter synthesized from tryptophan. *cis*-UCA was shown to mobilize intracellular calcium stores in cells that expressed 5-HT_{2A} (Walterscheid et al. 2006).

It is presently unknown on which cells 5-HT_{2A} is activated by *cis*-UCA. 5-HT_{2A} is encoded by the *HTR2A* gene which is mainly expressed in the brain. In the skin,

5-HT_{2A} has been reported to be expressed on Langerhans cells, mast cells and lymphocytes (Kim 2012) and to mediate the melanogenic effects of serotonin on melanocytes (Lee et al. 2011).

Keratinocytes are stimulated by *cis*-UCA independently of 5-HT_{2A}. Specifically, the treatment of human keratinocytes with *cis*-UCA led to increased secretion of prostaglandin E_2, TNF-α, and interleukin (IL)-6 despite absence of 5-HT_{2A} expression in keratinocytes (Kaneko et al. 2009). At least part of these effects were mediated by altered gene expression including strong upregulation of prostaglandin endoperoxide synthase 2 (PTGS2, also known as cyclooxygenase, COX-2) (Kaneko et al. 2008). These effects of *cis*-UCA depended on the formation of reactive oxygen species (Kaneko et al. 2011).

Peripheral blood mononuclear cells respond to lipopolysaccharide by the production of TNF-α in a process that can be suppressed by both *cis*-UCA and serotonin in vitro. However, only *cis*-UCA caused the production of prostaglandin and depended on it to exert its suppressive effect (Woodward et al. 2006), arguing against a common signaling mechanism of *cis*-UCA and serotonin in this experimental setting.

Most studies have suggested that *cis*-UCA, but not *trans*-UCA, is biologically active. However, there is also evidence for (direct) effects of *trans*-UCA on various cell types. In human dermal fibroblasts, *trans*-UCA induces cAMP (adenosine 3′,5′-cyclic monophosphate) formation by adenyl cyclase whereas *cis*-UCA suppresses cAMP formation (Palaszynski et al. 1992). Moreover, *trans*-UCA may contribute to the regulation of Langerhans cells (Schwarz et al. 2012). Therefore, despite many years of studies of UCA, it is not fully clear whether UV is required to "activate" UCA in terms of facilitating specific effects on cells.

4.4.3 Immunosuppressive Activity of cis-*UCA*

UV irradiation can suppress the immune system both locally and systemically (Kripke et al. 1992; Ullrich 2005; Schwarz and Schwarz 2011). This phenomenon has been observed in humans as well as other mammalian species such as mouse (De Fabo and Noonan 1983) and opossum (Ley et al. 2000) but not in lizards (Cope et al. 2001). UV-induced immunosuppression contributes to skin cancer but also represents a therapeutic approach for the treatment of autoimmune diseases. Regulatory T-cells, Langerhans cells, and cytokines are important mediators of immunosuppression in response to UV irradiation but the initiating event is the absorption of UV radiation. UV absorption by DNA and the resulting DNA damage are crucial for UV-induced immunosuppression (Schwarz et al. 2002). Accordingly, absorption of incident UV by skin chromophores such as UCA reduces DNA damage (Barresi et al. 2011) and, therefore, should decrease UV-induced immunosuppression. The effect of UCA-mediated UV absorption on immunosuppression has not been quantified yet. However, UV absorption by UCA itself has a second effect on the immune system, and this effect is opposite to the protection from UV damage. UV causes the isomerization of *trans*-UCA to *cis*-UCA, and *cis*-UCA acts as an immunosuppressive agent.

cis-UCA can mimic both local and systemic immunosuppressive effects of UV (Noonan and De Fabo 1992; Norval et al. 1995). Investigations of these effects were mainly based on the administration of exogenous *cis*-UCA. Other studies have used an antibody to neutralize endogenous UC-induced *cis*-UCA (el-Ghorr and Norval 1995). Another experimental setting might be the investigation of UV-induced immunosuppression in individuals (histidinemics) that have strongly reduced amounts of epidermal UCA due to defects in histidase. When histidinemic mice and wildtype mice were irradiated on the shaved back with doses of UV that yielded minimal skin damage, systemic suppression of contact hypersensitivity (CHS) was induced in wild-type mice but not histidinemic mice, indicating that endogenous UCA acts as the epidermal photoreceptor for UV-induced immunosuppression (De Fabo et al. 1983). Importantly, these studies need to be repeated in larger numbers of mice and investigations of the underlying mechanisms are warranted.

The mechanism by which *cis*-UCA induces immunosuppression is not fully understood at present. According to one hypothesis, *cis*-UCA activates the 5-HT_{2A} receptor on Langerhans cells and/or mast cells which are potent modulators of immune responses. In this scenario, *cis*-UCA signaling is independent from DNA damage-induced immunosuppression. Another hypothesis is based on the report that *cis*-UCA activates reactive oxygen species production in keratinocytes (Sreevidya et al. 2010). Subsequently, also pre-mutagenic DNA damage in the form of 8-oxo-deoxyguanosine (8-oxo-dG) is increased by *cis*-UCA, and this reaction can be blocked by an 5-HT_{2A} receptor antagonist. Furthermore, treatment with 5-HT_{2A} receptor antagonist accelerates nucleotide excision repair after UV irradiation, indicating that *cis*-UCA suppresses DNA repair (Sreevidya et al. 2010). These findings are compatible with the concept that UV-induced *cis*-UCA contributes to immune suppression (as well as photocarcinogenesis) mainly by the production of reactive oxygen which induces DNA damage and inhibits nucleotide excision repair (Langie et al. 2007). Intriguingly, the cytokine IL-12 reverses UV-induced immune suppression, at least in part, by activating DNA repair (Schwarz et al. 2002) and IL-12 also counteracts the inhibitory effects of *cis*-UCA on antigen presentation by Langerhans cells (Beissert et al. 2001).

4.4.4 Use of UCA as a Therapeutic Agent

UCA was used for the prevention of UVB photodamage for many years. It was discontinued as a component of cosmetic products because of reports that showed enhanced UV photocarcinogenesis in mice treated with topical UCA (Reeve et al. 1989; Andersen 1995). While immunosuppressive effects of *cis*-UCA were mainly responsible for the end of UCA-containing cosmetics, the same effects are considered a useful activity for the treatment of atopic dermatitis and ocular inflammation. A series of preclinical and clinical studies of UCA as a therapeutic agent have been conducted recently (Laihia et al. 2012; Peltonen et al. 2014; Jauhonen et al. 2015). Chemical conjugation of UCA with other substances may extend the applications of UCA. However, further investigations will be necessary to test the therapeutic potential of UCA and its derivatives.

4.5 Conclusions

UCA formation is controlled by (1) the supply of histidine which is derived from filaggrin, (2) the activity of histidase which depends on *HAL* gene expression and pH. The pH also affects the solubility of UCA, the binding of UCA to proteins and the UV absorption spectrum of UCA. Endogenous UCA contributes significantly to the UV absorption capacity of the stratum corneum and represents the most important natural sunscreen of the outermost layers of the skin. Because of its localization, UCA is prone to loss into the environment via elution. UVB irradiation causes isomerization between *trans*-UCA and *cis*-UCA. The latter has immunosuppressive activities and represents a marker of UV exposure. Its roles as UV chromophore and signaling molecule make UCA an attractive target for further studies in skin biology.

References

Alm J, Holmgren G, Larsson A, Schimpfessel L (1981) Histidinaemia in Sweden: report on a neonatal screening programme. Clin Genet 20:229–233

Andersen FA (1995) Final report on the safety assessment of urocanic acid. J Am Coll Toxicol 14:386–423

Baden HP, Pathak MA (1967) The metabolism and function of urocanic acid in skin. J Invest Dermatol 48:11–17

Baden HP, Hori Y, Pathak MA, Levy HL (1969a) Epidermis in histidinemia. Arch Dermatol 100:432–435

Baden HP, Sviokla S, Maderson PF (1969b) A comparative study of histidase activity in amphibian, avian, reptilian and mammalian epidermis. Comp Biochem Physiol 30:889–894

Barresi C, Stremnitzer C, Mlitz V, Kezic S, Kammeyer A, Ghannadan M, Posa-Markaryan K, Selden C, Tschachler E, Eckhart L (2011) Increased sensitivity of histidinemic mice to ultraviolet B radiation suggests a crucial role of endogenous urocanic acid in photoprotection. J Invest Dermatol 131:188–194

Beissert S, Rühlemann D, Mohammad T, Grabbe S, El-Ghorr A, Norval M, Morrison H, Granstein RD, Schwarz T (2001) IL-12 prevents the inhibitory effects of cis-urocanic acid on tumor antigen presentation by Langerhans cells: implications for photocarcinogenesis. J Immunol 167:6232–6238

Brand LM, Harper AE (1976) Histidine ammonia-lyase from rat liver. Purification, properties, and inhibition by substrate analogues. Biochemistry 15:1814–1821

Brookman J, Chacón JN, Sinclair RS (2002) Some photophysical studies of cis- and trans-urocanic acid. Photochem Photobiol Sci 1:327–332

Brusilow SW, Ikai K (1968) Urocanic acid in sweat: an artifact of elution from the epidermis. Science 160:1257–1258

Bulfield G, Kacser H (1975) Histamine and histidine levels in the brain of the histidinaemic mutant mouse. J Neurochem 24:403–405
Campos AM, Cárcamo C, Silva E, García S, Lemp E, Alarcón E, Edwards AM, Günther G, Lissi E (2008) Distribution of urocanic acid isomers between aqueous solutions and n-octanol, liposomes or bovine serum albumin. J Photochem Photobiol B 90:41–46
Colburn NH, Lau S, Head R (1975) Decrease of epidermal histidase activity by tumor-promoting phorbol esters. Cancer Res 35:3154–3159
Cope RB, Fabacher DL, Lieske C, Miller CA (2001) Resistance of a lizard (the green anole, Anolis carolinensis; Polychridae) to ultraviolet radiation-induced immunosuppression. Photochem Photobiol 74:46–54
De Fabo EC, Noonan FP (1983) Mechanism of immune suppression by ultraviolet irradiation in vivo. I. Evidence for the existence of a unique photoreceptor in skin and its role in photoimmunology. J Exp Med 158:84–98
De Fabo E, Noonan F, Fisher M, Burns J, Kacser H (1983) Further evidence that the photoreceptor mediating UV-induced systemic immune suppression is urocanic acid. J Invest Dermatol 80:319 (Abstract)
De Fabo EC, Webber LJ, Ulman EA, Broemeling LD (1997) Dietary L-histidine regulates murine skin levels of trans-urocanic acid, an immune-regulating photoreceptor, with an unanticipated modulation: potential relevance to skin cancer. J Nutr 127:2158–2164
de Fine Olivarius F, Wulf HC, Crosby J, Norval M (1996) The sunscreening effect of urocanic acid. Photodermatol Photoimmunol Photomed 12:95–99
de Fine Olivarius F, Wulf HC, Crosby J, Norval M (1998) Urocanic acid isomers and photosensitivity in healthy children. Br J Dermatol 139:605–609
Denecker G, Hoste E, Gilbert B, Hochepied T, Ovaere P, Lippens S, Van den Broecke C, Van Damme P, D'Herde K, Hachem JP, Borgonie G, Presland RB, Schoonjans L, Libert C, Vandekerckhove J, Gevaert K, Vandenabeele P, Declercq W (2007) Caspase-14 protects against epidermal UVB photodamage and water loss. Nat Cell Biol 9:666–674
Eckhart L, Schmidt M, Mildner M, Mlitz V, Abtin A, Ballaun C, Fischer H, Mrass P, Tschachler E (2008) Histidase expression in human epidermal: regulation by differentiation status and all-trans retinoic acid. J Dermatol Sci 50:209–215
el-Ghorr AA, Norval M (1995) A monoclonal antibody to cis-urocanic acid prevents the ultraviolet-induced changes in Langerhans cells and delayed hypersensitivity responses in mice, although not preventing dendritic cell accumulation in lymph nodes draining the site of irradiation and contact hypersensitivity responses. J Invest Dermatol 105:264–268
Espinós C, Pineda M, Martínez-Rubio D, Lupo V, Ormazabal A, Vilaseca MA, Spaapen LJ, Palau F, Artuch R (2009) Mutations in the urocanase gene UROC1 are associated with urocanic aciduria. J Med Genet 46:407–411
Ferguson J, Johnson BE (1986) Photosensitivity due to retinoids: clinical and laboratory studies. Br J Dermatol 115:275–283
Fluhr JW, Elias PM, Man MQ, Hupe M, Selden C, Sundberg JP, Tschachler E, Eckhart L, Mauro TM, Feingold KR (2010) Is the filaggrin-histidine-urocanic acid pathway essential for stratum corneum acidification? J Invest Dermatol 130:2141–2144
Forbes D, Johnston L, Gardner J, MacCallum SF, Campbell LE, Dinkova-Kostova AT, McLean WH, Ibbotson SH, Dawe RS, Brown SJ (2016) Filaggrin genotype does not determine the skin's threshold to UV-induced erythema. J Allergy Clin Immunol. doi:10.1016/j.jaci.2015.11.022
Fujitaka M, Eguchi T, Sakura N, Ueda K (1993) Measurement of histidase activity in human fingernail by reversed-phase HPLC. Clin Chim Acta 215:227–232
Gers-Balag H, Müller A, Sauermann G, Mann T (1997) The influence of sunscreens on the loss of urocanic acid during bathing. J Invest Dermatol 108:667 (Abstract)
Gibbs NK, Tye J, Norval M (2008) Recent advances in urocanic acid photochemistry, photobiology and photoimmunology. Photochem Photobiol Sci 7:655–667
Gill SC, von Hippel PH (1989) Calculation of protein extinction coefficients from amino acid sequence data. Anal Biochem 182:319–326

Gilmour JW, Vestey JP, Norval M (1993) The effect of UV therapy on immune function in patients with psoriasis. Br J Dermatol 129:28–38

Hanson KM, Simon JD (1998) Epidermal trans-urocanic acid and the UV-A-induced photoaging of the skin. Proc Natl Acad Sci USA 95:10576–10578

Heenen M, Giacomoni PU, Golstein P (2001) Individual variations in the correlation between erythemal threshold, UV-induced DNA damage and sun-burn cell formation. J Photochem Photobiol B 63:84–87

Hug DH, Dunkerson DD, Hunter JK (1999) The degradation of L-histidine and trans- and cis-urocanic acid by bacteria from skin and the role of bacterial cis-urocanic acid isomerase. J Photochem Photobiol B 50:66–73

Hunter A (1912) On urocanic acid. J Biol Chem 11:537–545

Ijland SA, Noonan FP, Ceryak S, Steenvoorden DP, Bouscarel B, Hug D, Beijersbergen van Henegouwen GM, De Fabo EC (1998) Urocanic acid does not photobind to DNA in mice irradiated with immunosuppressive doses of UVB. Photochem Photobiol 67:222–226

Imamura I, Watanabe T, Hase Y, Sakamoto Y, Fukuda Y, Yamamoto H, Tsuruhara T, Wada H (1984) Histamine metabolism in patients with histidinemia: determination of urinary levels of histamine, N tau-methylhistamine, imidazole acetic acid, and its conjugate(s). J Biochem 96:1925–1929

Jaffe M (1874) Ueber einen neuen Bestandtheil des Hundeharns. Berichte der deutschen chemischen Gesellschaft 7:1669–1673

Jauhonen HM, Kari E, Pylkkänen L, Poutanen J, Laihia J, Kaarniranta K, Leino L (2015) A randomized phase I clinical study of cis-urocanic acid eye drops in healthy adult subjects. Acta Ophthalmol 93:368–376

Jones CD, Barton AK, Crosby J, Norval M, Gibbs NK (1996) Investigating the red shift between in vitro and in vivo urocanic acid photoisomerization action spectra. Photochem Photobiol 63:302–305

Joo KM, Han JY, Son ED, Nam GW, Chung HY, Jeong HJ, Cho JC, Lim KM (2012) Rapid, simultaneous and nanomolar determination of pyroglutamic acid and cis-/trans-urocanic acid in human stratum corneum by hydrophilic interaction liquid chromatography (HILIC)-electrospray ionization tandem mass spectrometry. J Chromatogr B Analyst Technol Biomed Life Sci 897:55–63

Kacser H, Bulfield G, Wallace ME (1973) Histidinaemic mutant in the mouse. Nature 244:77–79

Kammeyer A, Eggelte TA, Bos JD, Teunissen MBM (1999) Urocanic acid isomers are good hydroxyl radical scavengers: a comparative study with structural analogues and with uric acid. Biochim Biophys Acta 1428:117–120

Kammeyer A, Eggelte TA, Overmars H, Bootsma A, Bos JD, Teunissen MBM (2001) Oxidative breakdown and conversion of urocanic acid isomers by hydroxyl radical generating systems. Biochim Biophys Acta 1526:277–285

Kaneko K, Smetana-Just U, Matsui M, Young AR, John S, Norval M, Walker SL (2008) cis-Urocanic acid initiates gene transcription in primary human keratinocytes. J Immunol 181:217–224

Kaneko K, Travers JB, Matsui MS, Young AR, Norval M, Walker SL (2009) cis-Urocanic acid stimulates primary human keratinocytes independently of serotonin or platelet-activating factor receptors. J Invest Dermatol 129:2567–2573

Kaneko K, Walker SL, Lai-Cheong J, Matsui MS, Norval M, Young AR (2011) cis-Urocanic acid enhances prostaglandin E2 release and apoptotic cell death via reactive oxygen species in human keratinocytes. J Invest Dermatol 131:1262–1271

Kawasaki H, Nagao K, Kubo A, Hata T, Shimizu A, Mizuno H, Yamada T, Amagai M (2012) Altered stratum corneum barrier and enhanced percutaneous immune responses in filaggrin-null mice. J Allergy Clin Immunol 129:1538–1546

Kezic S, Kammeyer A, Calkoen F, Fluhr JW, Bos JD (2009) Natural moisturizing factor components in the stratum corneum as biomarkers of filaggrin genotype: evaluation of minimally invasive methods. Br J Dermatol 161:1098–1104

Kim K (2012) Neuroimmunological mechanism of pruritus in atopic dermatitis focused on the role of serotonin. Biomol Ther (Seoul) 20:506–512

Kinuta M, Kinuta K, Yamada H, Abe T, Yoshida Y, Araki K, Li SA, Otsuka A, Nakanishi A, Moriyama Y, Takei K (2003) Formation of S-[2-carboxy-1-(1H-imidazol-4-yl) ethyl] glutathione, a new metabolite of L-histidine, from cis-urocanic acid and glutathione by the action of glutathione S-transferase. Electrophoresis 24:3212–3218

Krien PM, Kermici M (2000) Evidence for the existence of a self-regulated enzymatic process within the human stratum corneum - an unexpected role for urocanic acid. J Invest Dermatol 115:414–420

Kripke ML, Cox PA, Alas LG, Yarosh DB (1992) Pyrimidine dimers in DNA initiate systemic immunosuppression in UV-irradiated mice. Proc Natl Acad Sci USA 89:7516–7520

Kurogochi Y, Fukui Y, Nakagawa T, Yamamoto I (1957) A note on cis-urocanid acid. Jpn J Pharmacol 6:147–152

Laihia JK, Taimen P, Kujari H, Leino L (2012) Topical cis-urocanic acid attenuates oedema and erythema in acute and subacute skin inflammation in the mouse. Br J Dermatol 167:506–513

Langie SA, Knaapen AM, Houben JM, van Kempen FC, de Hoon JP, Gottschalk RW, Godschalk RW, van Schooten FJ (2007) The role of glutathione in the regulation of nucleotide excision repair during oxidative stress. Toxicol Lett 168:302–309

Lam WK, Cleary MA, Wraith JE, Walter JH (1996) Histidinaemia: a benign metabolic disorder. Arch Dis Child 74:343–346

Lee HJ, Park MK, Kim SY, Park Choo HY, Lee AY, Lee CH (2011) Serotonin induces melanogenesis via serotonin receptor 2A. Br J Dermatol 165:1344–1348

Levy HL, Baden HP, Shih VE (1969) A simple indirect method of detecting the enzyme defect in histidinemia. J Pediat 75:1056–1058

Ley RD, Reeve VE, Kusewitt DF (2000) Photobiology of Monodelphis domestica. Dev Comp Immunol 24:503–516

Mehler AH, Tabor H (1953) Deamination of histidine to form urocanic acid in liver. J Biol Chem 201:775–784

Miajlovic H, Fallon PG, Irvine AD, Foster TJ (2010) Effect of filaggrin breakdown products on growth of and protein expression by *Staphylococcus aureus*. J Allergy Clin Immunol 126:1184–1190

Mildner M, Jin J, Eckhart L, Kezic S, Gruber F, Barresi C, Stremnitzer C, Buchberger M, Mlitz V, Ballaun C, Sterniczky B, Födinger D, Tschachler E (2010) Knockdown of filaggrin impairs the diffusion barrier function and increases the UV sensitivity in a human skin model. J Invest Dermatol 130:2286–2294

Mlitz V, Strasser B, Jaeger K, Hermann M, Ghannadan M, Buchberger M, Alibardi L, Tschachler E, Eckhart L (2014) Trichohyalin-like proteins have evolutionarily conserved roles in the morphogenesis of skin appendages. J Invest Dermatol 134:2685–2692

Mohammad T, Morrison H, HogenEsch H (1999) Urocanic acid photochemistry and photobiology. Photochem Photobiol 69:115–135

Moodycliffe AM, Norval M, Kimber I, Simpson TJ (1993) Characterization of a monoclonal antibody to cis-urocanic acid: detection of cis-urocanic acid in the serum of irradiated mice by immunoassay. Immunology 79:667–672

Noonan FP, De Fabo EC (1992) Immunosuppression by ultraviolet B radiation: initiation by urocanic acid. Immunol Today 13:250–254

Norval M (2006) The mechanisms and consequences of ultraviolet-induced immunosuppression. Prog Biophys Mol Biol 92:108–118

Norval M, Gibbs NK, Gilmour J (1995) The role of urocanic acid in UV-induced immunosuppression: recent advances (1992–1994). Photochem Photobiol 62:209–217

Palaszynski EW, Noonan FP, De Fabo EC (1992) cis-urocanic acid down-regulates the induction of adenosine 3′,5′-cyclic monophosphate by either trans-urocanic acid or histamine in human dermal fibroblasts in vitro. Photochem Photobiol 55:165–171

Peltonen JM, Pylkkänen L, Jansén CT, Volanen I, Lehtinen T, Laihia JK, Leino L (2014) Three randomised phase I/IIa trials of 5% cis-urocanic acid emulsion cream in healthy adult subjects and in patients with atopic dermatitis. Acta Derm Venereol 94:415–420

Reaven EP, Cox AJ (1965) Histidine and keratinization. J Invest Dermatol 45:422–431

Reeve VE, Greenoak GE, Canfield PJ, Boehm-Wilcox C, Gallagher CH (1989) Topical urocanic acid enhances UV-induced tumour yield and malignancy in the hairless mouse. Photochem Photobiol 49:459–464

Reilly JT, Troester KA, Tyner TT, Vitale DA, Risher TR (2010) Inhibition of histidine ammonia lyase by 8-methoxypsoralen and psoralen-oxidized photoproducts. Photochem Photobiol 86:1272–1277

Safer D, Brenes M, Dunipace S, Schad G (2007) Urocanic acid is a major chemoattractant for the skin-penetrating parasitic nematode Strongyloides stercoralis. Proc Natl Acad Sci USA 104:1627–1630

Sastry CM, Whitmore SE, Breysse PN, Morison WL, Strickland PT (2005) The effect of clinical UVA/B exposures on urinary urocanic acid isomer levels in individuals with caucasian type (II/III) skin types. Dermatol Online J 11:1

Schwarz T, Schwarz A (2011) Molecular mechanisms of ultraviolet radiation-induced immunosuppression. Eur J Cell Biol 90:560–564

Schwarz A, Stander S, Berneburg M, Bohm M, Kulms D, van Steeg H, Grosse-Heitmeyer K, Krutmann J, Schwarz T (2002) Interleukin-12 suppresses ultraviolet radiation-induced apoptosis by inducing DNA repair. Nat Cell Biol 4:26–31

Schwarz A, Eckhart L, Tschachler E, Schwarz T (2012) The function of Langerhans cells is intrinsically regulated by urocanic acid. J Invest Dermatol 132 (Suppl 2):S118–S123 (Abstract)

Schwede TF, Rétey J, Schulz GE (1999) Crystal structure of histidine ammonia-lyase revealing a novel polypeptide modification as the catalytic electrophile. Biochemistry 38:5355–5361

Scott IR (1981) Factors controlling the expressed activity of histidine ammonia-lyase in the epidermis and the resulting accumulation of urocanic acid. Biochem J 194:829–838

Scott IR, Harding CR, Barrett JG (1982) Histidine-rich protein of the keratohyalin granules. Source of the free amino acids, urocanic acid and pyrrolidone carboxylic acid in the stratum corneum. Biochim Biophys Acta 719:110–117

Shen L, Ji HF (2008) Theoretical investigation of the photosensitization mechanisms of urocanic acid. J Photochem Photobiol B 91:96–98

Shimizu K, Andoh T, Yoshihisa Y, Shimizu T (2015) Histamine released from epidermal keratinocytes plays a role in α-melanocyte-stimulating hormone-induced itching in mice. Am J Pathol 185:3003–3010

Sreevidya CS, Fukunaga A, Khaskhely NM, Masaki T, Ono R, Nishigori C, Ullrich SE (2010) Agents that reverse UV-induced immune suppression and photocarcinogenesis affect DNA repair. J Invest Dermatol 130:1428–1437

Suchi M, Sano H, Mizuno H, Wada Y (1995) Molecular cloning and structural characterization of the human histidase gene (HAL). Genomics 29:98–104

Tabachnik J (1957) Urocanic acid, the major acid soluble UV absorbing compound in guinea pig epidermis. Arch Biochem Biophys 70:295–297

Tanabe M, Sakura N (1989) Hyperhistaminemia in patients with histidinemia due to increased decarboxylation of histidine. Clin Chim Acta 186:11–17

Taylor RG, Lambert MA, Sexsmith E, Sadler SJ, Ray PN, Mahuran DJ, McInnes RR (1990) Cloning and expression of rat histidase. Homology to two bacterial histidases and four phenylalanine ammonia-lyases. J Biol Chem 265:18192–18199

Taylor RG, Grieco D, Clarke GA, McInnes RR, Taylor BA (1993) Identification of the mutation in murine histidinemia (his) and genetic mapping of the murine histidase locus (Hal) on chromosome 10. Genomics 16:231–240

Thyssen JP, Thuesen B, Huth C, Standl M, Carson CG, Heinrich J, Krämer U, Kratzsch J, Berg ND, Menné T, Johansen JD, Carlsen BC, Schwab S, Thorand B, Munk M, Wallaschofski H, Heickendorff L, Meldgaard M, Szecsi PB, Stender S, Bønnelykke K, Weidinger S, Bisgaard H, Linneberg A (2012) Skin barrier abnormality caused by filaggrin

(FLG) mutations is associated with increased serum 25-hydroxyvitamin D concentrations. J Allergy Clin Immunol 130:1204–1207

Thyssen JP, Bikle DD, Elias PM (2014) Evidence that loss-of-function filaggrin gene mutations evolved in northern Europeans to favor intracutaneous vitamin D3 production. Evol Biol 41:388–396

Torres N, Martinez L, Aleman G, Bourges H, Tovar AR (1998) Histidase expression is regulated by dietary protein at the pretranslational level in rat liver. J Nutr 128:818–824

Tye J, Walter JH, Griffiths CEM, Gibbs NK (2008) A lack of epidermal urocanic acid in histidinaemic skin influences ultraviolet B-induced CD1a+ Langerhans cell trafficking. Br J Dermatol 158:885 (Abstract)

Ullrich SE (2005) Mechanisms underlying UV-induced immune suppression. Mutat Res 571:185–205

Walterscheid JP, Nghiem DX, Kazimi N, Nutt LK, McConkey DJ, Norval M, Ullrich SE (2006) Cis-urocanic acid, a sunlight-induced immunosuppressive factor, activates immune suppression via the 5-HT2A receptor. Proc Natl Acad Sci USA 103:17420–17425

Widhalm K, Virmani K (1994) Long-term follow-up of 58 patients with histidinemia treated with a histidine-restricted diet: no effect of therapy. Pediatrics 94:861–866

Wondrak GT, Jacobson MK, Jacobson EL (2006) Endogenous UVA-photosensitizers: mediators of skin photodamage and novel targets for skin photoprotection. Photochem Photobiol Sci 5:215–237

Woodward EA, Prele CM, Finlay-Jones JJ, Hart PH (2006) The receptor for cis-urocanic acid remains elusive. J Invest Dermatol 126:1191–1193

Wright AF, Bulfield G, Arfin SM, Kacser H (1982) Comparison of the properties of histidine ammonia-lyase in normal and histidinemic mutant mice. Biochem Genet 20:245–263

Yarosh DB, Gettings SD, Alas LG, Kibitel JT, San RH, Wagner VO 3rd, McEwen GN Jr (1992) The biological interaction of cis and trans-urocanic acid with DNA. Photodermatol Photoimmunol Photomed 9:121–126

Yokoya S, Tokuhiro E, Suwa S, Maesaka H (1983) Measurement of the skin urocanic acid content in normal and histidinemic infants. Eur J Pediatr 140:330–332

Yu B, Li AH, Muzny D, Veeraraghavan N, de Vries PS, Bis JC, Musani SK, Alexander D, Morrison AC, Franco OH, Uitterlinden A, Hofman A, Dehghan A, Wilson JG, Psaty BM, Gibbs R, Wei P, Boerwinkle E (2015) Association of rare loss-of-function alleles in HAL, serum histidine: Levels and incident coronary heart disease. Circ Cardiovasc Genet 8:351–355

Zannoni VG, La Du BN (1963) Determination of histidine alpha-deaminase in human stratum corneum and its absence in histidinaemia. Biochem J 88:160–162

Zenisek A, Kral JA (1953) The occurrence of urocanic acid in human sweat. Biochim Biophys Acta 12:479–480

Zenisek A, Kral JA, Hais IM (1955) Sun-screening effect of urocanic acid. Biochim Biophys Acta 18:589–591

Zhang Y, Wang W, Chen J, Zhang K, Gao F, Gao B, Zhang S, Dong M, Besenbacher F, Gong W, Zhang M, Sun F, Feng W (2013) Structural insights into the intrinsic self-assembly of Par-3 N-terminal domain. Structure 21:997–1006

Zhang XX, Ritchie SR, Rainey PB (2014) Urocanate as a potential signaling molecule for bacterial recognition of eukaryotic hosts. Cell Mol Life Sci 71:541–547

Chapter 5
The Skin Extracellular Matrix as a Target of Environmental Exposure: Molecular Mechanisms, Prevention and Repair

Kieran T. Mellody, Mike Bell and Michael J. Sherratt

Abstract The dermal extracellular matrix (ECM) undergoes age-related remodelling which leads to wrinkle formation and increased tissue fragility. In healthy young individuals structural ECM assemblies, such as collagens and elastin, are ordered into larger scale structures (collagen fibril bundles and elastic fibres), which mediate the mechanical properties of the dermis. Equally important however, are the less abundant extracellular accessory molecules that regulate complex processes such as cell migration, wound healing and which also orchestrate complex ECM protein-to-protein interactions. These structures and molecular interactions are perturbed in extrinsically aged skin. Using bioinformatics alongside established molecular investigations opens up exciting new ways to understand skin ageing and may help to identify novel biomarkers. In this chapter we propose a mechanism whereby UVR-induced damage of key ECM molecules drives elastosis. We discuss how: i) the amino acid composition of proteins can be used to predict their susceptibility to damage by ultraviolet radiation (UVR) and ii) other environmental factors, such as smoking and air pollution may contribute towards premature skin ageing. Finally this chapter reviews the latest topical applications and systemic therapies that may be able to reverse the consequences of damage to the ECM in ageing.

Keywords Skin · Ageing · Extracellular matrix · Ultraviolet radiation · Sunscreens · Anti-ageing formulations

K.T. Mellody · M.J. Sherratt (✉)
Centre for Tissue Injury and Repair, Institute of Inflammation and Repair, The University of Manchester, 1.529 Stopford Building, Oxford Road, Manchester M13 9PT, UK
e-mail: michael.sherratt@manchester.ac.uk

M. Bell
Walgreens Boots Alliance, Thane Road, Nottingham, UK

G.T. Wondrak (ed.), *Skin Stress Response Pathways*,
DOI 10.1007/978-3-319-43157-4_5

5.1 Introduction

Extracellular matrix (ECM) components perform key mechanical roles in the skin including resisting tensile (fibrillar collagens) and compressive (proteoglycans and hyaluronic acid) forces, and conferring elasticity (elastic fibres). With chronological age, and in particular with exposure to exogenous agents such as ultraviolet radiation (UVR), these components undergo architectural and structural remodelling which, in turn, is associated with the outward signs of ageing (wrinkles) and with increased skin stiffness and fragility (Agache et al. 1980; Baranoski 2000; Warren et al. 1991). Crucially, there is now a large and compelling body of evidence that highlights the important role played by ECM components in general and by elastic fibre components in particular in maintaining tissue homeostasis (Marastoni et al. 2008). As a consequence, it is likely that accumulated environmental damage to ECM components, by exposure to UVR for example, will not only affect the mechanical properties of the tissue, but may also precipitate further remodelling due to the release of sequestered cytokines and proteases (Watson et al. 2014). In this chapter, we briefly review the composition and function of cutaneous ECM components (in all three layers of the skin) before discussing the effects of environmental factors and the causative molecular mechanisms which may be involved in promoting skin ageing. We then consider current and future strategies to prevent and crucially, to repair damage accrued by ECM proteins.

5.2 The Extracellular Matrix: Composition and Architecture in Young, Healthy Skin

The skin is composed of three distinct tissue layers: the epidermis, dermis and hypodermis. Compared with the highly cellular and relatively thin epidermis, the thicker dermis undergoes profound remodelling as a consequence of exposure to environmental factors such as UVR (Yaar and Gilchrest 2007). The dermis is composed primarily of structural ECM molecules including fibrillar collagens, proteoglycans and elastin. It is this latter protein which, in combination with associated proteins and assemblies, forms both functional elastic fibres and the histological hallmark of photo-damage, solar elastosis. Given the key role which elastic fibre associated proteins, such as fibrillin microfibrils and fibulin-5, play in maintaining tissue function, in this section we consider not only collagen and elastin but also the influence of "minor" dermal ECM components (Ramirez and Sakai 2010).

5.2.1 Collagens

Currently there are 28 different types of collagens encoded by more than 44 separate genes, which assemble into a wide variety of supramolecular structures (Mienaltowski and Birk 2014). All collagens are characterised by the presence of at least one sequence of repeating Glycine-X-Y residues where the X and Y are typically proline and hydroxyproline respectively (Ramshaw et al. 1998). Collagen monomers are, in turn, assembled from three alpha chains in which the aligned Gly-X-Y repeats form a triple helical domain that is stabilised by the hydroxylation of proline (Birk and Bruckner 2005). The major structural fibrillar collagens such as collagen I, II and III are composed of an uninterrupted helical region which comprises the entire molecule in the processed form. Other sub-families such as the FACIT collagens (Fibril Associated with Interrupted Triple Helices) and the network forming collagens (e.g. collagen IV, VI and VIII) contain discontinuous triple helical regions and/or substantial non-helical (globular) domains. Although some collagens (e.g. collagen II in cartilage) are confined to specific tissues, many collagens are ubiquitously expressed.

The most abundant collagens found in the skin are the interstitial fibrillar collagens, types I, III and V. These collagens form fibrils which range in diameter from 80 to 180 nm (ovine skin) and which are commonly arranged into large fibril bundles throughout the dermis (Fang et al. 2012). The most abundant non-fibrillar collagen in skin and in many other tissues is collagen VI. The beaded microfibrillar networks formed by this collagen encircles dermal collagen I fibrils and are thought to play a role in mediating matrix assembly and fibroblast phenotype (Sabatelli et al. 2011; Theocharidis et al. 2015). Other dermal collagens exhibit more localised distributions. Collagen IV for example, assembles into a sheet structure that forms the basal lamina. Collagen XVII stabilises basement membranes including the dermal epidermal junction (DEJ) by assembling into hemi desmosomes that anchor the epidermis to the dermis. Similarly, collagen VII anchors the dermis to the DEJ (Abreu-Velez and Howard 2012; Chanut-Delalande et al. 2004; Craven et al. 1997; Loffek et al. 2014).

5.2.2 *Proteoglycans and Glycosaminoglycans*

Proteoglycans are proteins that are heavily modified by glycosaminoglycan (GAG) side chains with the exception of hyaluronic acid (HA) which does not contain a protein core. The most abundant proteoglycan in skin is decorin, a member of the small leucine rich proteoglycan family (SLRPs) which is modified with a single GAG chain. It regulates the early stages of collagen fibril formation adorning the length of mature collagen fibrils, protecting them against proteolysis (Ruehland et al. 2007; Stuart et al. 2011; Yamaguchi et al. 1990). Other proteoglycans present in skin include versican, a constituent of blood vessels in the dermis, perlecan which is localised to the basement membrane, cell-surface expressed glypians and syndecans, and HA which is localised to the epidermis (Maquart and Monboisse 2014; Papakonstantinou et al. 2012; Wang et al. 2007). The GAG chains on HA readily bind water molecules to help maintain stratum corneum hydration and barrier function. HA is also an important molecule for wound healing and fibroblast migration (Papakonstantinou et al. 2012). The age-related decrease in epidermal localised HA is thought to contribute towards skin dehydration and loss of skin elasticity. The use of HA fillers injected into the skin not only decreases the clinical appearance of wrinkles but also restores dermal matrix components by stimulating de novo collagen synthesis (Wang et al. 2007).

5.2.3 *Elastic Fibres*

The mature elastic fibre system is a multi-component assembly that includes fibrillin microfibrils and elastin fibres that endow dynamic tissues such as skin, with passive elastic recoil and resilience (Baldwin et al. 2013). In the papillary dermis, 'candelabra-like' structures, consisting primarily of fibrillin microfibrils, intercalate with the DEJ. Deeper in the reticular dermis, these fibrillin microfibrils form an outer mantle around a highly cross-linked elastin core that together forms the mature elastic fibre system (Kielty et al. 2002; Sakai et al. 1986).

Elastin is a multi-domain, highly hydrophilic protein which is encoded by a single gene on chromosome 7q11.23. Elastogenic cells, such as fibroblasts within the skin, secrete the soluble precursor, tropoelastin, which is subsequently processed (by the amine oxidase: lysyl oxidase [LOX]) to the cross-linked, insoluble mature fibre (Lucero and Kagan 2006). Functionally, the N-terminus of elastin endows the protein with its elastic recoil whilst the C-terminus and a recently identified central region of the protein are actively involved in $\alpha V\beta 3$ and $\alpha V\beta 5$ integrin-mediated cell adhesion and signalling respectively (Bax et al. 2009; Lee et al. 2014). Importantly however, elastic fibre assembly does not occur in isolation but is dependent on the presence of fibrillin microfibrils.

Fibrillins are large glycoproteins ($\sim$340 kDa) that are encoded by three separate genes (FBN 1-3) on distinct chromosomes. Fibrillin-1, which is the most abundant isoform in adult tissues, forms the major component of the insoluble fibrillin-rich microfibrils localised within the dermis. Fibrillins-2 and -3 are typically expressed in early development, although fibrillin-2 is also expressed by keratinocytes and is present at low levels within the DEJ in adult tissue (Brinckmann et al. 2010; Haynes et al. 1997). The fibrillins are composed mainly of repeating calcium binding epidermal growth factor-like (cbEGF) domains. Fibrillin monomers polymerise to form insoluble fibrillin-rich microfibrils that exhibit a characteristic 'beads on a string' appearance with a regular inter-bead periodicity of $\sim$56 nm. Microfibril assembly occurs pericellularly and is dependent upon integrin binding, fibronectin, heparin and heparin sulphate (Bax et al. 2003; Kinsey et al. 2008; Massam-Wu et al. 2010; Sabatier et al. 2014).

In addition to acting as a molecular scaffold for tropoelastin deposition in elastogenesis, coacervation studies have further highlighted the importance of fibrillin in anchoring and directing the alignment of tropoelastin molecules prior to cross-linking (Clarke et al. 2005). Further, the interaction of microfibrils with cells and the latent transforming growth factor beta (TGFβ) growth factor binding proteins (LTBP) and the Latency associated peptide (LAP) complex suggest fibrillin microfibrils also may orchestrate elastogenesis by regulating TGFβ availability within the ECM space (Kaartinen and Warburton 2003; Massam-Wu et al. 2010).

Aberrant TGFβ signalling and disruption to elastic fibres assembly during prenatal and neonatal development is a hallmark of Marfan syndrome (MFS) caused by mutations in the fibrillin-1 gene (Gigante et al. 1999; Neptune et al. 2003). However, it is not clear if microfibrils also regulate elastic fibre assembly in adult tissue or if their composition changes as part of the ageing process. This is why our laboratory is focussed on understanding how photodamaged fibrillin microfibrils affect the mature elastic fibre system in skin and if their composition changes in ageing. Interestingly, although fibrillin microfibrils play an important role in determining tissue function and maintaining homeostasis they constitute only relatively a small proportion of the organic material within the dermis.

5.2.4 The Importance of "Minor" Components

The "major" components of the dermal ECM, in terms of their relative abundance, are important in maintaining normal skin function. As a consequence, attention has focussed almost exclusively on widely expressed proteins, such as collagen I and to a lesser extent elastin, and on the GAG chain of HA as key biomarkers of damage and targets for repair. However, there is compelling evidence that less abundant and hence "minor" ECM components play central roles in mediating the architecture of large ECM assemblies and in controlling cell-mediated tissue homeostasis. In the case of fibrillar collagens, for example, the SLRP decorin controls collagen fibril diameter and packing. The importance of this supra-molecular architecture to maintaining skin function is evident in the decorin knockout mouse which suffers from increased skin fragility (Danielson et al. 1997). However, decorin is not the only mediator of collagen fibril structure. Other fibril associated SLRPs such as biglycan, fibromodulin, versican, collagens (XII and XVI) and the ECM glycoprotein periostin may be equally important in maintaining tissue structure (Grassel and Bauer 2013; Maruhashi et al. 2010). In addition to its structural role, decorin, in common with elastic fibre associated fibrillin microfibrils, is a negative regulator of TGFβ (Stuart et al. 2011; Yamaguchi et al. 1990).

As discussed previously, fibrillin microfibrils sequester and therefore play a role in regulating the availability of TGFβ within the ECM (Massam-Wu et al. 2010). Fibrillin-1 mutations that cause MFS can alter protein structure and function, rendering the molecule susceptible to proteolysis and perturbing TGFβ signalling (Habashi et al. 2006; Kirschner et al. 2011; Mellody et al. 2006). A central region of the fibrillin-1 gene, often referred to as the neonatal region (exons 24-32), is prone to a cluster of mutations that result in an early lethal form of MFS which is associated with profound skin wrinkling (Tiecke et al. 2001). Tables 5.1 and 5.2 summarise the molecular interactions and potential function of both "major" and "minor" dermal components which play important roles in modifying cell behaviour, regulating matrix-to-matrix interactions and inducing protease expression. The abundant fibrillar collagens endow the skin with tensile strength and together with the minor collagens also regulate many other cellular and extracellular processes such as cell

Table 5.1 Dermal extracellular matrix proteins

Major component		Structure	Functions and interactions	ROS/UVR susceptibility (% 1° sequence)	Crosslink susceptibility (% 1° sequence)
Fibrillar collagens	I	Forms fibrils	Provides tensile strength and rigidity. Involved in fibroblast migration	4.20	8.91
	III	Forms fibrils	Important in skin development and collagen I fibrillogenesis	5.47	8.39
	V	Forms fibrils	Predominant at the core of fibril bundles. Provides a scaffold for collagen I fibrillogenesis	4.89	9.27
	VII	Forms fibrils	Major component of the basement membrane. Anchors the epidermis to the dermis	4.17	10.55
Non-fibrillar collagens	IV	Forms sheet structure	Adhesion molecule within the DEJ. Provides a scaffold for ECM molecules	5.95	8.55
	XVII	Transmembrane protein	Component of hemidesmosomes. Essential for organisation of the basement membrane and directs keratinocyte migration in wound healing	7.28	8.55
	VI	Forms beaded microfilaments	Regulates cellular functions and provides structural support to cells	7.40	11.58
	XII	Associates with collagen fibrils	Regulates the organisation and mechanical properties of collagen fibril bundles	7.86	10.23

(continued)

Table 5.1 (continued)

Major component		Structure	Functions and interactions	ROS/UVR susceptibility (% 1° sequence)	Crosslink susceptibility (% 1° sequence)
	XIII		Involved in angiogenesis	5.16	11.30
	XIV	Associates with collagen fibrils	Induces skin fibroblast quiescence and differentiation	8.26	8.82
	XVI	Associates with microfibrils	Component of hemidesmosomes and induces metalloproteinase expression. May be a fibrillin-1 microfibril component within the papillary dermis	5.81	9.48
	XXII		Component of the hair follicle basement membrane and interacts with cell surface integrins	4.63	10.69

Human skin collagens. Fibrillar and non-fibrillar collagens are major components of the ECM in skin. Collagens not only provide structural support to skin but are also involved in a wide-range of molecular interactions as shown. Primary sequence analyses of the collagens predict that they are protected against UV and ROS-induced damage but are susceptible to crosslinking

migration (collagen I) (Li et al. 2004), angiogenesis (collagen XVIII) (Zatterstrom et al. 2000) and metalloproteinase expression (collagen XVI) (Bedal et al. 2014) (Table 5.1). Equally important are the non-collagenous proteins, many present in low abundance, which also exhibit a wide range of molecular interactions from collagen fibrillogenesis (decorin and biglycan) (Bielefeld et al. 2011; Zhang et al. 2009), wound healing (fibronectin) (Bielefeld et al. 2011) to cytokine regulation (fibrillin), thus highlighting the dynamic nature of the ECM (Table 5.2). Whilst the dermis is enriched in structural ECM proteins (in particular fibrillar collagens and elastin), ECM proteins are also found in both the hypodermis and epidermis.

5.2.5 *Non-dermal Extracellular Matrix Proteins*

We have previously shown that two LTBP isoforms and the ECM cross-linking lysyl oxidase-like enzyme (LOXL-1) are expressed in the human epidermis (Langton et al. 2012). This enzyme is also expressed epidermally in the mouse and there is little evidence in the literature of expression in the dermis (Liu et al. 2004).

Table 5.2 Non-collagenous proteins in human skin

Major component		Structure	Functions and interactions	ROS/UVR susceptibility (% 1° sequence)	Crosslink susceptibility (% 1° sequence)
Elastin		Forms elastic fibres	Secreted as soluble precursor, tropoelastin. Provides elastic recoil and regulates cell signalling	2.50	5.92
Fibrillins		Forms microfibrils	Regulate TGFβ and bind elastin	24.81	8.00
LTBPs		Large latent complex	Regulates TGFβ bioavailability. Binds fibrillin-rich microfibrils and influences cell function	19.39	8.66
Fibronectin		Supermolecular fibres	Binds to integrins and is essential for wound healing. Regulates fibrillin assembly	13.08	8.45
Fibulins		Associates with microfibrils	Cell-signalling and important in elastogenesis. Crosslinks tropoelastin to LOX	21.06	7.66
PGs	Perlecan	Heparan sulphate proteoglycan	Basement membrane associated PG involved in angiogenesis. Bridges laminin and collagen IV networks	13.78	7.46
	Aggrecan	Large chondroitin sulphate proteoglycan	Interacts with fibulin-1 and is involved in the dermal wound healing response	7.09	4.42
	Versican	Large chondroitin sulphate proteoglycan	Involved in hair follicle formation and cell migration, adhesion, proliferation and signalling	8.47	7.38

(continued)

Table 5.2 (continued)

Major component		Structure	Functions and interactions	ROS/UVR susceptibility (% 1° sequence)	Crosslink susceptibility (% 1° sequence)
SLRPs	Decorin	Chondroitin/dermatan sulphate proteoglycan	Collagen fibrillogenesis, protection from proteolysis. Inter-molecular bridges. Negatively regulates TGFβ signalling and modulates cell adhesion	9.04	11.37
	Biglycan	Chondroitin/dermatan sulphate proteoglycan	Cell signalling molecule which interacts with TGFβ and BMP. Involved in collagen fibrillogenesis	11.75	11.46
Lysyl oxidase family of proteins		Copper and quinone dependent enzymes	Involved in the covalent crosslinking of collagen and elastin in the ECM. May regulate gene transcription	17.62	9.95
MAGP1 (Microfibrillar-associated prot. 2)		Associated with fibrillin microfibrils	Associates with fibrillin-rich microfibrils and modifies their function. Binds active TGFβ and is involved in thermoregulation	18.67	8.43
Tenascin C			Anti-adhesion molecule. Expressed in tissue injury and stimulates fibronectin mediated cell-migration	13.54	9.13
Tenascin X			Cell-matrix interactions and modulates collagen fibrillogenesis and elastin fibre assembly	11.57	9.53

Many of the non-collagenous molecules are present in low abundance but are important in maintaining tissue integrity in skin. They, like the collagenous molecules, are implicated in many biological processes that highlight the dynamic nature of the ECM. Primary sequence analyses of these molecules predict them to be more susceptible to UV and ROS-induced damage compared with collagens

The role played by these proteins in the epidermis is unclear: although LTBPs commonly associate with fibrillin microfibrils and LOX enzymes contribute to elastic fibre assembly the epidermis itself is devoid of mature elastic fibres. The location of these proteins in basal keratinocytes suggests that epidermal cells may synthesise key proteins in the papillary dermis. The final layer of the skin, the hypodermis, is comprised primarily of white adipose tissue containing pre-adipocytes, adipocytes, macrophages and fibroblasts. The ECM content of this layer is sparse and the UVR exposure is likely to be low (Askew 2002). However, it is now becoming clear that the hypodermis is susceptible to longer wavelength UVR, becoming thinner in photoexposed regions of the body and that adipose tissue may regulate collagen and elastic fibre abundance in the dermis via the expression of matrix metalloproteinase-9 (MMP9) (Fenske and Lober 1986; Sherratt 2015).

5.3 Skin Remodelling by Environmental Factors

There are two broadly accepted categories of skin ageing: intrinsic and extrinsic. Intrinsic ageing refers to the naturally occurring degenerative process that causes fine wrinkling and a gradual loss of elasticity and dermal matrix proteins with the passage of time (El-Domyati et al. 2002). These degenerative processes may be due to systemic ageing mechanisms such as telomere shortening, cellular senescence and oxidative stress and aberrant glycation which are thought to affect multiple organ systems (Holliday 2006). In contrast, the second category of skin ageing, extrinsic ageing, is characterised by the formation of coarse wrinkles, mottled pigmentation and a marked loss of elasticity and resilience (El-Domyati et al. 2002; Yaar and Gilchrest 2007). These outward manifestations are accompanied by profound and localised remodelling of the dermal matrix [for a comprehensive review see (Naylor et al. 2011)]. In the latter part of this section we discuss the potential role played by smoking and environmental pollution in mediating extrinsic ageing, but first we concentrate on the major causative factor: UVR. The term photo aged is often used to describe chronically UV-exposed skin but this usage implies that UVR-exposure promotes remodelling via the same processes which induce intrinsic ageing. However, given the marked compositional, architectural and functional differences between intrinsically aged and "photo aged" skin, it seems more appropriate to refer to the process of photo damage rather than photo ageing.

5.3.1 Ultraviolet Radiation Exposure and Skin Photo-Damage

The key molecular targets and potential mediators of UVR-induced dermal remodelling are depicted in Fig. 5.1. In severely photoaged skin there is both a widespread loss of fibrillar collagens (I and III) throughout the dermis and a

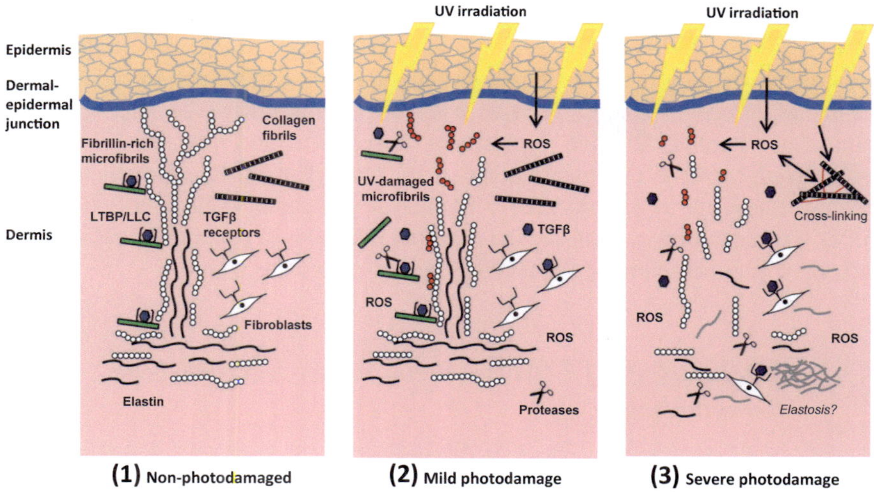

Fig. 5.1 Molecular mechanisms and consequences of chronic UVR-exposure. *1* Ordered fibrillin—rich microfibrils, originating in the reticular dermis, form candelabra-like structures at the dermal-epidermal junction. As well as providing a template for elastin deposition, fibrillin—rich microfibrils regulate TGF β bioavailability within the ECM by binding the LTBP/LLC complex. *2* In early photodamage the fibrillin-rich microfibrils are diminished from the upper dermis. The generation of ROS by cells in the epidermis in response to UV may activate dermal proteases to target microfibrils and disrupt LTBP/LLC binding resulting in aberrant TGF-β/fibroblast signalling. In addition, chromophoric amino acids within the primary sequence of the LTBP/LLC may render the assembly susceptible to damage by UV. Further, the complex may be displaced by proteolytic fibrillin fragments competing for binding sites along the length of remaining intact microfibrils. *3* Crosslinking of collagen fibrils, driven by ROS, occurs in extensive photodamage. The crosslinking of collagen may also drive ROS formation resulting in increased protease activity and degradation of fibrillin-rich microfibrils. It has yet to be elucidated if TGF β/fibroblast signalling results in the *de novo* deposition of elastin (elastosis) or the aggregation of resident mature dermal elastic fibres in photodamage

localised loss of collagen VII anchoring fibrils at the DEJ (El-Domyati et al. 2002; Talwar et al. 1995). In contrast, in the same tissue, dermal GAG content (in particular HA and chondroitin sulphate containing GAGs) is increased and co-localised with the elastic fibre network (Bernstein et al. 1996). It has become clear that this complex elastic fibre network is particularly sensitive to UVR-exposure [for a comprehensive review see (Naylor et al. 2011)]. For example, mildly photo-damaged skin is characterised by the loss of both the fibrillin microfibril candelabra-like structures (oxytalan fibres) and fibulin-5 in the papillary dermis whilst chronic UVR exposure induces profound dermis-wide changes in elastic fibre architecture (Kadoya et al. 2005; Watson et al. 1999). In such severely photo-damaged skin, the ordered arrangements of elastic and elaunin fibres in the reticular dermis (which differ in their proportion of elastin and fibrillin) and of fibrillin-microfibril containing oxytalan fibres in the papillary dermis is replaced by a disordered mass of elastin and fibrillin-rich "elastotic" material. This remodelling of the dermal ECM occurs in parallel with epidermal thickening and a flattening of the rete ridges which normally characterise the DEJ in many sun-protected sites (El-Domyati et al. 2002). However, the extent to which changes in dermal composition and architecture drive outward changes in skin appearance (specifically the formation of deep wrinkles) remains unknown. Furthermore, the relative contributions of potential causative mechanisms of dermal remodelling remain (such as UV-activation of the elastin promoter or by protease-mediated disruption of the existing elastic fibres network) are still under investigation (Sellheyer 2003; Uitto 2008). The next section discusses the potential roles played by cellular and acellular pathways in remodelling of the chronically sun-exposed dermis.

5.3.2 Mechanisms of Ultraviolet Radiation Induced Skin Remodelling

It is now well established that UV-exposure induces the expression of multiple proteases including many ECM-degrading matrix metalloproteinases (MMPs), but it is also evident that the substrate specificity of these enzymes is low [for a comprehensive review see (Watson et al. 2014)]. MMPs-1 and -9 for example, whose expression is upregulated in UVR exposed skin, can, collectively, degrade collagens I, III, IV and VII, elastin and the ubiquitous adhesive glycoprotein fibronectin (Chakraborti et al. 2003; Fisher et al. 1996). As a consequence, if these enzymes were the main mediators of photo damage then the early stages of UVR-exposure would be characterised by disruption of the DEJ (collagen IV and VII), the dermal fibrillar collagen matrix (collagens I and III), the elastic fibre system (elastin) and cell-matrix adhesion (fibronectin). However, as we have discussed in the previous section, it is components of the elastic fibre system, and in particular fibrillin microfibril bundles which appear to act as sensitive biomarkers of both mild and severe photo damage. We therefore proposed in 2010 that the amino acid composition of fibrillin-microfibrils (which are rich in UV-absorbing disulphide bonded Cys residues) would render them particularly susceptible to damage from direct UVR exposure and in 2014, that photoageing/photodamage may be due to both cellular and acellular pathways (the selective multi-hit model) (Sherratt et al. 2010; Watson et al. 2014).

We were not the first group to recognise the potential for UVR to damage extracellular dermal proteins either directly or via the production of reactive oxygen species (ROS), a process known as photosensitization (Pattison et al. 2011). Compelling evidence for the role of photosensitization in photoageing was provided by Sander and colleagues who characterised the UVR-dose dependent accumulation of oxidation-induced protein carbonyls in the acutely exposed human papillary dermis (Sander et al. 2002). Crucially however, the main protein targets of this oxidative damage were not identified. It has been generally assumed that the major structural proteins (fibrillar collagens and elastin) will be targets of UVR and ROS and there are numerous in vitro studies which report the UV-mediated degradation of collagen [i.e. (Jariashvili et al. 2012)]. In our 2014 review we related the UVR doses used in these in vitro studies to the minimal erythemal dose (MED) which will cause reddening of the skin (Watson et al. 2014). It was clear from this analysis that fibrillar collagen are readily degraded by non-physiological UV wavelengths (UVC) and doses (2–4 orders of magnitude greater than the MED). In contrast, we have shown that physiologically relevant UV sources and doses (up to an MED of UVA and UVB containing solar simulated radiation: SSR) have minimal effect on the structure and/or electrophoretic mobility of proteins (collagens I and VI, tropoelastin and α-lens crystallin) which are largely devoid of the UVA chromophoric amino acid residues (Cys, Trp and Tyr). In the same study, however, we also demonstrated that: (i) UVA chromophore-rich proteins (fibrillin-1 microfibrils, fibronectin β- and γ-lens crystallins) are susceptible to the same low SSR doses and that (ii) UV-exposed tissues are enriched in Cys, Tyr and Trp-containing proteins (Hibbert et al. 2015). This latter observation lead us to propose that UV-chromophore-rich proteins may act as endogenous sunscreens, protecting deeper components from UV-exposure.

5.3.3 Infrared Radiation and Tobacco Smoke

Although it is the most intensively studied, UVR is not the only environmental factor which is thought to promote skin ageing. In common with UVR, chronic exposure to infrared radiation (IR: ranging in wavelength from 760 nm to 1 mm) may also be associated with dermal elastosis and additionally with epidermal remodelling [for a comprehensive overview the reader is referred to two excellent reviews (Akhalaya et al. 2014; Schieke et al. 2003)]. The mechanisms which induce these changes in IR exposed skin remain to be fully characterised but exposure to IR can upregulate MMP-1 expression in cultured dermal fibroblasts, dysregulate TGFβ signalling and may promote oxidative stress (Akhalaya et al. 2014; Grether-Beck et al. 2014; Karu 1999; Schieke et al. 2002). In addition to radiation (UV and IR), the structure and function of human skin may be affected by the exogenous chemicals found in tobacco smoke.

The phenomenon of the deeply wrinkled “smoker’s face” is often reported but not universally accepted and may be influenced by the ethnicity of the subjects (Daniell 1971; O’Hare et al. 1999). The histological consequences of smoking in skin are also contentious. In UVR-exposed facial skin, smoking is associated with enhanced solar elastosis (Boyd et al. 1999). In order to separate the effects of UVR-exposure from the systemic effects of smoking, Allen and co-workers (in a predominantly non-Caucasian population) and more recently Knuutinen and colleagues examined the histological distribution of elastic fibres in upper-inner arm skin but were unable to identify any smoking-related differences (Allen et al. 1973; Knuutinen et al. 2002). In contrast, immuno-histochemical studies have identified non-elastosis-like deposition of elastin and increased elastic fibre deposition in the upper inner arm and foreskin respectively of smokers (Frances et al. 1991; Just et al. 2005; Rosado et al. 2012). The apparent absence of fibrillar collagen remodelling in the skin of smokers suggests that, in common with photo ageing/photo damage, the elastic fibre system, once again is particularly susceptible to environmental factors. What is also becoming clear is a link between the particulate matter associated with air pollution and premature skin ageing (Krutmann et al. 2013).

5.3.4 Identifying Biomarkers of Ageing

It is clear that not all skin components are equally susceptible to the effects of environmental factors such as UVR, IR and tobacco smoke. We have published evidence for the differential degradation of key ECM proteins by environmentally attainable UV exposures and the ability of bioinformatics approaches (applied to the entire human proteome) to identify potential targets (Hibbert et al. 2015; Sherratt et al. 2010; Watson et al. 2014). However, the composition of skin is complex and proteins are not the only molecules that can act as UV chromophores. Young and more recently Wondrak and colleagues have published excellent reviews which discuss the chromophoric (and in some cases photosensitization) abilities of DNA, porphyrins and flavins, vitamin K and B6 derivatives, bilirubin, NAD(P)H, urocanic acid and advanced glycation end products (AGEs) (Wondrak et al. 2006; Young 1997). The role of these latter age-associated post-translational modifications in mediating the targeted degradation of proteins is intriguing. Not all proteins are equally prone to non-enzymatic cross-linking with glucose and the number of free Lys residues may play an important role in determining susceptibility (Bailey 2001). Once formed, AGEs on elastin and collagen can act as photosensitizers driving H_2O_2 production and inhibiting fibroblast proliferation (Wondrak et al. 2003). The complexity of skin and the interactions with UVR suggest that multiple agents may be required to protect against photo-oxidative stress and to promote protective cellular responses (Wondrak 2007).

5.4 Preventing and Repairing Environmental Damage

As local exposure to UVR is associated with profound changes in skin appearance and function, most cutaneous anti-ageing strategies employ topical formulations containing putative active ingredients which are intended to perform preventative and/or reparative roles. These ingredients may block UVR, act as antioxidants, modify protease activity or promote the deposition of new ECM components. In this section we discuss the efficacy of these ingredients and also consider the potential role of physical methods and systemic treatments in preventing and repairing environmental damage to skin. We have not however addressed the potential role of botanical extracts in treating skin ageing as the efficacy and mode of action of such complex mixtures is difficult to determine.

5.4.1 Topical Agents

5.4.1.1 Sunscreens

The topical application of sunscreens is the first-line of defence against UVR-induced photo damage (Yaar and Gilchrest 2007). Organic sunscreens absorb photons and convert the energy to heat or light. In contrast, inorganic applications often contain oxide minerals, such as TiO_2 or ZnO, which scatter and reflect UVR. However, the photo degradation of organic compounds and the use of minerals in products can result in the formation of ROS and may also be linked to skin cancer (Shibata et al. 2007; Tran and Salmon 2011). For this reason antioxidants, such as tocopherol (vitamin E) acetate and polyphenolic molecules, are commonly added to formulations to counteract the effects of ROS. The use of more photo stable compounds in sunscreens not only helps to prevent the generation of ROS but also improves the efficacy of the products (Marrot et al. 2004). However, some of these ingredients have also been found to be associated with contact dermatitis in predisposed individuals (Manova et al. 2014). Modern day UV filter sunscreens commonly combine both organic and inorganic ingredients to improve photo protection but there are issues surrounding the environmental impact of these compounds (Ma et al. 2014; Tovar-Sanchez et al. 2013).

5.4.1.2 Regulated Anti-ageing Treatments

Topical retinoids, such as tretinoin and isotretinoin, are vitamin A derivatives used to improve the clinical appearance of photoaged skin. Retinoids bind nuclear retinoic acid and retinoid X receptors (RARs, RXRs) to augment gene activity, although their precise cellular and molecular mechanism of action remains unclear (Xiao et al. 1995). A number of early studies to test the efficacy and safety of retinoids reported improvement in photoaged features such as coarse wrinkling, sallowness and actinic lentigines (Kligman et al. 1986; Leyden et al. 1989). These improvements are marked by changes to the cutaneous microenvironment including all-trans retinoic acid (*t*-RA) induced increase in the abundance of collagens I and III and the deposition of both fibrillin microfibrils and collagen VII anchoring fibrils at the DEJ (Griffiths et al. 1993; Watson et al. 2001; Woodley et al. 1990). In the UK all-trans retinoic acid is classified as a prescription only drug and is prohibited as a cosmetic ingredient in all major markets. As a consequence there is a need for non-prescription (also known as over-the-counter [OTC]) reparative treatments.

5.4.1.3 Over-the-Counter Anti-ageing Formulations

This section briefly summarises the use of over the counter (OTC) formulations in repairing age and sun-exposure induced skin damage. The reader is referred to Bradley et al. (2015) for a comprehensive review (Bradley et al. 2015). Although many OTC formulations incorporate retinyl esters, as they require bio-conversion to their active form, their efficacy may be limited. For example, retinyl propionate alone was ineffective at reducing wrinkles after nearly 12 months continuous use in a double blinded placebo randomised controlled trial on 80 subjects (Green et al. 1998). Most anti-ageing preparations, therefore, use active ingredient blends/complexes. Those containing retinyl palmitate, for example, have been shown to induce clinical and histological improvements when combined with other anti-ageing ingredients (e.g. peptides and Vitamin C) (Watson et al. 2008, 2009). Other retinoid derivatives such as D-d-tocopheryl retinoate may also increase collagen I and HA synthesis, but their efficacy has only been demonstrated in small populations (Okano et al. 2006). In addition to vitamin A derived retinoids, OTC formulations may contain other vitamins and their derivatives. For example, L-ascorbic acid acts as both an antioxidant and a promoter of collagen and elastic fibre synthesis and the expression of ECM protease inhibitors (Geesin et al. 1986, 1988; Maia Campos et al. 2008; Murad et al. 1981; Nusgens et al. 2001; Raschke et al. 2004). Vitamin E has been shown to upregulate the expression of both enzymatic and non-enzymatic antioxidants in a murine model of photoageing but its efficacy in humans and reparative capacity remains unknown (Lopez-Torres et al. 1998).

Osmolytes are organic molecules that are not only important in maintaining cell isotonicity but can also protect against ROS. A study by Warskulat et al. (2004), found that keratinocytes increased osmolyte (Taurine, Betaine and Myoinositol) uptake in response to UV-B exposure and proposed that this mechanism formed part of the cellular defence against oxidative stress (Warskulat et al. 2004). Taurine, which is present in the skin, has also been shown to protect keratinocytes against UV-induced apoptosis (Janeke et al. 2003). Ectoin is a bacteria synthesised osmolyte that also exhibits photo protective properties in human skin (Buenger and Driller 2004). The findings of these studies and others have increased the use of osmolytes in photoprotective personal care products. Co-enzyme Q10 is another antioxidant which is often found in anti-ageing formulations. There is evidence that prolonged use of co-enzyme Q10-containing cream can reduce skin wrinkling, epidermal oxidation, cellular ROS and MMP-1 expression and increase human dermal fibroblast proliferation and synthesis of basement membrane ECM components (Hoppe et al. 1999; Muta-Takada et al. 2009).

5.4.1.4 Peptides and Matrikines

Many OTC formulations contain small peptides that are thought to induce ECM deposition. It has been reasoned that naturally occurring processed ECM fragments termed matrikines can act as signalling molecules that stimulate matrix deposition (Maquart et al. 1993). Published experimental evidence for the efficacy of matrikines in repairing photodamaged skin is minimal but this may reflect the commercial sensitivities which influence research into topical anti-ageing agents. One exception is the procollagen derived pentameric peptide lys-thr-thr-lys-ser (KTTKS) which stimulates expression of fibrillar collagens in vitro and is associated with improvements in facial wrinkles (albeit in association with palmitoyl (Katayama et al. 1993; Robinson et al. 2005). A combination of peptides (pal-GQPR and collagen II derived pal-GHK) can promote wound healing when administered with copper and pal-GHK alone can stimulate collagen deposition in vitro and affect collagen architecture in UVA irradiated ex vivo skin (Lintner and Peschard 2000; Maquart et al. 1993, 1988). However, the dermal matrix is not composed of fibrillar collagens alone. The amino acid sequence GEKG (Gly-Glu-Lys-Gly) is present in several ECM proteins and hence has been indented as a matrikine which may induce not only collagen I expression but also the synthesis of other ECM components including HA and fibronectin (Farwick et al. 2011).

5.4.1.5 Formulations and the Importance of Synergistic Effects

In practice, the putative active ingredients discussed above are not commonly applied in isolation but as part of a formulation in which discrete components may act synergistically to enhance biological activity. These synergistic effects have been most intensively studied in the case of vitamins. Vitamins C and,E for example, when applied topically to UV irradiated skin, reduce both erythema and DNA damage (thymidine dimer formation) (Lin et al. 2003). These synergistic effects may manifest clinically, as a reduction in wrinkles and histologically by promoting repair of the elastic fibre system following application of madecassoside and ascorbic acid combination (Haftek et al. 2008). The reader is referred to our recent 2015 review for a more comprehensive discussion (Bradley et al. 2015). As effective as topical agents have proven to be, there are alternative approaches which also show promise.

5.4.2 Systemic Treatments, Physical Methods and Devices

For a comprehensive review of the many treatments available the reader is referred to Ganceviciene et al. (2012). Briefly, oral supplements are popular as, if effective, they have the potential to improve not only skin appearance but also functionality of the whole body. However, despite many commercially available products, the clinical evidence supporting their effectiveness is generally lacking or very weak, especially when they are targeted at, for the most part, a healthy population. Vitamins C and E together with carotenoids are the most extensively studied antioxidant supplements. Ingestion of tomato paste and olive oil for 10 weeks was shown to reduce UV induced erythema and fibrillin-1 microfibril breakdown but the photoprotective effects of such antioxidants would be small compared to the effects of topical sunscreens. For an improvement in photoaged appearance, clinical evidence from placebo controlled double blinded trials has been generated in post-menopausal subjects. A 6 month double blind placebo controlled trial performed on 80 subjects with an oral supplement that included soy extract, fish protein polysaccharides, vitamins C and E (Imedeen Prime Renewal^{TM}) showed improvements in several clinical grading parameters from 3 months (Skovgaard et al. 2006). However, the magnitude of these benefits, whilst statistically significant, was small.

In the clinic, a wide range of non-surgical (e.g. Botox, dermal fillers, chemical peels) and surgical interventions (e.g. liposuction) are available. Botulinum toxin A (Botox) reduces dynamic wrinkle appearance by promoting muscle relaxation. To compensate for loss of facial volume in age, injectable fillers based on collagen or hyaluronic acid are most often used. For hyperpigmentation such as facial solar lentigines, chemical peels which vary in their strength and therefore depth of effect (e.g. glycolic acid up to 70 % as a superficial peel; CO_2 laser for deep peel) are more likely used. Dermabrasion is an alternative approach to renew the skin surface but with an added benefit of increasing collagen production in the generated repair zone. Lasers can also be used for treatment of pigment and vascular irregularities. In conclusion whilst these treatments show promise, in many cases their efficacy and mechanism of action, remains to be determined.

5.5 Conclusions and Future Directions

Although ECM proteins play important and well-recognised roles in mediating the mechanical and biochemical functions of the dermis, it is becoming increasingly clear that these functions are not confined solely to the "major" components such as collagen I and elastin. Some of these less abundant "minor" components (which perform cell-signalling roles and help to organise the matrix) may also be highly susceptible to degradation by UVR and ROS as might proteins which undergo post-translational modification with advanced glycation end products. We have proposed that this susceptibility may in some cases be beneficial allowing the proteins to act as endogenous sunscreens and antioxidants. However UVR is not the only potential mediator of environmental damage and increasingly there is interest in the effects of IR and factors such as tobacco smoke. The damage caused by these factors may be prevented and or repaired by the application of topical agents. The action of many of these agents remains poorly defined and is a key area of research.

Acknowledgments This work was supported by a programme Grant from Walgreens Boots Alliance, Nottingham, UK. The authors would like to thank Mr. Matiss Ozols for his contributions to the calculating UVR/ROS and cross-link susceptibility as reported in Tables 5.1 and 5.2.

References

Abreu-Velez AM, Howard MS (2012) Collagen IV in normal skin and in pathological processes. North Am J Med Sci 4:1–8

Agache PG, Monneur C, Leveque JL, Derigal J (1980) Mechanical-properties and youngs modulus of human-skin in vivo. Arch Dermatol Res 269:221–232

Akhalaya MY, Maksimov GV, Rubin AB, Lademann J, Darvin ME (2014) Molecular action mechanisms of solar infrared radiation and heat on human skin. Ageing Res Rev 16:1–11

Allen HB, Johnson BL, Diamond SM (1973) Smokers wrinkles. Jama J Am Med Assoc 225:1067–1069

Askew EW (2002) Work at high altitude and oxidative stress: antioxidant nutrients. Toxicology 180:107–119

Bailey AJ (2001) Molecular mechanisms of ageing in connective tissues. Mech Ageing Dev 122:735–755

Baldwin AK, Simpson A, Steer R, Cain SA, Kielty CM (2013) Elastic fibres in health and disease. Expert Rev Mol Med 15:30

Baranoski S (2000) Skin tears: the enemy of frail skin. Adv Skin Wound Care 13:123–126

Bax DV, Bernard SE, Lomas A, Morgan A, Humphries J, Shuttleworth CA, Humphries MJ, Kielty CM (2003) Cell adhesion to fibrillin-1 molecules and microfibrils is mediated by alpha (5)beta(1) and alpha(v)beta(3) integrins. J Biol Chem 278:34605–34616

Bax DV, Rodgers UR, Bilek MMM, Weiss AS (2009) Cell adhesion to tropoelastin is mediated via the C-terminal GRKRK motif and integrin alpha(V)beta(3). J Biol Chem 284:28616–28623

Bedal KB, Grassel S, Oefner PJ, Reinders J, Reichert TE, Bauer R (2014) Collagen XVI induces expression of MMP9 via modulation of AP-1 transcription factors and facilitates invasion of oral squamous cell carcinoma. Plos One 9

Bernstein EF, Underhill CB, Hahn PJ, Brown DB, Uitto J (1996) Chronic sun exposure alters both the content and distribution of dermal glycosaminoglycans. Br J Dermatol 135:255–262

Bielefeld KA, Amini-Nik S, Whetstone H, Poon R, Youn A, Wang J, Alman BA (2011) Fibronectin and beta-catenin act in a regulatory loop in dermal fibroblasts to modulate cutaneous healing. J Biol Chem 286:27687–27697

Birk DE, Bruckner P (2005) Collagen suprastructures. In: Collagen, vol 247. Springer, Berlin, pp 185–205

Boyd AS, Stasko T, King LE, Cameron GS, Pearse AD, Gaskell SA (1999) Cigarette smoking-associated elastotic changes in the skin. J Am Acad Dermatol 41:23–26

Bradley EJ, Griffiths CEM, Sherratt MJ, Bell M, Watson REB (2015) Over-the-counter anti-ageing topical agents and their ability to protect and repair photoaged skin. Maturitas 80:265–272

Brinckmann J, Hunzelmann N, Kahle B, Rohwedel J, Kramer J, Gibson MA, Hubmacher D, Reinhardt DP (2010) Enhanced fibrillin-2 expression is a general feature of wound healing and sclerosis: potential alteration of cell attachment and storage of TGF-beta. Lab Invest 90:739–752

Buenger J, Driller H (2004) Ectoin: an effective natural substance to prevent UVA-induced premature photoaging. Skin Pharmacol Physiol 17:232–237

Chakraborti S, Mandal M, Das S, Mandal A, Chakraborti T (2003) Regulation of matrix metalloproteinases: an overview. Mol Cell Biochem 253:269–285

Chanut-Delalande H, Bonod-Bidaud C, Cogne S, Malbouyres M, Ramirez F, Fichard A, Ruggiero F (2004) Development of a functional skin matrix requires deposition of collagen V heterotrimers. Mol Cell Biol 24:6049–6057

Clarke AW, Wise SG, Cain SA, Kielty CM, Weiss AS (2005) Coacervation is promoted by molecular interactions between the PF2 segment of fibrillin-1 and the domain 4 region of tropoelastin. Biochemistry 44:10271–10281

Craven NM, Watson REB, Jones CJP, Shuttleworth CA, Kielty CM, Griffiths CEM (1997) Clinical features of photodamaged human skin are associated with a reduction in collagen VII. Br J Dermatol 137:344–350

Daniell HW (1971) Smokers wrinkles—study in epidemiology of crows feet. Ann Intern Med 75:873–880
Danielson KG, Baribault H, Holmes DF, Graham H, Kadler KE, Iozzo RV (1997) Targeted disruption of decorin leads to abnormal collagen fibril morphology and skin fragility. J Cell Biol 136:729–743
El-Domyati M, Attia S, Saleh F, Brown D, Birk DE, Gasparro F, Ahmad H, Uitto J (2002) Intrinsic aging vs. photoaging: a comparative histopathological, immunohistochemical, and ultrastructural study of skin. Exp Dermatol 11:398–405
Fang M, Liroff KG, Turner AS, Les CM, Orr BG, Holl MMB (2012) Estrogen depletion results in nanoscale morphology changes in dermal collagen. J Invest Dermatol 132:1791–1797
Farwick M, Grether-Beck S, Marini A, Maczkiewitz U, Lange J, Koehler T, Lersch P, Falla T, Felsner I, Brenden H et al (2011) Bioactive tetrapeptide GEKG boosts extracellular matrix formation: in vitro and in vivo molecular and clinical proof. Exp Dermatol 20:602–604
Fenske NA, Lober CW (1986) Structural and functional changes of normal aging skin. J Am Acad Dermatol 15:571–585
Fisher GJ, Datta SC, Talwar HS, Wang Z-Q, Varani J, Kang S, Voorhees JJ (1996) Molecular basis of sun-induced premature skin ageing and retinoid antagonism. Nature 379:335–339
Frances C, Boisnic S, Hartmann DJ, Dautzenberg B, Branchet MC, Lecharpentier Y, Robert L (1991) Changes in the elastic tissue of the non-sun-exposed skin of cigarette smokers. Br J Dermatol 125:43–47
Ganceviciene R, Liakou AI, Theodoridis A, Makrantonaki E, Zouboulis CC (2012) Skin anti-aging strategies. Dermato-endocrinology 4:308–319
Geesin J, Murad S, Pinnell SR (1986) Ascorbic-acid stimulates collagen production without altering intracellular degradation in cultured human-skin fibroblasts. Biochim Biophys Acta 886:272–274
Geesin JC, Darr D, Kaufman R, Murad S, Pinnell SR (1988) Ascorbic-acid specifically increases type-I and type III procollagen messenger-RNA levels in human-skin fibroblasts. J Invest Dermatol 90:420–424
Gigante A, Chillemi C, Greco F (1999) Changes of elastic fibers in musculoskeletal tissues of Marfan syndrome: a possible mechanism of joint laxity and skeletal overgrowth. J Pediatr Orthop 19:283–288
Grassel S, Bauer RJ (2013) Collagen XVI in health and disease. Matrix Biol 32:64–73
Green C, Orchard G, Cerio R, Hawk JLM (1998) A clinicopathological study of the effects of topical retinyl propionate cream in skin photoageing. Clin Exp Dermatol 23:162–167
Grether-Beck S, Marini A, Jaenicke T, Krutmann J (2014) Photoprotection of human skin beyond ultraviolet radiation. Photodermatol Photoimmunol Photomed 30:167–174
Griffiths CEM, Russman AN, Majmudar G, Singer RS, Hamilton TA, Voorhees JJ (1993) Restoration of collagen formation in photodamaged human skin by tretinoin (retinoic acid). N Engl J Med 329:530–535
Habashi JP, Judge DP, Holm TM, Cohn RD, Loeys BL, Cooper TK, Myers L, Klein EC, Liu GS, Calvi C et al (2006) Losartan, an AT1 antagonist, prevents aortic aneurysm in a mouse model of Marfan syndrome. Science 312:117–121
Haftek M, Mac-Mary S, Le Bitoux M-A, Creidi P, Seite S, Rougier A, Humbert P (2008) Clinical, biometric and structural evaluation of the long-term effects of a topical treatment with ascorbic acid and madecassoside in photoaged human skin. Exp Dermatol 17:946–952
Haynes SL, Shuttleworth CA, Kielty CM (1997) Keratinocytes express fibrillin and assemble microfibrils: implications for dermal matrix organization. Br J Dermatol 137:17–23
Hibbert SA, Watson RE, Gibbs NK, Costello P, Baldock C, Weiss AS, Griffiths CE, Sherratt MJ (2015) A potential role for endogenous proteins as sacrificial sunscreens and antioxidants in human tissues. Redox Biol 5:101–113
Holliday R (2006) Aging is no longer an unsolved problem in biology. In: Rattan S, Kristensen P, Clark BFC (eds) Understanding and modulating aging, vol 1067, pp 1–9

Hoppe U, Bergemann J, Diembeck W, Ennen J, Gohla S, Harris I, Jacob J, Kielholz J, Mei W, Pollet D et al (1999) Coenzyme Q(10), a cutaneous antioxidant and energizer. Biofactors 9:371–378

Janeke G, Siefken W, Carstensen S, Springmann G, Bleck O, Steinhart H, Hoger P, Wittern KP, Wenck H, Stab F et al (2003) Role of taurine accumulation in keratinocyte hydration. J Invest Dermatol 121:354–361

Jariashvili K, Madhan B, Brodsky B, Kuchava A, Namicheishvili L, Metreveli N (2012) UV damage of collagen: insights from model collagen peptides. Biopolymers 97:189–198

Just M, Monso E, Ribera M, Lorenzo JC, Morera J, Ferrandiz C (2005) Relationships between lung function, smoking and morphology of dermal elastic fibres. Exp Dermatol 14:744–751

Kaartinen V, Warburton D (2003) Fibrillin controls TGF-beta activation. Nat Genet 33:331–332

Kadoya K, Sasaki T, Kostka G, Timpl R, Matsuzaki K, Kumagai N, Sakai LY, Nishiyama T, Amano S (2005) Fibulin-5 deposition in human skin: decrease with ageing and ultraviolet B exposure and increase in solar elastosis. Br J Dermatol 153:607–612

Karu T (1999) Primary and secondary mechanisms of action of visible to near-IR radiation on cells. J Photochem Photobiol B Biol 49:1–17

Katayama K, Armendarizborunda J, Raghow R, Kang AH, Seyer JM (1993) A pentapeptide from type-I procollagen promotes extracellular-matrix production. J Biol Chem 268:9941–9944

Kielty CM, Sherratt MJ, Shuttleworth CA (2002) Elastic fibres. J Cell Sci 115:2817–2828

Kinsey R, Williamson MR, Chaudhry S, Mellody KT, McGovern A, Takahashi S, Shuttleworth CA, Kielty CM (2008) Fibrillin-1 microfibril deposition is dependent on fibronectin assembly. J Cell Sci 121:2696–2704

Kirschner R, Hubmacher D, Iyengar G, Kaur J, Fagotto-Kaufmann C, Bromme D, Bartels R, Reinhardt DP (2011) Classical and neonatal marfan syndrome mutations in fibrillin-1 cause differential protease susceptibilities and protein function. J Biol Chem 286:32810–32823

Kligman AM, Grove GL, Hirose R, Leyden JJ (1986) Tpocial tretinoin for photoaged skin. J Am Acad Dermatol 15:836–859

Knuutinen A, Kallioinen M, Vahakangas K, Oikarinen A (2002) Smoking and skin: a study of the physical qualities and histology of skin in smokers and non-smokers. Acta Dermato-Venereol 82:36–40

Krutmann J (2003) Premature skin aging by ultraviolet radiation and other environmental hazards. The molecular basis. Hautarzt 54:809–817

Langton AK, Sherratt MJ, Griffiths CEM, Watson REB (2012) Differential expression of elastic fibre components in intrinsically aged skin. Biogerontology 13:37–48

Lee P, Bax DV, Bilek MMM, Weiss AS (2014) A novel cell adhesion region in tropoelastin mediates attachment to integrin alpha(V)beta(5). J Biol Chem 289:1467–1477

Leyden JJ, Grove GL, Grove MJ, Thorne EG, Lufrano L (1989) Treatment of photodamaged facial skin with topical tretinoin. J Am Acad Dermatol 21:638–644

Li W, Fan J, Chen M, Guan S, Sawcer D, Bokoch GM, Woodley DT (2004) Mechanism of human dermal fibroblast migration driven by type I collagen and platelet-derived growth factor-BB. Mol Biol Cell 15:294–309

Lin JY, Selim MA, Shea CR, Grichnik JM, Omar MM, Monteiro-Riviere NA, Pinnell SR (2003) UV photoprotection by combination topical antioxidants vitamin C and vitamin E. J Am Acad Dermatol 48:866–874

Lintner K, Peschard O (2000) Biologically active peptides: from a laboratory bench curiosity to a functional skin care product. Int J Cosmet Sci 22:207–218

Liu XQ, Zhao Y, Gao JG, Pawlyk B, Starcher B, Spencer JA, Yanagisawa H, Zuo J, Li TS (2004) Elastic fiber homeostasis requires lysyl oxidase-like 1 protein. Nat Genet 36:178–182

Loffek S, Hurskainen T, Jackow J, Sigloch FC, Schilling O, Tasanen K, Bruckner-Tuderman L, Franzke CW (2014) Transmembrane collagen XVII modulates integrin dependent keratinocyte migration via PI3K/Rac1 signaling. Plos One 9:11

Lopez-Torres M, Thiele JJ, Shindo Y, Han D, Packer L (1998) Topical application of alpha-tocopherol modulates the antioxidant network and diminishes ultraviolet-induced oxidative damage in murine skin. Br J Dermatol 138:207–215

Lucero HA, Kagan HM (2006) Lysyl oxidase: an oxidative enzyme and effector of cell function. Cell Mol Life Sci 63:2304–2316

Ma H, Wallis LK, Diamond S, Li S, Canas-Carrell J, Parra A (2014) Impact of solar UV radiation on toxicity of ZnO nanoparticles through photocatalytic reactive oxygen species (ROS) generation and photo-induced dissolution. Environ Pollut 193:165–172

Maia Campos PMBG, Goncalves GMS, Gaspar LR (2008) In vitro antioxidant activity and in vivo efficacy of topical formulations containing vitamin C and its derivatives studied by non-invasive methods. Skin Res Technol 14:376–380

Manova E, von Goetz N, Hungerbuhler K (2014) Ultraviolet filter contact and photocontact allergy: consumer exposure and risk assessment for octocrylene from personal care products and sunscreens. Br J Dermatol 171:1368–1374

Maquart FX, Monboisse JC (2014) Extracellular matrix and wound healing. Pathol Biol 62:91–95

Maquart FX, Pickart L, Laurent M, Gillery P, Monboisse JC, Borel JP (1988) Stimulation of collagen-synthesis in fibroblast-cultures by the tripeptide-copper complex glycyl-L-histidyl-L-lysine-L-lysine-Cu2+. Febs Lett 238:343–346

Maquart FX, Bellon G, Chaqour B, Wegrowski J, Patt LM, Trachy RE, Monboisse JC, Chastang F, Birembaut P, Gillery P et al (1993) In-vivo stimulation of connective-tissue accumulation by the tripeptide copper complex glycyl-L-histidyl-L-lysine-Cu2+ in rat experimental wounds. J Clin Invest 92:2368–2376

Marastoni S, Ligresti G, Lorenzon E, Colombatti A, Mongiat M (2008) Extracellular matrix: a matter of life and death. Connect Tissue Res 49:203–206

Marrot L, Belaidi JP, Lejeune F, Meunier JR, Asselineau D, Bernerd F (2004) Photostability of sunscreen products influences the efficiency of protection with regard to UV-induced genotoxic or photoageing-related endpoints. Br J Dermatol 151:1234–1244

Maruhashi T, Kii I, Saito M, Kudo A (2010) Interaction between periostin and BMP-1 promotes proteolytic activation of lysyl oxidase. J Biol Chem 285:13294–13303

Massam-Wu T, Chiu M, Choudhury R, Chaudhry SS, Baldwin AK, McGovern A, Baldock C, Shuttleworth CA, Kielty CM (2010) Assembly of fibrillin microfibrils governs extracellular deposition of latent TGF beta. J Cell Sci 123:3006–3018

Mellody KT, Freeman LJ, Baldock C, Jowitt TA, Siegler V, Raynal BDE, Cain SA, Wess TJ, Shuttleworth CA, Kielty CM (2006) Marfan syndrome-causing mutations in fibrillin-1 result in gross morphological alterations and highlight the structural importance of the second hybrid domain. J Biol Chem 281:31854–31862

Mienaltowski MJ, Birk DE (2014) Structure, physiology, and biochemistry of collagens. In: Halper J (ed) Progress in heritable soft connective tissue diseases, vol 802. Springer, Berlin, pp 5–29

Murad S, Grove D, Lindberg KA, Reynolds G, Sivarajah A, Pinnell SR (1981) Regulation of collagen synthesis by ascorbic acid. Proc Natl Acad Sci USA Biol Sci 78:2879–2882

Muta-Takada K, Terada T, Yamanishi H, Ashida Y, Inomata S, Nishiyama T, Amano S (2009) Coenzyme Q(10) protects against oxidative stress-induced cell death and enhances the synthesis of basement membrane components in dermal and epidermal cells. Biofactors 35:435–441

Naylor EC, Watson REB, Sherratt MJ (2011) Molecular aspects of skin ageing. Maturitas 69:249–256

Neptune ER, Frischmeyer PA, Arking DE, Myers L, Bunton TE, Gayraud B, Ramirez F, Sakai LY, Dietz HC (2003) Dysregulation of TGF-beta activation contributes to pathogenesis in Marfan syndrome. Nat Genet 33:407–411

Nusgens BV, Humbert P, Rougier A, Colige AC, Haftek M, Lambert CA, Richard A, Creidi P, Lapiere CM (2001) Topically applied vitamin C enhances the mRNA level of collagens I and III, their processing enzymes and tissue inhibitor of matrix metalloproteinase 1 in the human dermis. J Invest Dermatol 116:853–859

O'Hare PM, Fleischer AB, D'Agostino RB, Feldman SR, Hinds MA, Rassette SA, McMichael AJ, Williford PM (1999) Tobacco smoking contributes little to facial wrinkling. J Eur Acad Dermatol Venereol 12:133–139

Okano Y, Obayashi K, Yahagi S, Kurihara K, Kaburagi S, Kurata Y, Masaki H (2006) Improvement of wrinkles by an all-trans-retinoic acid derivative, D-delta-tocopheryl retinoate. J Dermatol Sci: S65–S74

Papakonstantinou E, Roth M, Karakiulakis G (2012) Hyaluronic acid: a key molecule in skin aging. Dermatoendocrinol 4:253–258

Pattison D, Rahmanto A, Davies M (2011) Photo-oxidation of proteins. Photochem Photobiol Sci 11:38–53

Ramirez F, Sakai LY (2010) Biogenesis and function of fibrillin assemblies. Cell Tissue Res 339:71–82

Ramshaw JAM, Shah NK, Brodsky B (1998) Gly-X-Y tripeptide frequencies in collagen: a context for host-guest triple-helical peptides. J Struct Biol 122:86–91

Raschke T, Koop U, Dusing HJ, Filbry A, Sauermann K, Jaspers S, Wenck H, Wittern KP (2004) Topical activity of ascorbic acid: from in vitro optimization to in vivo efficacy. Skin Pharmacol Physiol 17:200–206

Robinson LR, Fitzgerald NC, Doughty DG, Dawes NC, Berge CA, Bissett DL (2005) Topical palmitoyl pentapeptide provides improvement in photoaged human facial skin. Int J Cosmet Sci 27:155–160

Rosado JP, Favorito LA, Cavalcanti AGL, Costa WS, Cardoso LEM, Sampaio FJB (2012) Structural alterations of foreskin caused by chronic smoking may explain high levels of urethral reconstruction failure using foreskin flaps. Int Braz J Urol 38:529–535

Ruehland C, Schonherr E, Robenek H, Hansen U, Iozz RV, Bruckner P, Seidler DG (2007) The glycosaminoglycan chain of decorin plays an important role in collagen fibril formation at the early stages of fibrillogenesis. FEBS J 274:4246–4255

Sabatelli P, Gara SK, Grumati P, Urciuolo A, Gualandi F, Curci R, Squarzoni S, Zamparelli A, Martoni E, Merlini L et al (2011) Expression of the collagen VI alpha 5 and alpha 6 chains in normal human skin and in skin of patients with collagen VI-related myopathies. J Invest Dermatol 131:99–107

Sabatier L, Djokic J, Hubmacher D, Dzafik D, Nelea V, Reinhardt DP (2014) Heparin/heparan sulfate controls fibrillin-1, -2 and -3 self-interactions in microfibril assembly. Febs Lett 588:2890–2897

Sakai LY, Keene DR, Engvall E (1986) Fibrillin, a new 350-kD glycoprotein, is a component of extracellular microfibrils. J Cell Biol 103:2499–2509

Sander CS, Chang H, Salzmann S, Muller CSL, Ekanayake-Mudiyanselage S, Elsner P, Thiele JJ (2002) Photoaging is associated with protein oxidation in human skin in vivo. J Invest Dermatol 118:618–625

Schieke SM, Stege H, Kurten V, Grether-Beck S, Sies H, Krutmann J (2002) Infrared-A radiation-induced matrix metalloproteinase 1 expression is mediated through extracellular signal-regulated kinase 1/2 activation in human dermal fibroblasts. J Invest Dermatol 119:1323–1329

Schieke SM, Schroeder P, Krutmann J (2003) Cutaneous effects of infrared radiation: from clinical observations to molecular response mechanisms. Photodermatol Photoimmunol Photomed 19:228–234

Sellheyer K (2003) Pathogenesis of solar elastosis: synthesis or degradation? J Cutan Pathol 30:123–127

Sherratt MJ (2015) Body mass index and dermal remodelling. Exp Dermatol

Sherratt MJ, Bayley CP, Reilly SM, Gibbs NK, Griffiths CEM, Watson REB (2010) Low-dose ultraviolet radiation selectively degrades chromophore-rich extracellular matrix components. J Pathol 222:32–40

Shibata T, Sakai N, Fukuda K, Ebina Y, Sasaki T (2007) Photocatalytic properties of titania nanostructured films fabricated from titania nanosheets. Phys Chem Chem Phys 9:2413–2420

Skovgaard GRL, Jensen AS, Sigler ML (2006) Effect of a novel dietary supplement on skin aging in post-menopausal women. Eur J Clin Nutr 60:1201–1206

Stuart K, Paderi J, Snyder PW, Freeman L, Panitch A (2011) Collagen-binding peptidoglycans inhibit MMP mediated collagen degradation and reduce dermal scarring. Plos One 6:7

Talwar HS, Griffiths CEM, Fisher GJ, Hamilton TA, Voorhees JJ (1995) Reduced type-I and type-III procollagens in photodamaged adult human skin. J Invest Dermatol 105:285–290

Theocharidis G, Drymoussi Z, Kao AP, Barber AH, Lee DA, Braun KM, Connelly JT (2015) Type VI collagen regulates dermal matrix assembly and fibroblast motility. J Invest Dermatol

Tiecke F, Katzke S, Booms P, Robinson PN, Neumann L, Godfrey M, Mathews KR, Scheuner M, Hinkel GK, Brenner RE et al (2001) Classic, atypically severe and neonatal Marfan syndrome: twelve mutations and genotype-phenotype correlations in FBN1 exons 24-40. Eur J Hum Genet 9:13–21

Tovar-Sanchez A, Sanchez-Quiles D, Basterretxea G, Benede JL, Chisvert A, Salvador A, Moreno-Garrido I, Blasco J (2013) Sunscreen products as emerging pollutants to coastal waters. Plos One 8:8

Tran DT, Salmon R (2011) Potential photocarcinogenic effects of nanoparticle sunscreens. Australas J Dermatol 52:1–6

Uitto J (2008) The role of elastin and collagen in cutaneous aging: intrinsic aging versus photoexposure. J Drugs Dermatol JDD 7:s12–s16

Wang F, Garza LA, Kang S, Varani J, Orringer JS, Fisher GJ, Voorhees JJ (2007) In vivo stimulation of de novo collagen production caused by cross-linked hyaluronic acid dermal filler injections in photodamaged human skin. Arch Dermatol 143:155–163

Warren R, Gartstein V, Kligman AM, Montagna W, Allendorf RA, Ridder GM (1991) Age, sunlight, and facial skin: a histologic and quantitative study. J Am Acad Dermatol 25:751–760

Warskulat U, Reinen A, Grether-Beck S, Krutmann J, Haussinger D (2004) The osmolyte strategy of normal human keratinocytes in maintaining cell homeostasis. J Invest Dermatol 123:516–521

Watson REB, Griffiths CEM, Craven NM, Shuttleworth CA, Kielty CM (1999) Fibrillin-rich microfibrils are reduced in photoaged skin. Distribution at the dermal-epidermal junction. J Invest Dermatol 112:782–787

Watson REB, Craven NM, Kang SW, Jones CJP, Kielty CM, Griffiths CEM (2001) A short-term screening protocol, using fibrillin-1 as a reporter molecule, for photoaging repair agents. J Invest Dermatol 116:672–678

Watson REB, Long SP, Bowden JJ, Bastrilles JY, Barton SP, Griffiths CEM (2008) Repair of photoaged dermal matrix by topical application of a cosmetic 'antiageing' product. Br J Dermatol 158:472–477

Watson REB, Ogden S, Cotterell LF, Bowden JJ, Bastrilles JY, Long SP, Griffiths CEM (2009) A cosmetic 'anti-ageing' product improves photoaged skin: a double-blind, randomized controlled trial. Br J Dermatol 161:419–426

Watson REB, Gibbs NK, Griffiths CEM, Sherratt MJ (2014) Damage to skin extracellular matrix induced by UV exposure. Antioxid Redox Signal 21:1063–1077

Wondrak GT (2007) Let the sun shine in: mechanisms and potential for therapeutics in skin photodamage. Curr Opin Invest Drugs 8:390–400

Wondrak GT, Roberts MJ, Cervantes-Laurean D, Jacobson MK, Jacobson EL (2003) Proteins of the extracellular matrix are sensitizers of photo-oxidative stress in human skin cells. J Invest Dermatol 121:578–586

Wondrak GT, Jacobson MK, Jacobson EL (2006) Endogenous UVA-photosensitizers: mediators of skin photodamage and novel targets for skin photoprotection. Photochem Photobiol Sci 5:215–237

Woodley DT, Zelickson AS, Briggaman RA, Hamilton TA, Weiss JS, Ellis CN, Voorhees JJ (1990) Treatment of photoaged skin with topical tretinoin increases epidermal-dermal anchoring fibrils—a preliminary report. Jama J Am Med Assoc 263:3057–3059

Xiao JH, Durand B, Chambon P, Voorhees JJ (1995) Endogenous retinoic acid receptor (RAR)-retinoid X receptor (RXR) heterodimers are the major functional forms regulating retinoid-responsive elements in adult human keratinocytes. Binding of ligands to RAR only is sufficient for RAR-RXR heterodimers to confer ligand-dependent activation of hRAR beta 2/RARE (DR5). J Biol Chem 270:3001–3011

Yaar M, Gilchrest BA (2007) Photoageing: mechanism, prevention and therapy. British J Dermatol 157:874–887

Yamaguchi Y, Mann DM, Ruoslahti E (1990) Negative regulation of transforming growth-factor-beta by the proteoglycan decorin. Nature 346:281–284

Young AR (1997) Chromophores in human skin. Phys Med Biol 42:789–802

Zatterstrom UK, Felbor U, Fukai N, Olsen BR (2000) Collagen XVIII/endostatin structure and functional role in angiogenesis. Cell Struct Funct 25:97–101

Zhang G, Chen S, Goldoni S, Calder BW, Simpson HC, Owens RT, McQuillan DJ, Young MF, Iozzo RV, Birk DE (2009) Genetic evidence for the coordinated regulation of collagen fibrillogenesis in the cornea by decorin and biglycan. J Biol Chem 284:8888–8897

Chapter 6
Nitric Oxide Derivatives and Skin Environmental Exposure to Light: From Molecular Pathways to Therapeutic Opportunities

Christoph V. Suschek

Abstract The role of nitric oxide in human skin physiological as well as pathophysiological has been under investigation since first reports of cutaneous nitric oxide synthase (NOS)-expression in human skin tissue in. Already in the first years on NO research it became obvious that NO plays a pivotal role in the dermal response to environmental stimuli like ultraviolet radiation, heat, and cold. Additionally to enzymatically produced NO a range of non-enzymatic pathways for NO generation has been identified. Substantial quantities of NO radicals are continuously generated in the human skin, and formation of NO can be enhanced 3–5 fold by illumination with UVA light, especially in the outer skin. This phenomenon is attributed to the photolysis of photolabile nitroso compounds, which play an outstanding role in mammalian physiology. Previous work has shown that human skin is quite rich in these compounds, which attain local concentrations far higher than found in the blood circulation under normal conditions. Both are known to deliver free NO radicals upon UVA photolysis even at the modest UVA fluxes as found in sunlight at sea level. Accordingly, the degree of exposure of skin to ambient light will significantly affect the NO status of human skin, which plays an outstanding role in the regulation of local hemodynamic parameters, inflammation, infection, wound healing, and protection from the injurious effects of UV radiation.

Keywords UV radiation · UVA · UVB · Nitric oxide (NO) · Nitric oxide synthase (NOS) · Human skin tissue · Oxidative stress · Reactive oxygen species (ROS) · Skin physiology

---

C.V. Suschek (✉)
Department of Trauma and Hand Surgery, Medical Faculty
of the Heinrich-Heine-University Düsseldorf, Moorenstraße 5,
40225 Düsseldorf, Germany
e-mail: suschek@hhu.de

G.T. Wondrak (ed.), *Skin Stress Response Pathways*,
DOI 10.1007/978-3-319-43157-4_6

6.1 Nitric Oxide in Human Skin Physiology

6.1.1 Enzymatic Nitric Oxide Formation in Human Skin

Nitric oxide (NO) can be enzymatically produced from the amino acid L-arginine by at least three isoforms of nitric oxide synthases (NOS). The endothelial and neuronal isoforms (eNOS or nNOS) are constitutively expressed and regulated tightly by phosphorylation and binding of Calmodulin. NO released by these two isoforms usually acts as an intercellular signaling molecule mediating time-restricted events such as neurotransmission or vasorelaxation. In contrast, the third, by pro-inflammatory cytokines inducible isoform (iNOS) was initially found in activated macrophages. All NOS isoforms show moderate homology with cytochrome P450 reductase and exist in their active form as homodimers of two identical subunits, and produce NO via a five-electron oxidation of a nitrogen atom of the guanidinium group of L-arginine and O_2. The enzymatic reaction has been described to be one of the most complicated enzymatic activities currently known and the exact mechanism of NO synthesis is still not completely understood. Further, it is important to mention that the three members of the NOS enzyme family are encoded by different genes located on different chromosomes (Knowles and Moncada 1994).

Regarding the both constitutively expressed NO synthases, in human skin the nNOS is expressed in epidermal keratinocytes and melanocytes of the stratum

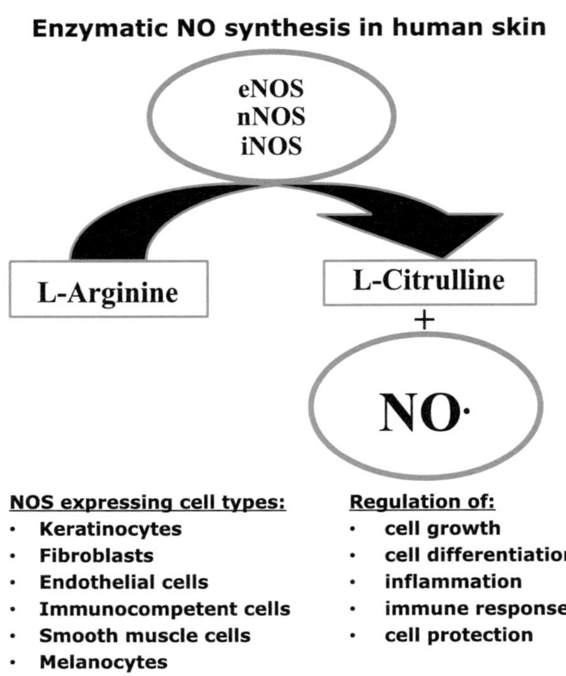

Fig. 6.1 Enzymatic NO synthesis in human skin

basale (Fig. 6.1), whereas the eNOS isoform appears to be delimited to endothelial cells and fibroblasts. In contrast, the expression of the inducible NOS isoform can be stimulated by pro-inflammatory stimuli in all cutaneous cell types, including keratinocytes, Langerhans cells, endothelial cells, melanocytes, and fibroblasts. As indicated, iNOS expression is predominantly associated with inflammation and strongly depends on the presence of pro-inflammatory mediators, mainly Interleukin-1-beta (IL1β), Tumor Necrosis Factor-alpha (TNFα), and/or gamma-Interferon (γIFN). In contrast, glucocorticosteroids, cyclophilins, and retinoids as well as the so called anti-inflammatory Th2-cytokines, i.e. Transforming Growth Factor-beta (TGFβ), Interleukin-4, and/or Interleukin-10 represent effective inhibitors of iNOS mRNA expression as well as enzyme activity (Bruch-Gerharz et al. 1998a, b).

In addition to NOS-generated NO formation from its specific substrate L-arginine, NO also can be released by non-enzymatic pathways from nitroso-compounds as well as higher nitrogen oxides such nitrite or nitrate. Mechanisms and relevance of cutaneous enzyme-independent NO formation will be discussed in detail below in this chapter (Paunel et al. 2005).

6.1.2 Antimicrobial and Antiviral Effects of Nitric Oxide

Due to its radically properties NO may effectively serve as an agent of cutaneous non-specific host defense. Thus, NO exerts antimicrobial effects on diverse microorganisms including fungi, yeast, bacteria, viruses, and protozoa (Weller et al. 1996, 2001). Thus, as the front line against the invasion by pathogens, the constitutive and steady production of NO on the skin's surface is likely to play an important role. In patients with psoriasis, the constitutive induction of iNOS and elevated NO synthesis may be responsible for the relatively high protection against infection seen in this disease (Weller et al. 1997). Although infectious bacterial as well as viral pathogens stimulate iNOS-derived NO production, which seems to limit their progression, pathogen-induced NO overproduction may promote severe inflammation, which, in certain cases, results in epidermal necrolysis and damage to peripheral nerve terminals. Sometimes, the induction of iNOS appears to be uncontrolled and results in excessive inflammation with serious consequences. In an experimental model of *herpes simplex*-induced pneumonia, the administration of NOS inhibitors improved survival and pulmonary compliance (Adler et al. 1997). This observation suggests that the improvement was mediated by the attenuation of the inflammatory response. Important targets for the antiviral effect of NO include the inhibition of reverse transcriptase and zinc finger domains necessary for DNA-binding and transcription, viral ribonucleotide reductase, and viral envelope (Kröncke et al. 1997, 2000).

6.1.3 Role of Nitric Oxide in Cutaneous Wound Healing

NO plays a pivotal role in the regulation of wound healing-relevant biological processes. The positive effects of L-arginine supplementation and NO donors, coupled to the negative effects of NOS inhibitors or the deletion of the iNOS or eNOS genes, have provided unambiguous evidence of a key role for NO (Frank et al. 2002). The expression of iNOS is stimulated in wound tissue, particularly in the basal keratinocytes adjacent to the wound (Frank et al. 1998). One of the key functions of NO in wound healing seems to be its modulatory activity on proliferation and differentiation of keratinocytes and fibroblasts, which helps to promote wound contraction and reepithelialization. One study has noted that low concentrations (0.01–0.25 mM) of NO stimulate cell division, whereas high concentrations (>10 mM) are cytostatic (Krischel et al. 1998). Interestingly, it seems to be the influence of the superoxide anion in the cell that determines the mitogenic capacity of the NO signal (Vallette et al. 1998). Together, they form Peroxynitrite, which dose-dependently inhibits proliferation. Removal of this anion reduces the inhibitory effect. The likely importance of NO-modulated cytokine signaling in the wound healing process has been noted by others and of particular interest seem to be the NO-induced activation of TGFβ and enhancement of IL-1β and IL-8 production. NO is also known to stimulate epithelial cells to produce and release of chemokines and other growth mediators such as vascular endothelial growth factor (VEGF), epidermal growth factor (EGF) and keratinocyte growth factor (KGF). KGF is released by IL-1β activated fibroblasts and stimulates the proliferation and migration of keratinocytes. In addition, high levels of VEGF are found at the hyperproliferative epithelium of the wound, which appears to be important for keratinocyte proliferation and angiogenesis (Frank et al. 1999, 2002).

Beside its role as modulator of cell growth and proliferation, NO also is an effective modulatory agent of collagen metabolism by fibroblasts. The inhibition of NOS by competitive inhibitors has been shown to reduce collagen synthesis and the tensile strength of regenerating tissue was significantly reduced in eNOS-knockout mice, as compared to the wild-type. Primary dermal fibroblasts obtained from iNOS-knockout mice have been shown to synthesize less collagen compared to wild-type cells, but their production can be augmented by the addition of NO donors (Shi et al. 2001). Concordant with this positive effect of NO, topical estrogen, perhaps acting via a stimulatory effect on NOS activity, has been found to accelerate the process of wound healing in the aged skin (Ashcroft et al. 1999). Furthermore, in the context of NO as wound healing regulating agent it is mentionable that animals and humans instinctively lick injured skin to promote healing and reduce infection. Benjamin et al. proposed that licking of wounds promote the release of nitric oxide from nitrite in the saliva (Benjamin et al. 1997).

6.1.4 Role of Nitric Oxide in Regulation of Cutaneous Blood Flow

The constitutive release of NO by microvascular endothelial cells plays an important role in regulation of the resting blood flow rate. In a rat animal model local or systemic application of NOS activity inhibitors significantly reduced flow rates in the skin (Goldsmith et al. 1996; Kellogg et al. 1998). The vasoconstricting effect of NOS inhibition is enhanced in locally warmed skin (Goldsmith et al. 1996). In contrast, when the whole body is warmed, intradermal injections of NOS inhibitors have relatively little effect. This is due to a neurally mediated vasodilatation reflex, involving the release of calcitonin gene-related peptide (CGRP) as well as NO (Goldsmith et al. 1996; Kellogg et al. 1999). Although CGRP has intrinsic vasodilatatory activity, NO release is required for a complete vasodilator response (Kellogg et al. 1998). Thus, NOS responds rapidly to local changes in temperature and neurogenic signals with an increase in NO production that has a direct effect on the vasculature. In unstimulated endothelial cells, at normal temperatures, it is likely that the primary regulator of NOS is blood flow shear stress (Corson et al. 1996), although circulating cytokines, steroids, and peptide hormones will also play a part. In the response to heat, it is possible that the vanilloid receptor family of cationic channels, which allow the entry of Ca^{2+} into the cell, may be important in controlling the activity of constitutive NOS. Members of this heat-sensitive family of channels are expressed by neurons and keratinocytes. In conclusion, the constitutive release of NO in the skin is involved in setting the rate of resting blood flow, via a cGMP-dependent relaxation of the vascular smooth muscle (Weller 2003). In addition, it seems reasonable to hypothesize that NO is involved in localized or diffuse erythematous eruptions of the skin, caused environmental factors like ultraviolet radiation (UVR), drugs, toxins, bacterial or viral infections. On the other hand, a local deficiency of NO contributes to vasospasms in circumscribed regions of the skin, as for example in the cold-induced vasoconstrictive processes of Raynaud's disease (Anggard 1994).

6.2 UV Radiation—Skin Interaction

6.2.1 Penetration of UVA into Human Skin

The optical properties of skin tissue vary significantly with depth, due to inhomogeneity in the distribution of absorbing chromophores and endogenous scatters. Upon normal incidence, a significant fraction of incident light is reflected due to the significant contrast in refractive index between air and stratum corneum. Strong scattering in deeper layers of the skin causes additional emission from the skin, in particular by the collagen fibers in the dermis. Optical remittance from skin is defined as the sum of the primary surface reflection and the secondary scattering from deeper layers. The absorption of UVA and VIS (300–700 nm) is dominated by the melanin content of stratum corneum and epidermis. Accordingly, the skin of black people has far higher absorbance and far lower remittance than that of fair skinned Caucasians. In healthy stratum corneum and epidermis the scattering of radiation remains small, and epidermal transmittance of fair Caucasian skin is quite good for UVA, VIS and near infrared irradiation. For more in-depth information to this topic see also (Suschek et al. 2010).

The optical properties of the underlying dermis are significantly different from stratum corneum: The reflective index is lower, and it is highly scattering due to the presence of copious collagen fibers with a size distribution spanning all wavelengths of light. The strong scattering by fibrous collagen makes that incident radiation propagates diffusively rather than as a collimated wave front. The dermis does not contain melanin but has significant UVA-VIS absorption by the presence of oxy-hemoglobin, bilirubin and beta-carotene. Accordingly, the properties of this layer depend on the degree of vascularization. For a typical UVA wavelength of 350–360 nm, the penetration depth is estimated to be around 70 μm (Anderson and Parrish 1981). This distance is the depth where the light intensity is reduced by a factor of 1/e–0.37. It should be kept in mind that the light intensity at this depth is not negligible but still a significant 37 % of the incoming light. The light intensity is reduced to the insignificant 1 % level only deeper than four penetration depths (in this case ca. 300–400 μm). In other words, nearly all UVA is absorbed in the outer half millimeter of skin. This region comprises the full stratum corneum and epidermis, the upper horizontal plexus as well as the upper layers of the dermis. In particular, substantial UVA intensities penetrate the region of the dermal microcirculation of the upper horizontal plexus (located between epidermis and dermis). It implies that the microcirculation has access to the photoproducts generated by UVA irradiation in skin. This is not the case for shorter wavelengths of UVB, where the far higher extinction coefficients of the outer epidermal layers provide effective screening. For more in-depth information to this topic see also (Suschek et al. 2010).

6.2.2 *Physiological Effects of UV Irradiation*

A prominent effect of UVA on DNA is the formation of cyclobutane pyrimidine dimers (CPD's) and other bipyrimidine photoproducts. Both may inhibit DNA synthesis and gene transcription. In addition, UV irradiation of the skin induces the release of a plethora of biologically active molecules. Some of these are created photochemically, by the modification of various proteins, carbohydrates, and lipids, whereas others are induced or released in consequence. Amongst the important diffusible transmitters released by UV-activated keratinocytes are IL1β, IL-6, IL-8, IL-10, TNFα, TGFα, TGFβ1, prostaglandin E_2 (PGE_2), endothelin-1, and the pro-opiomelanocortin peptides. UV irradiation also directly activates certain transmembrane receptors, such as the epidermal growth factor (EGF) receptor and the keratinocyte growth factor (KGF) receptor, which go on to activate downstream pathways and initiate the production of peroxide and reactive oxygen species (ROS). Additionally, irradiation of cultured endothelial cells or cultured keratinocytes by UVB led to dose-dependent increase in NO and cGMP (Deliconstantinos et al. 1992, 1995).

In the present literature, the effect of UV on iNOS expression is still controversial. On the one hand UVB was shown to suppress iNOS mRNA expression at 4 and 12 h after UVB irradiation, suggesting that the enhancement of NO production observed after UVB irradiation in murine keratinocytes may be explained in part by the upregulation of nNOS expression, but not iNOS expression (Sasaki et al. 2000). On the other hand UVB radiation was shown to down regulate iNOS expression induced by IFNγ or TNFα in the murine keratinocyte. Controversially, UVB was reported to induce a de novo expression of iNOS mRNA and NO generation in cultured keratinocyte cell lines (Seo et al. 2002). Both UVA and UVB are potent promoters of endothelial iNOS expression in human skin endothelial cells (Suschek et al. 2001b, 2004). The growing body of data attests that the endogenous generation of NO plays a significant role in the response to UV (Fig. 6.2).

Finally, in addition to NOS-generated NO, light exposure may release free NO from a range of photolabile S-nitroso-compounds found in biological tissues like S-nitroso-glutathione (GS-NO) or S-nitroso-albumin (van Faassen and Vanin 2007). O-nitroso and C-nitroso compounds may similarly be photolysed. Visible illumination of strongly absorbing nitrosyl-iron (Fe^{2+}–NO and Fe^{3+}–NO) complexes has high quantum yield for release of the nitrosyl ligand as free NO radical. In normal situations, only the upper layers of skin or the retinal tissues of the eye will be exposed to significant light intensities. The first case will be considered in detail below.

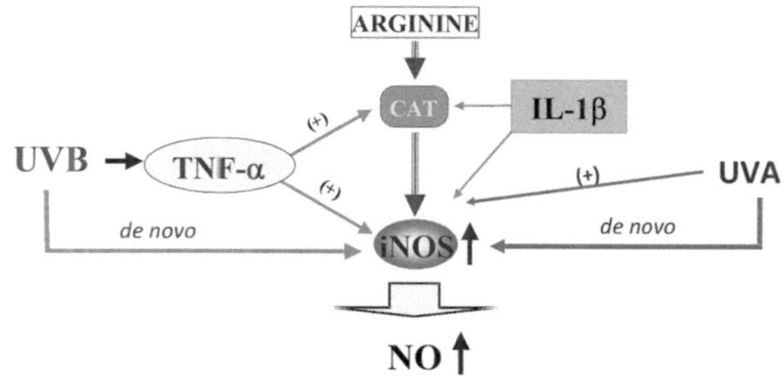

Fig. 6.2 UVB induces human iNOS promoter activity, protein expression in vascular endothelia of human skin and strongly augments cytokine-induced iNOS expression and activity by mechanisms comprising the involvement of CAT-2 and/or TNF-α-dependent effects on CAT-2- and iNOS-mRNA expression, respectively

6.3 Nitric Oxide in UV-Exposed Skin

6.3.1 Role of Nitric Oxide in UV-Induced Cutaneous Erythema

It is well known that UV radiation dose-dependently induces erythema formation. Typically, UV-induced erythema arises after a delay of about 4–24 h. At this, the erythemal threshold of human skin is in the case of UVB (22 mJ cm^{-2}) approximately three orders of magnitude lower than that for UVA (60 J cm^{-2}). Thus, human skin seems to be very sensitive to small quantities of energy in the UVB region. More interestingly, cutaneous application of NOS inhibitors prevented from UV-induced erythema formation and abolished the characteristic erythemal increase in blood flow, even when application occurred 30 min before the predicted onset of erythema (Warren et al. 1993).

A comparable result was found in human volunteers, where the intradermal injection of a NOS inhibitor attenuated the erythemal increase of blood flow (Warren 1994) and produced a long-lasting (24 h) pallor around the UVB irradiated injection site (Weller et al. 1996). In addition to the erythema reducing effects of NOS inhibitors, NO acts in concert with prostaglandin E_2 (PGE_2), since the NOS inhibitor-induced block was lost at high doses of UVB, when a stronger stimulation of PGE_2 occurs (Rhodes et al. 2001). Deliconstantinos et al. (1992, 1995) and others (Suschek et al. 2001b, 2004) have proposed that UV irradiation augments both the activity and expression of nNOS and eNOS.

In addition, UV irradiation was also found to induce the expression and therefore activity of iNOS. In normal skin, iNOS is detectable at about 6 h after UV exposure. The dermal iNOS content becomes highest after approx. 24 h and slowly returns to resting levels after 72 h. Although UVA irradiation by itself promotes iNOS expression (Suschek et al. 2001b, 2004), local cytokine release is likely to contribute significantly (Lee et al. 2000; Suschek et al. 2004). The experimental inhibition of constitutive NOS during the exposure to UV has been found to inhibit the induction of iNOS (Lee et al. 2000). Therefore, in the early stages of UV exposure there would appear to be a positive feedback effect of NO on iNOS induction. The rise in intracellular calcium that occurs upon UV stimulation appears to be the principal activator of the constitutive NOS. This calcium flux is also essential for ROS production via the UV-activated EGF receptor. We note that the kinetics for UV-induced erythema appears to correlate closely with the expression of iNOS (Szabo et al. 2001). Thus, the cutaneous production of NO appeared to be a central component of the delayed-onset erythema. It seems plausible that the iNOS isoform is the source of this NO, but definite proof is lacking at the moment.

6.3.2 Regulative Effects of Nitric Oxide on UV-Modulated Cutaneous Immune Response

Acute UV exposure makes a weighty impact on cutaneous immune response. Thus UV more or less reversibly suppresses both contact hypersensitivity and delayed-type hypersensitivity, and thus might lead to a temporally limited development of antigen-specific suppressor cells especially Langerhans cells, which number strongly decay in UV irradiated human epidermis (Cals-Grierson and Ormerod 2004). Strongly implicated in this response is the release of calcitonin gene-related peptide (CGRP) from peripheral neurons and cytokine stimulation, particularly TNFα and IL-10 (Suschek et al. 2004; Townley et al. 2002). The elevated NO synthesis following iNOS induction after UV exposure might exert further complex effects on the immune system and in models of skin transplantation. Enhanced iNOS-driven NO levels are associated with rejection of skin grafts, whereby application of specific iNOS inhibitors led to improved graft survival rates, and it appears in this situation that the inhibition of NO enhances the release of anti-inflammatory Th2-cytokines (IL-10 and IL-4) and reduces the release of pro-inflammatory Th1-cytokines (IL-2 and INFγ), thereby favoring tolerance (Holan et al. 2002).

6.3.3 Impact of Nitric Oxide on UV-Induced Cutaneous Inflammation

A large body of work indicates that elevated levels of NO are pro-inflammatory and many similarities exist between UV-induced erythema and inflammation (Cals-Grierson and Ormerod 2004). The exposure of skin to UV irradiation or to chemical irritants results in higher levels of NO synthesis and the production of pro-inflammatory cytokines (Warren et al. 1993). Application of an NO-releasing emulsion to the skin of human volunteers evoked local inflammation and other inflammatory events, including the loss of Langerhans cells and the induction of apoptosis in keratinocytes (Ormerod et al. 1999). If the production of NO in the skin was blocked, then the inflammatory response was lessened. In guinea pig skin, the inflammatory response—as detected in the form of edema formation—to an intradermal injection of bradykinin, histamine or platelet-activation factor was attenuated by the co-injection of a NOS inhibitor (Teixeira et al. 1993). In iNOS knock-out mice experimentally induced inflammation was less severe than in wild-type mice. Normally, inflammation is self-regulating. This is partly due to NO-induced nitrosylation of the inflammation-related transcription factor NF-κB, which prevents the transcription factor from binding to the iNOS promoter, but other points of feedback may also be involved.

A lot of recent research has focused on the role of reactive oxygen species (ROS) and particularly superoxide (O_2^-), which in combination with NO, forms peroxynitrite. In vitro experiments have confirmed that this highly reactive molecule can cause the nitrosation of tyrosine (Ormerod et al. 1999), DNA strand breakage, and activation of the poly(ADP–ribose) polymerase pathway of necrotic cell death (Szabo et al. 2001). When the self-regulation of inflammation breaks down, severe and sometimes life-threatening dermatoses can occur. The Stevens–Johnson syndrome, an inflammatory skin condition with toxic epidermal necrolysis, is notable for its persistent upregulation of iNOS mRNA (Lerner et al. 2000).

Paradoxically, UV irradiation of inflammatory skin conditions can suppress iNOS expression (Sur et al. 2002). In experiments on keratinocytes and macrophages, UVB irradiation interfered with the binding of the iNOS-related transcription factors NF-κB and Stat-1 to DNA and inhibited the induction of iNOS by IFNγ.

6.3.4 Protective Effects of Nitric Oxide Against UV-Induced Injuries

The cellular response to intracellular NO concentration increases seems to depend to a significant extent on the redox potential of the cell, which is itself influenced by the resting levels of NO. For example, in human neuroblastoma cells NO induces thioredoxin expression via a protein-kinase-G (PKG)-dependent pathway, which helps to protect the cells from oxidative stress and apoptosis, whereas higher levels of NO can promote apoptotic cell death (Kröncke et al. 1997). The protective effects of NO in the skin have been demonstrated by experiments on iNOS or eNOS deficient mice, which show significantly higher numbers of apoptotic skin cells following UV irradiation, than in wild-type mice (Weller et al. 2003). The mechanism of this protective action is still uncertain. An induction of Bcl-2 expression and inhibition of caspase activation have been suggested by some studies (Suschek et al. 1999), but this fails to explain the rapid timescale of the response. Also evoked is the inhibition of ROS-mediated lipid peroxidation (Suschek et al. 2001a) and indeed, lipid peroxidation is widely used as in vivo measure of UV-induced oxygen free radical production, a reaction suppressed by the NO donor sodium nitroprusside and enhanced by L-NAME, an effective NOS inhibitor (Lee et al. 2000).

Studies with chemical probes implicate the involvement of H_2O_2, super oxide radical ($O_2^{\cdot-}$), hydroxyl radical ($OH^{\cdot}$) and an important role for singlet oxygen ($^1O_2$) in UVA-mediated cytotoxicity (Suschek et al. 1999, 2001a) (Fig. 6.3). In biological environments singlet oxygen is highly reactive with a sufficiently long half-life to reach specific compartments. All reactive oxygen species (ROS) are potentially harmful to cells. Exposure to ROS results in progressive cell damage by oxidative modification of various bio-molecules including the peroxidation of lipid membranes (Sies 1986). Previously published data suggest that NO radicals may terminate radical-chain reaction (Suschek et al. 2001a). This role is supported by the tendency of cellular NO to partition preferably in the apolar lipid or protein compartments. In these compartments, the local NO concentration is about an order of

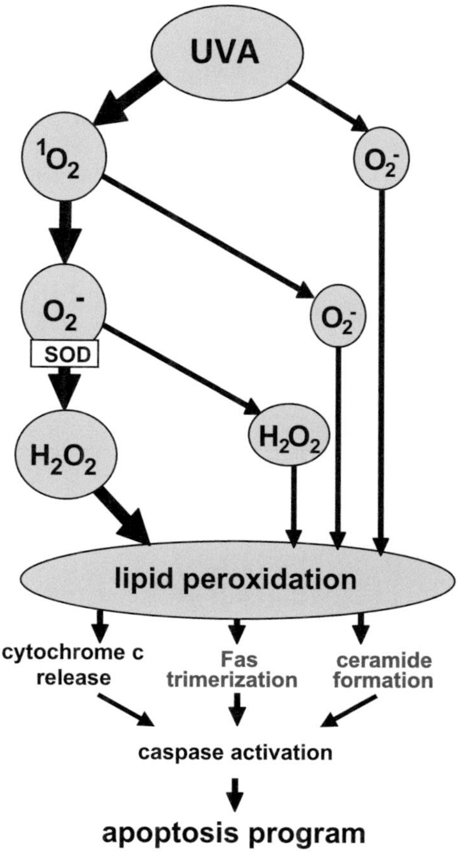

Fig. 6.3 Pathways of UVA-induced and ROS-mediated apoptosis

magnitude higher than in the aqueous phase. Lipid peroxidation represents a late step in UVA-induced apoptosis as a prerequisite for mitochondrial cytochrome c leakage, the initiation step for the mitochondrial pathway of apoptosis (Suschek et al. 2001a). Lipid peroxidation results from the net abstraction of an allylic hydrogen atom of an unsaturated fatty acid by an initiating radical species. The lipid radical generated then reacts with O_2 resulting in an alkylperoxy radical (LOO˙) which can then react with neighboring lipid to form another lipid radical that can also react with O_2 and so on. Thus, a single initiating event can lead to the destruction/modification of numerous lipid molecules resulting in loss of membrane integrity. Indeed, the reaction of NO with LOO˙ species predominates over the slower initiation of secondary peroxidation propagation reactions by LOO˙ with vicinal unsaturated lipids. When inhibiting lipid peroxidation propagation reactions, NO undergoes an initial termination reaction with organic peroxyl radicals to form organic peroxynitrates (LOONO) (Miranda et al. 2000).

Furthermore, it had been repeatedly shown that NO regulates the expression of a wide range of genes including protective stress response genes such as vascular

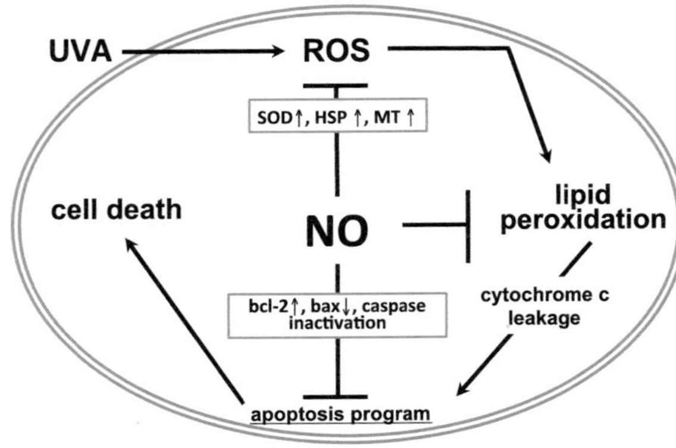

Fig. 6.4 Protective role of NO in UVA-induced and ROS-mediated cell death of human skin cells

endothelial growth factor (VEGF), heme oxygenase (HO)-1 and Bcl-2 (Suschek et al. 2003b) (Fig. 6.4). But the involvement of a "NO-specific" cGMP-mediated pathway cannot be excluded.

6.4 Enzyme-Independent Nitric Oxide Generation in Human Skin

6.4.1 Nitric Oxide Derivates in Human Skin

The action of NO is largely determined by its high diffusion rate (D $\sim$ 3300 $\mu m^2\ s^{-1}$ at 37 °C) and its ability to penetrate cell membranes. The diffusion coefficient is about 1.4-fold higher than that of O_2 or CO, and thus the diffusion distance in tissues for NO has been calculated to be that of many cell diameters (up to 500 μm). NO penetrates not only biological membranes but also diffuses readily into the core of native and oxidized low-density lipoprotein. Within tissues, some of the NO may react with thiols leading to the formation of comparatively more stable S-nitro-thiols (RS-NOs). However, it should be noted that NO, though a radical, is a very inefficient nitrosating agent by itself. Even at supraphysiological concentrations, NO will not S-nitrosate thiols to any significant extent. However, the presence of trace metal ions like iron and copper may greatly enhance the nitrosation rates via more complicated radical reaction pathways (van Faassen and Vanin 2007). RS-NOs like S-nitrosoalbumin, S-nitrosoglutathione or S-nitrosocysteine have been detected and quantified in vivo (Feelisch et al. 2002) and are thought to be responsible for some of the well-documented physiological processes that previously had been attributed to NO itself (Stamler et al. 1992). Furthermore, S- and N-nitroso compounds (RS-NOs or RN-NOs) as well as the oxidation products nitrite or nitrate represent important products of the NO metabolism in human skin (Fig. 6.5). Concentrations of up to 15 μM nitrite and 7 μM RS-NO were detected in human skin, representing more than 25- and 360-times higher concentrations of these compounds than found in plasma of healthy volunteers (Paunel et al. 2005).

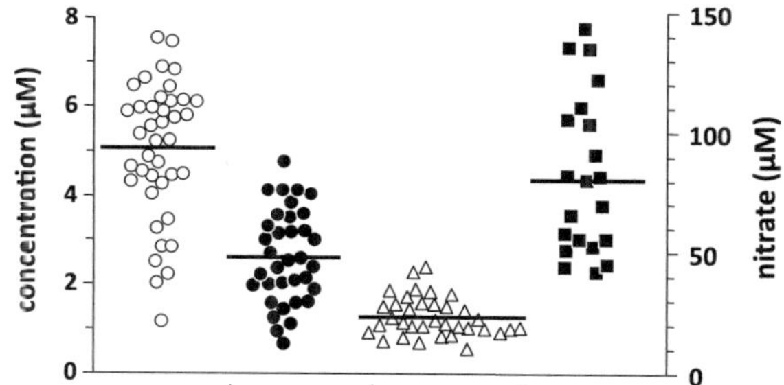

Fig. 6.5 Nitric oxide derivates in human skin tissue

	NO_2^-	RS-NO	RN-NO	NO_3^-	
Skin	**5.1±1.6**	**2.6±1.0**	**1.3±0.4**	**82.4 ±33.6**	**µM**
Serum	**0.20 ±0.02**	**0.007 ±0.001**	**0.032 ±0.005**	**14.4 ±1.7**	
Ratio	**25**	**370**	**40**	**6**	**-fold**

Sweat has been reported to contain concentrations of up to 40 µM nitrate (which continuously is reduced to nitrite by commensal bacteria) and 10 µM nitrite, which appears to reflect the rate of cutaneous NO formation (Weller et al. 1996). However, under normal sun- and heat-exposed conditions the sweat secretion will undergo rapid evaporation, and deposit its nitrate and nitrite content on the skin surface. Consequently, challenge of normal human skin with UVA light at doses equivalent to only 3–5 min of sun exposure in the Central European summer (according to an UVA radiant power of approximately 5 mW cm^{-2}) leads to a significant non-enzymatic NO formation due to photolysis of nitrite and/or RS-NOs (Fig. 6.6).

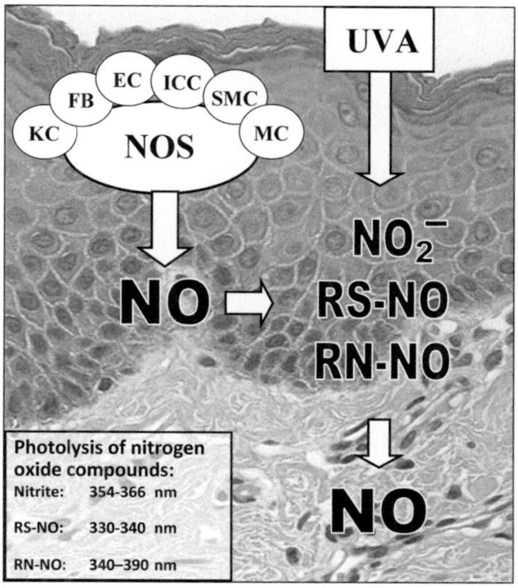

Fig. 6.6 Mechanisms of cutaneous NO formation

This enzyme-independent NO formation was detected directly above the skin surface as NO gas, but was also verified within cultured cells of intact healthy skin tissue (Paunel et al. 2005). Interestingly, cutaneous UVA-induced NO formation was comparable or higher than found with maximally iNOS-activated human keratinocyte cultures (Bruch-Gerharz et al. 2003).

The adult human skin has a total weight of about 10–12 kg and provides the largest pool of NO derivatives like nitrite or RS-NOs. Since NO has been found to play important roles in regulating skin pigmentation, as well as growth and differentiation of keratinocytes, it appears likely that photodecomposition of intradermal nitrite and RS-NOs as well as of extradermal nitrite has physiological significance. This may affect processes in human skin like melanogenesis or may confer protection from UV-induced cell damage (Suschek et al. 1999, 2003b).

It is known that circulating levels of NO-related products in plasma can be influenced by dietary intake of nitrate or nitrite. Thus, Mowbray et al. propose that dietary NO derivates may also offer a source for manipulation of cutaneous NO-related products and an individual's dietary consumption of green leafy vegetables may in part influence their cutaneous response to UV radiation (Mowbray et al. 2008). It is well known that vegetarians are at reduced risk of developing hypertension and other cardiovascular diseases, and it has been speculated that the high nitrate/nitrite content of many vegetables may contribute to these cardioprotective effects. In analogy to these observations, the findings described by Mowbray et al. strongly implicate an analogous role for nitrite/nitrate containing nutrients in the protection against the injurious inflammatory or carcinogenic properties of pro-oxidative environmental stimuli like UVA radiation.

6.4.2 *UVA-Induced Photolysis of Nitrite In Vitro*

UV-Photolysis of nitrite and nitrate has been known for a long time and been studied in a large variety of contexts spanning from atmospheric chemistry to advanced oxidation technologies for detoxication of hazardous organic pollutants. The primary photolytic reaction releases an oxygen radical ($O^{\cdot -}$) that is rapidly protonated to the hydroxyl radical $OH^{\cdot}$.

The main reactions are tabulated below (Treinin and Hayon 1970; Zafiriou and Bonneau 1987):

$$NO_2^- + h\nu \rightarrow NO^{\cdot} + O^{\cdot -} \tag{6.1}$$

$$O^{\cdot -} + H_2O \leftrightarrow {}^{\cdot}OH + {}^{-}OH \; (pK_a = 11.9) \tag{6.2}$$

$$NO^{\cdot} + {}^{\cdot}OH \rightarrow HNO_2 \rightarrow NO_2^- + H^+ \tag{6.2b}$$

$$NO_2^- + {}^{\cdot}OH \rightarrow NO_2^{\cdot} + OH^- \tag{6.3}$$

$$NO_2^{\cdot} + NO^{\cdot} \rightarrow N_2O_3 \tag{6.4}$$

$$N_2O_3 + H_2O \rightarrow 2NO_2^- + 2H^+ \tag{6.5}$$

The threshold for both reactions is around 410 nm, corresponding to a photon energy of 3.0 eV. The secondary reactions between nitrite and the hydroxyl radical generate nitrogen dioxide radicals ($NO_2^{\cdot}$), N_2O_4, and nitrate (Mack and Bolton 1999). Obviously, a certain quantity of gaseous nitrogen oxides (e.g. NO, $NO_2^{\cdot}$) is released by these pathways and may be lost from the solution. The interest in the photolysis of nitrite for detoxification of fluid waste is based on the high reactivity of the hydroxyl radical towards organic compounds. In the presence of biological materials, or even inside tissues, the hydroxyl intermediates have a plethora of reaction partners and give rise to a large variety of end products and initiate autocatalytic oxidations as in unsaturated lipids. The photoexcitation of nitrite rests on an intense UVC $\pi \rightarrow \pi^*$ transition at 205 nm (ε_{205} = 5500 $(Mcm)^{-1}$) and a much weaker $\pi \rightarrow \pi^*$ transition in the UVA at 354 nm (ε_{354} = 22.5 $(Mcm)^{-1}$). For photolysis under solar illumination, this weak UVA absorption has highest relevance. Recent in vitro experiments (Anastasio and Chu 2009) reported significant quantum yields for hydroxyl formation from nitrite anions and nitrous acid at room temperature under illumination at 366 nm. We note that protonation enhances the NO-quantum yield of nitrite by an order of magnitude. Accordingly, acidification significantly accelerates the photogeneration of hydroxyl radicals by shifting the equilibrium from nitrite to nitrous acid.

6.4.3 UVA-Induced Photolysis of Nitrite In Vivo

In the 1960s Furchgott and associates accidentally made the observation that daylight irradiation of vessels induces dilation, a phenomenon called photorelaxation (Ehrreich and Furchgott 1968). This effect was markedly potentiated by addition of nitrite (Matsunaga and Furchgott 1989), indicating that under certain circumstances nitrite may exhibit relaxation activities comparable to NO. Indeed, studies in environmental chemistry revealed that both the nitrite anion as well as nitrous acid in aqueous solutions undergo photodecomposition when irradiated with UV light at 200–400 nm, resulting in the release of free NO radicals (Fischer and Warneck 1996). The N–O-bond of the nitrite ion in aqueous solution will be disrupted by energy of light at 340–360 nm.

UVA-induced photodecomposition of nitrite results in a modest but sustained release of NO radicals. In contrast, irradiation of RS-NOs leads to a much higher release of NO due to the far higher extinction coefficient of this species. Under high UVA intensities the release of NO is short-lived due to rapid depletion of RS-NO (photobleaching). It should be noted that neither nitrate nor N-nitrosated species (RN-NOs), contribute to UVA-provoked NO release from human skin (Paunel et al. 2005).

Detailed analysis of the mechanism of light-induced nitrite decomposition in human skin revealed the formation of very reactive and potentially cytotoxic radical species like $NO_2^{\cdot}$. The radical $NO_2^{\cdot}$ recombines rapidly with NO to N_2O_3 which is a very efficient nitrosating agent, in particular for thiols. Via this reaction, $NO_2^{\cdot}$ decreases the yield of free NO from UVA-induced nitrite decomposition. In the presence of thiols like glutathione, however, the NO-trapping capacity of $NO_2^{\cdot}$ (Kirsch et al. 2002) will be counteracted via three reactions. First, N_2O_3 efficiently nitrosates thiols to RS-NO, which by itself is efficiently photolysed to NO and thiyl radicals ($RS^{\cdot}$) under illumination by UVA. Secondly, $NO_2^{\cdot}$ will directly be reduced to nitrite by thiolates like GS^-, and thirdly, $RS^{\cdot}$ reacts efficiently with GS-NO to yield NO and a disulfide (RS-SR). In contrast, simple recombination of $GS^{\cdot}$ and $NO^{\cdot}$ has not been observed. Therefore, reaction of thiols with both $NO_2^{\cdot}$ and with N_2O_3 will increase the formation of NO (Kirsch et al. 2002). The reaction of thiolate anions with $NO_2^{\cdot}$ is about 10 times faster than the reaction with N_2O_3 (Kirsch et al. 2002).

The preceding discussion shows that photolysis of nitrite initiates complex radical reaction chemistry of various nitrogen oxides. Photolysis of nitrite is concomitant with release of hydroxyl radicals ($OH^{\cdot}$). In some cases, radical oxygen species may initiate self-sustained radical chain reactions (Halliwell and Gutteridge 1989). Lipid peroxidation of unsaturated membrane bilayers is a well-studied example of hydroxyl damage (Halliwell and Gutteridge 1989). Therefore, the release of hydroxyl radicals poses a very significant threat of cellular damage due to the initiation of secondary radical reactions. The formation of hydroxyl and secondary lipid radicals under UVA illumination of human skin samples was explicitly demonstrated by spin trapping (Herrling et al. 2002). The radical adducts had highest concentration on the outer apical skin surface and could be detected to a depth of ca. 0.5 mm.

The photolytic quantum yield for NO release is not just a given intra-molecular property but profoundly affected by environmental factors. For example, the NO quantum yield for nitrite anions is ca. 0.03 in the presence of hydroxyl scavengers, but goes down to zero in ultrapure water, where the photolytic products have no alternative to recombining into nitrite. Similarly, the NO quantum yield of S-nitrosothiols may be significantly enhanced by the presence of photosensitizers. The presence of compounds with long-lived photoexcited spin triplet states in particular will have profound effect on the photolytic quantum yield of NO. Such spin triplet states are characteristic for phosphorescent compounds, and they are routinely found in biological settings. This should be kept in mind when extrapolating in vitro results to a physiological setting like human skin.

6.4.4 *Nitric Oxide Emanating from Human Skin Is Enhanced by UVA*

Using a collection chamber with an UVA transparent front window for the accumulation of gases from a small area of healthy human skin 80 ± 50 ppb NO in argon had accumulated after 2 min (Suschek et al. 2010). This is still a fairly low concentration: For comparison NO levels in exhaled breath are of 17–19 ppb in adults, thousand fold higher 5–50 ppm in breathing air used for clinical inhalation therapy and the still higher levels of 300–700 ppm in fresh cigarette smoke (Suschek et al. 2010).

The yields from the chamber allowed a rough estimate of the total quantity of NO emanating from human skin, and amounts of basal NO release were calculated to be 68 ± 40 fmol NO s^{-1} cm^{-2}. For a human adult with 2 m^2 skin surface a total release of 120 ± 70 μmol NO gas per day into the ambient air was estimated (Suschek et al. 2010). This quantity is more than two orders of magnitude smaller than the daily nitrate plus nitrite uptake of up to 180 mg per day. Therefore it is small compared to the total nitrogen turnover in humans and may be easily missed from the total metabolic nitrogen balance. We note that the basal release of 68 ± 40 fmol NO s^{-1} cm^{-2} is only a firm lower bound for basal NO production in skin, since some NO will be lost by reaction pathways other than escape to the air. Plausibly, we estimate the total basal NO production 3–4 fold higher at 0.2–0.3 pmol NO s^{-1} cm^{-2} (Suschek et al. 2010).

Under illumination with a low-pressure UVA source (18 mW cm^{-2}) with narrow band emission at 365 ± 10 nm, the release of gaseous NO was enhanced threefold: After 120 s, the collection chamber had accumulated a quantity of 260 ± 100 ppb NO in argon. This amounts to a NO flux of 213 ± 80 fmol s^{-1} cm^{-2} from the skin (Suschek et al. 2010). The total $UVA_{365\ nm}$ dose of 2.2 J cm^{-2} corresponded to a sun exposure time of approx. 30 min in a temperate climate zone. Again, we note that the UVA-induced release of 213 ± 80 fmol NO s^{-1} cm^{-2} is a firm lower bound for induced NO production in skin, since a part of NO will be lost by reaction pathways other than escape from the skin into the air. Therefore, we estimated the total UVA-induced NO production 3–4 fold higher at 0.6–0.9 pmol NO s^{-1} cm^{-2} (Suschek et al. 2010).

Given that UVA penetrates up to 300–400 μm deep into human skin, and presuming that the epidermal store of stable NO products are not continuously replenished, a single hour of sun exposure would be enough to deplete the 5–8 μM of photolabile NO derivates (Paunel et al. 2005) in human skin. In reality, this is unlikely to happen since the pool of NO derivates in skin is dynamically coupled to the much larger pool in the blood circulation. It seems improbable that a moderate sun exposure could lead to a depletion of the mentioned NO "prodrugs" in the upper skin regions and thus may impair the skin-protective effects of non-enzymatic NO formation. As shown by Mowbray et al. (2008) the concentration of NO-related products in the superficial dermis does not only represent the limited amount of oxidation products of cutaneous NOS generated NO, as postulated by Paunel et al.

(2005). The endodermal NO stores appear coupled to the levels of NO-related products circulating in blood. As the levels of NO-related products in plasma can be influenced by dietary intake of nitrate or nitrite, Mowbray et al. postulate that dietary NO derivates may offer a pathway for manipulation of cutaneous NO-related products via the consumption of green leafy vegetables. This should ultimately affect the release of NO in skin under UV radiation (Suschek et al. 2010).

6.5 Relevance of Light-Induced Non-enzymatic Nitric Oxide Generation in Human Skin

6.5.1 Local Effects

The factors and mechanisms controlling the efflux of NO from skin are not yet precisely known. Human skin contains naturally occurring photolabile NO donors. Their activation by exposure of skin to sunlight causes non-enzyme-derived high-output NO formation. Nitrite content and acidity of the apical skin surface are definitely important parameters. Previous publications noted highly significant protection against UVA-induced cell damage and death conferred by high-output NO-formation (Suschek et al. 1999, 2001b) (Fig. 6.4). Accordingly, non-enzymatic NO production has biological relevance and appears to act as an intrinsic UVA screen in human skin. The non-enzymatic NO formation is always available and bridges the time delay between acute UV-challenge and the induction of iNOS and melanin (Suschek et al. 2001b).

In the last 20 years an ongoing discussion in the NO research field tries to typify the (patho)physiological character of NO. The cellular response to intracellular NO concentration-increases seems to depend to a significant extent on the redox potential of the cell, which is itself influenced by the resting levels of NO. In human skin cells and tissues even supra physiological high NO concentrations were shown to protect cells from oxidative stress and UVA-induced apoptosis (Suschek et al. 2003a). Contrary, in other cell systems NO had been shown to promote apoptosis even at “physiological” concentrations, earning it the epithet “the Janus-faced molecule” (Kröncke et al. 1997, 1998). In recent years we noted similar characteristics for nitrite. For instance, nitrite protected cultured rat endothelial cells against UVA-induced cell injury (Suschek et al. 2003b) and reduced the susceptibility of human skin fibroblasts to UVA-induced cell death (Oplander et al. 2008). On the other side, high nitrite concentrations (100 μM) significantly promoted UVA-induced cell death in cultured human skin fibroblasts due to the simultaneous generation of highly toxic $OH^{\cdot}$ and $NO_2^{\cdot}$ radicals, i.e. typical photoproducts of nitrite (Oplander et al. 2007). Therefore, photolysis of nitrite has a Janus-faced character as well. It combines beneficial release of cutaneous NO with harmful production of $OH^{\cdot}$ and $NO_2^{\cdot}$ radicals. We recall that the presence of physiological levels of nitrite (5 μM) enhanced the UVA and UVB damage to free calf thymus DNA by an order of magnitude in vitro (Suzuki and Inukai 2006).

With regard to potential therapeutic applications, it is natural to think of methods to suppress the harmful aspects while retaining the benefits. Neutralization of the noxious $OH^{\cdot}$ and $NO_2^{\cdot}$ radicals by scavenging is an obvious proposition. As shown recently, an antioxidative intervention represents a successful strategy for protection from UVA/nitrite-induced injuries (Oplander et al. 2007). Ascorbic acid enhances UVA-induced NO formation from nitrite and effectively protects from UVA/nitrite-induced cell damage (Kirsch et al. 2002). Interestingly, protection against UVA/nitrite-induced cell death was also achieved by exogenously applied nitric oxide (Oplander et al. 2007). These findings indicate that the balance between NO and ROS during UVA decides between cellular death or survival. This balance is clearly redox dependent and may be modulated by external agents. Proof of principle is found in the skin care sections of every supermarket: Cosmetic self-tanning agents like dihydroxyacetone (DHA) or erythrulose act by promoting UVA-induced radical formation and subsequent darkening of melanin by oxidation. Sunscreens and antioxidant creams aim at shifting the balance in opposite direction. Scavenging of $OH^{\cdot}$ or $NO_2^{\cdot}$ and enhancement of NO will favor cell protection.

6.5.2 Systemic Effects

Apart from its effects on stroke, renal failure and peripheral arterial disease, systemic arterial hypertension is a major risk factor for cardiovascular complications, including coronary artery disease, heart failure and sudden cardiac death.

Interestingly, mean systolic and diastolic pressures and the prevalence of hypertension vary throughout the world. Many data suggest a linear rise in blood pressure at increasing distances from the equator. Similarly, blood pressure is higher in winter than summer. Previously, it has been hypothesized that reduced epidermal vitamin D_3 photosynthesis associated with decreased UV light intensity at distances from the equator, alone or when coupled with decreased dietary calcium and vitamin D, may be associated with reduced vitamin D stores and increased parathyroid hormone secretion (Rostand 1997). These changes may stimulate growth of vascular smooth muscle and enhance its contractility by affecting intracellular calcium, adrenergic responsiveness, and/or endothelial function. Thus, UV light intensity and efficiency of epidermal vitamin D_3 photosynthesis may contribute to geographic and racial variability in blood pressure and the prevalence of hypertension (Rostand 1997).

However, there might exist another or additional supporting mechanism (Fig. 6.7), respectively, by which ambient electromagnetic radiation may affect blood pressure. As already mentioned above Robert Furchgott and his colleagues noted as long ago as 1961 that exposure to sun light relaxed isolated arterial preparations (Furchgott et al. 1961). The vascular photo relaxation was wavelength dependent to UV radiation, and photo relaxation was markedly potentiated by

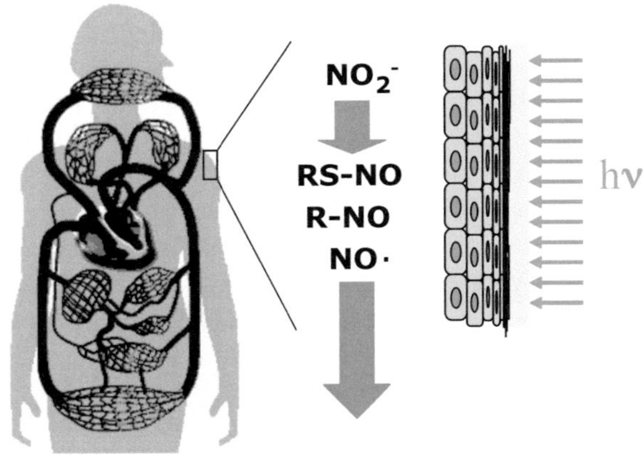

Fig. 6.7 Local and/or systemic effects

solutions containing nitrite (Furchgott 1991; Furchgott and Jothianandan 1991; Wigilius et al. 1990), indicating that under certain circumstances nitrite may exhibit relaxing activities comparable to NO.

Indeed, Oplander et al. could show that UVA-irradiation of healthy human skin significantly increased intra-cutaneous nitric oxide and S-nitrosothiol concentrations due to decomposition of cutaneous photo-labile NO-derivates with the result of significantly enhanced concentration of plasma nitroso compounds and a pronounced decrease in systemic blood pressure (Oplander et al. 2009). The observation of systemic UVA-response can be plausibly explained by a mechanism comprising three elementary steps. First, UVA liberates nitric oxide from photo-labile intra-cutaneous NO metabolites. Second, a fraction of the highly mobile NO diffuses towards the outer surface where it escapes into the ambient atmosphere (This fraction is detectable with the airtight skin chamber mentioned above). Another NO fraction diffuses to deeper tissue layers, where it enters the capillary vessels and enhances local levels of RS-NO. These nitrosated species might be low molecular weight like glutathione-S-NO or protein bound high molecular weight like albumin-S-NO. Third, the fairly stable nitroso compounds are distributed via the blood circulation where it may elicit a systemic response like a drop in blood pressure. We note that the vasodilating and hypotensive properties of S-nitrosothiols are well documented (Rassaf and Kelm 2007).

These systemic effects significantly correlated with increased concentrations of nitroso compounds in the systemic circulation. As the observed effects were attributed to photolysis of cutaneous nitrite, UVA-induced physiological responses might be enhanced by loading the skin with photo-labile NO derivates prior to irradiation. Alternatively, endogenous photo-sensitive NO derivates may be modulated by control over dietary nitrate and nitrite intake (Larsen et al. 2006; Lundberg et al. 2008). These findings reveal the impact of light as an environmental parameter contributing to the phenomenon of "French paradox" and thus might have potential for the therapeutic applications in diseases with hypertension. It is well known that vegetarians have smaller risk of developing hypertension and other cardiovascular diseases, and it has been speculated that the high nitrate/nitrite content of many vegetables may contribute to these cardioprotective effects.

6.6 Mechanism and Relevance of Nitrite Photolysis by Blue Light

Beside UVA radiation also electromagnetic radiation within the blue spectrum (420–490 nm) is able to generate NO via photodecomposition of the nitrite ion as well as of S-nitroso thiols in aqueous solutions. In analogy to UVA, blue light was shown also to induce non-enzymatic NO formation from photo-labile NO precursors in human skin tissue in vitro and in vivo, which was characterized by a significantly enhanced migration of nitrite-derived NO from the apical side of irradiated skin to deeper regions of skin tissue, increased intracutaneous formation of S-nitroso compounds, and significantly augmented local blood flow due to vasodilation of the concerned dermal blood vessels (Oplander et al. 2013). In analogy to UVA, these observations of a local hemodynamic response of blue light can be plausibly explained by a mechanism comprising two elementary steps. First, blue light liberates nitric oxide from photo-labile intra-cutaneous NO metabolites. Second, a fraction of the highly mobile NO diffuses to deeper tissue layers, where it enters the capillary vessels, and exerts NO-specific biological responses.

Blue light at wavelengths of 420 and 453 nm is close in wavelength to UVA and therefore relatively energy-rich but without the pronounced reactive oxygen species (ROS)-generating properties of UVA radiation. With human skin cell cultures exposure to light at 453 nm was shown to be nontoxic up to a fluence of 500 J cm^{-2} (Liebmann et al. 2010; Oplander et al. 2011). In contrast, with UVA in most cases the appearance of light-induced injuries already appeared at doses of 10–30 J cm^{-2} (Oplander et al. 2007, 2008; Suschek et al. 1999, 2001b). Furthermore, even at therapeutically non-relevant high doses of 200 J cm^{-2} blue light (453 nm) did not induce DNA strand breaks, whereas with 100 J cm^{-2} of UVA a strongly positive TUNEL signal could be observed.

Experimental energies of activation for the decomposition of S-nitroso compounds (RS-NOs) have been reported by different groups to range from +23 to +34 kcal mol^{-1} (Koppenol 2012; Zhao et al. 2005). Therefore, in vitro irradiation of solutions with visible light in the range from 410 nm up to 590 nm, which corresponds to a radiation energy range from +69.7 to approx. +48.5 kcal mol^{-1}, leads to significant photodecomposition of S-nitroso-albumin. On the other side, the finding of photo-decomposition of the nitrite ion by blue light is unexpected, because for the nitrite ion the calculated energy of the transition state (+87.4 kcal mol^{-1}) and the N–O bonding energy (+93.3 kcal mol^{-1}) are predicted to be notably higher than the radiation energies corresponding to 420 or 453 nm (+68 or 63 kcal mol^{-1}), respectively. Thus, blue-light induced NO formation from nitrite has to follow fundamentally different mechanisms than the well-known of UVA-induced nitrite decomposition (Oplander et al. 2010). Indeed, blue-light induced nitrite decomposition needs the presence of cupric ion (Cu^{2+}) traces. Moreover, decomposition of nitrite by blue light is essentially dependent on the formation and presence of the reduced cuprous form, on Cu^{1+}. In copper-decontaminated pure aqueous solutions or in the presence of Cu^{1+}-specific chelators photo-decomposition of nitrite is completely absent (Oplander et al. 2013).

By studying the absorption spectra of a number of heavy-metal nitrite salts (Ni^{2+}, Ag^{+}, Pb^{2+} Cd^{2+}, Ti^{+}) Maria et al. found near 425 nm a further absorption maximum, which corresponds to the spin-forbidden transition from the ground singlet state to the first excited triplet state of the nitrite ion (Maria et al. 1968a, 1969). Furthermore, in the presence of Cu^{2+} aqueous nitrite solutions exhibit also an apparent absorption increase near 425 nm, whereas neither Fe^{2+}- nor Fe^{3+}-containing nitrite solutions showed a comparable shift in the UV-vis absorption spectrum. Thus, copper salts catalyze under blue-light exposure the spin-forbidden formation of the intermediate triplet-nitrite ($^3NO_2^-$) (Maria et al. 1968b, 1969):

$$Cu^{2+} + NO_2^- \rightarrow \left[Cu^{2+} NO_2^-\right] + 63 \text{ kcal mol}^{-1} \rightarrow \left[Cu^{2+\,3}NO_2^-\right] \qquad (6.6)$$

The postulated step in Eq. 6.6 represents experimentally accepted data. The lifetime of the triplet state of nitrite in solution is very sensitive to the nature of the associated metal ion, varying from $\sim 10^{-1}$ s in $NaNO_2$ to 10^{-4} s in $Pb(NO_2)_2$ (Maria et al. 1968a). Thus, transitions metal do double duty because they accelerate under blue-light irradiation the spin-forbidden formation of $^3NO_2^-$ and they accelerate the decay of this intermediate. Nevertheless, the lifetime of the triplet molecule is, of course, short but high enough to allow principally a $^3NO_2^-$-derived chemistry. On the basis of the accepted electron affinity of 55.35 kcal mol^{-1} for NO_2 (Richardson et al. 1974) and a value of 177.6 kcal mol^{-1} for the ionization potential of Cu^{1+}, partial transfer of the electron from NO_2^- towards Cu^{2+} would certainly be energetically feasible with the excited $^3NO_2^-$ state. Such a proposed ligand to metal charge transfer has previously been shown to play a role in thallium (Tl) sensitized photolysis of the nitrite ion in Tl–NO_2 complex-containing solutions (Cunningham et al. 1985), which exhibit comparable thermodynamic values to copper-nitrite complexes. The following mechanisms of Cu^{1+}-mediated nitrite reduction could be similar to the mechanism as outlined in Eqs. 6.7–6.9.

$$\left[Cu^{2+\,3}NO_2^-\right] \rightarrow Cu^{1+} + NO_2 \qquad (6.7)$$

$$2\ NO_2 + H_2O \rightarrow NO_2^- + NO_3^- + 2\ H^+ \qquad (6.8)$$

$$Cu^{1+} + NO_2^- \rightarrow \left[Cu^{1+} NO_2^-\right] + H^+ \rightarrow Cu^{2+} + H_2O + NO \qquad (6.9)$$

Nevertheless, the astute reader must ask the question whether these conclusions and proposed mechanisms of blue light-induced NO formation in vitro or in human skin specimens can be transferred to the in vivo situation. It is well accepted that in a biological milieu free copper ions are sparingly soluble under physiological conditions and attach to ceruloplasmin, albumin, transcuprein, and other copper-amino acid complexes, which function as copper transport forms in vivo. As protein-bound copper ions loose their catalytic properties for blue light-induced nitrite reduction, it seems to be very unlikely that photodecomposition of nitrite might play a significant role within human skin tissue. Nevertheless, on skin surface as well as in sweat nitrite at concentration of up to 12 μM, and free copper concentrations of approx. 10 μM have been detected. Thus, on human skin surface the prerequisite for successful NO formation from nitrite is given. Furthermore, application of nitrite/Cu^{2+}-containing liniments prior to light exposure could be used to exponentiate epicutaneous NO formation. Indeed, due to the excellent diffusion properties of NO, epicutaneous NO generation by blue light led to a rapid translocation of nitric oxide from the apical part of the skin and to a significant accumulation of NO derivates even in deeper tissue regions beneath the irradiated skin area, finally resulting in an up to 10-fold increased plasma concentration of vasoactive NO derivates in the epidermal as well as dermal layer of human skin, i.e. S-nitrosothiols RS-NOs (Oplander et al. 2013). In the case of UVA the dermal fraction of S-nitrosated compounds predominantly represented S-nitroso-albumin, which due to absent circulation activity in the skin specimens reflect the blood or serum filling of cutaneous microvasculature (Oplander et al. 2009). Functioning as a transport form for nitric oxide, S-nitroso-albumin will favor its rapid local but also systemic distribution as well as its vaso-availability. S-nitroso-albumin has been previously proposed to act as a reservoir of NO within the circulation, transporting and releasing NO into vascular beds to cause vasodilation. Because blue light has been shown to penetrate the epidermis and reaching dermal regions down to 1.5 mm, by exposure to blue light the entire potential for cutaneous as well as intra-vasal dermal photo-labile RS-NOs can be retrieved for non-enzymatic NO formation. We therefore postulate that the observed effects of blue light on local increases in vasodilation and blood flow predominantly were due to photodecomposition of RS-NOs. Of course, principally every other kind of visible light with the respective energy intake would be able to contribute to NO formation via photodecomposition of RS-NOs. Nevertheless, in order to reach comparable NO yields already with green light many-fold higher irradiances than that of a blue light-emitting LED array would have to be used (Oplander et al. 2013).

It is important to mention that under otherwise identical conditions blue light-induced NO accumulation in human skin tissue is comparable to that found in human skin after UVA exposure. In both cases the resulted NO derivate concentrations are sufficient to induce significant increases in local blood flow or even reduction in systemic blood pressure (Oplander et al. 2009, 2012). Thus, concerning the potency for intracutaneous NO generation from RS-NOs, blue light is comparable to UVA-induced effects. These findings reveal the impact and relevance of visible, especially blue light as an environmental parameter with therapeutic potential for local or systemic hemodynamic disorders that might arise from insufficient availability of NO or its bio-active NO derivates, respectively (Fig. 6.7).

References

Adler H, Beland JL, Del-Pan NC, Kobzik L, Brewer JP, Martin TR, Rimm IJ (1997) Suppression of herpes simplex virus type 1 (HSV-1)-induced pneumonia in mice by inhibition of inducible nitric oxide synthase (iNOS, NOS2). J Exp Med 185:1533–1540

Anastasio C, Chu L (2009) Photochemistry of nitrous acid (HONO) and nitrous acidium ion (H2ONO) in aqueous solution and ice. Environ Sci Technol 43:1108–1114

Anderson RR, Parrish JA (1981) The optics of human-skin. J. Invest Dermatol 77:13–19

Anggard E (1994) Nitric oxide: mediator, murderer, and medicine. Lancet 343:1199–1206

Ashcroft GS, Greenwell-Wild T, Horan MA, Wahl SM, Ferguson MW (1999) Topical estrogen accelerates cutaneous wound healing in aged humans associated with an altered inflammatory response. Am J Pathol 155:1137–1146

Benjamin N, Pattullo S, Weller R, Smith L, Ormerod A (1997) Wound licking and nitric oxide. Lancet 349:1776

Bruch-Gerharz D, Ruzicka T, Kolb-Bachofen V (1998a) Nitric oxide and its implications in skin homeostasis and disease—a review. Arch Dermatol Res 290:643–651

Bruch-Gerharz D, Ruzicka T, Kolb-Bachofen V (1998b) Nitric oxide in human skin: current status and future prospects. J. Invest Dermatol 110:1–7

Bruch-Gerharz D, Schnorr O, Suschek C, Beck KF, Pfeilschifter J, Ruzicka T, Kolb-Bachofen V (2003) Arginase 1 overexpression in psoriasis: limitation of inducible nitric oxide synthase activity as a molecular mechanism for keratinocyte hyperproliferation. Am J Pathol 162: 203–211

Cals-Grierson MM, Ormerod AD (2004) Nitric oxide function in the skin. Nitric Oxide 10: 179–193

Corson MA, James NL, Latta SE, Nerem RM, Berk BC, Harrison DG (1996) Phosphorylation of endothelial nitric oxide synthase in response to fluid shear stress. Circ Res 79:984–991

Cunningham ML, Johnson JS, Giovanazzi SM, Peak MJ (1985) Photosensitized production of superoxide anion by monochromatic (290–405 nm) ultraviolet irradiation of NADH and NADPH coenzymes. Photochem Photobiol 42:125–128

Deliconstantinos G, Villiotou V, Fassitsas C (1992) Ultraviolet-irradiated human endothelial cells elaborate nitric oxide that may evoke vasodilatory response. J Cardiovasc Pharmacol 20(Suppl 12):S63–S65

Deliconstantinos G, Villiotu V, Stravides JC (1995) Release by ultraviolet B (u.v.B.) radiation of nitric oxide (NO) from human keratinocytes: a potential role for nitric oxide in erythema production. Br J Pharmacol 114:1257–1265

Ehrreich SJ, Furchgott RF (1968) Relaxation of mammalian smooth muscles by visible and ultraviolet radiation. Nature 218:682–684

Feelisch M, Rassaf T, Mnaimneh S, Singh N, Bryan NS, Jourd'Heuil D, Kelm M (2002) Concomitant S-, N-, and heme-nitros(yl)ation in biological tissues and fluids: implications for the fate of NO in vivo. Faseb J 16:1775–1785

Fischer M, Warneck P (1996) Photodecomposition of nitrite and undissociated nitrous acid in aqueous solution. J Phys Chem 100:18749–18756

Frank S, Madlener M, Pfeilschifter J, Werner S (1998) Induction of inducible nitric oxide synthase and its corresponding tetrahydrobiopterin-cofactor-synthesizing enzyme GTP-cyclohydrolase I during cutaneous wound repair. J. Invest. Dermatol. 111:1058–1064

Frank S, Stallmeyer B, Kampfer H, Kolb N, Pfeilschifter J (1999) Nitric oxide triggers enhanced induction of vascular endothelial growth factor expression in cultured keratinocytes (HaCaT) and during cutaneous wound repair. FASEB J. 13:2002–2014

Frank S, Kampfer H, Wetzler C, Pfeilschifter J (2002) Nitric oxide drives skin repair: novel functions of an established mediator. Kidney Int 61:882–888

Furchgott RF (1991) Endothelium-dependent relaxation, endothelium-derived relaxing factor and photorelaxation of blood vessels. Semin Perinatol 15:11–15

Furchgott RF, Jothianandan D (1991) Endothelium-dependent and -independent vasodilation involving cyclic GMP: relaxation induced by nitric oxide, carbon monoxide and light. Blood Vessels 28:52–61

Furchgott RF, Ehrreich SJ, Greenblatt E (1961) The photoactivated relaxation of smooth muscle of rabbit aorta. J Gen Physiol 44:499–519

Goldsmith PC, Leslie TA, Hayes NA, Levell NJ, Dowd PA, Foreman JC (1996) Inhibitors of nitric oxide synthase in human skin. J Invest Dermatol 106:113–118

Halliwell B, Gutteridge J (1989) Free radicals in biology and medicine, 2nd edn. Oxford University Press, Oxford

Herrling T, Zastrow L, Fuchs J, Groth N (2002) Electron spin resonance detection of UVA-induced free radicals. Skin Pharmacol Appl Skin Physiol 15:381–383

Holan V, Krulova M, Zajicova A, Pindjakova J (2002) Nitric oxide as a regulatory and effector molecule in the immune system. Mol Immunol 38:989–995

Kellogg DL Jr, Crandall CG, Liu Y, Charkoudian N, Johnson JM (1998) Nitric oxide and cutaneous active vasodilation during heat stress in humans. J Appl Physiol 85:824–829

Kellogg DL Jr, Liu Y, Kosiba IF, O'Donnell D (1999) Role of nitric oxide in the vascular effects of local warming of the skin in humans. J Appl Physiol 86:1185–1190

Kirsch M, Korth HG, Sustmann R, de Groot H (2002) The pathobiochemistry of nitrogen dioxide. Biol Chem 383:389–399

Knowles RG, Moncada S (1994) Nitric oxide synthases in mammals. Biochem J 298(Pt 2): 249–258

Koppenol WH (2012) Nitrosation, thiols, and hemoglobin: energetics and kinetics. Inorg Chem 51:5637–5641

Krischel V, Bruch-Gerharz D, Suschek C, Kröncke K-D, Ruzicka T, Kolb-Bachofen V (1998) Biphasic effect of exogenous nitric oxide on proliferation and differentiation in skin derived keratinocytes but not fibroblasts. J Invest Dermatol 111:286–291

Kröncke KD, Suschek CV, Kolb-Bachofen V (2000) Implications of inducible nitric oxide synthase expression and enzyme activity. Antioxid Redox Signal 2:585–605

Kröncke KD, Fehsel K, Kolb-Bachofen V (1997) Nitric oxide: cytotoxicity versus cytoprotection–how, why, when, and where? Nitric Oxide 1:107–120

Kröncke KD, Fehsel K, Kolb-Bachofen V (1998) Inducible nitric oxide synthase in human diseases. Clin Exp Immunol 113:147–156

Larsen FJ, Ekblom B, Sahlin K, Lundberg JO, Weitzberg E (2006) Effects of dietary nitrate on blood pressure in healthy volunteers. N Engl J Med 355:2792–2793

Lee SC, Lee JW, Jung JE, Lee HW, Chun SD, Kang IK, Won YH, Kim YP (2000) Protective role of nitric oxide-mediated inflammatory response against lipid peroxidation in ultraviolet B-irradiated skin. Br J Dermatol 142:653–659

Lerner LH, Qureshi AA, Reddy BV, Lerner EA (2000) Nitric oxide synthase in toxic epidermal necrolysis and Stevens-Johnson syndrome. J Invest Dermatol 114:196–199

Liebmann J, Born M, Kolb-Bachofen V (2010) Blue-light irradiation regulates proliferation and differentiation in human skin cells. J Invest Dermatol 130:259–269

Lundberg JO, Weitzberg E, Gladwin MT (2008) The nitrate-nitrite-nitric oxide pathway in physiology and therapeutics. Nat Rev Drug Discov 7:156–167

Mack J, Bolton J (1999) Photochemistry of nitrite and nitrate in aqueous solution: a review. J Photochem Photobiol, B A128:1–13

Maria HJ, Armstrong AT, McGlynn SP (1968a) Luminescence of inorganic nitrite salts. J Chem Phys 48:4694–4697

Maria HJ, Wahlborg A, McGlynn SP (1968b) Triplet state of the nitrite molecule-ion. J Chem Phys 49:4925–4928

Maria HJ, Armstrong AT, McGlynn SP (1969) Spin polarization in the triplet state of silver nitrite. J Chem Phys 50:2777–2778

Matsunaga K, Furchgott RF (1989) Interactions of light and sodium nitrite in producing relaxation of rabbit aorta. J Pharmacol Exp Ther 248:687–695

Miranda KM, Espey MG, Jourd'heuil D, Grisham MB, Fukuto J, Feelisch M, Wink DA (2000) The chemical biology of nitric oxide. In: Ignarro LJ (eds) Nitric oxide: biology and pathobiology. Academic Press, San Diego, pp 41–56
Mowbray M, McLintock S, Weerakoon R, Lomatschinsky N, Jones S, Rossi AG, Weller RB (2008) Enzyme-Independent NO stores in human skin: quantification and influence of UV radiation. J Invest Dermatol 129:834–842
Oplander C, Cortese MM, Korth HG, Kirsch M, Mahotka C, Wetzel W, Pallua N, Suschek CV (2007) The impact of nitrite and antioxidants on ultraviolet-A-induced cell death of human skin fibroblasts. Free Radic Biol Med 43:818–829
Oplander C, Wetzel W, Cortese MM, Pallua N, Suschek CV (2008) Evidence for a physiological role of intracellularly occurring photolabile nitrogen oxides in human skin fibroblasts. Free Radic Biol Med 44:1752–1761
Oplander C, Volkmar CM, Paunel-Gorgulu A, van Faassen EE, Heiss C, Kelm M, Halmer D, Murtz M, Pallua N, Suschek CV (2009) Whole body UVA irradiation lowers systemic blood pressure by Release of nitric oxide from intracutaneous photolabile nitric oxide derivates. Circ Res Sep 24 [Epub ahead of print]
Oplander C, Baschin M, Faassen EE, Born M, Moller M, Pallua N, Suschek CV (2010) A new method for sustained generation of ultra-pure nitric oxide-containing gas mixtures via controlled UVA-photolysis of nitrite solutions. Nitric Oxide Biol, Chem
Oplander C, Hidding S, Werners FB, Born M, Pallua N, Suschek CV (2011) Effects of blue light irradiation on human dermal fibroblasts. J Photochem Photobiol, B 103:118–125
Oplander C, Romer A, Paunel-Gorgulu A, Fritsch T, van Faassen EE, Murtz M, Bozkurt A, Grieb G, Fuchs P, Pallua N, Suschek CV (2012) Dermal application of nitric oxide in vivo: kinetics, biological responses, and therapeutic potential in humans. Clin Pharmacol Ther 91:1074–1082
Oplander C, Deck A, Volkmar CM, Kirsch M, Liebmann J, Born M, van Abeelen F, van Faassen EE, Kröncke KD, Windolf J, Suschek CV (2013) Mechanism and biological relevance of blue-light (420–453 nm)-induced nonenzymatic nitric oxide generation from photolabile nitric oxide derivates in human skin in vitro and in vivo. Free Radic Biol Med 65:1363–1377
Ormerod AD, Copeland P, Hay I, Husain A, Ewen SW (1999) The inflammatory and cytotoxic effects of a nitric oxide releasing cream on normal skin. J Invest Dermatol 113:392–397
Paunel AN, Dejam A, Thelen S, Kirsch M, Horstjann M, Gharini P, Murtz M, Kelm M, de Groot H, Kolb-Bachofen V, Suschek CV (2005) Enzyme-independent nitric oxide formation during UVA challenge of human skin: characterization, molecular sources, and mechanisms. Free Radic Biol Med 38:606–615
Rassaf T, Kelm M (2007) Nitrite and nitrosospecies in blood and tissue: approaching the gap between bench and bedside. In: van Faassen EE, Vanin AF (eds) Radicals for life: the various forms of nitric oxide. Elsevier, Amsterdam, pp 269–288
Rhodes LE, Belgi G, Parslew R, McLoughlin L, Clough GF, Friedmann PS (2001) Ultraviolet-B-induced erythema is mediated by nitric oxide and prostaglandin E2 in combination. J Invest Dermatol 117:880–885
Richardson JH, Stephenson LM, Brauman JI (1974) Photodetachment of NO_2—; experimental evidence for a new isomer. Chem Phys Lett 25:318–320
Rostand SG (1997) Ultraviolet light may contribute to geographic and racial blood pressure differences. Hypertension 30:150–156
Sasaki M, Yamaoka J, Miyachi Y (2000) The effect of ultraviolet B irradiation on nitric oxide synthase expression in murine keratinocytes. Exp Dermatol 9:417–422
Seo SJ, Choi HG, Chung HJ, Hong CK (2002) Time course of expression of mRNA of inducible nitric oxide synthase and generation of nitric oxide by ultraviolet B in keratinocyte cell lines. Br J Dermatol 147:655–662
Shi HP, Most D, Efron DT, Tantry U, Fischel MH, Barbul A (2001) The role of iNOS in wound healing. Surgery 130:225–229
Sies H (1986) Biochemistry of oxidative stress. Angew Chem Int Ed 25:1058–1071

Stamler JS, Simon DI, Osborne JA, Mullins ME, Jaraki O, Michel T, Singel DJ, Loscalzo J (1992) S-nitrosylation of proteins with nitric oxide: synthesis and characterization of biologically active compounds. Proc Natl Acad Sci USA 89:444–448

Sur R, Heck DE, Mariano TM, Jin Y, Murphy WJ, Laskin JD (2002) UVB light suppresses nitric oxide production by murine keratinocytes and macrophages. Biochem Pharmacol 64:1469–1481

Suschek CV, Krischel V, Bruch-Gerharz D, Berendji D, Krutmann J, Kröncke K-D, Kolb-Bachofen V (1999) Nitric oxide fully protects against UVA-induced apoptosis in tight correlation with Bcl-2 up-regulation. J Biol Chem 274:6130–6137

Suschek CV, Briviba K, Bruch-Gerharz D, Sies H, Kröncke KD, Kolb-Bachofen V (2001a) Even after UVA-exposure will nitric oxide protect cells from reactive oxygen intermediate-mediated apoptosis and necrosis. Cell Death Differ 8:515–527

Suschek CV, Bruch-Gerharz D, Kleinert H, Forstermann U, Kolb-Bachofen V (2001b) Ultraviolet al radiation induces nitric oxide synthase-2 expression in human skin endothelial cells in the absence of proinflammatory cytokines. J Invest Dermatol 117:1200–1205

Suschek CV, Schnorr O, Hemmrich K, Aust O, Klotz LO, Sies H, Kolb-Bachofen V (2003a) Critical role of L-arginine in endothelial cell survival during oxidative stress. Circulation 107:2607–2614

Suschek CV, Schroeder P, Aust O, Sies H, Mahotka C, Horstjann M, Ganser H, Murtz M, Hering P, Schnorr O, Kröncke KD, Kolb-Bachofen V (2003b) The presence of nitrite during UVA irradiation protects from apoptosis. Faseb J 17:2342–2344

Suschek CV, Mahotka C, Schnorr O, Kolb-Bachofen V (2004) UVB radiation-mediated expression of inducible nitric oxide synthase activity and the augmenting role of co-induced TNF-alpha in human skin endothelial cells. J Invest Dermatol 123:950–957

Suschek CV, Oplander C, van Faassen EE (2010) Non-enzymatic NO production in human skin: effect of UVA on cutaneous NO stores. Nitric Oxide 22:120–135

Suzuki T, Inukai M (2006) Effects of nitrite and nitrate on DNA damage induced by ultraviolet light. Chem Res Toxicol 19:457–462

Szabo E, Virag L, Bakondi E, Gyure L, Hasko G, Bai P, Hunyadi J, Gergely P, Szabo C (2001) Peroxynitrite production, DNA breakage, and poly(ADP-ribose) polymerase activation in a mouse model of oxazolone-induced contact hypersensitivity. J Invest Dermatol 117:74–80

Teixeira MM, Williams TJ, Hellewell PG (1993) Role of prostaglandins and nitric oxide in acute inflammatory reactions in guinea-pig skin. Br J Pharmacol 110:1515–1521

Townley SL, Grimbaldeston MA, Ferguson I, Rush RA, Zhang SH, Zhou XF, Conner JM, Finlay-Jones JJ, Hart PH (2002) Nerve growth factor, neuropeptides, and mast cells in ultraviolet-B-induced systemic suppression of contact hypersensitivity responses in mice. J Invest Dermatol 118:396–401

Treinin A, Hayon E (1970) Absorption spectra and reaction kinetics of NO2, N2O3, and N2O4 in aqueous solution. J Am Chem Soc 92:5821–5828

Vallette G, Tenaud I, Branka JE, Jarry A, Sainte-Marie I, Dreno B, Laboisse CL (1998) Control of growth and differentiation of normal human epithelial cells through the manipulation of reactive nitrogen species. Biochem J 331(Pt 3):713–717

van Faassen EE, Vanin AF (2007) Low-molecular-weight S-nitrosothiols. In: van Faassen EE, Vanin AF (eds) Radicals for life: the various forms of nitric oxide. Elsevier, Amsterdam, pp 173–199

Warren JB (1994) Nitric oxide and human skin blood flow responses to acetylcholine and ultraviolet light. FASEB J 8:247–251

Warren JB, Loi RK, Coughlan ML (1993) Involvement of nitric oxide synthase in the delayed vasodilator response to ultraviolet light irradiation of rat skin in vivo. Br J Pharmacol 109:802–806

Weller R (2003) Nitric oxide: a key mediator in cutaneous physiology. Clin Exp Dermatol 28:511–514

Weller R, Pattullo S, Smith L, Golden M, Ormerod A, Benjamin N (1996) Nitric oxide is generated on the skin surface by reduction of sweat nitrate. J Invest Dermatol 107:327–331

Weller R, Dykhuizen R, Leifert C, Ormerod A (1997) Nitric oxide release accounts for the reduced incidence of cutaneous infections in psoriasis. J Am Acad Dermatol 36:281–282

Weller R, Price RJ, Ormerod AD, Benjamin N, Leifert C (2001) Antimicrobial effect of acidified nitrite on dermatophyte fungi, Candida and bacterial skin pathogens. J Appl Microbiol 90:648–652

Weller R, Schwentker A, Billiar TR, Vodovotz Y (2003) Autologous nitric oxide protects mouse and human keratinocytes from ultraviolet B radiation-induced apoptosis. Am J Physiol Cell Physiol 284:C1140–C1148

Wigilius IM, Axelsson KL, Andersson RG, Karlsson JO, Odman S (1990) Effects of sodium nitrite on ultraviolet light-induced relaxation and ultraviolet light-dependent activation of guanylate cyclase in bovine mesenteric arteries. Biochem Biophys Res Commun 169:129–135

Zafiriou OC, Bonneau R (1987) Wavelength-dependent quantum yield of OH radical formation from photolysis of nitrite ion in water. Photochem Photobiol 45:723–727

Zhao YL, McCarren PR, Houk KN, Choi BY, Toone EJ (2005) Nitrosonium-catalyzed decomposition of s-nitrosothiols in solution: a theoretical and experimental study. J Am Chem Soc 127:10917–10924

Chapter 7
Melanocortin 1 Receptor (MC1R) as a Global Regulator of Cutaneous UV Responses: Molecular Interactions and Opportunities for Melanoma Prevention

Erin M. Wolf Horrell and John A. D'Orazio

Abstract UV radiation is a pervasive environmental agent that affects the skin in complex ways. It benefits human health by its contribution to the biosynthesis of vitamin D in the skin, however it also is a major carcinogen responsible for millions of skin cancers diagnosed each year. One of the most important physiologic responses recruited with UV exposure is the melanocortin signaling axis. This pathway, initiated by melanocortins such as melanocyte stimulating hormone (α-MSH) or adrenocorticotropic hormone (ACTH), is dependent on the signaling function of the melanocortin 1 receptor (MC1R), a G_s protein-coupled cell surface receptor found on melanocytes in the skin. MC1R mediates its downstream UV-protective responses through activation of adenylyl cyclase and production of the second messenger cAMP. In melanocytes, cAMP stimulation leads to improved survival and UV-defensive sequelae. Here, we review how MC1R signaling protects melanocytes from UV-induced malignant degeneration, focusing on recent insights into molecular links between MC1R signaling and the nucleotide excision repair (NER) genome maintenance pathway. Finally, we highlight how insights into the MC1R UV protective response may facilitate the development of rational melanoma-protective strategies.

Keywords Melanocyte · Melanoma · UV radiation · Mutation · MC1R · Melanocortin · Skin cancer · ATR · cAMP · PKA · DNA repair

E.M. Wolf Horrell
Department of Physiology, University of Kentucky College of Medicine, Lexington, USA

J.A. D'Orazio (✉)
Departments of Pediatrics, Toxicology and Cancer Biology, Physiology, and Pharmacology and Nutritional Sciences, University of Kentucky College of Medicine, Markey Cancer Center, 800 Rose Street, Combs 204, Lexington, KY 40536-0096, USA
e-mail: jdorazio@uky.edu

G.T. Wondrak (ed.), *Skin Stress Response Pathways*,
DOI 10.1007/978-3-319-43157-4_7

7.1 Introduction

Diagnosed in almost 70,000 Americans per year, melanoma is the most lethal skin cancer and claims the lives of nearly 10,000 people each year in the US (Simard et al. 2012). Like other skin cancer, melanoma has a clear association with UV and incidence increases with age due to the cumulative effects of mutations over time. Melanoma, which is derived from melanocytes, accounts for approximately 4 % of skin tumors but accounts for about three quarters of all deaths by skin cancer (Narayanan et al. 2010). Melanoma metastasizes relatively quickly and once it has spread is difficult to control. In contrast, the keratinocyte-derived skin malignancies (basal cell carcinomas and squamous cell carcinomas) are diagnosed more often but are much less deadly because most remain confined to their primary site of origin and are amenable to local control measures such as surgical resection. Because melanoma incidence has been increasing for many years (Linos et al. 2009), our research focuses on understanding early events in melanoma carcinogenesis in order to reduce melanoma morbidity and mortality through the development of rational interventions. Abundant molecular and epidemiologic data link melanoma to UV (Hodis et al. 2012; Lawrence et al. 2013; Shain et al. 2015), and it is estimated that UV causes nearly 65 % of melanomas (Pleasance et al. 2010). Risk of melanoma is also heavily influenced by skin complexion, with more darkly pigmented individuals being relatively protected from disease. A major reason why darkly pigmented people are protected from melanoma is the abundance of melanin in the epidermis which acts as a "built-in sunblock" to physically interfere with UV penetration into the skin. However it is now evident that certain pigment-regulating genes also influence melanocytic UV responses in melanin-independent ways that heavily influence UV mutagenesis, which is the focus of this chapter. Since UV signature mutations are frequently found in melanoma, it follows that resistance to UV-induced DNA changes is of paramount importance to melanoma risk.

7.2 The Skin

The great majority of melanomas are thought to initiate in the skin. The largest organ of the body, the skin accounts for approximately 16 % of total body mass. Skin is a complex tissue made up of two primary layers—the epidermis and the dermis—along with numerous specialized cells and structures of epithelial, mesenchymal, glandular and neurovascular components. The epidermis, derived from embryonic ectoderm, is the outermost layer of the skin and serves as the main protective barrier for the body's interaction with the external environment. The epidermis is critically important to resisting environmental stressors such as foreign microorganisms, chemical and physical agents and UV. The epidermis is mainly

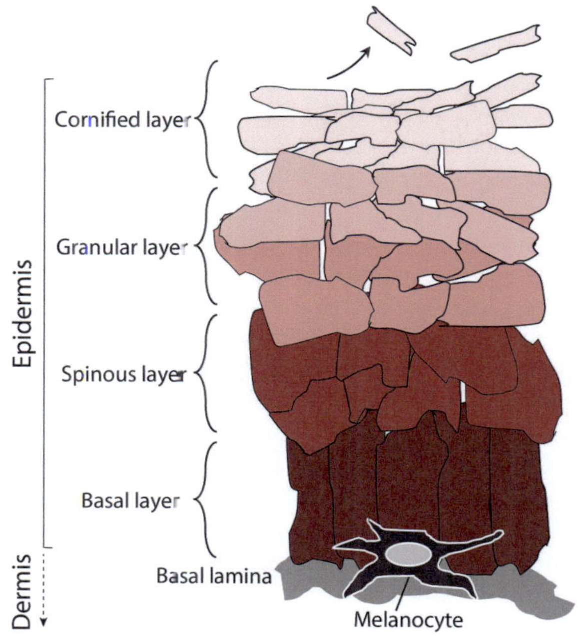

Fig. 7.1 Structure of the epidermis. The outermost layer of the skin is the epidermis, a self-renewing tissue composed mainly of keratinocytes in various stages of terminal differentiation. Nascent keratinocytes are produced in the basal layer (stratum basale). As they move outward through the epidermis, displaced by newly formed cells below, they differentiate into cytokeratin-rich cells linked to each other by tight junctions to form an effective physico-chemical barrier layer. Keratinocytes receive melanin pigments made from melanocytes, the pigment producing cells in the skin

made up of keratinocytes, which are epithelial cells organized into distinct layers defined largely by intercellular associations, nucleation and differential cytokeratin expression (Fig. 7.1). Keratinocytes are the most abundant cells in the epidermis and are characterized by their expression of cytokeratins and formation of desmosomes and tight junctions that together make the skin highly resistant to environmental stressors and pathogens. The dermis, derived from mesoderm, underlies and supports the epidermis and harbors cutaneous structures including hair follicles, nerves, sebaceous glands and sweat glands. Dermal immune cells and fibroblasts actively participate in many physiologic cutaneous responses. The dermis is separated from the epidermis by a basement membrane known as the basal layer which is where epidermal melanocytes are positioned. Epidermal keratinocytes, derived from keratinocyte stem cells in the basal layer, differentiate as they move outward toward the surface of the skin, accumulating cytokeratins, losing their nuclei and adhering to each other. As they mature, keratinocytes also accumulate melanin pigments that block incoming UV radiation from penetrating the epidermis to reach cells deep in the skin.

Although the majority of epidermal melanin may be in keratinocytes, it is not made by keratinocytes. Rather, melanin is exclusively synthesized in melanocytes which are neural crest-derived dendritic cells found in dermal hair follicles as well as in the interfollicular epidermis in the basal layer. Melanocytes intimately associate with several maturing keratinocytes by way of their dendritic processes. Through this interaction, keratinocytes and melanocytes signal each other through contact-dependent and paracrine interactions and melanin pigments are passed from melanocytes to keratinocytes. It has been estimated that an epidermal melanocyte may be functionally associated with as many as fifty keratinocytes in what has been termed an "epidermal melanin unit" (Nordlund 2007). In melanocytes, pigment is made in discreet intracellular organelles known as melanosomes which are membrane bound and contain the necessary enzymes and ion channels needed for melanogenesis. As melanin accumulates, melanosomes are transported away from perinuclear regions of the melanocytes along dendrites for eventual transfer to keratinocytes in the epidermal melanin unit. Rather than being released by exocytosis into the extracellular milieu, melanin is transferred to keratinocytes still packaged in melanosomes that are actively exported from melanocytes and taken up intact by neighboring keratinocytes (Yamaguchi and Hearing 2009). Once inside the keratinocytes, melanosomes accumulate in a cell-polarized manner to "shield" keratinocyte nuclei by accumulating on the side of the cell facing the outside of the skin where UV would enter. Interestingly, most inherited pigmentary defects are caused not by melanocyte deficiency but rather by mutations in melanogenic enzymes such as tyrosinase that causes oculocutaneous albinism type 1 (Scherer and Kumar 2010). Thus, the total number of melanocytes in the skin is similar regardless of an individual's complexion.

7.3 Melanocytes

Melanocytes are pigment producing cells derived from melanoblasts in embryonic development. After leaving the neural crest which develops in paravertebral/spinal locations, melanoblasts migrate through the mesenchyme to position themselves in dermal hair follicles and in the basal layer of the epidermis (Sommer 2011). Melanoblast survival and differentiation into melanocytes is dependent upon cell signaling events including stem cell factor-cKit and endothelin-endothelin B receptor interactions (Grichnik et al. 1998; Hou et al. 2004) as well as expression of the microphthalmia (Mitf) transcription factor (Widlund and Fisher 2003). Developmental defects in these signaling pathways lead to pigmentation defects such as piebaldism and Waardenburg syndrome. Cutaneous melanocytes in the basal layer at the epidermal/dermal junction play a major role in pigmentation of the skin. Indeed melanocytes are the only pigment-producing cell in the skin. Outside the skin, melanocytes are found in the leptomeninges, cochlea, retinal pigment epithelium, substantia nigricans and locus coerulus where they serve important homeostatic mechanisms to these tissues. The great majority of melanomas, however, are thought to derive from melanocytes in the basal layer of the epidermis. Because they are long-lived terminally differentiated cells, melanocytes are highly susceptible to environmental carcinogens including UV radiation, heavy metal and chemicals. Accordingly, because of their position in the skin, melanocytes must be able to repair DNA damage to prevent mutations and carcinogenesis lest they undergo carcinogenic transformation. To that end, melanocytes have innate and inducible protective mechanisms to prevent and repair environmental-induced damage to preserve genomic maintenance. We and others have observed that the melanocortin signaling axis, discussed in depth below, significantly enhances the ability of melanocytes to resist UV damage and mutagenesis (Bohm et al. 2005; Abdel-Malek et al. 2006, 2009; Hauser et al. 2006; Song et al. 2009; Kadekaro et al. 2012; Jagirdar et al. 2013; Jarrett et al. 2014, 2015; Swope et al. 2014).

7.4 Melanin

Perhaps more than anything else, melanocytes are recognized for their production of melanin pigments. These pigments are physiologically critical to UV resistance since they are able to absorb UV energy and in so doing, prevent UV photons from entering the deep layers of the skin (Miyamura et al. 2007). Melanin is a heterogeneous bioaggregate made up of pigmented chemical species derived from the amino acid tyrosine. It exists in two major forms: (1) a brown/black pigment known as eumelanin that is abundantly expressed in the skin of individuals with dark UV-protected skin complexion, and (2) a reddish/blonde sulfated pigment called pheomelanin that is the main melanin species in fair-skinned UV-sensitive individuals (Slominski et al. 2004). Eumelanin and pheomelanin are both formed from the sequential oxidation and cyclization of tyrosine, with their synthetic pathways diverging after the formation of DOPAquinone. Since the amount of epidermal eumelanin is among the most important determinants of UV sensitivity and skin cancer risk, much attention has been made on the physiologic factors that regulate its production. Melanocytic eumelanin production is largely regulated by the amount of cAMP second messenger in melanocytes which is largely determined by the signaling activity of the melanocortin 1 receptor (MC1R) (Nasti and Timares 2015). Thus, fair-skinned people who are almost always UV-sensitive and have high risk of skin cancer have a high incidence of inherited loss-of-function polymorphisms in the MC1R and as a result express low levels of epidermal eumelanin. Skin cells of such individuals receive much more UV than those of darker-skinned individuals who, because of more epidermal UV-blocking eumelanin, have built-in "sunblock" in their skin.

7.5 Skin Complexion

Epidermal pigmentation is a multigenic phenotype and is among the most important determinants of UV sensitivity and cancer risk. Largely determined by epidermal eumelanin levels, skin pigmentation directly predicts how much cellular damage will be realized by UV. Many genes regulate basal pigmentation, with many associated with melanin synthesis or melanosome structure/function (Scherer and Kumar 2010). Many pigment-relevant genes were first identified through the study of color phenotype in mice and other model organisms. Since tyrosinase catalyzes the first two chemical reactions seminal for the production of either eumelanin or pheomelanin, its deficiency results in albinism wherein neither pigment is made to any significant degree. As a result, individuals with albinism are exceptionally sun-sensitive and burn with minimal doses of UV. In contrast, defects in other melanogenic enzymes cause dilutional pigmentary effects rather than total melanin loss. Finally, mutations in key melanocyte survival/differentiation regulators result in profound melanocyte-defect phenotypes such as piebaldism caused by loss-of-function of the c-Kit tyrosine kinase receptor (Tomita and Suzuki 2004).

7.6 Fitzpatrick Pigmentation Phenotype

The "Fitzpatrick Scale", developed in the 1970s by Dr. T.B. Fitzpatrick, to describe skin tone, is comprised of six pigmentation categories that describe a person's pigmentary phototype basted on skin color and sensitivity to UV radiation (Fig. 7.2). A semi-quantitative measurement of UV sensitivity is the "minimal erythematous dose" (MED) which reflects how much UV is required to result in skin inflammation. MED is generally calculated 24–48 h after UV exposure and is assessed using clinical indications of inflammation—erythema (redness) and edema (swelling)—as endpoints. Because eumelanin is an efficient UV blocker, more UV is generally needed to "burn" skin of dark pigmentation as compared to light-colored skin, and MED will accordingly be higher in dark-skinned individuals (Fig. 7.3).

The capacity to "tan" after UV exposure is an important physiologic cutaneous reaction to UV exposure. This adaptive pigmentary response is a well-regulated mechanism that is recruited into action following exposure to UV. It involves the proliferation of melanocytes and keratinocytes as well as increases in the production and accumulation of eumelanin in the epidermis. In this way, the skin protects itself against further UV insult. The tanning response is dependent on the function of the MC1R (D'Orazio et al. 2006), and people with inherited loss-of-function MC1R alleles tend to be particularly sun-sensitive. Thus, persons of skin phototypes I and II are quick to sunburn, tend not to be able to tan and are at higher risk for melanoma and other skin cancers when compared to people of higher Fitzpatrick phototype.

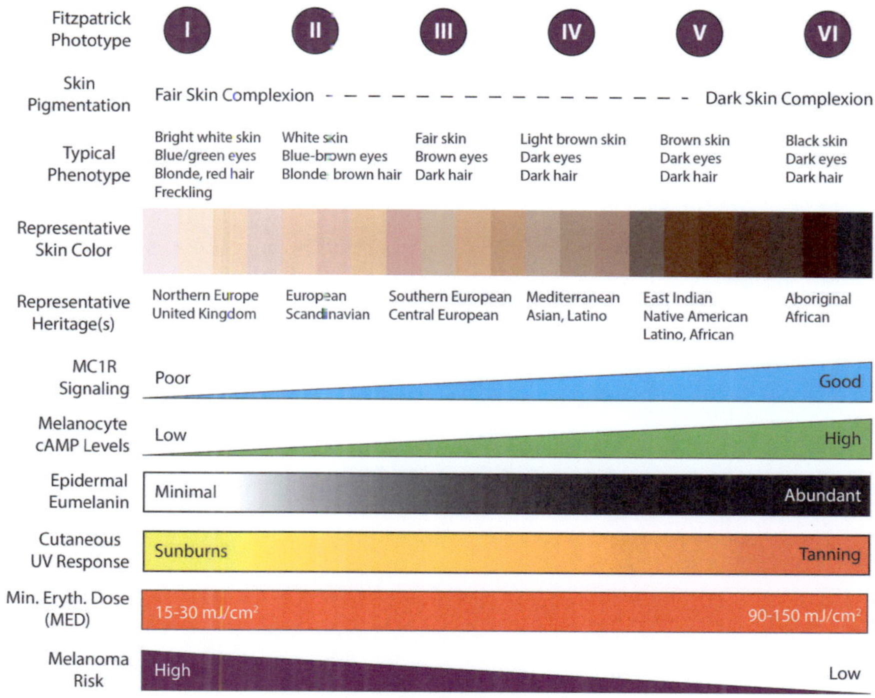

Fig. 7.2 Skin pigmentation, Fitzpatrick scale, MED and UV sensitivity. Skin complexion can be described by Fitzpatrick phototype, with individuals of least pigmentation having phototype I and persons of darkest complexion having phototype VI. Though pigmentation is determined by many genes, skin complexion and UV responses are heavily regulated by the MC1R signaling and epidermal eumelanin composition. Robust MC1R signaling leads to induction of cAMP in melanocytes which promotes eumelanin production responsible for a vigorous tanning response (adaptive pigmentation) and better protection from subsequent UV insults. Skin cancer risk, including melanoma, is heavily influenced by skin pigmentation and MC1R signaling

7.7 UV Radiation

UV radiation is a common and pervasive environmental carcinogen. Humans receive UV from ambient sunlight and increasingly from artificial UV sources such as indoor tanning devices. Though UV offers important health benefits including cutaneous production of vitamin D from cholesterol precursors (Holick 2008), excess exposure to UV causes many health consequences including photoaging, wrinkling, inflammation and cancer (Krutmann et al. 2012). UV is part of the electromagnetic spectrum, with wavelengths situated between the visible light and gamma radiation. Most ambient sunlight that strikes the Earth's surface is made up of a blend of UV-A and UV-B radiation in an approximate 9:1 ratio. UV-A has the longest wavelengths (315–400 nm) but the least energy of all UV. Nonetheless, UV-A can penetrate deeply into the skin, well into the dermis. UV-B radiation

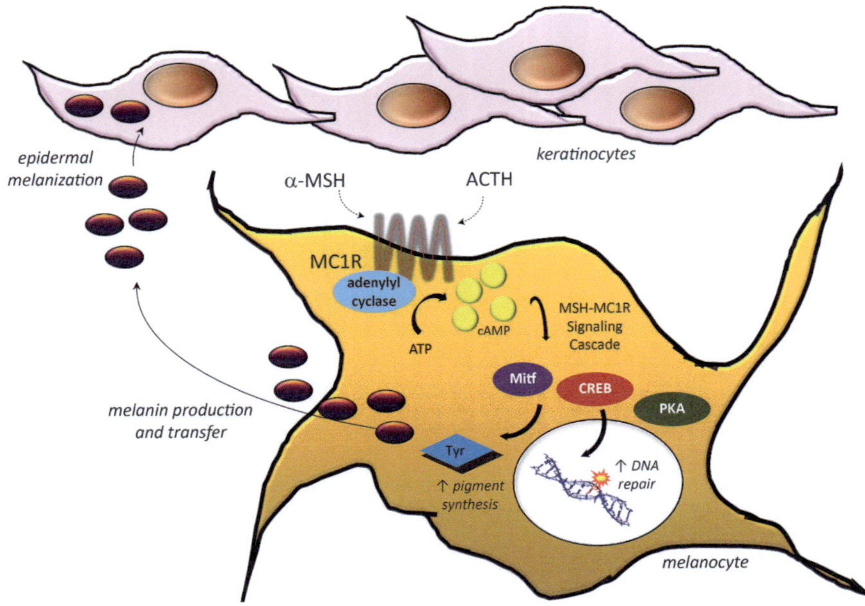

Fig. 7.3 Melanocortin—MC1R signaling axis. One of the most important ways in which the skin protects itself from UV damage is through increasing its melanin content after UV exposure. This process, commonly known as "tanning", is regulated by the melanocortin signaling axis. Melanocortins (α-MSH, ACTH) bind MC1R to activate adenylyl cyclase and stimulate cAMP production. cAMP activates the CREB and Mitf transcription factor network and increases the activity of PKA. Pigment enzymes such as tyrosinase are subsequently up-regulated and eumelanin production in melanosomes is increased. Melanin is transferred to neighboring keratinocytes to lay down a UV-protective layer of pigment in the epidermis. In the absence of effective MC1R signaling (e.g. in persons with loss-of-function MC1R alleles), these pathways are blunted and the skin does not tan effectively. Such individuals are also at higher risk for melanoma, in part because of sub-optimal DNA repair which permits the accumulation of UV signature mutations that contribute to malignant degeneration of melanocytes

(280–315 nm) is the highest energy component of ambient sunlight and can also penetrate into the skin and have significant physiologic impact on skin cells.

Indoor tanning and purposeful UV exposure represent an increasing risk factor for melanoma. With the successful marketing and increasing commercial availability of indoor tanning, the regular use of indoor tanning salons has skyrocketed in America. Whereas only 1 % of the US population had ever used a tanning bed 30 years ago, now over 25 % of Americans have used indoor tanning (Choi et al. 2010). The US tanning industry caters to nearly 30 million clients, employs roughly 100,000 workers and makes billions of dollars each year. Indeed, a significant percentage of the population regularly seeks out artificial UV in the form of indoor tanning with people starting to tan in adolescence and young adulthood. Because the UV administered from such sources can be up to ten times more powerful than ambient sunlight and can deliver both UVA and UVB radiation, indoor tanning represents an increasingly important source of human UV exposure (Nilsen et al. 2011). Moreover, indoor tanning machines are poorly regulated and vary widely with respect to UV composition and strength. Indoor tanning is now unequivocally linked to increase risk of many forms of skin cancer including basal cell and squamous cell carcinomas, the most commonly diagnosed skin cancers. With respect to melanoma, lifetime risk increases by 75 % if people engage in artificial tanning before the age of 35 years (Fisher and James 2010). Most experts conclude the risks of indoor tanning and purposeful UV exposure far outweigh their potential health benefits. Indeed, decreasing UV radiation exposure may be the single best way to reduce incidence of melanoma and other skin cancers.

UV affects DNA directly through the absorption of UV energy by nucleotides in the double helix as well as indirectly through the generation of free radicals and subsequent oxidative damage to nucleotide bases in chromatin. The 5-6 double bond of pyrimidines seems especially vulnerable to UV-induced cleavage. When this occurs between neighboring cytosines or thymidines, abnormal covalent bonds can result to form two major "photolesions": [6,4]-photoproducts or cyclopyrimidine dimers. Each is highly mutagenic, mispairing with abnormal bases during replication to cause permanent base changes in the genome to yield "UV signature mutations" (particularly C-to-T transitions) (Brash 2015). Recently, UV photolesions have also been reported to be formed as a result of free radical damage even after UV exposure has ended—so called "dark photolesions" (Premi et al. 2015). A day's worth of sun exposure may result in up to 100,000 UV photolesions in every skin cell (Hoeijmakers 2009). Fortunately, melanocytes and other skin cells have a DNA repair pathway—nucleotide excision repair (NER)—to fix UV photodimers before they have the opportunity to result in a permanent somatic mutation in the genome.

7.8 Cutaneous Responses to UV

The skin responds to UV with a coordinated series of physiologic changes to limit cellular damage and to prevent further injury. Cutaneous response is proportional to the UV dose realized by the skin and is determined by strength of UV radiation, time of exposure and degree of photoprotection afforded by epidermal melanin. UV penetration into the skin elicits a variety of cellular events including release of cytokines, recruitment of immune cells, epidermal thickening and up-regulation of pigment synthesis to protect the skin from further UV insult. Above a certain dose threshold, UV induces inflammation, manifested by pain, erythema (redness) and edema (swelling). UV-induced inflammation, commonly referred to as "sunburn," is mediated by a variety of cytokines, vasoactive and neuroactive mediators in the skin. UV exposure causes an initial erythema that worsens over a period of 24–72 h due to vasodilation mediated in part by nitric oxide production by keratinocytes. Neutrophils infiltrate the dermis for several hours after UV exposure and promote inflammation through degranulation and production of free radicals.

The inflammatory response in the skin following exposure to UV radiation is complex, involving induction of pro-inflammatory cytokines and induction of an immunosuppressive phenotype. UV results in the production of TNF-alpha, IL-1β, and IL-10 by keratinocytes and IL-1α/β, IL-6, IL-8, and TNFα by melanocytes [reviewed in (Ullrich and Byrne 2012)]. These pro-inflammatory cytokines exert paracrine and autocrine effects locally and systemically. Above a certain UV threshold, keratinocytes die by apoptosis as manifested by the accumulation of "sunburn cells" (apoptotic keratinocytes) in UV-exposed skin (Lippens et al. 2009). UV induces a variety of other physiologic changes in the skin, including keratinocyte proliferation and stratum corneum thickening. The hyperkeratosis phenotype is a protective mechanism to prevent damage from subsequent UV radiation (Scott et al. 2012). Thus, UV causes a variety of physiologic changes in the skin, many of which lead to inflammation, photoaging and cancer.

7.9 Melanocortin—MC1R Signaling Axis

One of the most widely recognized effects of UV exposure on the skin is the up-regulation of melanin production, commonly referred to as "tanning". The tanning response occurs in two distinct stages: immediate pigment darkening and delayed tanning. The initial darkening is due to redistribution of pre-formed melanin granules while the delayed tanning response results from synthesis of new melanin pigment. The melanization response is largely under the control of the MC1R signaling cascade. There are three main known categories of MC1R ligands: positive melanocortin agonists adrenocorticotropic releasing hormone (ACTH) and alpha-melanocyte stimulating hormone (α-MSH), the negative agonist agouti signaling protein (ASIP), and the neutral antagonist beta-defensin 3 (βD3). MC1R agonists up-regulate melanin synthesis whereas MC1R antagonists either inhibit MC1R signaling directly or compete with MC1R agonists for MC1R binding.

The two major melanocortins—ACTH and α-MSH—are cleavage products from the pro-opiomelanocortin (POMC) protein. Besides basal POMC production by the pituitary, POMC can be made in the skin and UV exposure promotes its expression from keratinocytes in a cellular damage- and p53-dependent manner (Cui et al. 2007). The melanocortins bind to the MC1R with high affinity to promote a variety of survival and differentiation events in melanocytes. The MC1R is a G_s protein-coupled receptor (GPCR) and binding of MC1R by either ACTH or α-MSH activates adenylyl cyclase to induce cAMP second messenger generation. In turn, cAMP accumulation leads to a variety of signaling events including stimulation of the activity of protein kinase A (PKA) and increased expression and enhanced activity of the cAMP responsive binding element (CREB) and microphthalmia (Mitf) transcription factors (Yamaguchi and Hearing 2009). Many melanogenic biosynthetic enzymes and regulators are influenced by cAMP signaling and the CREB and Mitf pathways including tyrosinase, dopachrome tautomerase, and pmel17. Similar to other GPCRs, the MC1R has seven transmembrane helical domains with an extracellular N-terminus and intracellular C-terminus (Garcia-Borron et al. 2005).

The MC1R is a highly polymorphic protein with many variants (Kennedy et al. 2001), some of which are associated with the red hair color (RHC) phenotype (Box et al. 1997). Of the alleles associated with the RHC phenotype, there are those that are strongly associated with RHC ('R' alleles: D84E, R151C, R160 W, and D294H) and those that are weakly associated with RHC phenotype ('RHC' alleles: V60L, V92M, R163Q) (Duffy et al. 2004). Mutations in MC1R affect either MC1R function or prevent relocation to the plasma membrane (Beaumont et al. 2005). Individuals with loss-of-function MC1R polymorphisms are highly susceptible to developing melanoma for at least three reasons: (1) they burn easily and accumulate a greater degree of UV damage, (2) they cannot repair UV damage as efficiently and are more susceptible to UV-induced mutations, and (3) they cannot tan and therefore do not protect their skin from future exposure to UV radiation. Pharmacologic manipulation of the MC1R signaling axis in individuals with defective MC1R signaling is a potential mechanism to prevent UV-induced damage and melanoma development.

7.10 MC1R Antagonists

There are two major proteins that bind to MC1R and antagonize MC1R signaling and downstream cAMP accumulation: agouti signaling protein (ASIP) and beta-defensin 3 (βD3). ASIP is a potent MC1R antagonist, decreasing basal MC1R signaling and antagonizing melanocortin effects on melanocytes by functioning as a competitive inhibitor to α-MSH (Sviderskaya et al. 2001). Binding of ASIP to MC1R causes a decrease in the pigment enzymes levels of tyrosinase related protein 1 and 2 and a decrease in tyrosinase activity, all of which diminishes eumelanin production (Suzuki et al. 1997). The effects of ASP (the mouse homolog to human ASIP) on pigment are evident in mice with the lethal yellow mutation in *ASP* that overexpress agouti and exhibit a blonde pheomelanotic coat color as a result (Jordan and Jackson 1998). Importantly, the effect of ASIP on mouse coat color is dependent on a functional MC1R confirming agouti's role as an MC1R regulatory ligand (Ollmann et al. 1998).

βD3, like ASIP, antagonizes melanocortin signaling through MC1R. βD3 is a member of the defensin family, a group of small antimicrobial proteins that exhibit innate antibacterial and antifungal properties (Arnett and Seveau 2011). In 2007, Barsh and coworkers determined that in addition to its role in the immune response, βD3 could affect pigmentation through interactions with MC1R. The group determined that black coat color of certain dog breeds was due to dominant overexpression of the canine homolog of βD3 (CBD103) rather than loss-of-function MC1R mutations (Candille et al. 2007). Although the role of βD3 at MC1R remains somewhat controversial with one report suggesting it may act as a weak MC1R agonist (Beaumont et al. 2012), most experimental results suggest that βD3 functions as a neutral MC1R antagonist (Swope et al. 2012; Jarrett et al. 2015). Thus, unlike ASIP which down-regulates ligand-independent MC1R signaling, βD3 appears to act as competitive inhibitor for both the melanocortins and ASIP and therefore regulates skin pigmentation. The induction of βD3 following inflammatory stimuli is well established (Kaiser and Diamond 2000), however, the regulation following UV exposure is unclear. In vivo exposure of human subjects to UV radiation resulted in an increase in βD3 gene and protein expression (Glaser et al. 2009), however these results were not confirmed in an ex vivo setting suggesting the damage response initiated by UV radiation was not sufficient to induce βD3 expression (Wolf Horrell and D'Orazio 2014). The induction of the inflammatory response may be critical for the induction of βD3 following UV radiation which may be relevant in the setting of sunburns: if cutaneous βD3 expression is upregulated with UV exposure, it may compete with melanocortin-MC1R interactions and inhibit induction of MC1R-mediated UV protective pathways.

7.11 Nucleotide Excision Repair (NER)

Skin cells repair UV-induced DNA damage through a highly coordinated genome maintenance pathway known as the nucleotide excision repair (NER) pathway. The NER pathway repairs bulky DNA lesions that distort the double helical backbone and/or interfere with transcription (Nouspikel 2009). It repairs lesions with high fidelity, reliant on the undamaged complementary strand for specificity and invoking at least eight essential proteins that function coordinately to carry out NER. We understand NER's importance by observing the natural history of xeroderma pigmentosum (XP) patients who lack NER because of inherited homozygous loss of any one of the eight essential NER factors: *XPA, ERCC1, ERCC3 (XP-B), XPC, ERCC2 (XP-D), DDB2 (XP-E), ERCC4 (XP-F), ERCC5 (XP-G) and POLH.* Although rare, XP is a UV hypersensitivity syndrome largely characterized by progressive skin degenerative changes in UV-exposed areas. Because they lack NER and cannot reverse DNA photodamage, XP patients are profoundly UV sensitive, burning easily with minimal sun exposure and developing disfiguring skin changes in childhood including abnormal pigmentation, cutaneous telangiectasias, scarring and atrophy. Their risk of melanoma and other skin cancers is roughly 3 logs higher than unaffected patients, with premalignant and true skin cancers frequently occurring in childhood—decades before their peak in the general population—despite their best attempts to avoid UV (DiGiovanna and Kraemer 2012).

NER is a complex pathway regulated by many more proteins than simply the eight core NER factors, and the reader is referred elsewhere for an in-depth review of NER (Scharer 2013). In general, NER can conceptualized in discreet stages.

DNA damage is recognized either because it physically distorts the double helix or because it interferes with RNA polymerase in actively transcribed genes. In either case, a multiprotein repair complex is recruited to the damaged site where the damaged strand is isolated, unwound, stabilized and nicked on either side of the damage. A 25–30 mer oligo containing the damage is excised and the resultant gap is filled in by DNA polymerase using the undamaged complementary strand as a template. Finally, DNA ligase seals the nicks to restore the DNA to its original undamaged state in a manner designed to preserve fidelity of sequence (Fig. 7.4).

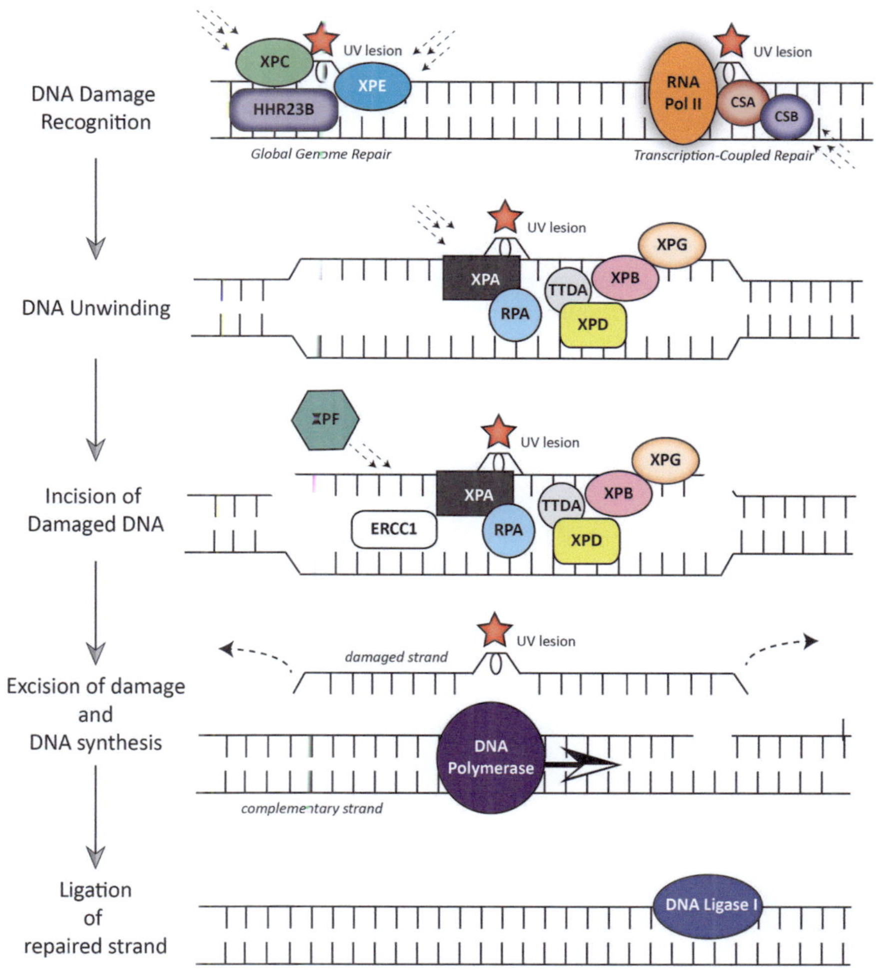

Fig. 7.4 Nucleotide excision repair (NER) pathway. At least eight core NER factors function in a coordinated manner to identify bulky DNA lesions, excise a 25–30 mer oligonucleotide harboring the damage and replace the excised region using the complementary strand to ensure fidelity of process. *Note* this is a highly simplified model of NER that does not show many accessory factors that regulate the repair process

While NER's importance to UV resistance and protection from malignancy is most clearly evident in XP patients, it is becoming evident that less penetrant NER polymorphisms may also impact cancer risk in the general population (Li et al. 2013). Since melanoma is heavily influenced by UV damage and mutagenesis, it follows that efficiency of NER is an important melanoma determinant.

7.12 MC1R and NER

NER efficiency is increased in melanocytes that have been stimulated by the MC1R/cAMP pathway. This was first demonstrated in human primary melanocyte lines wherein the clearance of UV photoproducts was improved by stimulating cells with melanocortins (Hauser et al. 2006). The benefit of MC1R was subsequently shown in whole skin of a congenic mouse model of humanized skin. Specifically, using *K14-Scf* transgenic mice that retain melanocytes in the interfollicular dermis because of constitutive expression of Kit ligand (stem cell factor), we found that repair of UV photoproducts was more efficient and more complete in *Mc1r*-intact (vs.-defective) animals. Moreover, when forskolin, a skin-permeable adenylyl cyclase stimulator, was applied to the skin of *Mc1r*-defective mice, their NER efficiency was greatly enhanced (Jarrett et al. 2014), showing that pharmacologic manipulation of cAMP in the skin could impact DNA repair of UV photolesions. These proof-of-concept experiments confirmed the important contribution of MC1R to NER in a genetically-defined system and, most importantly, suggested that NER can be pharmacologically boosted in Mc1r-defective UV-sensitive and melanoma-prone individuals.

Defining the mechanisms that link MC1R signaling to melanocytic DNA repair responses has been an active area of investigation. Recently, we reported that the key molecular event involved in MC1R-mediated augmentation of NER involves a post-translational modification of the global cell damage response protein "ataxia and rad3-related" (ATR) protein by PKA. We discovered that cAMP induction and activation of PKA, either through conventional melanocortin-MC1R interactions or through pharmacologic activation of adenylyl cyclase by forskolin, causes PKA to phosphorylate ATR on a serine at position 435. This event does not impact canonical ATR activation as defined by ATR-mediated phosphorylation of Chk1 and cell cycle arrest, but rather enhances the binding affinity of ATR for the xeroderma pigmentosum A (XPA) protein to facilitate NER (Fig. 7.5). With cAMP stimulation, XPA and pS435-ATR co-localize to UV photoproducts in a greatly accelerated and enhanced manner and NER is much more efficient and complete (Jarrett et al. 2014). Our group's efforts to determine how pS435-ATR is regulated and how it impacts NER are ongoing.

Melanocortin signaling may impact genome stability through other pathways beside PKA-mediated ATR phosphorylation and XPA recruitment. MC1R signaling, for example, promotes cellular antioxidant defenses, thereby endowing melanocytes with an improved ability to resist UV-mediated oxidative and free radical

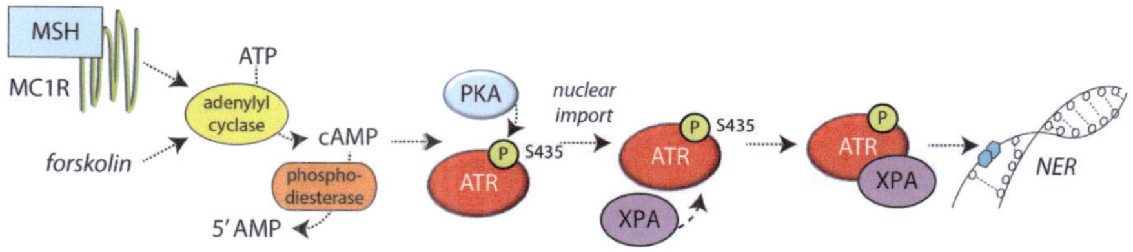

Fig. 7.5 MC1R augmentation of NER. Elevated levels of the second messenger cAMP can result from MC1R signaling (e.g. MSH), adenylyl cyclase activation (e.g. forskolin) or phosphodiesterase inhibition (e.g. rolipram). cAMP promotes the phosphorylation of ATR on the Ser 435 residue by PKA, which in turn facilitates ATR's nuclear import and association with the key NER factor XPA. Together, pS435-ATR and XPA translocate to sites of nuclear photodamage to accelerate NER in melanocytes

injury (Kadekaro et al. 2012). Furthermore, the cAMP signaling pathway may impact melanocytes by bolstering key DNA damage and repair factors besides XPA and ATR. The Abdel-Malek group found that MC1R stimulation promoted XPC expression, enhanced UV-induced phosphorylation of both ATR and ATM and increased phosphorylation of histone γH2AX (Swope et al. 2014). Smith and colleagues published that MC1R signaling resulted in increased expression of NR4A subfamily of nuclear receptors which were recruited to nuclear photodamage along with XPC and XPE (Jagirdar et al. 2013). Therefore the melanocortin-MC1R-cAMP signaling axis represents a multifaceted inducible pathway to protect melanocytes against UV injury and mutagenesis.

7.13 Future Directions: The Melanocortin-MC1R Axis as an Exploitable Melanoma Prevention Strategy

Inherited loss-of-function MC1R polymorphisms are common in the population, with some estimating up to 6–8 million Americans harboring double allele polymorphisms and millions more being hemizygous. Such persons tend to have fair complexions, are UV-sensitive (sunburn easily) and a four-fold or higher risk of melanoma (Kennedy et al. 2001). As we understand it, MC1R-mediated UV protection and melanoma resistance is proportional to the robustness of the cAMP response downstream of MC1R signaling. cAMP signaling positions melanocytes to resist UV damage and mutagenesis by stimulating production of melanin and by enhancing DNA repair through improving the efficiency of nucleotide excision repair (Fig. 7.6). In this way, persons with blunted MC1R signaling accumulate more UV damage because of diminished eumelanin production and less innate UV protection. Melanocytes in MC1R-defective individuals are also much less efficient at repairing UV photodamage because of a lack of the MC1R NER "boost". As a result, cells accumulate more UV-induced mutations and are more prone to carcinogenic transformation.

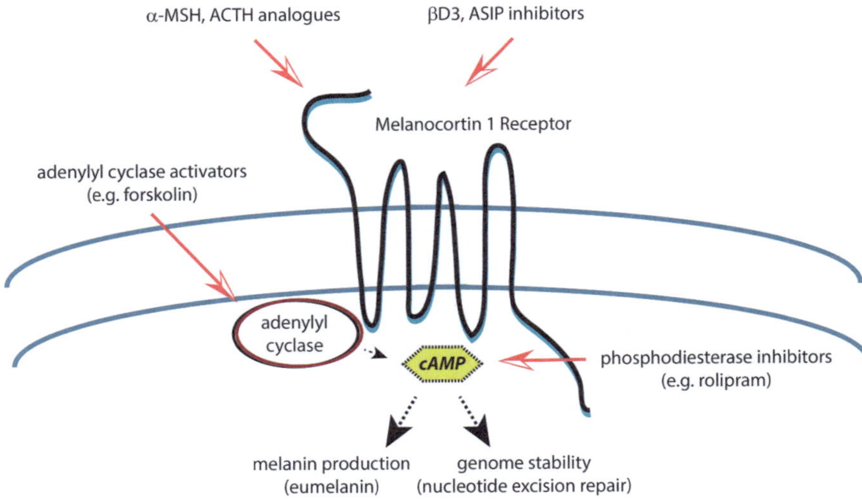

Fig. 7.6 Exploiting the MC1R-cAMP signaling axis for UV protection and melanoma prevention. Inducing cAMP in melanocytes, whether through up-regulating MC1R signaling with melanocortin analogs, activating adenylyl cyclase or inhibiting phosphodiesterases, would be expected to enhance pigment production and augment DNA repair, both of which would reduce UV-induced mutagenesis and cancer risk

Since a variety of pharmacologic strategies exist to impact cAMP signaling, it might be possible to reduce UV mutagenesis in melanocytes and reduce melanoma risk by exploiting the MC1R signaling axis. We previously showed that topical application of forskolin, a direct activator of adenylyl cyclase, rescued eumelanin production in fair-skinned and UV-sensitive *Mc1r*-defective animals (D'Orazio et al. 2006). This same animal model was used to show that topical application of rolipram, a phosphodiesterase-4 inhibitor, similarly rescued dark melanization of the skin (Khaled et al. 2010). In both cases, pharmacologic melanization of the skin protected against UV damage. Thus skin-permeable agents the increase cAMP in epidermal melanocytes are an effective way to mimic MC1R signaling in melanocytes and protect the skin against UV injury. Most recently, we published that topically-applied forskolin could also enhance clearance of UV photoproducts in the skin of these mice, essentially enhancing the level of repair to that of animals with intact Mc1r signaling (Jarrett et al. 2014). Together, these studies clearly prove the feasibility of pharmacologic manipulation of the cAMP signaling axis and subsequent protection of melanocytes against UV damage and mutagenesis.

Though applying general cAMP manipulators to the skin upregulates cAMP levels in epidermal melanocytes, this approach lacks specificity to induce signaling only in melanocytes. The effects of cAMP induction in other skin cells or in off-target tissues through systemic absorption are complex and likely to impede translational development. Melanocyte-directed approaches for cAMP stimulation would greatly enhance the potential translational appeal of this approach. To that end, targeted melanocyte-specific cAMP induction can be achieved through melanocortin analogues such as those reported by Abdel-Malek and colleagues (Abdel-Malek et al. 2006). Melanocortin effects would be expected to be restricted to cells expressing melanocortin receptors such as MC1R on melanocytes. This approach, while offering better melanocyte specificity, requires MC1R signaling function to be intact in order for cells to respond to melanocortins by upregulating cAMP. Persons with inherited defects in MC1R signaling—the very individuals most at risk for UV sensitivity and melanoma development—would probably not benefit much from melanocortin therapy since MC1R signaling is impaired. For these individuals, perhaps the only way to trigger cAMP in melanocytes may be a global pharmacologic approach. Clearly much more mechanistic and feasibility work needs to be done to understand the risks and benefits of pharmacologic cAMP manipulation in melanocytes and in the skin. Overall, however, the broad melanocortin-MC1R signaling axis remains an attractive and potentially exploitable pathway for the development of novel melanoma prevention strategies in at-risk populations.

Acknowledgments We acknowledge Dr. Stuart Jarrett for insights and key experimental discoveries seminal to our understanding of the molecular links between the melanocortin signaling axis and melanocyte UV resistance and DNA repair. We are grateful for support from the National Cancer Institute (R01 CA131075), the Melanoma Research Alliance (MRA) and the Regina Drury Endowment for Pediatric Research as well as T32CA165990 which supported E.W.H.

References

Abdel-Malek ZA, Kadekaro AL, Kavanagh RJ, Todorovic A, Koikov LN, McNulty JC, Jackson PJ, Millhauser GL, Schwemberger S, Babcock G, Haskell-Luevano C, Knittel JJ (2006) Melanoma prevention strategy based on using tetrapeptide alpha-MSH analogs that protect human melanocytes from UV-induced DNA damage and cytotoxicity. Faseb J 20 (9):1561–1563

Abdel-Malek ZA, Ruwe A, Kavanagh-Starner R, Kadekaro AL, Swope V, Haskell-Luevano C, Koikov L, Knittel JJ (2009) alpha-MSH tripeptide analogs activate the melanocortin 1 receptor and reduce UV-induced DNA damage in human melanocytes. Pigm Cell Melanoma Res 22 (5):635–644

Arnett E, Seveau S (2011) The multifaceted activities of mammalian defensins. Curr Pharm Des 17 (38):4254–4269

Beaumont KA, Newton RA, Smit DJ, Leonard JH, Stow JL, Sturm RA (2005) Altered cell surface expression of human MC1R variant receptor alleles associated with red hair and skin cancer risk. Hum Mol Genet 14(15):2145–2154

Beaumont KA, Smit DJ, Liu YY, Chai E, Patel MP, Millhauser GL, Smith JJ, Alewood PF, Sturm RA (2012) Melanocortin-1 receptor-mediated signalling pathways activated by NDP-MSH and HBD3 ligands. Pigm Cell Melanoma Res 25(3):370–374

Bohm M, Wolff I, Scholzen TE, Robinson SJ, Healy E, Luger TA, Schwarz T, Schwarz A (2005) alpha-Melanocyte-stimulating hormone protects from ultraviolet radiation-induced apoptosis and DNA damage. J Biol Chem 280(7):5795–5802

Box NF, Wyeth JR, O'Gorman LE, Martin NG, Sturm RA (1997) Characterization of melanocyte stimulating hormone receptor variant alleles in twins with red hair. Hum Mol Genet 6 (11):1891–1897

Brash DE (2015) UV signature mutations. Photochem Photobiol 91(1):15–26
Candille SI, Kaelin CB, Cattanach BM, Yu B, Thompson DA, Nix MA, Kerns JA, Schmutz SM, Millhauser GL, Barsh GS (2007) A -defensin mutation causes black coat color in domestic dogs. Science 318(5855):1418–1423
Choi K, Lazovich D, Southwell B, Forster J, Rolnick SJ, Jackson J (2010) Prevalence and characteristics of indoor tanning use among men and women in the United States. Arch Dermatol 146(12):1356–1361
Cui R, Widlund HR, Feige E, Lin JY, Wilensky DL, Igras VE, D'Orazio J, Fung CY, Schanbacher CF, Granter SR, Fisher DE (2007) Central role of p53 in the suntan response and pathologic hyperpigmentation. Cell 128(5):853–864
D'Orazio JA, Nobuhisa T, Cui R, Arya M, Spry M, Wakamatsu K, Igras V, Kunisada T, Granter SR, Nishimura EK, Ito S, Fisher DE (2006) Topical drug rescue strategy and skin protection based on the role of Mc1r in UV-induced tanning. Nature 443(7109):340–344
DiGiovanna JJ, Kraemer KH (2012) Shining a light on xeroderma pigmentosum. J Invest Dermatol 132(3 Pt 2):785–796
Duffy DL, Box NF, Chen W, Palmer JS, Montgomery GW, James MR, Hayward NK, Martin NG, Sturm RA (2004) Interactive effects of MC1R and OCA2 on melanoma risk phenotypes. Hum Mol Genet 13(4):447–461
Fisher DE, James WD (2010) Indoor tanning–science, behavior, and policy. N Engl J Med 363 (10):901–903
Garcia-Borron JC, Sanchez-Laorden BL, Jimenez-Cervantes C (2005) Melanocortin-1 receptor structure and functional regulation. Pigm Cell Res 18(6):393–410
Glaser R, Navid F, Schuller W, Jantschitsch C, Harder J, Schroder JM, Schwarz A, Schwarz T (2009) UV-B radiation induces the expression of antimicrobial peptides in human keratinocytes in vitro and in vivo. J Allergy Clin Immunol 123(5):1117–1123
Grichnik JM, Burch JA, Burchette J, Shea CR (1998) The SCF/KIT pathway plays a critical role in the control of normal human melanocyte homeostasis. J Invest Dermatol 111(2):233–238
Hauser JE, Kadekaro AL, Kavanagh RJ, Wakamatsu K, Terzieva S, Schwemberger S, Babcock G, Rao MB, Ito S, Abdel-Malek ZA (2006) Melanin content and MC1R function independently affect UVR-induced DNA damage in cultured human melanocytes. Pigm Cell Res 19(4):303–314
Hodis E, Watson IR, Kryukov GV, Arold ST, Imielinski M, Theurillat JP, Nickerson E, Auclair D, Li L, Place C, Dicara D, Ramos AH, Lawrence MS, Cibulskis K, Sivachenko A, Voet D, Saksena G, Stransky N, Onofrio RC, Winckler W, Ardlie K, Wagle N, Wargo J, Chong K, Morton DL, Stemke-Hale K, Chen G, Noble M, Meyerson M, Ladbury JE, Davies MA, Gershenwald JE, Wagner SN, Hoon DS, Schadendorf D, Lander ES, Gabriel SB, Getz G, Garraway LA, Chin L (2012) A landscape of driver mutations in melanoma. Cell 150(2):251–263
Hoeijmakers JH (2009) DNA damage, aging, and cancer. N Engl J Med 361(15):1475–1485
Holick MF (2008) Sunlight, UV-radiation, vitamin D and skin cancer: how much sunlight do we need? Adv Exp Med Biol 624:1–15
Hou L, Pavan WJ, Shin MK, Arnheiter H (2004) Cell-autonomous and cell non-autonomous signaling through endothelin receptor B during melanocyte development. Development 131 (14):3239–3247
Jagirdar K, Yin K, Harrison M, Lim W, Muscat GE, Sturm RA, Smith AG (2013) The NR4A2 nuclear receptor is recruited to novel nuclear foci in response to UV irradiation and participates in nucleotide excision repair. PLoS ONE 8(11):e78075
Jarrett SG, Wolf Horrell EM, Christian PA, Vanover JC, Boulanger MC, Zou Y, D'Orazio JA (2014) PKA-mediated phosphorylation of ATR promotes recruitment of XPA to UV-induced DNA damage. Mol Cell 54(6):999–1011
Jarrett SG, Wolf Horrell EM, Boulanger MC, D'Orazio JA (2015) Defining the contribution of MC1R physiological ligands to ATR phosphorylation at Ser435, a predictor of DNA repair in melanocytes. J Invest Dermatol

Jordan SA, Jackson IJ (1998) Melanocortin receptors and antagonists regulate pigmentation and body weight. BioEssays 20(8):603–606

Kadekaro AL, Chen J, Yang J, Chen S, Jameson J, Swope VB, Cheng T, Kadakia M, Abdel-Malek Z (2012) Alpha-melanocyte-stimulating hormone suppresses oxidative stress through a p53-mediated signaling pathway in human melanocytes. Mol Cancer Res 10(6):778–786

Kaiser V, Diamond G (2000) Expression of mammalian defensin genes. J Leukoc Biol 68(6):779–784

Kennedy C, ter Huurne J, Berkhout M, Gruis N, Bastiaens M, Bergman W, Willemze R, Bavinck JN (2001) Melanocortin 1 receptor (MC1R) gene variants are associated with an increased risk for cutaneous melanoma which is largely independent of skin type and hair color. J Invest Dermatol 117(2):294–300

Khaled M, Levy C, Fisher DE (2010) Control of melanocyte differentiation by a MITF-PDE4D3 homeostatic circuit. Genes Dev 24(20):2276–2281

Krutmann J, Morita A, Chung JH (2012) Sun exposure: what molecular photodermatology tells us about its good and bad sides. J Invest Dermatol 132(3 Pt 2):976–984

Lawrence MS, Stojanov P, Polak P, Kryukov GV, Cibulskis K, Sivachenko A, Carter SL, Stewart C, Mermel CH, Roberts SA, Kiezun A, Hammerman PS, McKenna A, Drier Y, Zou L, Ramos AH, Pugh TJ, Stransky N, Helman E, Kim J, Sougnez C, Ambrogio L, Nickerson E, Shefler E, Cortes ML, Auclair D, Saksena G, Voet D, Noble M, DiCara D, Lin P, Lichtenstein L, Heiman DI, Fennell T, Imielinski M, Hernandez B, Hodis E, Baca S, Dulak AM, Lohr J, Landau DA, Wu CJ, Melendez-Zajgla J, Hidalgo-Miranda A, Koren A, McCarroll SA, Mora J, Lee RS, Crompton B, Onofrio R, Parkin M, Winckler W, Ardlie K, Gabriel SB, Roberts CW, Biegel JA, Stegmaier K, Bass AJ, Garraway LA, Meyerson M, Golub TR, Gordenin DA, Sunyaev S, Lander ES, Getz G (2013) Mutational heterogeneity in cancer and the search for new cancer-associated genes. Nature 499(7457):214–218

Li C, Yin M, Wang LE, Amos CI Zhu D, Lee JE, Gershenwald JE, Grimm EA, Wei Q (2013) Polymorphisms of nucleotide excision repair genes predict melanoma survival. J Invest Dermatol 133(7):1813–1821

Linos E, Swetter SM, Cockburn MG, Colditz GA, Clarke CA (2009) Increasing burden of melanoma in the United States J Invest Dermatol 129(7):1666–1674

Lippens S, Hoste E, Vandenabeele P, Agostinis P, Declercq W (2009) Cell death in the skin. Apoptosis 14:549–569

Miyamura Y, Coelho SG, Wolber R, Miller SA, Wakamatsu K, Zmudzka BZ, Ito S, Smuda C, Passeron T, Choi W, Batzer J, Yamaguchi Y, Beer JZ, Hearing VJ (2007) Regulation of human skin pigmentation and responses to ultraviolet radiation. Pigm Cell Res 20(1):2–13

Narayanan DL, Saladi RN, Fox JL (2010) Ultraviolet radiation and skin cancer. Int J Dermatol 49 (9):978–986

Nasti TH, Timares L (2015) MC1R, eumelanin and pheomelanin: their role in determining the susceptibility to skin cancer. Photochem Photobiol 91(1):188–200

Nilsen LT, Aalerud TN, Hannevik M, Veierod MB (2011) UVB and UVA irradiances from indoor tanning devices. Photochem Photobiol Sci 10:1129–1136

Nordlund JJ (2007) The melanocyte and the epidermal melanin unit: an expanded concept. Dermatol Clin 25(3):271–281, vii

Nouspikel T (2009) DNA repair in mammalian cells: nucleotide excision repair: variations on versatility. Cell Mol Life Sci 66(6):994–1009

Ollmann MM, Lamoreux ML, Wilson BD, Barsh GS (1998) Interaction of Agouti protein with the melanocortin 1 receptor in vitro and in vivo. Genes Dev 12(3):316–330

Pleasance ED, Cheetham RK, Stephens PJ, McBride DJ, Humphray SJ, Greenman CD, Varela I, Lin ML, Ordonez GR, Bignell GR, Ye K, Alipaz J, Bauer MJ, Beare D, Butler A, Carter RJ, Chen L, Cox AJ, Edkins S, Kokko-Gonzales PI, Gormley NA, Grocock RJ, Haudenschild CD, Hims MM, James T, Jia M, Kingsbury Z, Leroy C, Marshall J, Menzies A, Mudie LJ, Ning Z,

Royce T, Schulz-Trieglaff OB, Spiridou A, Stebbings LA, Szajkowski L, Teague J, Williamson D, Chin L, Ross MT, Campbell PJ, Bentley DR, Futreal PA, Stratton MR (2010) A comprehensive catalogue of somatic mutations from a human cancer genome. Nature 463(7278):191–196

Premi S, Wallisch S, Mano CM, Weiner AB, Bacchiocchi A, Wakamatsu K, Bechara EJ, Halaban R, Douki T, Brash DE (2015) Photochemistry. Chemiexcitation of melanin derivatives induces DNA photoproducts long after UV exposure. Science 347(6224):842–847

Scharer OD (2013) Nucleotide excision repair in eukaryotes. Cold Spring Harb Perspect Biol 5 (10):a012609

Scherer D, Kumar R (2010) Genetics of pigmentation in skin cancer–a review. Mutat Res 705 (2):141–153

Scott TL, Christian PA, Kesler MV, Donohue KM, Shelton B, Wakamatsu K, Ito S, D'Orazio J (2012) Pigment-independent cAMP-mediated epidermal thickening protects against cutaneous UV injury by keratinocyte proliferation. Exp Dermatol 21(10):771–777

Shain AH, Yeh I, Kovalyshyn I, Sriharan A, Talevich E, Gagnon A, Dummer R, North J, Pincus L, Ruben B, Rickaby W, D'Arrigo C, Robson A, Bastian BC (2015) The genetic evolution of melanoma from precursor lesions. N Engl J Med 373(20):1926–1936

Simard EP, Ward EM, Siegel R, Jemal A (2012) Cancers with increasing incidence trends in the United States: 1999 through 2008. CA Cancer J Clin 62:118–128

Slominski A, Tobin DJ, Shibahara S, Wortsman J (2004) Melanin pigmentation in mammalian skin and its hormonal regulation. Physiol Rev 84(4):1155–1228

Sommer L (2011) Generation of melanocytes from neural crest cells. Pigm Cell Melanoma Res 24 (3):411–421

Song X, Mosby N, Yang J, Xu A, Abdel-Malek Z, Kadekaro AL (2009) Alpha-MSH activates immediate defense responses to UV-induced oxidative stress in human melanocytes. Pigm Cell Melanoma Res 22(6):809–818

Suzuki I, Tada A, Ollmann MM, Barsh GS, Im S, Lamoreux ML, Hearing VJ, Nordlund JJ, Abdel-Malek ZA (1997) Agouti signaling protein inhibits melanogenesis and the response of human melanocytes to alpha-melanotropin. J Invest Dermatol 108(6):838–842

Sviderskaya EV, Hill SP, Balachandar D, Barsh GS, Bennett DC (2001) Agouti signaling protein and other factors modulating differentiation and proliferation of immortal melanoblasts. Dev Dyn 221(4):373–379

Swope VB, Jameson JA, McFarland KL, Supp DM, Miller WE, McGraw DW, Patel MA, Nix MA, Millhauser GL, Babcock GF, Abdel-Malek ZA (2012) Defining MC1R regulation in human melanocytes by its agonist alpha-melanocortin and antagonists agouti signaling protein and beta-defensin 3. J Invest Dermatol 132(9):2255–2262

Swope V, Alexander C, Starner R, Schwemberger S, Babcock G, Abdel-Malek ZA (2014) Significance of the melanocortin 1 receptor in the DNA damage response of human melanocytes to ultraviolet radiation. Pigm Cell Melanoma Res 27(4):601–610

Tomita Y, Suzuki T (2004) Genetics of pigmentary disorders. Am J Med Genet C Semin Med Genet 131C(1):75–81

Ullrich SE, Byrne SN (2012) The immunologic revolution: photoimmunology. J Invest Dermatol 132(3 Pt 2):896–905

Widlund HR, Fisher DE (2003) Microphthalamia-associated transcription factor: a critical regulator of pigment cell development and survival. Oncogene 22(20):3035–3041

Wolf Horrell E, D'Orazio J (2014) UV-independent induction of beta defensin 3 in neonatal human skin explants. F1000Res 3:288

Yamaguchi Y, Hearing VJ (2009) Physiological factors that regulate skin pigmentation. BioFactors 35(2):193–199

Chapter 8
The Cutaneous Melanocyte as a Target of Environmental Stressors: Molecular Mechanisms and Opportunities

Laurent Marrot

Abstract Pigmentation is regarded as a natural way to protect skin against harmful impact of UV from sunlight. In fact, prevalence of sunburn or skin cancer (carcinoma and melanoma) is lower in individuals with dark skin, suggesting that melanin is an efficient sunscreen. However, UV-induced melanoma generally originates from pigmented cells or pigmented skin areas (nevi) and in vitro or in vivo data have shown that melanin and/or its precursors could also be a source of photo-oxidative stress. Pigmentation behaves thus like a two-edged sword. Despite this adverse biological context, melanocytes generally persist a long time in skin probably because of specific abilities to repair DNA, to manage oxidative stress and to resist apoptosis. In addition to sunlight, melanocytes can also be targeted by specific chemicals whose toxicity is linked to the melanogenic pathway. For instance, activation of phase I metabolism through AhR pathway can stimulate pigmentation whereas biochemical transformation of some phenols by tyrosinase can trigger melanocyte death. In conclusion, due to its very peculiar physiology, the melanocyte is a unique and delicate cell type in epidermis. Since its alteration can give rise to melanoma, one of the most dangerous cancers, a specific protection is required to ensure pigment cell homeostasis.

Keywords Epidermal melanocytes · Melanin · UV-induced pigmentation · p53 · Nrf2 · AhR · DNA photodamage

L. Marrot (✉)
Cutaneous Redox Homeostasis Research Unit, Department of Clinical and Biological Research, L'OREAL Advanced Research, 1 Avenue Eugene Schueller, 93600 Aulnay sous Bois, France
e-mail: lmarrot@rd.loreal.com

G.T. Wondrak (ed.), *Skin Stress Response Pathways*,
DOI 10.1007/978-3-319-43157-4_8

8.1 Introduction

Skin pigmentation in humans is considered a natural protection against environmental insults, particularly against the UV rays present in sunlight. Individuals with dark skin originate from latitudes where radiation in the UVB spectrum, the most harmful to reach the earth's surface, is most intense. Since the prevalence of sunburn and skin cancer in these individuals is low, it seems highly probable that their skin color is protective. Fair skinned individuals can adapt their pigmentation in accordance with UVB exposure: tanning is a response to UV stress, aimed at protecting skin from additional irradiation. The risk of skin cancer is significantly increased in individuals with red hair who are unable to tan and who develop erythema easily. The central player in this process is a highly specialized cell, the melanocyte, which is amazing for many reasons. Amazing firstly because of its embryogenic origin from the neural crest: melanoblasts, melanocyte precursor cells, migrate away from the neuroepithelium to populate the skin and the hair follicles. Amazing also because of its diverse localizations in the body: not only in the skin and hair, but also in the iris of the eye, the cochlea of the inner ear, the heart, the brain: Amazing finally because although it is supposed to provide skin protection, it can give rise to melanoma, one of the most dangerous cancers. A central issue in the pigmentation process is the production of melanins, biopolymers which are synthesized from tyrosine in several successive enzymatic reactions in specialized organelles named melanosomes. Paradoxically, melanin the "natural anti-UV sunscreen" is not itself very photostable and is moreover the result of a biochemical recipe which produces toxic compounds such as reactive quinones.

Melanocytes are located in a dispersed pattern at the dermal-epidermal junction and each melanocyte interacts with around 40 keratinocytes in the basal and suprabasal layers: this constitutes the "epidermal-melanin unit". Once melanization is completed, melanosomes are transferred to surrounding keratinocytes. Skin color does not depend on the number of melanocytes which is comparable in different skin phototypes, but rather on the number, size and distribution of melanosomes in the epidermis. In keratinocytes, melanin granules have been shown to accumulate over the nucleus, like a protective cap filtering out harmful UV radiation to prevent the induction of mutagenic DNA damage. Interestingly, melanocytes are particularly resistant to apoptosis, it is maybe why the limited epidermal population of melanocytes remains in the skin for a long time despite a limited mitotic index. Such a low renewal rate is an astonishing phenomenon considering that melanocytes are subject to several environmental aggressions. Their location deep in the epidermis is only partially protective against solar UVB. Although the shorter solar wavelengths of around 300 nm may be absorbed by keratin and melanin in the stratum corneum and stratum granulosum, it is highly probable that wavelengths over 310 nm penetrate significantly towards the dermal-epidermal junction. Moreover, melanocytes are daily exposed to significant doses of UVA (from 320 to 400 nm) which can reach the dermis. UVA exposure can produce a strong oxidative stress via photoactivation of endogenous chromophores, and even induces the production of mutagenic pyrimidine dimers (CPD). In addition to sunlight, melanocytes have also to deal with chemicals derived either from the skin surface when penetration is possible, or from systemic exposure through the blood. Chemicals used for medical treatments, products present in food and drink must be considered, as well as atmospheric pollutants which can enter the skin either from its surface when barrier function is impaired or from the blood following diffusion from the pulmonary alveoli.

This chapter deals firstly with the stress induced by sunlight in melanocytes in fair-skinned individuals with a particular focus on the ambiguous role of melanin. Then, the question of melanocyte susceptibility to chemicals will be addressed through complementary examples, including that of post-inflammatory hyperpigmentation as a response to external insults.

8.2 The Melanocyte and Sunlight: A Cooperative but High-Risk Relationship

8.2.1 UV-Induced Pigmentation as a Stress Response: The Omnipresence of p53

8.2.1.1 Photodamage in Keratinocytes Triggers a Preventive Paracrine Pathway Leading to Melanogenesis

The melanocyte-keratinocyte unit responds quickly to the impact of solar UV and skin tanning relies mainly on a paracrine pathway where keratinocytes "communicate" their stressed status to melanocytes. In the early 1990s, the role of melanocortins in human pigmentation, particularly α-MSH, was highlighted. α-MSH is derived from the precursor peptide POMC (pro-opiomelanocortin) which is synthesized in the epidermis and upregulated in response to exposure to sunlight. Melanocytes express a specific cell surface α-MSH receptor: the melanocortin-1 receptor (MC1R) which, as a G protein-coupled receptor, transduces a signaling pathway involving cAMP and protein kinase A (PKA). Pigmentation is mediated by activation of microphthalmia-associated transcription factor (MITF), one of the numerous pro-differentiation pathways controlled by MC1R. MITF modulates expression of genes involved in melanin biosynthesis such as tyrosinase TYR, and the tyrosinase related proteins TRP1 and TRP2 (DCT). This paracrine process ensures a rapid response to UV stress, even before damage to melanocytes reaches a critical level (for review, see García-Borrón et al. 2014; Cheli et al. 2009). The link between UV damage in keratinocyte DNA and pigmentation was further documented in the 2000s, when pigmentation was linked to p53 activation. In keratinocytes, the accumulation of DNA photodamage (mainly pyrimidine dimers (CPD)) triggers the stabilization and activation of p53 through its phosphorylation. This transcription factor controls the most important anti-genotoxic pathways:

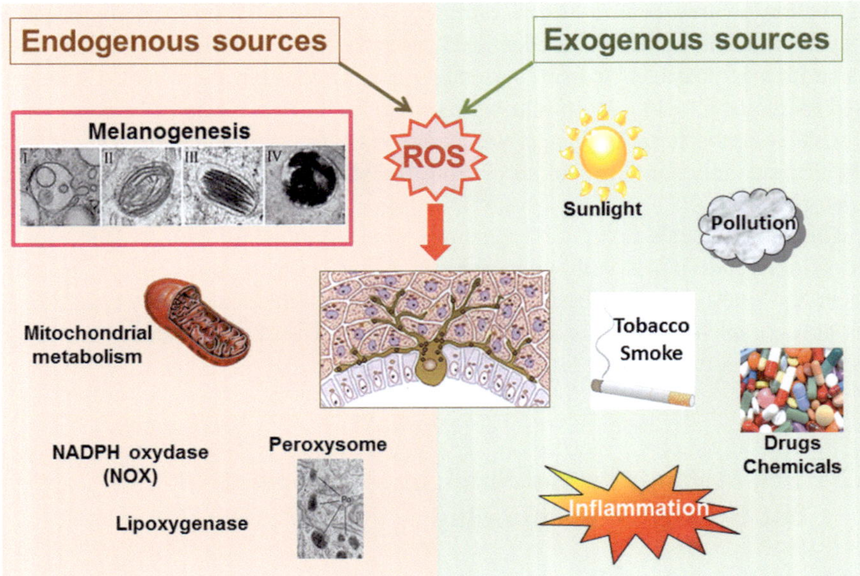

Fig. 8.1 Stressors targeting melanocyte: melanogenesis constitutes a peculiar additional source of stress compared to other epidermal cells

(i) cell cycle arrest and DNA repair are mobilized in order to prevent genomic degradation or (ii) apoptosis, programmed cell death, eliminates highly damaged cells. In the epidermis for instance, sunburn cells are apoptotic (for review see Marrot and Meunier 2008). Cui et al. demonstrated that p53 stimulates the POMC promoter and secretion by keratinocytes in response to UV. In fact, the tanning response to UVB exposure is only minimally present in p53 knockout mice, thus p53 functions as a sensor and effector of UV-induced pigmentation (Cui et al. 2007) (Fig. 8.1).

The peptide endothelin-1 (EDN1) was also shown to be upregulated in murine skin following UVB irradiation, and it interacts with specific G protein-coupled receptors (endothelin receptor: ENDR). END1 stimulates melanogenesis, proliferation, dendricity and MC1R expression in melanocytes. It was recently shown that UV-induced END1 expression in keratinocytes was directly and positively controlled by p53 transcriptional activity. In fact, END1 was significantly downregulated in the epidermis of p53 knockout mice (Hyter et al. 2012). Thus, END1 and POMC/α-MSH may have a synergistic effect aiming at increasing melanocyte activity in order to protect the epidermis from sunlight-induced genotoxic stress. P53 may drive this pigmentary adaptive response (Fig. 8.2).

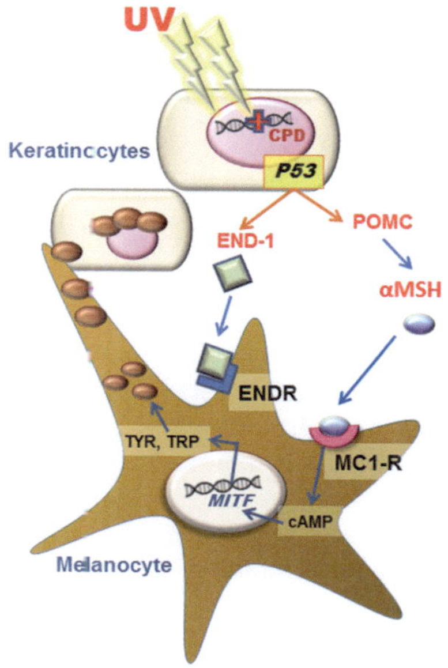

Fig. 8.2 Melanogenic paracrine pathways from keratinocytes in response to UV stress. Induction of photodamage (CPD) activates p53 in keratinocytes, and p53 stimulates secretion of POMC (which is cleaved to produce α-MSH) and endothelin-1 ET-1. ET-1/ENDR interaction triggers signaling pathways inside melanocyte leading to differentiation (melanogenesis, dendricity). α-MSH/MC1R interaction activates production of cAMP which in turn stimulates transcriptional activity of MITF. MITF upregulates the expression of melanogenic enzymes: melanogenesis takes place in melanosomes which are transferred to keratinocytes and protect their genomic DNA from further UV exposures (tanning process)

8.2.1.2 Melanogenesis: A Response also Directly Linked to DNA Damage in Melanocytes

Melanogenesis can be upregulated in cultured melanocytes exposed to UV, even in the absence of keratinocytes. In fact, intracellular signaling also contributes to the pigmentary response and an unexpected link between DNA damage and melanin production was reported some years ago. For instance, treatment of irradiated melanocytes with a liposome-encapsulated DNA repair enzyme which accelerated CPD excision stimulated melanogenesis (Gilchrest et al. 1993). The same team observed that addition of the dinucleotide pTpT to culture medium was associated with a pro-pigmenting effect which was confirmed in vivo after its application to guinea pig skin (Eller et al. 1996). Since pTpT was able to mimic the DNA segment excised during the repair of TT pyrimidine dimers, the authors speculated about the influence of DNA damage on melanogenesis. They finally demonstrated that pTpT targeted and disrupted structures of telomeres, leading to an artificial DNA damage response in which p53 was activated. The tanning response was thus largely mediated by p53: as proof, UV-induced pigmentation is reduced in p53 knockout mice. Melanogenesis together with improved DNA repair can thus be considered a SOS response by the skin against environmental genotoxicity and here again, p53 has a crucial influence (for review see Gilchrest et al. 2009).

8.2.2 Melanin: A Two-Edged Sword for Melanocytes

This concept of a two-edged sword was first proposed a few decades ago by Hill et al. when they observed that melanin could generate a significant oxidative stress under UV exposure (Hill et al. 1997). Several papers were published on this paradoxical behavior of our natural sunscreen. Reports were first based on in vitro experiments, but recent in vivo data confirmed that melanin could exacerbate UV stress. A scientific consensus seems to emerge and it reconciles the Janus face of pigmentation: cutaneous protection as a global process but a risk to the melanocyte itself, particularly in fair skin exposed to UV.

8.2.2.1 Intrinsic Pro-oxidant Potential of Melanin and Its Precursors

Melanogenesis involves several oxidation reactions, which potentially produce adverse biochemical effects (Fig. 8.3 and for review see Denat et al. 2014). For instance, tyrosinase oxidizes tyrosine firstly into dopa and then into dopaquinone, and this orthoquinone can react with nucleophilic compounds such as thiols or amino groups. Moreover, the generation of superoxide anions in association with tyrosinase activity has been reported in the literature (Koga et al. 1992; Tomita et al. 1984). Dihydroxy-indole (5,6-DHI) is oxidized into indolequinone and dihydroxy-indole carboxylic acid (5,6-DHICA). DHICA is converted into the corresponding quinone. Redox cycling from indoles to quinones can generate ROS (ultimately hydrogen peroxide H_2O_2) as reported by Nappi and Vass (1996). Polymerization of these quinones results finally in a black or brown eumelanin pigment whereas production of the reddish-brown pheomelanin requires the incorporation of cysteine: the resulting cysteinyldopa is converted into benzothiazine derivatives. It was suggested that cysteine consumption in pheo-melanogenesis may compete with glutathione synthesis and affect redox homeostasis in melanocytes (Morgan et al. 2013). Melanogenesis takes place inside melanosomes which ensures that toxic chemical intermediates are contained. However, melanosomes displaying structural abnormalities with partial leakage of their content were observed in dysplastic nevi and melanoma cells (Borovanský et al. 1991; Meyskens et al. 2001). Similarly, the diffusion of H_2O_2 into cytoplasm is highly probable, enabling the production of genotoxic hydroxyl radicals $^{\cdot}OH$. Miranda et al. showed that the rate of chromosomal aberrations (sister chromatid exchange) correlated with the concentration of tyrosine supplied to cultured melanocytes: stimulation of melanogenesis could thus damage chromosomes (Miranda et al. 1997). In line with this, Maresca et al. reported that catalase activity

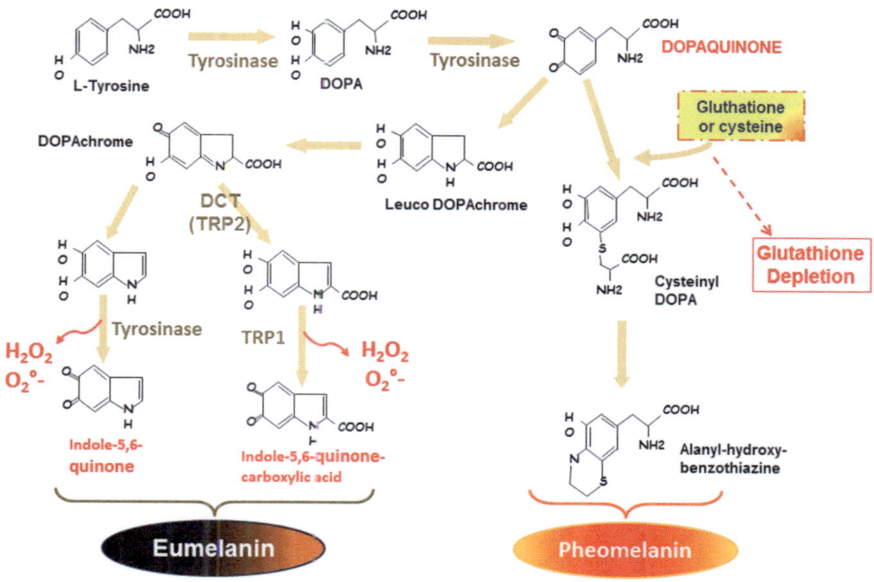

Fig. 8.3 The mammalian melanogenic pathway. Tyrosine-hydroxylase and dopa-oxidase activities of tyrosinase transform tyrosine into dopaquinone. Dopaquinone either react with cysteine to enter pheo-melanogenic pathway (red melanin) or is transformed into indole-quinone moieties to enter eu-melanogenic pathway (black or brown melanin). TRP2/DCT tautomerase activity prevents spontaneous decarboxylation of dopachrome which is converted into dihydroxy-indole-carboxylic acid. Possible contributions to oxidative stress generation or to impairment of redox homeostasis are mentioned in red in this scheme

(enzymatic protection against H_2O_2) correlated with melanogenic intensity. This natural protection against oxidative stress was thus required together with melanin production (Maresca et al. 2008). In dysplastic nevi in which melanocytes are hyperpigmented, melanosome sulphur and iron content was much higher than in normal melanocytes and an oxidative imbalance was observed using a specific probe for oxidative stress (Pavel et al. 2004). Smit et al. obtained similar results in melanocytes from pigmented dysplastic nevi, where an unusually high level of oxidative DNA damage was detected (Smit et al. 2008). Interestingly, a protective role was proposed for the melanogenic enzyme dopachrome tautomerase DCT/TRP2. TRP2 favors the production of DHICA (see Fig. 8.3), which is less toxic than DHI and TRP2 was reported to increase glutathione levels in amelanotic melanoma cells, providing protection against oxidative DNA damage and H_2O_2-induced cytotoxicity (Michard et al. 2008). TRP2, as a direct player in melanogenesis, could thus be the first "line of defense" against oxidative stress associated with pigmentation.

8.2.2.2 Melanin Photoreactivity: A Significant Source of Stress in Melanocytes Exposed to Sunlight

Early studies indicated that tanning confers only limited sun protection (a protection factor of less than 3 as reported by Cripps 1981), suggesting that melanin is not a perfect sunscreen. Moreover, melanin photochemistry is intriguing and appears sometimes to contradict its photoprotective role.

In Vitro Data

The phototoxicity of pheomelanin and its instability in the presence of UV light were reported in the literature some time ago. These properties are consistent with the vulnerability of individuals with red hair to sun damage (for review see Napolitano et al. 2014). However, the production of ROS by synthetic or natural black and brown pigments exposed to UV radiation has also been observed in vitro (Tomita et al. 1984; Korytowski et al. 1987; Kipp and Young 1999). These unexpected results were confirmed in cultured melanocytes irradiated with different UV spectra, using DNA damage as a marker. Noz et al. used the comet assay, which quantifies DNA breaks in individual cells, to compare the sensitivity of melanocytes from dysplastic nevi, common nevi and normal skin to UVB-induced DNA damage. The highest level of DNA damage (in the dark or under UVB) was observed in dysplastic nevus cells, the most highly pigmented cell type used in the experiments (Noz et al. 1996). Wenczl et al. obtained comparable data in UVA-exposed cells in which melanogenesis had been previously increased by adding tyrosine to the culture medium (Wenczl et al. 1998). Marrot et al. compared DNA damage in human fibroblasts, in melanocytes from different donors and in melanocytes activated by tyrosine. Here again, DNA damage induction correlated with melanin content (Marrot et al. 1999). Kvam and Tyrrell showed enhanced induction of 8-OHdG oxidative damage in the DNA of murine or human melanoma cells, when melanogenesis was activated prior to UVA exposure (Kvam and Tyrrell 1999).

In Vivo Data

Whether those in vitro data reflect an in vivo reality has been a matter of debate, since constitutive skin pigmentation unquestionably determines the incidence of skin cancer. In fact, squamous cell carcinomas and melanomas are respectively 50 or 13 times more common in Caucasians than in African Americans (Halder and Bridgeman-Shah 1995). In vivo, induction of DNA damage in the form of pyrimidine dimers is inversely correlated with ethnic pigmentation (Bykov et al. 2000; Kobayashi et al. 2001) or with skin color as assessed by individual typology angle (ITA) (Del Bino et al. 2006). However, could the resistance of dark skin to DNA photodamage be attributable solely to pigmentation? A 2005 review discussed the prevention of DNA photodamage by melanogenesis and concluded that the repair of DNA damage could correlate with skin phototype, i.e. repair would occur more rapidly in the dark-skinned type IV than in the fair-skinned type II (Agar and Young 2005) More recently, Miyamura et al. reported that UVA-induced tanning did not confer significant protection against UVB-induced pyrimidine dimers, and that other protective factors such as DNA repair might be linked to skin pigmentation (Miyamura et al. 2011). The deleterious impact of melanin in vivo was addressed by some results obtained using the Platyfish *Xiphophorus*. The action spectra of UV and visible light in the induction of melanoma were studied, and heavily pigmented hybrids appeared very sensitive to tumor induction in the UVA spectrum. The authors considered that the photoreactivity of melanin may play a role in increasing the risk of UV-induced cancer (Setlow et al. 1993). The action spectra of radical species generation by melanin in *Xiphophorus* assessed by EPR and that of melanoma induction were comparable, suggesting that ROS produced by pigment photoreactivity contributed to tumor formation (Wood et al. 2006). Takeushi et al. compared the impact of UVB/UVA radiation on the skin of black, yellow and albino mice (the hair follicles and the inter-follicular epidermis). Although the level of pyrimidine dimers was similar in the three mouse strains, UV-induced apoptosis was higher in the upper portion of the hair follicles in most pigmented animals, suggesting that melanin acts as a photocatalyst of ROS production in hair bulbs (Takeuchi et al. 2004). Yamaguchi et al. compared levels of apoptotic cells in the epidermis of fair-skinned and dark-skinned human volunteers exposed to erythemal UV doses. Seven-fold more apoptotic cells were detected in dark skin, although DNA damage induction (CPD) was lower than in fair skin (Yamaguchi et al. 2006). Recently, Noonan et al. confirmed the capacity of melanin to increase the risk of melanoma in vivo through generation of oxidative stress in melanocytes exposed to UVA. Using a HGF transgenic mouse previously developed as a model for UV induced melanoma (Noonan et al. 2001), they compared tumorigenesis in black and albino animals. Melanoma induction by UVA required the presence of melanin (i.e. the frequency of UVA-induced melanoma was higher in black mice than in albino ones) and UVA exposure of pigmented animals was followed by significant formation of 8-oxo-dG in melanocyte DNA (Noonan et al. 2012). Interestingly, in the skin of these transgenic mice, melanocytes were not confined to hair follicles but were scattered within the epidermis and dermis, and melanin transfer to keratinocytes was relatively inefficient. Therefore, the UV protection provided by the upper epidermis was limited, while melanin accumulated within melanocytes, where its presence probably promoted the generation of a significant oxidative stress on exposure to UVA. In a way, data obtained by Noonan et al. constituted an in vivo proof of concept for in vitro experiments conducted on UVA-irradiated cultured melanocytes. Premi et al. recently reported the induction of CPD in melanocytes, in the dark and several hours after exposure to UVA. This *a priori* improbable process relies on a chemiexcitation pathway which begins with the generation of peroxynitrite from UVA-induced ROS and RNS (reactive nitrogen species). Melanin precursors (or melanin degradation products) associated with peroxynitrite critically influence this process by catalyzing the formation of excited-state triplet carbonyl residues in the vicinity of nuclear DNA. These carbonyl entities can then transfer the required energy to pyrimidines for the formation of pyrimidine dimers in the absence of light (Premi et al. 2015). UVA and melanin can thus also contribute to the induction of UVB-like mutagenic lesions in melanocytes.

In conclusion, accumulating evidence suggests that melanogenesis combined with exposure to sunlight may constitute a serious risk factor for the development of skin cancer. Although this phenomenon mainly concerns lightly pigmented skin, it may not be neglected in photoprotection strategies.

8.3 Melanocytes as Targets of (Bio) Chemical Toxicity

8.3.1 AhR Activators

The Aryl hydrocarbon Receptor (AhR) is a cytoplasmic transcription factor which is activated by various chemical ligands (Fig. 8.4). It controls expression of some cytochrome P450 enzymes including CYP1A1 and CYP1B1 which are involved in the metabolism of compounds such as dioxin (TCCD), Polycyclic Aromatic Hydrocarbons (PAH, e.g. benzopyrene), indocarbinols, flavonoids. As monooxygenases, CYP1A1 and B1 reduce the hydrophobicity of chemicals but can also generate reactive metabolites (e.g. epoxides) which are either transformed into diols and glucuronides or are conjugated to glutathione before excretion. UVB radiation produces a tryptophan photoproduct, FICZ, which is also a very potent AhR activator at concentrations in the picomolar range (Fritsche et al. 2007). Since AhR is present in the epidermis, FICZ may constitute a chemical link between sunlight and skin metabolism. AhR activation produces reactive and potentially mutagenic intermediates, it is thus suspected that this pathway may promote tumorigenesis. AhR is expressed in all skin cells and may increase the development of carcinoma: the incidence of benzopyrene-induced skin cancer is lower in AhR-/- knockout mice (Shimizu et al. 2000). AhR is also expressed in melanocytes and may be responsible for the hypermelanosis that is generally reported in individuals exposed to dioxin, a powerful AhR activator. Dioxin or FICZ may stimulate melanin production in vitro by increasing the activity of melanogenic enzymes (TYR and TRP1) in an AhR-dependent process involving MITF (Luecke et al. 2010). Moreover, UVB-induced pigmentation was reduced in AhR-/- mice compared to wild type animals, confirming a possible involvement of AhR in tanning (Jux et al. 2011). Pigmentation was also increased in melanocytes treated with cigarette smoke extracts which contain PAH as potential AhR ligands (Nakamura et al. 2013) and in vivo, smoking is associated with lip and gingival hyperpigmentation (Haresaku et al. 2007). A paradoxical stress-induced depigmentation was reported in pityriasis versicolor, a skin disease caused by *Malassezia furfur*, a lipophilic yeast which is one of the flora resident on human skin. *M furfur* produces indole derivatives such as pityriacitrin,

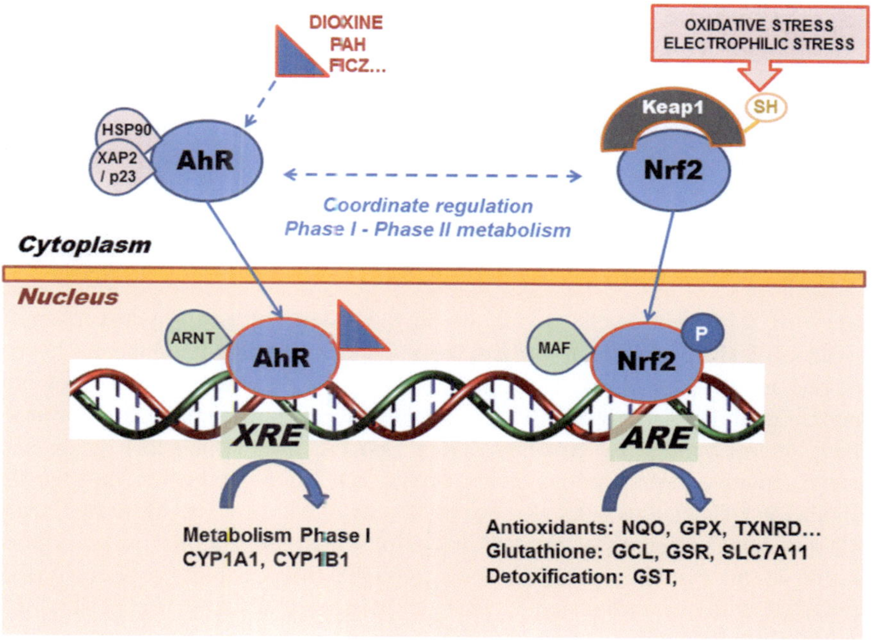

Fig. 8.4 AhR and Nrf2 pathways. Cytoplasmic AhR is maintained inactive in a multiprotein complex. Interaction with chemical ligands modifies AhR structure and facilitates its nuclear translocation where it binds the specific sequence XRE (xenobiotic responsive element). As a transcription factor, AhR controls expression of genes involved in phase I metabolism such as CYP1A1/B1 (for review see Denison et al. 2011). Nrf2 is repressed by Keap1, which contains thiol residues as redox sensors. After alteration of Keap1 conformation or after phosphorylation, Nrf2 translocates into the nucleus and binds the specific sequence ARE (antioxidant responsive element). Nrf2 controls and coordinates expression of a battery of genes encoding antioxidant and detoxifying enzymes (for review see Niture et al. 2014). Coordination of both AhR and Nrf2 activations ensures safe metabolism of xenobiotics since toxic metabolites are neutralized and excreted by Nrf2 pathway. In fact, a biochemical crosstalk between AhR and Nrf2 was recently described (Kalthoff et al. 2010)

indirubin or malassezin, some of which are potential AhR ligands (for review see Gaitanis et al. 2013). However, instead of triggering AhR-induced pigmentation, malassezin displayed a potent melanocytotoxicity in vitro (mainly apoptosis) which explains the occurrence of white spots in infected skin (Krämer et al. 2005). Zinc pyrithione (ZnPT) is a microbiocidal agent used as a topical antimicrobial. It targets *Malassezia* and thus behaves as an efficient antidandruff compound. Strikingly ZnPT also displayed toxic effects in melanocytes in vitro: it induced high expression of the stress marker HSP70, damaged genomic DNA and could finally trigger apoptosis (Lamore et al. 2010).

8.3.2 Phenol Compounds as Chemicals with Melanocyte-Specific Cytotoxicity

Melanocytes are generally resistant to the apoptosis induced by different kinds of stress; however some phenol compounds can produce a targeted toxicity leading to leukoderma, a vitiligo-like disease. Leukoderma symptoms include partial to complete depigmentation of the skin areas in contact with damaging products due to a significant decrease in the melanocyte population. Phenolic structures involved in this toxic process can be found in pharmaceutical products, cosmetic ingredients and food additives, such as for instance rhododenol (4-(4-hydroxyphenyl)-2-butanol) and the corresponding raspberry ketone, 4-tertiary-butylphenol, hydroquinone monomethyl-ether. These compounds may penetrate melanosomes and interfere with the melanogenic process as their structures resemble that of tyrosine. They are transformed by tyrosinase/TRP1 into quinones which then generate a strong oxidative stress through redox cycling and ROS production: in fact, the stimulation of melanogenesis aggravates this cytotoxic process. Moreover, these quinones bind protein thiol residues, some of which are essential for enzymatic activities. This cytotoxic process further highlights the possibility of specific risks associated with the melanogenic pathway (Manga et al. 2006; Ito et al. 2015; Nagata et al. 2015).

8.3.3 Mediators of Inflammatory Stress Can Lead to Hyperpigmentation

Post-inflammatory hyperpigmentation (PIH) appears as the hypermelanosis often associated with acne, contact dermatitis or atopic dermatitis, but also results from stresses such as phototoxic drug eruption, burns and even mechanical irritation. PIH is manifested more commonly in dark skin as pigmented macules involving the epidermis and sometimes the dermis. PIH can be stimulated by inflammatory mediators such as endothelin-1 or stem cell factor, in addition to ROS or nitric oxide released by inflammatory cells. Oxidation of arachidonic acid, a well-known by-product of the inflammatory process, generates the leukotrienes LTC4 and LTD4, the thromboxane TXB2 and the prostaglandins PGE1, PGE2 and PGF2α. These factors stimulate melanocytes in vitro: dendricity is increased in treated cells which transfer more melanin to surrounding keratinocytes. Various messengers (cAMP, cGMP, diacylglycerol) and effectors (MAPK, PKC, PKA) are mobilized and this complex network reflects the exquisite connection of melanocyte physiology with general skin status (Lamel et al. 2013; for review Costin and Hearing 2007). Solar lentigo (SL) is sometimes considered an interesting PIH paradigm exemplifying the connection between pigmentation and skin health (for review see

Cardinali et al. 2012). SL appears as pigmented lesions in photodamaged skin, which increase with chronological aging. The number of melanocytes in SL is comparable to that in healthy skin, however hyperpigmentation affects the epidermal basal layer. Pigmentary proteins/peptides (tyrosinase, POMC, endothelin-1 (ET-1) and its receptor (ETRB), stem cell factor (SCF)) as well as keratinocyte growth factor (KGF) are locally upregulated. It is considered by experts that melanogenesis is stimulated by local damage to skin resulting in the overproduction of ET-1, SCF or KGF. SCF and KGF may constitute soluble factors secreted by fibroblasts: sun-damaged dermis may thus contribute directly to hypermelanosis in SL (Kovacs et al. 2010). Recently, UVA-mediated bystander stress produced in melanocytes by keratinocytes or fibroblasts was shown to further increase oxidative effects in pigment cells (Redmond et al. 2014). More generally, the influence of dermis status on pigmentation is now well established and for instance photoaged fibroblasts can contribute to local hyperpigmentation (Hedley et al. 2002; Duval et al. 2014).

8.3.4 Drug-Induced Hyperpigmentation

A recent systematic review of 306 publications stated that it appears likely that drug-induced hyperpigmentation is caused by only a limited number of compounds (Krause 2013). The use of prostaglandin agonists in ocular treatment leads to hyperpigmentation of periorbital skin, consistent with the pro-pigmenting impact of prostaglandins in inflammation-induced hyperpigmentation. In line with this, PGF2α analogs, such as for instance Latanoprost, were shown to stimulate skin pigmentation after topical application in guinea pigs (Anbar et al. 2009). Some other chemicals which do not produce harmful effects in the dark can be photoactivated by UVA, and their phototoxicity sometimes triggers hyperpigmentation. Psoralens have been extensively studied in this regard as 8-methoxy-psoralen (8-MOP) and in particular 5-methoxy-psoralen (5-MOP) are used in combination with UVA exposure (PUVA therapy) to repigment vitiligo lesions. This pigmentary response is probably linked to skin damage through genotoxic activation of p53. In fact, under UVA exposure, 8MOP or 5MOP induce DNA adduct formation (mono-adducts and crosslinks) leading to p53 mutation: moreover p53 regulates tyrosinase gene expression (Gasparro 2000; Khlgatian et al. 2002). There is insufficient space to cite all the data published on modulation of pigmentation by various drugs (antibiotics such as fluoroquinolones or minocycline; amiodarone, phenothiazine), particularly on exposure to sunlight: here again, pigmentation appears closely linked to skin stress (for review see Dereure 2001).

8.4 Melanocyte-Specific Defensive Capabilities

Despite the limited number of melanocytes in the epidermis and their low mitotic index, and despite chronic exposures to sunlight and to other environmental stressors, skin pigmentation generally persists throughout life. A resistance to apoptosis may be one explanation for this striking longevity, which carries an associated risk of damage accumulation ultimately leading to senescence or transformation. Moreover, recent data suggest that pigment cells can improve their ability to repair DNA damage and to manage oxidative stress.

8.4.1 αMSH/MC1R Improves Anti-genotoxic Protection

MC1R activates the main pathway controlling UV-induced pigmentation. Fortunately, the MC1R-cAMP response also facilitates repair of DNA photodamage by enhancing nucleotide excision repair in melanocytes. Stimulation of MC1R contributes to p53 serine-15 phosphorylation mediated by the cAMP/PKA pathway. The resulting stabilization and activation of p53 improves DNA repair within melanocytes (Kadekaro et al. 2012). It was recently proposed that MC1R-cAMP signaling could even act upstream of the repair process by allowing PKA-mediated phosphorylation of ATR. ATR interacts with the XP repair factor to form a complex at sites of DNA photolesions and this accelerates excision repair of damaged DNA (Jarrett et al. 2014). In order to maintain the melanocyte population in skin, α-MSH also inhibits UV-induced cell death by increasing levels of the anti-apoptotic protein Bcl2. In fact, Bcl2 is a target for the transcription factor MITF which is activated by the MC1R-cAMP pathway. This mechanism could explain why melanocytes can survive acute UV doses and persist in photoexposed skin for decades (Böhm et al. 2005; Kadekaro et al. 2005). Overexposure to sun is generally associated with increased melanoma genesis but the molecular mechanisms involved remain unclear. Some oncogenes are frequently mutated in melanoma caused by chronic irradiation or non-chronic acute UV exposures (C-KIT and BRAF respectively). The risk of melanoma increased for BRAF mutants in a context of MC1R variants (Fink and Fisher 2013) or when p53 was also mutated (Viros et al. 2014). These results further highlight the influence of MC1R and p53 in the prevention of melanocyte transformation.

8.4.2 Adjustment of Endogenous Antioxidants

In the last decade, the transcription factor Nrf2 has aroused increasing interest because of its central role in controlling cellular redox homeostasis. In normal conditions, Nrf2 is maintained inactive as a protein complex with its repressor protein Keap1. In response to oxidative stress or in the presence of electrophiles, oxidation of Keap1 cysteine residues and/or Nrf2 phosphorylation leads to complex dissociation (Fig. 8.4). Nrf2 translocates into the nucleus where it interacts with the specific DNA ARE sequence (antioxidant responsive element). This pathway upregulates the expression of several downstream genes involved in antioxydation, preservation of glutathione homeostasis and detoxification. In our laboratory, we compared basal expression in the dark of around 200 genes involved in skin metabolism in melanocytes and keratinocytes in coculture (same culture medium) from the same donors (same genetic background). Most genes were expressed equally but some interesting differences could be observed as shown in Table 8.1 (Denat et al. manuscript in preparation). Higher levels of expression of NQO1/2, catalase and ferritin in melanocytes could be linked to a specific need for protection against quinones or H_2O_2 generated during melanogenesis.

Nrf2 is activated by UV (mainly UVA) or by natural electrophilic chemicals such as sulforaphane or lipoic acid. Interestingly, the panel of overexpressed genes in cells from the same donors differs between keratinocytes and melanocytes: for instance HO-1 is always upregulated in pigment cells (Marrot et al. 2008). In line with this, a recent study showed that downregulation of Nrf2 in immortalized human melanocyte cell line increased sensitivity to oxidative stress whereas upregulation of Nrf2 protected melanocytes from H_2O_2 toxicity. HO-1 was the most efficient Nrf2 downstream gene involved in this protection pathway (Jian et al. 2011). More recently, the same team observed that the Nrf2 pathway was impaired in melanocytes in vitiligo, and thus HO-1 expression was significantly reduced. This inability to adjust antioxidant status could explain the high sensitivity to H_2O_2 (Jian et al. 2014). In skin explants exposed to UVA or to 4 tertiary-butylphenol

Table 8.1 Relative expression of antioxidant genes in melanocytes and keratinocytes

	Overexpression in Melanocyte (M)	Overexpression in Keratinocyte (K)
Quinone detoxification	NQO-1 (×20) NQO-2 (×3)	–
ROS detoxification	Catalase (×4) Ferritin-FTL (×3) HO-1 (×7)	GPX-2 (×3) GPX-3 (×14)
ROS/RNS	NOX4 (×43)	NOS-1 (0 in M)
Glutathione metabolism	GST-A4 (×2) GST-M2 (×37) GST-M3 (0 in K)	GCLC (×4) GGT1 (×4)

Cells from the same donor (same genetic background) were co-cultured in two chambers separated by a membrane in the same dish (same culture medium). Duplicate experiments were performed with cells from two different donors. Messenger RNAs from melanocytes and keratinocytes were extracted separately and analyzed by quantitative RT-PCR. This table shows antioxidant genes overexpressed in one cell type versus the other. For instance, melanocytes displayed a higher expression of genes involved in protection against melanogenesis related oxidative stress (NQO1/2 against quinones, catalase and ferritin against H_2O_2 toxicity) (a melanocytotoxic compound), Ellasuity et al. showed that HO-1 was upregulated in melanocytes. This result was confirmed in cultured cells, and HO-1 overexpression may protect melanocytes from UVB-induced cytotoxicity (Elassiuty et al. 2011).

Importantly, α-MSH drives increased Nrf2 expression which in turn upregulates target genes such as HO-1, GCL or GST, and therefore α-MSH is also linked to antioxidant protection in melanocytes. Moreover, α-MSH also abolishes the inhibitory effect of UVB on Nrf2 therefore maintaining melanocyte capacity to manage oxidative stress even under high levels of exposure to sunlight (Kokot et al. 2009).

8.5 Conclusion: Molecular Opportunities

Melanocytes undoubtedly play a crucial role in the response of the skin to the environment. Paradoxically, melanocytes are present in skin in limited numbers, their basal proliferation rate is low, they are thought to remain active for decades, the process of melanogenesis carries risks for these cells, and their transformation leads to melanoma. Melanocyte protection is thus of huge importance and current knowledge offers several molecular opportunities. The avoidance of sunlight seems indispensable particularly when there is active melanogenesis. In order to ensure protection of the melanocyte genome against sunlight-induced DNA damage (pyrimidine dimers and oxidative breakage), photostable and broad-spectrum sunscreen formulations which provide significant UVA absorption are required (Marrot et al. 1999; Jean et al. 2001). Antioxidants are also generally recommended in photoprotection and a comprehensive approach to prevention might be secured by activation of the endogenous defenses controlled by Nrf2. Interestingly, it was recently reported that Nrf2 could also regulate melanogenesis by modulating the PI3 K/Akt signaling pathway or by reducing melanogenesis induced by UVA (Shin et al. 2014; Chaiprasongsuk et al. 2016) whereas NQO1, one the Nrf2 downstream genes, behaves as a positive regulator of the pigmentation process (Choi et al. 2010). Nrf2 is involved in the phase II detoxification process and interacts with other stress-related pathways such as AhR or NFkB (Hayes and Dinkova-Kostova 2014). Moreover, some Nrf2 inducers can kill melanoma cells but not normal melanocytes (Qiao et al. 2012): chemoprevention targeting melanocytes might thus be a promising strategy for skin protection against UV and toxic chemicals. Activation of the MC1R-cAMP pathway seems to be a very interesting way to prevent stress and also to repair damage in melanocytes responding to α-MSH. In fact, since MC1R is linked to Nrf2, α-MSH signaling may represent a valuable general preventive pathway. Once photodamage is induced, stimulation of DNA repair could be of huge interest as an anticancer approach since it has been reported that DNA repair capacity in melanoma patients is reduced. Melanocortin analog peptides have been reported to counteract the photodamaging effects of UV in vitro, sometimes better than α-MSH itself. However, their efficiency ex vivo (in human skin explants) or in clinical trials remains to be demonstrated: penetration of peptides into the deep epidermis is a difficult challenge (for review see Abdel-Malek et al. 2014). Another possibility would be to capitalize on natural α-MSH production by stimulating the production of p53 in keratinocytes in a way that is safe for the cell. Some chemical activators which interact with mdm2, the natural p53 repressor protein, have been studied for several years. For instance, the compound nutlin-3 can potentiate p53 activity in melanocytes in vitro (Kadekaro et al. 2012), and can reduce CPD and apoptosis in mouse skin in vivo (Lerche et al. 2010), even if its ability to decrease sunlight-induced carcinogenesis is not yet established (Lerche et al. 2012).

In conclusion, the protection of melanocytes is a concern that is relevant to cosmetic goals (tanning or lightening) as well as to therapeutic applications (vitiligo, melanoma). Knowledge in this field is increasing and suggests that skin pigment cells have a unique physiology and require very specific care.

Acknowledgments Dr V Facy and Dr F Laugier (L'Oréal Advanced Research) are deeply acknowledged for their help in preparing this manuscript.

References

Abdel-Malek ZA, Swope VB, Starner RJ, Koikov L, Cassidy P, Leachman S (2014) Melanocortins and the melanocortin 1 receptor, moving translationally towards melanoma prevention. Arch Biochem Biophys 563:4–12

Agar N, Young AR (2005) Melanogenesis: a photoprotective response to DNA damage? Mutat Res Fundam Mol Mech Mutagen 571(1-2 SPEC. ISS.):121–132

Anbar TS, Abdel-Raouf H, Awad SS, Ragaie MH, Abdel-Rahman AT (2009) The hair follicle melanocytes in vitiligo in relation to disease duration. J Eur Acad Dermatol Venereol 23 (8):934–939

Böhm M, Wolff I, Scholzen TE, Robinson SJ, Healy E, Luger TA, Schwarz T, Schwarz A (2005) α-Melanocyte-stimulating hormone protects from ultraviolet radiation-induced apoptosis and DNA damage. J Biol Chem 280(7):5795–5802

Borovanský J, Vedralová E, Hach P (1991) An estimate of melanosome concentration in pigment tissues. Pigment Cell Res 4(5–6):222–224

Bykov VJ, Marcusson JA, Hemminki K (2000) Effect of constitutional pigmentation on ultraviolet B-induced DNA damage in fair-skinned people. J Invest Dermatol 114(1):40–43

Cardinali G, Kovacs D, Picardo M (2012) Mechanisms underlying post-inflammatory hyperpigmentation: lessons from solar lentigo. Ann Dermatol Venereol 139(Suppl 4):S148–S152

Chaiprasongsuk A, Onkoksoong T, Pluemsamran T, Limsaengurai S, Panich U (2016) Photoprotection by dietary phenolics against melanogenesis induced by UVA through Nrf2-dependent antioxidant responses. Redox Biol 8:79–90

Cheli Y, Ohanna M, Ballotti R, Bertolotto C (2009) Fifteen-year quest for microphthalmia-associated transcription factor target genes. Pigm Cell Melanoma Res 23 (1):27–40

Choi W, Miyamura Y, Wolber R, Smuda C, Reinhold W, Liu H, Kolbe L, Hearing VJ (2010) Regulation of human skin pigmentation in situ by repetitive UV exposure: Molecular characterization of responses to UVA and/or UVB. J Invest Dermatol 130(6):1685–1696

Costin G, Hearing VJ (2007) Human skin pigmentation: melanocytes modulate skin color in response to stress. FASEB J 21(4):976–994

Cripps DJ (1981) Natural and artificial photoprotection. J Invest Dermatol 77(1):154–157

Cui R, Widlund HR, Feige E, Lin JY, Wilensky DL, Igras VE, D'Orazio J, Fung CY, Schanbacher CF, Granter SR, Fisher DE (2007) Central role of p53 in the suntan response and pathologic hyperpigmentation. Cell 128(5):853–864

Del Bino S, Sok J, Bessac E, Bernerd F (2006) Relationship between skin response to ultraviolet exposure and skin color type. Pigm Cell Res 19(6):606–614

Denat L, Kadekaro AL, Marrot L, Leachman SA, Abdel-Malek ZA (2014) Melanocytes as instigators and victims of oxidative stress. J Invest Dermatol 134(6):1512–1518

Denison MS, Soshilov AA, He G, DeGroot DE, Zhao B (2011) Exactly the same but different: promiscuity and diversity in the molecular mechanisms of action of the aryl hydrocarbon (dioxin) receptor. Toxicol Sciences 124(1):1–22

Dereure O (2001) Drug-induced skin pigmentation. American J Clin Dermatol 2(4):253–262

Duval C, Cohen C, Chagnoleau C, Flouret V, Bourreau E, Bernerd F (2014) Key regulatory role of dermal fibroblasts in pigmentation as demonstrated using a reconstructed skin model: impact of photo-aging. PLoS ONE 9(12)

Elassiuty YE, Klarquist J, Speiser J, Yousef RM, El Refaee AA, Hunter NS, Shaker OG, Gundeti M, Nieuweboer-Krobotova L, Caroline Le Poole I (2011) Heme oxygenase-1 expression protects melanocytes from stress-induced cell death: implications for vitiligo. Exp Dermatol 20(6):496–501

Eller MS, Ostrom K, Gilchrest BA (1996) DNA damage enhances melanogenesis. Proc Natl Acad Sci USA 93(3):1087–1092

Fink EC, Fisher DE (2013) BRAF and MC1R in Melanoma: different in Head and Neck Tumors? J Invest Dermatol 133(4):878–880

Fritsche E, Schäfer C, Calles C, Bernsmann T, Bernshausen T, Wurm M, Hübenthal U, Cline JE, Hajimiragha H, Schroeder P, Klotz L-, Rannug A, Fürst P, Hanenberg H, Abel J, Krutmann J (2007) Lightening up the UV response by identification of the arylhydrocarbon receptor as a cytoplasmatic target for ultraviolet B radiation. Proc Natl Acad Sci USA 104(21):8851–8856

Gaitanis G, Velegraki A, Mayser P, Bassukas ID (2013) Skin diseases associated with malassezia yeasts: Facts and controversies. Clin Dermatol 31(4):455–463

García-Borrón JC, Abdel-Malek Z, Jiménez-Cervantes C (2014) MC1R, the cAMP pathway, and the response to solar UV: extending the horizon beyond pigmentation. Pigm Cell Melanoma Res 27(5):699–720

Gasparro FP (2000) The role of PUVA in the treatment of psoriasis: Photobiology issues related to skin cancer incidence. Am J Clin Dermatol 1(6):337–348

Gilchrest BA, Zhai S, Eller MS, Yarosh EB, Yaar M (1993) Treatment of human melanocytes and S01 melanoma cells with the DNA repair enzyme T4 endonuclease V enhances melanogenesis after ultraviolet irradiation. J Invest Dermatol 101(5):666–672

Gilchrest BA, Eller MS, Yaar M (2009) Telomere-mediated effects on melanogenesis and skin aging. J Invest Dermatol Symp Proc 14(1):25–31

Halder RM, Bridgeman-Shah S (1995) Skin cancer in african americans. Cancer 75(2 Suppl.):667–673

Haresaku S, Hanioka T, Tsutsui A, Watanabe T (2007) Association of lip pigmentation with smoking and gingival melanin pigmentation. Oral Dis 13(1):71–76

Hayes JD, Dinkova-Kostova A (2014) The Nrf2 regulatory network provides an interface between redox and intermediary metabolism. Trends Biochem Sci 39(4):199–218

Hedley SJ, Layton C, Heaton M, Chakrabarty KH, Dawson RA, Gawkrodger DJ, Mac Neil S (2002) Fibroblasts play a regulatory role in the control of pigmentation in reconstructed human skin from skin types I and II. Pigm Cell Res 15(1):49–56

Hill HZ, Li W, Xin P, Mitchell DL (1997) Melanin: A two edged sword? Pigm Cell Res 10 (3):158–161

Hyter S, Coleman DJ, Ganguli-Indra G, Merrill GF, Ma S, Yanagisawa M, Indra AK (2012) Endothelin-1 is a transcriptional target of p53 in epidermal keratinocytes and regulates ultraviolet-induced melanocyte homeostasis. Pigm Cell Melanoma Res 26(2):247–258

Ito S, Okura M, Nakanishi Y, Ojika M, Wakamatsu K, Yamashita T (2015) Tyrosinase-catalyzed metabolism of rhododendrol (RD) in B16 melanoma cells: Production of RD-pheomelanin and covalent binding with thiol proteins. Pigm Cell Melanoma Res 28(3):295–306

Jarrett SG, Horrell EMW, Christian PA, Vanover JC, Boulanger MC, Zou Y, D'Orazio JA (2014) PKA-mediated phosphorylation of ATR promotes recruitment of XPA to UV-induced DNA damage. Mol Cell 54(6):999–1011

Jean S, De Méo M, Sabatier A-, Laget M, Hubaud J-, Verrando P, Duménil G (2001) Evaluation of sunscreen protection in human melanocytes exposed to UVA or UVB irradiation using the alkaline comet assay. Photochem Photobiol 74(3):417–423

Jian Z, Li K, Liu L, Zhang Y, Zhou Z, Li C, Gao T (2011) Heme oxygenase-1 protects human melanocytes from H2O 2-induced oxidative stress via the Nrf2-ARE pathway. J Invest Dermatol 131(7):1420–1427

Jian Z, Li K, Song P, Zhu G, Zhu L, Cui T, Liu B, Tang L, Wang X, Wang G, Gao T, Li C (2014) Impaired activation of the Nrf2-ARE signaling pathway undermines H_2O_2-induced oxidative stress response: a possible mechanism for melanocyte degeneration in vitiligo. J Invest Dermatol 134(8):2221–2230

Jux B, Kadow S, Luecke S, Rannug A, Krutmann J, Esser C (2011) The aryl hydrocarbon receptor mediates UVB radiation-induced skin tanning. J Invest Dermatol 131(1):203–210

Kadekaro AL, Kavanagh R, Kanto H, Terzieva S, Hauser J, Kobayashi N, Schwemberger S, Cornelius J, Babcock G, Shertzer HG, Scott G, Abdel-Malek ZA (2005) α-Melanocortin and endothelin-1 activate antiapoptotic pathways and reduce DNA damage in human melanocytes. Cancer Res 65(10):4292–4299

Kadekaro AL, Chen J, Yang J, Chen S, Jameson J, Swope VB, Cheng T, Kadakia M, Abdel-Malek Z (2012) Alpha-melanocyte-stimulating hormone suppresses oxidative stress through a p53-mediated signaling pathway in human melanocytes. Mol Cancer Res 10(6): 778–786

Kalthoff S, Ehmer U, Freiberg N, Manns MP, Strassburg CP (2010) Interaction between oxidative stress sensor Nrf2 and xenobiotic-activated aryl hydrocarbon receptor in the regulation of the human phase II detoxifying UDP-glucuronosyltransferase 1A10. J Biol Chem 285(9):5993–6002

Khlgatian MK, Hadshiew IM, Asawanonda P, Yaar M, Eller MS, Fujita M, Norris DA, Gilchrest BA (2002) Tyrosinase gene expression is regulated by p53. J Invest Dermatol 118 (1):126–132

Kipp C, Young AR (1999) The soluble eumelanin precursor 5,6-dihydroxyindole-2-carboxylic acid enhances oxidative damage in human keratinocyte DNA after UVA irradiation. Photochem Photobiol 70(2):191–198

Kobayashi N, Katsumi S, Imoto K, Nakagawa A, Miyagawa S, Furumura M, Mori T (2001) Quantitation and visualization of ultraviolet-induced DNA damage using specific antibodies: Application to pigment cell biology. Pigm Cell Res 14(2):94–102

Koga S, Nakano M, Tero-Kubota S (1992) Generation of superoxide during the enzymatic action of tyrosinase. Arch Biochem Biophys 292(2):570–575

Kokot A, Metze D, Mouchet N, Galibert M-, Schiller M, Luger TA, Böhm M (2009) α-Melanocyte-stimulating hormone counteracts the suppressive effect of UVB on Nrf2 and nrf-dependent gene expression in human skin. Endocrinology 150(7):3197–3206

Korytowski W, Pilas B, Sarna T, Kalyanaraman B (1987) Photoinduced generation of hydrogen peroxide and hydroxyl radicals in melanins. Photochem Photobiol 45(2):185–190

Kovacs D, Cardinali G, Aspite N, Cota C, Luzi F, Bellei B, Briganti S, Amantea A, Torrisi MR, Picardo M (2010) Role of fibroblast-derived growth factors in regulating hyperpigmentation of solar lentigo. Br J Dermatol 163(5):1020–1027

Krämer H-, Podobinska M, Bartsch A, Battmann A, Thoma W, Bernd A, Kummer W, Irlinger B, Steglich W, Mayser P (2005) Malassezin, a novel agonist of the aryl hydrocarbon receptor from the yeast malassezia furfur, induces apoptosis in primary human melanocytes. ChemBioChem 6(5):860–865

Krause W (2013) Drug-induced hperpigemntation: A systematic review. JDDG J German Soc Dermatol 11(7):644–652
Kvam E, Tyrrell RM (1999) The role of melanin in the induction of oxidative DNA base damage by ultraviolet A irradiation of DNA or melanoma cells. J Invest Dermatol 113(2):209–213
Lamel SA, Rahvar M, Maibach HI (2013) Postinflammatory hyperpigmentation secondary to external insult: An overview of the quantitative analysis of pigmentation. Cutaneous Ocul Toxicol 32(1):67–71
Lamore SD, Cabello CM, Wondrak GT (2010) The topical antimicrobial zinc pyrithione is a heat shock response inducer that causes DNA damage and PARP-dependent energy crisis in human skin cells. Cell Stress Chaperones 15(3):309–322
Lerche CM, Thomsen BM, Wulf HC, Gniadecki R (2010) Topical nutlin-3 potentiates the UVB-induced p53 response and reduces DNA photodamage and apoptosis in mouse epidermal keratinocytes in vivo. J Clin Exp Dermatol Res 1:106
Lerche CM, Philipsen PA, Poulsen T, Gniadecki R, Wulf HC (2012) Topical nutlin-3a does not decrease photocarcinogenesis induced by simulated solar radiation in hairless mice. Photodermatol Photoimmunol Photomed 28(4):207–212
Luecke S, Backlund M, Jux B, Esser C, Krutmann J, Rannug A (2010) The aryl hydrocarbon receptor (AHR), a novel regulator of human melanogenesis. Pigm Cell Melanoma Res 23 (6):828–833
Manga P, Sheyn D, Yang F, Sarangarajan R, Boissy RE (2006) A role for tyrosinase-related protein 1 in 4-tert-butylphenol-induced toxicity in melanocytes: Implications for vitiligo. Am J Pathol 169(5):1652–1662
Maresca V, Flori E, Briganti S, Mastrofrancesco A, Fabbri C, Mileo AM, Paggi MG, Picardo M (2008) Correlation between melanogenic and catalase activity in in vitro human melanocytes: a synergic strategy against oxidative stress. Pigm Cell Melanoma Res 21(2):200–205
Marrot L, Meunier JR (2008) Skin DNA photodamage and its biological consequences. J Am Acad Dermatol 58(5 SUPPL. 2):S139–S148
Marrot L, Belaidi J-, Meunier J-, Perez P, Agapakis-Causse C (1999) The human melanocyte as a particular target for UVA radiation and an endpoint for photoprotection assessment. Photochem Photobiol 69(6):686–693
Marrot L, Jones C, Perez P, Meunier JR (2008) The significance of Nrf2 pathway in (photo)-oxidative stress response in melanocytes and keratinocytes of the human epidermis. Pigm Cell Melanoma Res 21(1):79–88
Meyskens FL Jr, Farmer P, Fruehauf JP (2001) Redox regulation in human melanocytes and melanoma. Pigm Cell Res 14(3):148–154
Michard Q, Commo S, Belaidi J-, Alleaume A-, Michelet J-, Daronnat E, Eilstein J, Duche D, Marrot L, Bernard BA (2008) TRP-2 specifically decreases WM35 cell sensitivity to oxidative stress. Free Radic Biol Med 44(6):1023–1031
Miranda M, Ligas C, Amicarelli F, D'Alessandro E, Brisdelli F, Zarivi O, Poma A (1997) Sister chromatid exchange (SCE) rates in human melanoma cells as an index of mutagenesis. Mutagenesis 12(4):233–236
Miyamura Y, Coelho SG, Schlenz K, Batzer J, Smuda C, Choi W, Brenner M, Passeron T, Zhang G, Kolbe L, Wolber R, Hearing VJ (2011) The deceptive nature of UVA tanning versus the modest protective effects of UVB tanning on human skin. Pigm Cell Melanoma Res 24 (1):136–147
Morgan AM, Lo J, Fisher DE (2013) How does pheomelanin synthesis contribute to melanomagenesis?: two distinct mechanisms could explain the carcinogenicity of pheomelanin synthesis. BioEssays 35(8):672–676
Nagata T, Ito S, Itoga K, Kanazawa H, Masaki H (2015) The mechanism of melanocytes-specific cytotoxicity induced by phenol compounds having a prooxidant effect, relating to the appearance of leukoderma. BioMed Res Int 2015
Nakamura M, Ueda Y, Hayashi M, Kato H, Furuhashi T, Morita A (2013) Tobacco smoke-induced skin pigmentation is mediated by the aryl hydrocarbon receptor. Exp Dermatol 22(8):556–558

Napolitano A, Panzella L, Monfrecola G, d'Ischia M (2014) Pheomelanin-induced oxidative stress: bright and dark chemistry bridging red hair phenotype and melanoma. Pigm Cell Melanoma Res 27(5):721–733

Nappi AJ, Vass E (1996) Hydrogen peroxide generation associated with the oxidations of the eumelanin precursors 5,6-dihydroxyindole and 5,6-dihydroxyindole-2-carboxylic acid. Melanoma Res 6(5):341–349

Niture SK, Khatri R, Jaiswal AK (2014) Regulation of Nrf2-an update. Free Rad Biol Med 66:36–44

Noonan FP, Recio JA, Takayama H, Duray P, Anver MR, Rush WL, De Fabo EC, Merlino G (2001) Neonatal sunburn and melanoma in mice. Nature 413(6853):271–272

Noonan FP, Zaidi MR, Wolnicka-Glubisz A, Anver MR, Bahn J, Wielgus A, Cadet J, Douki T, Mouret S, Tucker MA, Popratiloff A, Merlino G, De Fabo EC (2012) Melanoma induction by ultraviolet A but not ultraviolet B radiation requires melanin pigment. Nat Commun 3

Noz KC, Bauwens M, Van Buul PPW, Vrolijk H, Schothorst AA, Pavel S, Tanke HJ, Vermeer BJ (1996) Comet assay demonstrates a higher ultraviolet B sensitivity to DNA damage in dysplastic nevus cells than in common melanocytic nevus cells and foreskin melanocytes. J Invest Dermatol 106(6):1198–1202

Pavel S, Van Nieuwpoort F, Van Der Meulen H, Out C, Pizinger K, Cetkovská P, Smit NPM, Koerten HK (2004) Disturbed melanin synthesis and chronic oxidative stress in dysplastic naevi. Eur J Cancer 40(9):1423–1430

Premi S, Wallisch S, Mano CM, Weiner AB, Bacchiocchi A, Wakamatsu K, Bechara EJH, Halaban R, Douki T, Brash DE (2015) Chemiexcitation of melanin derivatives induces DNA photoproducts long after UV exposure. Science 347(6224):842–847

Qiao S, Lamore SD, Cabello CM, Lesson JL, Muñoz-Rodriguez JL, Wondrak GT (2012) Thiostrepton is an inducer of oxidative and proteotoxic stress that impairs viability of human melanoma cells but not primary melanocytes. Biochem Pharmacol 83(9):1229–1240

Redmond RW, Rajadurai A, Udayakumar D, Sviderskaya EV, Tsao H (2014) Melanocytes are selectively vulnerable to UVA-mediated bystander oxidative signaling. J Invest Dermatol 134 (4):1083–1090

Setlow RB, Grist E, Thompson K, Woodhead AD (1993) Wavelengths effective in induction of malignant melanoma. Proc Natl Acad Sci USA 90(14):6666–6670

Shimizu Y, Nakatsuru Y, Ichinose M, Takahashi Y, Kume H, Mimura J, Fujii-Kuriyama Y, Ishikawa T (2000) Benzo[a]pyrene carcinogenicity is lost in mice lacking the aryl hydrocarbon receptor. Proc Natl Acad Sci U S A 97(2):779–782

Shin J, Kim MY, Sohn K, Jung S, Lee H, Lim JW, Kim S, Lee Y, Im M, Seo Y, Kim CD, Lee J, Lee Y, Yoon T (2014) Nrf2 negatively regulates melanogenesis by modulating PI3 K/Akt signaling. PLoS ONE 9(4)

Smit NPM, Van Nieuwpoort FA, Marrot L, Out C, Poorthuis B, Van Pelt H, Meunier J-, Pavel S (2008) Increased melanogenesis is a risk factor for oxidative DNA damage—study on cultured melanocytes and atypical nevus cells. Photochem Photobiol 84(3):550–555

Takeuchi S, Zhang W, Wakamatsu K, Ito S, Hearing VJ, Kraemer KH, Brash DE (2004) Melanin acts as a potent UVB photosensitizer to cause an atypical mode of cell death in murine skin. Proc Natl Acad Sci USA 101(42):15076–15081

Tomita Y, Hariu A, Kato C, Seiji M (1984) Radical production during tyrosinase reaction, dopa-melanin formation, and photoirradiation of dopa-melanin. J Invest Dermatol 82 (6):573–576

Viros A, Sanchez-Laorden B, Pedersen M, Furney SJ, Rae J, Hogan K, Ejiama S, Girotti MR, Cook M, Dhomen N, Marais R (2014) Ultraviolet radiation accelerates BRAF-driven melanomagenesis by targeting TP53. Nature 511(7510):478–482

Wenczl E, Van Der Schans GP, Roza L, Kolb RM, Timmerman AJ, Smit NPM, Pavel S, Schothorst AA (1998) (Pheo)melanin photosensitizes UVA-induced DNA damage in cultured human melanocytes. J Invest Dermatol 111(4):678–682

Wood SR, Berwick M, Ley RD, Walter RB, Setlow RB, Timmins GS (2006) UV causation of melanoma in xiphophorus is dominated by melanin photosentisized oxidant production. Proc Natl Acad Sci USA 103(11):4111–4115
Yamaguchi Y, Takahashi K, Zmudzka BZ, Kornhauser A, Miller SA, Tadokoro T, Berens W, Beer JZ, Hearing VJ (2006) Human skin responses to UV radiation: pigment in the upper epidermis protects against DNA damage in the lower epidermis and facilitates apoptosis. FASEB J 20(9):1486–1488

Chapter 9
The Role of Epidermal p38 Signaling in Solar UV Radiation-Induced Inflammation: Molecular Pathways and Preventive Opportunities

Jin Mo Park and Yasuyo Sano

Abstract Excessive exposure to sunlight poses a multitude of health risks, ranging from sunburn and premature skin aging to impaired immunity and skin cancer. Ultraviolet radiation is the component of sunlight that gives rise to these detrimental consequences. Inflammation is a key process underlying both acute skin damage and the long-term deleterious effects exerted by ultraviolet radiation. The protein kinase p38α, the most widely expressed p38 isoform in mammalian tissues, is activated by and mediates cellular responses to environmental stress such as ultraviolet radiation. Recent studies have shown that p38α signaling in epithelial cells of the skin, or keratinocytes, is essential for ultraviolet radiation-induced skin inflammation; mice with keratinocyte-specific p38α ablation exhibit a marked decrease in vascular changes, neutrophil infiltration, and other manifestations of inflammation. Mechanistically, p38α signaling drives the expression of a multitude of keratinocyte genes with a known function in inflammation. Small-molecule p38α inhibitors hold potential for suppressing ultraviolet radiation-induced skin inflammation and pathology, particularly if administered topically. A deeper understanding of the signaling events upstream and downstream of p38α in keratinocytes will help devised effective strategies for preventing the detrimental effects of solar ultraviolet radiation.

Keywords p38 · p38α · Protein kinase · Signaling · Ultraviolet radiation · Skin · Inflammation · Keratinocyte · Epidermis · Skin aging · Skin cancer · p38 inhibitors

---

J.M. Park (✉) · Y. Sano
Cutaneous Biology Research Center, Massachusetts General Hospital and Harvard Medical School, 149 Thirteenth Street, Charlestown, MA 02129, USA
e-mail: jmpark@cbrc2.mgh.harvard.edu

G.T. Wondrak (ed.), *Skin Stress Response Pathways*,
DOI 10.1007/978-3-319-43157-4_9

9.1 UV Radiation-Induced Skin Inflammation and Pathology

The stratified epithelium of the skin, or the epidermis, is a singular tissue in which cells are directly exposed to solar ultraviolet radiation (UVR). Epithelial cells constituting the epidermis—keratinocytes—elicit changes in intracellular signaling and gene expression in response to UVR exposure. These responses not only produce cell-autonomous effects such as the senescence, differentiation, and death of keratinocytes, but also lead to inflammation and other non-cell-autonomous consequences with local and systemic impacts. UVR-induced inflammation in itself is a protective response, promoting the repair of UVR-damaged skin and affording heightened antimicrobial defense until disrupted epidermal barrier function is restored. If not dampened or terminated in a timely manner, however, inflammation produces deleterious effects ranging from sunburn and impaired T cell immunity to premature skin aging and skin cancer (Yaar and Gilchrest 2007; Hart et al. 2011; Elmets and Athar 2013).

Ultraviolet B radiation (UVB), 290–315 nm in wavelength, is a component of sunlight that mainly contributes to the formation of cyclobutane pyrimidine dimers (CPD) and (6-4) pyrimidine-pyrimidone photoproducts (6-4PP) in DNA (Pfeifer and Besaratinia 2012). In addition, UVB-induced reactive oxygen species results in the generation of oxidized nucleosides in DNA, with the most prominent products being 8-hydroxy-2′-deoxyguanosine (8-OHdG), which tautomerizes to 8-oxo-7,8-dihydro-2′-deoxyguanosine (8-oxo-dG) (Pfeifer and Besaratinia 2012). Similar photoproducts and oxidized nucleosides can be formed in RNA. Ultraviolet A radiation (UVA), 315–400 nm in wavelength, is not as effective as UVB in forming CPD and 6-4PP, but able to generate reactive oxygen species and oxidized nucleosides (Pfeifer and Besaratinia 2012). Photons of UVB have a limited penetration into the skin and can only inflict direct damage on epidermal cells. Keratinocytes incurring DNA lesions undergo apoptosis, which is characterized by caspase activation and the fragmentation and condensation of chromosomal DNA. Presumably depending on the extent of DNA damage, UVR-exposed keratinocytes may also undergo necrosis, bringing about plasma membrane leakage and passive release of intracellular molecules (Caricchio et al. 2003). There are multiple forms of necrotic cell death, including RIPK3-dependent necroptosis and caspase-1/11-dependent pyroptosis. It remains to be determined which form of necrosis is involved in the death of UVR-damaged keratinocytes.

UVR-damaged skin exhibits the cardinal signs of inflammation: redness (erythema), swelling (edema), heat, and pain. Erythema and edema are attributable to vasodilation and vascular leakage, respectively. In addition, the inflammatory response to UVR entails neutrophil infiltration and epidermal hyperplasia (acanthosis). All of these acute conditions resolve as the injury heals and inflammation subsides. Chronicity of UVR-induced inflammation, on the other hand, leads to longer-lasting or even permanent tissue anomalies (e.g. loss of dermal elastic fibers, hyperplastic and dysplastic lesions) that are associated with tissue aging, and herald

Table 9.1 Tissue changes associated with UVR-induced skin inflammation

Cytological, histological, and functional feature	Markers and assays	Underlying molecular process
DNA lesions	Cyclobutane pyrimidine dimer (CPD)	DNA photoproduct formation
	(6-4) photoproduct (6-4PP)	DNA photoproduct formation
	8-Hydroxy-2′-deoxyguanosine (8-OHdG)/ 8-oxo-7,8-dihydro-2′-deoxyguanosine (8-oxo-dG)	Nucleoside oxidation
Epidermal cell death	TUNEL	Apoptotic DNA fragmentation
	Cleaved caspase-3	Caspase activation
Acanthosis	Keratin K14/K5	Basal layer-specific keratin
	Ki67	Cell proliferation
	BrdU incorporation	DNA synthesis
Neutrophil infiltration	Gr-1/Ly6G	Neutrophil-specific surface molecule
	Neutrophil elastase	Neutrophil-specific enzyme
	Myeloperoxidase	Neutrophil-specific enzyme
Edema and vascular leakage	Skin thickness	Edema formation
	Tissue coloration by intravenously injected dye (e.g. Evans blue)	Vascular permeability increase
Epidermal permeability	Transepidermal water loss	Epidermal barrier disruption

non-melanoma and melanoma skin cancer. Prevention of excessive and prolonged inflammatory responses in UVR-exposed skin is therefore thought to be important for not only alleviating the immediate skin-damaging effects of solar radiation but also mitigating its long-term sequelae. Table 9.1 summarizes well-established molecular markers for detecting tissue changes associated with UVR-induced skin inflammation.

9.2 Activation of p38 Signaling by UV Radiation

Reversible protein phosphorylation mediated by protein kinases and phosphatases is crucial to signal transduction. The mitogen-activated protein kinase pathways mediated by ERK, JNK and p38 family members play a pivotal role in linking

Table 9.2 Cellular sensors for molecular signatures of UVR exposure that serve to induce inflammatory responses

Receptor protein	Molecules or events sensed	Reference
Innate immune receptors		
NLRP3 inflammasome	Intracellular Ca^{2+}	Feldmeyer et al. (2007)
Toll-like receptor 3	UVB-damaged noncoding RNA	Bernard et al. (2012)
Toll-like receptor 4	HMGB1	Bald et al. (2014)
STING	Oxidized DNA	Gehrke et al. (2013)
Nuclear receptors		
Aryl hydrocarbon receptor	6-Formylindolo[3,2-*b*]carbazole	Fritsche et al. (2007)
Vitamin D receptor	1α,25-Dihydroxyvitamin D_3	Biggs et al. (2010)
Miscellaneous		
Serotonin receptor 5-HT_{2A}	*Cis*-urocanic acid	Walterscheid et al. (2006)
Ion channel TRPV4	Unknown	Moore et al. (2013)

extracellular stimuli to cellular responses during the inflammatory response. The protein kinase p38α is the most abundant and ubiquitously expressed among the four mammalian p38 isoforms (p38α, p38β, p38γ, and p38δ). p38α was discovered based on its binding affinity for a group of anti-inflammatory compounds (Lee et al. 1994) and also due to its activation by environmental stress and pro-inflammatory stimuli (Han et al. 1994; Rouse et al. 1994; Freshney et al. 1994). Therefore, the involvement of p38α signaling in inflammatory responses seemed apparent from the moment of its discovery. p38α signaling is activated by UVR in organisms ranging from single-celled eukaryotes to mammals (Price et al. 1996; Iordanov et al. 1997; Degols and Russell 1997; Han et al. 1998). In keeping with the extent of UVB penetration into the skin, UVB-induced p38 activation in mouse skin is confined to epidermal cells (Sano and Park 2014).

A multitude of inflammation-related signaling pathways involve p38 as an intracellular module: p38 activity is induced in response to pro-inflammatory cytokines, microbial products, and injurious environmental insults. It remains obscure what upstream events connect UVB irradiation with the p38 signaling module. Certain biochemical signatures of UVR-damaged epidermis likely trigger a signaling cascade that culminates in p38 activation. Besides generating photoproducts and oxidized nucleosides in nucleic acids, UVR catalyzes various other chemical reactions, producing cholecalciferol (Holick 1981), *cis*-urocanic acid (De Fabo and Noonan 1983), and 6-formylindolo[3,2-*b*]carbazole (Fritsche et al. 2007), among others. These products, serving as signatures of UVR exposure, may initiate epidermal signaling processes leading to p38 activation. Numerous studies have shown that sensors for such signature molecules are required for inducing inflammatory responses in UVR-exposed skin although the implication of p38 in those specific settings remains to be determined. Table 9.2 provides a list of sensors for photoproducts, oxidized cell components, and other signatures associated with UVR exposure that may function as cues for inflammatory responses. These sensors include receptors of the innate immune system that detect microbe- and tissue damage-associated molecules, nuclear receptors for lipophilic ligands, and other functionally heterogeneous proteins.

The p38 signaling pathway impinges on gene expression. Among the substrate proteins phosphorylated by p38 or its downstream protein kinases (e.g. MAP kinase-activated protein kinases, or MKs) are DNA-binding transcription factors, transcriptional coactivators and corepressors, nucleosomal constituents, and regulators of mRNA stability and translation. The MKs functioning downstream of p38 include MK2 and MK3, mitogen- and stress-activated kinase 1 (MSK1) and MSK2, and MAPK-interacting kinase 1 (Mnk1) and Mnk2 (Arthur and Ley 2013). p38 and its MKs exert modulation upon substrate proteins via phosphorylation-dependent changes in their activity, turnover, and subcellular location. Several studies have reported UVR-responsive MK activation in cultured keratinocytes and mouse epidermis (Chen and Bowden 1999; Nomura et al. 2001; Kim et al. 2005b; Terazawa et al. 2015), yet it remains to be determined whether MKs play an indispensable role in relaying p38-transmitted signals in UVR-exposed cells and, if so, how they contribute to UVR-induced skin inflammation.

9.3 The Effects of Loss of p38 Signaling on Skin Inflammation

The embryonic lethality of p38α-null mice (Tamura et al. 2000; Adams et al. 2000; Allen et al. 2000; Mudgett et al. 2000) precluded the investigation of the effects of p38α deficiency using mouse models of inflammation. These limitations hampered advances in understanding the physiological role of p38α in adult skin until conditional p38α knockout mice were generated in which p38α gene ablation was restricted to specific cell types in skin. Small-molecule inhibitor studies revealed that p38 inhibition alleviated skin inflammation and pathology in mice exposed to UVB (Hildesheim et al. 2004; Kim et al. 2005b), providing key evidence linking p38 signaling and UVB-induced inflammation in mammalian skin. These studies, however, left unclear which p38 isoform mediates the effects of UVB and in which cell type p38 signaling serves this function. Moreover, the off-target effects of p38 inhibitors (Godl et al. 2003; Karaman et al. 2008) limited the interpretation of the results.

Genetic ablation of p38α in skin cells provided definitive evidence for its role in UVB-induced inflammatory responses. Mice with keratinocyte-specific ablation of p38α expression exhibited marked decreases in inflammation-associated tissue changes following UVB exposure: loss of p38α in keratinocytes prevented UVB-induced vasodilation, vascular leakage, neutrophil infiltration, and acanthosis (Kim et al. 2008; Sano and Park 2014). Despite these effects, p38α-deficient keratinocytes incurred UVB-induced DNA lesions and apoptosis to extents comparable to wild-type cells (Sano and Park 2014), indicating that p38α did not play a significant role in generating or repairing UVB-inflicted damage but served to initiate or amplify inflammatory responses following the damage. In contrast to keratinocyte-specific

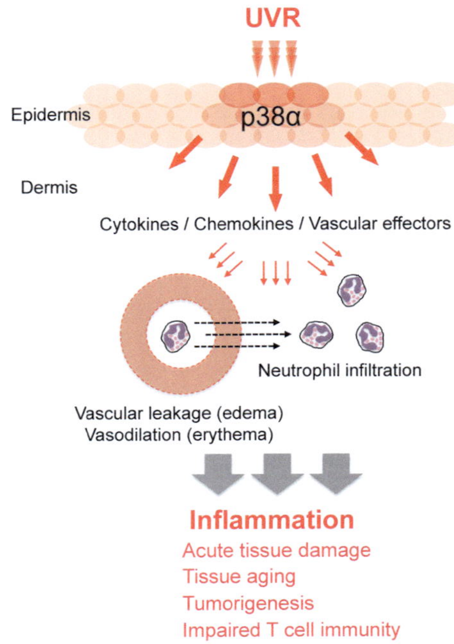

Fig. 9.1 UVR-induced inflammatory responses in the skin epidermal keratinocyte-derived factors play a key role in UVR-induced p38α-dependent skin inflammation, which not only causes acute tissue damage but also exerts long-term detrimental effects such as tissue aging, tumorigenesis, and impaired immunity

p38α knockout mice, mice lacking p38α in myeloid cells, such as macrophages and neutrophils, developed more severe skin inflammation upon UVB exposure (Kim et al. 2008), illustrating that p38α exerted both pro-inflammatory or anti-inflammatory functions in UVB-induced inflammation depending on the cell type in which it is expressed and functioning. In addition to epithelial cells, the mouse epidermis harbors hematopoietic-derived cells, Langerhans cells and dendritic epidermal T cells, which can be accessed by photons of UVB and thus have potential to mount direct cellular responses to solar UVR. Ablation of p38α expression in these cell types, however, did not affect UVB-induced skin inflammation (Sano and Park 2014). Taken together, the findings from conditional p38α knockout studies showed that p38α signaling served to promote inflammation in the epithelial compartment of UVB-exposed epidermis (Fig. 9.1). Synthetic or natural chemical agents that interfere with p38α signaling in keratinocytes but not myeloid cells likely suppress UVB-induced skin inflammation as well as prevent the pathology it brings about.

9.4 Molecular Targets of p38 Signaling in the Skin Epithelium

Consistent with the important role of epithelial p38α signaling in evoking inflammatory responses in UVR-exposed skin, p38α signaling has been shown to drive the expression of UVR-inducible genes in keratinocytes. A DNA microarray

Table 9.3 p38α target genes expressed in mouse keratinocytes

Functional category	Gene	Gene product
Eicosanoid biosynthesis	*Ptgs2*	Cyclooxygenase-2 (COX-2)
	Alox12b	Arachidonate 12-lipoxygenase (12R-LOX)
Cytokine and growth factor signaling	*Csf2*	Granulocyte-macrophage colony stimulating factor (GM-CSF)
	Il1a	Interleukin-1A (IL-1α)
	Il1f5	IL-1 family, member 5 (IL-1F5)
	Il1f6	IL-1 family, member 6 (IL-1F6)
	Areg	Amphiregulin
	Ereg	Epiregulin
	Hbegf	Heparin-binding EGF-like growth factor (HB-EGF)
Leukocyte recruitment	*Cxcl2*	Chemokine (C-X-C motif) ligand 2
	Cxcl3	Chemokine (C-X-C motif) ligand 3
	Ccl3	Chemokine (C-C motif) ligand 3
Antimicrobial defense	*Defb3*	Defensin-β3
	Lcn2	Lipocalin-2
	S100a8	S100 calcium binding protein A8
	S100a9	S100 calcium binding protein A9
Proteolysis	*Mmp13*	Matrix metallopeptidase-13
	Spink5	Serine peptidase inhibitor, Kazal type 5
	Slpi	Secretory leukocyte peptidase inhibitor
Cornified envelope formation	*Lce*	Late cornified envelope (multiple members)
	Sprr	Small proline-rich protein (multiple members)
	Cnfn	Cornifelin
	Flg	Filaggrin
	Lor	Loricrin
	Tgm1	Transglutaminase-1

experiment that compared gene expression in wild-type and p38α-deficient mouse keratinocytes revealed that the expression of numerous inflammation-related genes was induced by UVB and dependent on p38α signaling (Sano and Park 2014). The p38α target genes thus identified, as summarized in Table 9.3, included those representing the following functional categories: eicosanoid-synthesizing enzymes, cytokines, chemokines, growth factors, antimicrobial proteins, proteolytic enzymes/inhibitors, and cornified envelope components. This gene repertoire accounts for attenuated inflammation in mice lacking p38α in keratinocytes. Most importantly, cyclooxygenese-2 (COX-2) and the chemokine CXCL2, both encoded by p38α target genes, have established roles in vasodilation/vascular leakage and neutrophil infiltration, respectively. Other genes whose expression in keratinocytes

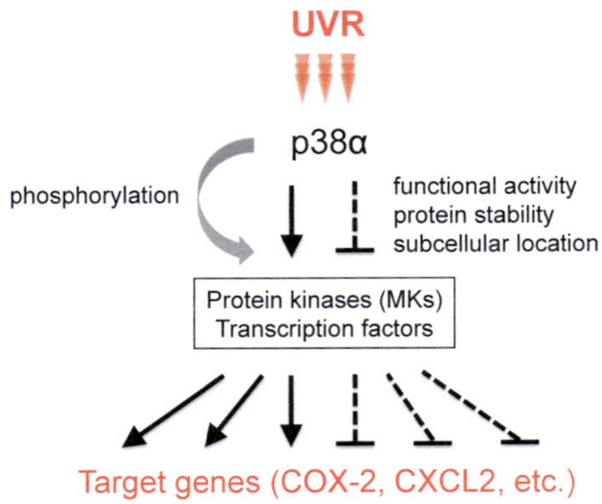

Fig. 9.2 UVR-induced intracellular signaling and gene expression in keratinocytes p38α serves as a key signal transducer for UVR-induced gene expression. p38α phosphorylates and thereby modulates the activity, stability, and subcellular location of downstream protein kinases and transcription factors that are crucial for target gene expression. This modulation likely involves both positive and negative regulatory effects (*solid arrows* and *dotted lines*, respectively) resulting from phosphorylation by p38α

depends on p38α may also participate in UVR-induced inflammation, and contribute to other aspects of inflammation-associated skin pathology (Fig. 9.2).

COX-2 is a key enzyme driving the biosynthesis of prostaglandins, eicosanoid lipid messengers that serve pleiotropic inflammation-related functions. Unlike its paralog, COX-1, whose expression is largely constitutive, COX-2 is transcriptionally induced in response to inflammatory stimuli. COX activity is inhibited by what is collectively known as non-steroidal anti-inflammatory drugs (NSAIDs). Pharmacological COX-2 inhibition by NSAIDs or COX-2-selective inhibitors has been shown to suppress UVB-induced skin inflammation in mice and humans (Takiwaki et al. 1994; Wilgus et al. 2000). Furthermore, COX-2-null mice and mice lacking COX-2 expression in keratinocytes exhibited decreases in edema, acanthosis, and other signs of inflammation following UVB exposure (Sano and Park 2014; Jiao et al. 2014). These findings, obtained from both pharmacological inhibition and genetic ablation studies, highlight COX-2 as a key mediator of UVR-induced inflammation that functions downstream of p38α in keratinocytes.

9.5 Synthetic and Natural Compounds Inhibiting p38 Signaling

Numerous small-molecule compounds inhibiting p38α alone or both p38α and p38β have been investigated in clinical settings. These clinical studies evaluated the efficacy of p38 inhibitors against rheumatoid arthritis, chronic obstructive pulmonary disease,

Crohn's disease, and inflammatory pain (Arthur and Ley 2013). In several of these studies, p38α inhibition showed some efficacy but resulted in adverse effects including hepatic, dermatologic, and gastrointestinal toxicity (Salgado et al. 2014). These undesired effects may arise from disrupting the homeostatic or anti-inflammatory functions of p38α. In keeping with this idea, loss of p38α in certain cell types gives rise to abnormal tissue homeostasis or uncontrolled inflammatory reactions in mice (Ventura et al. 2007; Otsuka et al. 2010; Caballero-Franco et al. 2013). In particular, p38α signaling in myeloid cells has been shown to exert anti-inflammatory functions in various modes of inflammation including UVR-induced skin inflammation (Kim et al. 2008; Ritprajak et al. 2012; Guma et al. 2012). These regulatory functions rely, at least in part, on p38α/MSK-dependent anti-inflammatory gene expression in macrophages (Kim et al. 2008). Therefore, while pharmacological p38α inhibition may produce favorable effects on UVR-inflamed skin via interference with epithelial p38α signaling, this benefit could be offset or outweighed by detrimental effects resulting from perturbed p38α function in myeloid cells. Topical inhibitor treatment may provide some selectivity; epidermal keratinocytes would have better access to topical p38α inhibitors than myeloid cells, which mainly exist in the dermis.

Whereas synthetic small-molecule inhibitors often achieve a state of complete loss of target function with their potent inhibitory effects, inhibitors derived from natural sources are likely to exert more moderate inhibition and spare residual target function. This may be advantageous when p38α is considered as a target for preventing UVB-induced inflammation: ideally, natural compounds or extracts should be able to inhibit p38α signaling to such as extent as to suppress inflammatory responses but not to ablate it so completely as to perturb the beneficial physiological functions served by p38α. Numerous plant- and microbial-derived compounds have been identified that suppress p38 signaling and exert anti-inflammatory effects in vivo (Kim et al. 2005a; Kalhan et al. 2008; Sur et al. 2008; Paul et al. 2009; Yogianti et al. 2014).

Not all of the p38 pathway inhibitors identified in a cell culture-based screening platform would suppress UVR-induced skin inflammation and pathology when topically administered. The epidermal permeability barrier poses a major obstacle for the delivery of chemicals via topical route (Schmieder et al. 2015), and impedes dermatological applications of otherwise promising bioactive agents. Besides, relaxed target specificity is inherent with nearly all natural bioactive agents; most of them likely affect signaling pathways other than the intended target and may produce undesired physiological effects. All in all, in order to be used for the prevention of sunlight-induced skin pathology, p38α inhibitors should meet multiple criteria: they should be amenable for transepidermal delivery and effectively suppress UVR-induced skin inflammation, yet without disrupting beneficial physiological functions through on-target or off-target mechanisms. These criteria should be considered at the outset of efforts to test or screen candidate molecules.

9.6 Future Perspectives

Recent progresses in understanding the signaling mechanisms essential for UVR-induced inflammation have brought new opportunities to prevent the harmful effects of solar radiation. Inhibition of epithelial p38α signaling, a key molecular event driving inflammatory responses in UVR-exposed skin, has emerged as a means of realizing such opportunities. Several unanswered questions still remain, however, about the p38α-dependent epithelial response to UVR. First of all, it is unclear how p38α activity is switched on in epidermal cells following UVR exposure. Specifically, the nature of biochemical signals that serve as cues for p38α activation remains to be determined: is it photoproducts, oxidized molecules, or signatures of stressed or injured cells (e.g. molecular "patterns" associated with senescent, dying or dead cells) that trigger the signaling cascade? Questions also exist about the mechanisms by which p38α signaling drives the induction of COX-2 and other inflammatory mediators in keratinocytes. The role of MKs and transcription factors functioning downstream of p38α in this response has not been rigorously investigated. Finally, the precise role of UVR-inducible p38α target genes in inflammation remains to be established. Besides COX-2 and CXCL2, many other keratinocyte genes are expressed in a p38α-dependent manner, but their contribution to UVR-induced skin inflammation is not immediately apparent. There will be greater opportunities to devise effective strategies for preventing the detrimental effects of solar UVR as these knowledge voids are filled.

References

Adams RH, Porras A, Alonso G, Jones M, Vintersten K, Panelli S, Valladares A, Perez L, Klein R, Nebreda AR (2000) Essential role of p38α MAP kinase in placental but not embryonic cardiovascular development. Mol Cell 6:109–116

Allen M, Svensson L, Roach M, Hambor J, McNeish J, Gabel CA (2000) Deficiency of the stress kinase p38alpah results in embryonic lethality: characterization of the kinase dependence of stress responses of enzyme-deficient embryonic stem cells. J Exp Med 191:859–870

Arthur JS, Ley SC (2013) Mitogen-activated protein kinases in innate immunity. Nat Rev Immunol 13:679–692

Bald T, Quast T, Landsberg J, Rogava M, Glodde N, Lopez-Ramos D, Kohlmeyer J, Riesenberg S, van den Boorn-Konijnenberg D, Hömig-Hölzel C et al (2014) Ultraviolet-radiation-induced inflammation promotes angiotropism and metastasis in melanoma. Nature 507:109–113

Bernard JJ, Cowing-Zitron C, Nakatsuji T, Muehleisen B, Muto J, Borkowski AW, Martinez L, Greidinger EL, Yu BD, Gallo RL (2012) Ultraviolet radiation damages self noncoding RNA and is detected by TLR3. Nat Med 18:1286–1290

Biggs L, Yu C, Fedoric B, Lopez AF, Galli SJ, Grimbaldeston MA (2010) Evidence that vitamin D_3 promotes mast cell-dependent reduction of chronic UVB-induced skin pathology in mice. J Exp Med 207:455–463

Caballero-Franco C, Choo MK, Sano Y, Ritprajak P, Sakurai H, Otsu K, Mizoguchi A, Park JM (2013) Tuning of protein kinase circuitry by p38α is vital for epithelial tissue homeostasis. J Biol Chem 288:23788–23797

Caricchio R, McPhie L, Cohen PL (2003) Ultraviolet B radiation-induced cell death: critical role of ultraviolet dose in inflammation and lupus autoantigen redistribution. J Immunol 171: 5778–5786

Chen W, Bowden GT (1999) Activation of p38 MAP kinase and ERK are required for ultraviolet-B induced c-fos gene expression in human keratinocytes. Oncogene 18:7469–7476

De Fabo EC, Noonan FP (1983) Mechanism of immune suppression by ultraviolet irradiation in vivo. I. Evidence for the existence of a unique photoreceptor in skin and its role in photoimmunology. J Exp Med 158:84–98

Degols G, Russell P (1997) Discrete roles of the Spc1 kinase and the Atf1 transcription factor in the UV response of Schizosaccharomyces pombe. Mol Cell Biol 17:3356–3363

Elmets CA, Athar M (2013) Milestones in photocarcinogenesis. J Invest Dermatol 133:E13–E17

Feldmeyer L, Keller M, Niklaus G, Hohl D, Werner S, Beer HD (2007) The inflammasome mediates UVB-induced activation and secretion of interleukin-1β by keratinocytes. Curr Biol 17:1140–1145

Freshney NW, Rawlinson L, Guesdon F, Jones E, Cowley S, Hsuan J, Saklatvala J (1994) Interleukin-1 activates a novel protein kinase cascade that results in the phosphorylation of Hsp27. Cell 78:1039–1049

Fritsche E, Schäfer C, Calles C, Bernsmann T, Bernshausen T, Wurm M, Hübenthal U, Cline JE, Hajimiragha H, Schroeder P et al (2007) Lightening up the UV response by identification of the arylhydrocarbon receptor as a cytoplasmatic target for ultraviolet B radiation. Proc Natl Acad Sci U S A 104:8851–8856

Gehrke N, Mertens C, Zillinger T, Wenzel J, Bald T, Zahn S, Tüting T, Hartmann G, Barchet W (2013) Oxidative damage of DNA confers resistance to cytosolic nuclease TREX1 degradation and potentiates STING-dependent immune sensing. Immunity 39:482–495

Godl K, Wissing J, Kurtenbach A, Habenberger P, Blencke S, Gutbrod H, Salassidis K, Stein-Gerlach M, Missio A, Cotten M et al (2003) An efficient proteomics method to identify the cellular targets of protein kinase inhibitors. Proc Natl Acad Sci U S A 100:15434–15439

Guma M, Hammaker D, Topolewski K, Corr M, Boyle DL, Karin M, Firestein GS (2012) Antiinflammatory functions of p38 in mouse models of rheumatoid arthritis: advantages of targeting upstream kinases MKK-3 or MKK-6. Arthritis Rheum 64:2887–2895

Han J, Lee JD, Bibbs L, Ulevitch RJ (1994) A MAP kinase targeted by endotoxin and hyperosmolarity in mammalian cells. Science 265:808–811

Han ZS, Enslen H, Hu X, Meng X, Wu IH, Barrett T, Davis RJ, Ip YT (1998) A conserved p38 mitogen-activated protein kinase pathway regulates Drosophila immunity gene expression. Mol Cell Biol 18:3527–3539

Hart PH, Gorman S, Finlay-Jones JJ (2011) Modulation of the immune system by UV radiation: more than just the effects of vitamin D? Nat Rev Immunol 11:584–596

Hildesheim J, Awwad RT, Fornace AJ Jr (2004) p38 Mitogen-activated protein kinase inhibitor protects the epidermis against the acute damaging effects of ultraviolet irradiation by blocking apoptosis and inflammatory responses. J Invest Dermatol 122:497–502

Holick MF (1981) The cutaneous photosynthesis of previtamin D3: a unique photoendocrine system. J Invest Dermatol 77:51–58

Iordanov M, Bender K, Ade T, Schmid W, Sachsenmaier C, Engel K, Gaestel M, Rahmsdorf HJ, Herrlich P (1997) CREB is activated by UVC through a p38/HOG-1-dependent protein kinase. EMBO J 16:1009–1022

Jiao J, Mikulec C, Ishikawa TO, Magyar C, Dumlao DS, Dennis EA, Fischer SM, Herschman H (2014) Cell-type-specific roles for COX-2 in UVB-induced skin cancer. Carcinogenesis 35:1310–1319

Kalhan R, Smith LJ, Nlend MC, Nair A, Hixon JL, Sporn PH (2008) A mechanism of benefit of soy genistein in asthma: inhibition of eosinophil p38-dependent leukotriene synthesis. Clin Exp Allergy 38:103–112

Karaman MW, Herrgard S, Treiber DK, Gallant P, Atteridge CE, Campbell BT, Chan KW, Ciceri P, Davis MI, Edeen PT et al (2008) A quantitative analysis of kinase inhibitor selectivity. Nat Biotechnol 26:127–132

Kim SO, Kundu JK, Shin YK, Park JH, Cho MH, Kim TY, Surh YJ (2005a) [6]-Gingerol inhibits COX-2 expression by blocking the activation of p38 MAP kinase and NF-κB in phorbol ester-stimulated mouse skin. Oncogene 24:2558–2567

Kim AL, Labasi JM, Zhu Y, Tang X, McClure K, Gabel CA, Athar M, Bickers DR (2005b) Role of p38 MAPK in UVB-induced inflammatory responses in the skin of SKH-1 hairless mice. J Invest Dermatol 124:1318–1325

Kim C, Sano Y, Todorova K, Carlson BA, Arpa L, Celada A, Lawrence T, Otsu K, Brissette JL, Arthur JS et al (2008) The kinase p38α serves cell type-specific inflammatory functions in skin injury and coordinates pro- and anti-inflammatory gene expression. Nat Immunol 9:1019–1027

Lee JC, Laydon JT, McDonnell PC, Gallagher TF, Kumar S, Green D, McNulty D, Blumenthal MJ, Heys JR, Landvatter SW et al (1994) A protein kinase involved in the regulation of inflammatory cytokine biosynthesis. Nature 372:739–746

Moore C, Cevikbas F, Pasolli HA, Chen Y, Kong W, Kempkes C, Parekh P, Lee SH, Kontchou NA, Yeh I et al (2013) UVB radiation generates sunburn pain and affects skin by activating epidermal TRPV4 ion channels and triggering endothelin-1 signaling. Proc Natl Acad Sci USA 110:E3225–E3234

Mudgett JS, Ding J, Guh-Siesel L, Chartrain NA, Yang L, Gopal S, Shen MM (2000) Essential role for p38α mitogen-activated protein kinase in placental angiogenesis. Proc Natl Acad Sci USA 97:10454–10459

Nomura M, Kaji A, Ma WY, Zhong S, Liu G, Bowden GT, Miyamoto KI, Dong Z (2001) Mitogen- and stress-activated protein kinase 1 mediates activation of Akt by ultraviolet B irradiation. J Biol Chem 276:25558–25567

Otsuka M, Kang YJ, Ren J, Jiang H, Wang Y, Omata M, Han J (2010) Distinct effects of p38α deletion in myeloid lineage and gut epithelia in mouse models of inflammatory bowel disease. Gastroenterology 138:1255–1265

Paul S, Rimando AM, Lee HJ, Ji Y, Reddy BS, Suh N (2009) Anti-inflammatory action of pterostilbene is mediated through the p38 mitogen-activated protein kinase pathway in colon cancer cells. Cancer Prev Res 2:650–657

Pfeifer GP, Besaratinia A (2012) UV wavelength-dependent DNA damage and human non-melanoma and melanoma skin cancer. Photochem Photobiol Sci 11:90–97

Price MA, Cruzalegui FH, Treisman R (1996) The p38 and ERK MAP kinase pathways cooperate to activate Ternary Complex Factors and c-fos transcription in response to UV light. EMBO J 15:6552–6563

Ritprajak P, Hayakawa M, Sano Y, Otsu K, Park JM (2012) Cell type-specific targeting dissociates the therapeutic from the adverse effects of protein kinase inhibition in allergic skin disease. Proc Natl Acad Sci USA 109:9089–9094

Rouse J, Cohen P, Trigon S, Morange M, Alonso-Llamazares A, Zamanillo D, Hunt T, Nebreda AR (1994) A novel kinase cascade triggered by stress and heat shock that stimulates MAPKAP kinase-2 and phosphorylation of the small heat shock proteins. Cell 78:1027–1037

Salgado E, Maneiro JR, Carmona L, Gomez-Reino JJ (2014) Safety profile of protein kinase inhibitors in rheumatoid arthritis: systematic review and meta-analysis. Ann Rheum Dis 73:871–882

Sano Y, Park JM (2014) Loss of epidermal p38α signaling prevents UVR-induced inflammation via acute and chronic mechanisms. J Invest Dermatol. 134:2231–2240

Schmieder S, Patel P, Krishnamurthy K (2015) Research Techniques Made Simple: Drug Delivery Techniques, Part 1: Concepts in Transepidermal Penetration and Absorption. J Invest Dermatol 135:1–5

Sur R, Babad JM, Garay M, Liebel FT, Southall MD (2008) Anti-inflammatory activity of sertaconazole nitrate is mediated via activation of a p38-COX-2-PGE2 pathway. J Invest Dermatol 128:336–344

Takiwaki H, Shirai S, Kohno H, Soh H, Arase S (1994) The degrees of UVB-induced erythema and pigmentation correlate linearly and are reduced in a parallel manner by topical anti-inflammatory agents. J Invest Dermatol 103:642–646

Tamura K, Sudo T, Senftleben U, Dadak AM, Johnson R, Karin M (2000) Requirement for p38α in erythropoietin expression: a role for stress kinases in erythropoiesis. Cell 102:221–231

Terazawa S, Mori S, Nakajima H, Yasuda M, Imokawa G (2015) The UVB-stimulated expression of transglutaminase 1 is mediated predominantly via the NFκB signaling pathway: new evidence of its significant attenuation through the specific interruption of the p38/MSK1/NFκBp65 Ser276 Axis. PLoS ONE 10:e0136311

Ventura JJ, Tenbaum S, Perdiguero E, Huth M, Guerra C, Barbacid M, Pasparakis M, Nebreda AR (2007) p 38α MAP kinase is essential in lung stem and progenitor cell proliferation and differentiation. Nat Genet 39:750–758

Walterscheid JP, Nghiem DX, Kazimi N, Nutt LK, McConkey DJ, Norval M, Ullrich SE (2006) Cis-urocanic acid, a sunlight-induced immunosuppressive factor, activates immune suppression via the 5-HT2A receptor. Proc Natl Acad Sci U S A 103:17420–17425

Wilgus TA, Ross MS, Parrett ML, Oberyszyn TM (2000) Topical application of a selective cyclooxygenase inhibitor suppresses UVB mediated cutaneous inflammation. Prostaglandins Other Lipid Mediat 62:367–384

Yaar M, Gilchrest BA (2007) Photoageing: mechanism, prevention and therapy. Br J Dermatol 157:874–887

Yogianti F, Kunisada M, Nakano E, Ono R, Sakumi K, Oka S, Nakabeppu Y, Nishigori C (2014) Inhibitory effects of dietary Spirulina platensis on UVB-induced skin inflammatory responses and carcinogenesis. J Invest Dermatol 134:2610–2619

Chapter 10
UV-Induced Chemokines as Emerging Targets for Skin Cancer Photochemoprevention

Scott N. Byrne and Gary M. Halliday

Abstract The ultraviolet (UV) radiation contained in sunlight is a complete carcinogen because it can damage DNA, suppress anti-tumour immunity and enhance metastasis of skin cancers. A major way in which UV affects cancer cells and anti-tumour immunity is by modulating the expression of cytokines and chemokines. Knowing this has allowed us to develop and deploy revolutionary biologics that target these UV-induced molecules. This so called "photochemoprevention" can involve topical or oral intervention by biologically active compounds that prevent or repair the damage caused by UV radiation. Many of the successful photochemoprevention strategies involve protection from UV induction of chemokines and cytokines. This chapter will discuss which cutaneous cytokines/chemokines are affected by UV exposure and highlight the ways in which targeting these molecules is providing us with new therapeutic options for preventing and treating skin cancer.

Keywords Chemokines · Cytokines · CXCR4 · Immune suppression · Interleukins · Metastasis · Nicotinamide · Platelet activating factor · Prostaglandin E2 · Skin cancer · Stem cell factor · Stromal derived factor · Sunlight · Tumour necrosis factor · Ultraviolet radiation · Vitamin D

S.N. Byrne (✉)
Infectious Diseases and Immunology, Charles Perkins Centre, Sydney Medical School, University of Sydney, Level 5 (East), Charles Perkins Centre Hub (D17), Sydney, NSW 2006, Australia
e-mail: scott.byrne@sydney.edu.au

S.N. Byrne · G.M. Halliday
Dermatology Research Laboratories, Bosch Institute, Sydney Medical School, University of Sydney, Sydney, Australia

G.T. Wondrak (ed.), *Skin Stress Response Pathways*,
DOI 10.1007/978-3-319-43157-4_10

10.1 Introduction

Exposure to solar ultraviolet (UV) radiation is the prime cause of skin cancer. UV initiates skin carcinogenesis by damaging DNA while simultaneously suppressing adaptive immunity to enable UV-induced tumours to evade immunological destruction (Halliday 2005). UV also promotes the growth and metastasis of established skin cancers (Bald et al. 2014). A major way in which UV affects cancer cells and anti-tumour immunity is by modulating the expression of cytokines. In so doing, sunlight can influence all of the key events required for carcinogenesis including tumour initiation, promotion, immune evasion, invasion *and* metastasis. Revelation of the biological mechanisms responsible for UV radiation causing the skin damage that leads to skin cancer is revealing photochemoprevention strategies. Photochemoprevention is topical or oral intervention by biologically active compounds that prevent or repair the damage caused by UV radiation. UV-induced cytokines are a promising new molecular target for photochemoprevention.

Cytokines are secreted proteins that exert their biological effects by binding to specific cell-surface receptors. They can act locally in an autocrine and/or paracrine manner, or systemically to affect distant cells in an endocrine manner. Solar ultraviolet (UV) radiation (280–400 nm), particularly UVB (280–320 nm), is well known for its capacity to modulate the expression of cytokines in the skin including interleukin (IL)-1 (Kupper et al. 1987), IL-6 (Chung et al. 1996), IL-4, IL-10 and tumour necrosis factor (TNF) (Rivas and Ullrich 1994) as well as IL-33 (Byrne et al. 2011). Cytokines that modulate the chemotaxis of cells are commonly referred to as *chemo*tactic cyto*kines*, or ***chemokines***. More than 50 different chemokines have been identified that bind specific G protein coupled receptors (Griffith et al. 2014). By establishing chemokine gradients, these small proteins can recruit receptor-expressing cells to sites of inflammation and tissue damage. Chemokines also play a key role in the homeostatic control of cellular traffic (Zlotnik and Yoshie 2012). More recently, the traditional chemoattractant view of chemokines has expanded to include an appreciation that some chemokines, especially C-X-C-motif ligand 12 (CXCL12/Stromal cell derived factor (SDF)-1α), play important roles in cell growth and differentiation (Zlotnik 2006). It is now recognised that a major way UV suppresses immunity and promotes skin-carcinogenesis is by altering the expression of chemokines and their receptors. The arrival of new biologics that target both cytokines/chemokines and their receptors is allowing for the development of new therapeutic options and approaches for preventing and treating skin cancer.

10.2 Cutaneous Cytokines/Chemokines Affected by UV Exposure

10.2.1 TNF Family Members

One of the earliest cytokines identified as being involved in UV-induced immune suppression and skin carcinogeneis was tumour necrosis factor-α (TNF) (Oxholm et al. 1988; Kock et al. 1990). Exposure to UV can trigger the production of TNF from keratinocytes (Kock et al. 1990), or the release of pre-formed TNF from dermal mast cells (Alard et al. 1999). UV-induced TNF plays a key role in cutaneous immune suppression, in part by affecting the prevalence and activity of dermal mast cells (Hart et al. 1998) as well as altering the migration of immunoregulatory epidermal Langerhans cells (LC) to skin-draining lymph nodes (Vermeer and Streilein 1990; Yoshikawa et al. 1992; Moodycliffe et al. 1994). While polymorphisms in TNF correlate with the ability of UV to cause skin cancer (Vincek et al. 1993), this may not be mediated via TNF-suppression of anti-tumour immunity (Allen et al. 1998). TNF acts locally in the skin as a growth factor and immune modulator as well as a potent chemoattractant for neutrophils (Malaviya et al. 1996). Indeed, IL-4-producing immune regulatory neutrophils are rapidly (within 24 h) recruited to sites of UV-exposure in humans (Teunissen et al. 2002). This recruitment may also be mediated by UV-induced IL-8 (CXCL8) (Singh et al. 1995; Strickland et al. 1997), a well known neutrophil chemoattractant (Ribeiro et al. 1991).

TNF-α is just one of 19 currently identified TNF family members. More recently, TNFSF11; better known as Receptor activator of NF-κB ligand (RANKL), was shown to be upregulated in UV-exposed skin (Loser et al. 2006). Epidermal expression of RANKL is driven in part by UV-induced 1,25-dihydroxyvitamin D_3 ($1{,}25(OH)_2D_3$), the active form of vitamin D_3. Like TNF itself, RANKL activated immune regulatory LC migrate to local skin draining lymph nodes where they mediate the induction of CD4+CD25+ regulatory T cells (T_{Regs}). Other TNF family members including TNFSF4 (OX40 Ligand) (Yoshiki et al. 2010), TNFSF5 (CD40 Ligand) (Ito et al. 2003) and TNFSF18 (GITR Ligand) (Maeda et al. 2008) are also upregulated by UV. In contrast to activation of these TNF family members, UVB has also been shown to downregulate other TNF family members and their receptors, particularly TNFSF6 (CD95/Fas Ligand) and TNFSF10 receptors (TNF-related apoptosis-inducing ligand or "TRAIL" receptors) (Bachmann et al. 2001). Indeed, TRAIL is expressed in normal skin, but not chronically sun-damaged skin or non-melanoma skin cancer (Ständer and Schwarz 2005). Considering the important role of these TNF family members in mediating apoptosis this may be a mechanism by which UV contributes to skin carcinogenesis. Thus, TNF and its related family members are a key cytokine/chemokine targeted by UV that leads to immune suppression and carcinogenesis. Anti-human TNF monoclonal antibodies are being used to treat a range of inflammatory conditions including rheumatoid arthritis and psoriasis. This TNF-targeting pharmacological

Table 10.1 Biologics that target established and emerging UV-induced cytokines/chemokines

Cytokine/Chemokine	Pharmacological agent	Description/Mode of action
TNF	**Etanercept** (Enbrel)	Fusion protein of the Fc portion of IgG_1 and the extracellular domain of the TNF receptor (p75)
	Adalimumab (Humira)	Fully humanized anti-TNFα monoclonal antibody
	Denosumab (Prolia, XGEVA)	Fully humanized anti-RANKL monoclonal antibody
IL-1	**Anakinra** (Kineret)	Recombinant IL-1 receptor antagonist (IL-1Ra)
	DZ13	*cJUN*-mRNA targeting DNAzyme
	SB-485232	Recombinant human IL-18 (currently in Phase II clinical trials) (Golab and Stoklosa 2005)
	Soluble IL-33 receptor (sST2)	IL-33 "decoy" receptor (acts to inhibit IL-33 activity)
	Allopurinol (Zyloprim)	Structural isomer of hypoxanthine and inhibitor of xanthine oxidase. Blocks uric acid production and hence may inhibit formation of the NALP3 inflammasome required for bioactive IL-1 family members
IL-6	**Tocilizumab** (Actemra)	Fully humanized anti-IL-6R monoclonal antibody
CXCL12	**AMD3100** (Mozobil)	CXCR4 antagonist
PAF	**Rupatadine**	Dual histamine (H_1) and PAF receptor antagonist
S1P	**K6PC-5**	a short-chain pseudo-ceramide that directly activates sphingosine kinase 1
CCL5	**Maraviroc** (Selzentry)	CCR5 antagonist

agent, and others like it (Table 10.1), may also prove useful in the prevention and treatment of skin cancer.

10.2.2 IL-1 Family Members

Interleukin (IL)-1 is another pro-inflammatory cytokine that is released in skin and into the circulation upon UV-exposure (Gahring et al. 1984; Kupper et al. 1987; Oxholm et al. 1988; Schwarz et al. 1988; Konnikov et al. 1989; Kondo et al. 1994). UV kinetically up-regulates not only the expression of IL-1α (early) and IL-1β (later) (Kondo et al. 1994) but also the IL-1 receptor (Grewe et al. 1996). Simultaneously, UV *reduces* keratinocyte expression of the natural IL-1 antagonist, IL-1F3 (IL-1ra) (Lew et al. 1995). This combination of events significantly increases the bioavailability and inflammatory activity of IL-1, which can trigger LC migration to the lymph nodes independently of TNF (Byrne et al. 2001) and reduce IL-2 and enhance IL-4 production (Araneo et al. 1989). In this way UV-induced IL-1 contributes to immune suppression by affecting T_{Reg} activation, effector T cell proliferation and differentiation. Surprisingly, via its downstream effects on endogenous TNF release, IL-1 is also known for its ability to enhance UV-induced apoptosis independently of the UV dose (Kothny-Wilkes et al. 1999). Immune suppressive prostaglandin (PG)-E_2 is also synthesised in response to UV-induced IL-1 (Pentland and Mahoney 1990). Thus, the founding member of the IL-1 superfamily makes a major contribution to UV-induced apoptosis, inflammation, immune suppression and skin carcinogenesis. It will be interesting to see if novel approaches including DNAzymes that inhibit the downstream targets of IL-1-mediated inflammation (Fahmy et al. 2006) can be used to prevent and treat skin cancer. Indeed, catalytically cleaving c-*JUN* mRNA with the DNAzyme DZ13 cures mice of transplanted UV-induced skin tumours (Cai et al. 2012). In Phase I clinical trials of patients with nodular basal-cell carcinoma, DZ13 was safe and even resulted in a decrease of histological tumour depth in more than half of those treated (Cho et al. 2013).

IL-1F4 (IL-18) is another member of the IL-1 super family that is activated by UV via a reactive oxygen-mediated process (Cho et al. 2002). In contrast to IL-1α and IL-1β, IL-18 does not enhance apoptosis, inflammation or immune suppression. Rather, IL-18 can *reduce* the DNA damage caused by UV (Schwarz et al. 2006) meaning it may work in a similar way as IL-12 (Schwarz et al. 2002) to protect from UV-immune suppression and carcinogenesis. Indeed, loss of IL-18 is a marker of UV-induced melanoma in pre-clinical animal models and humans (Hacker et al. 2008).

IL-33 is a recently described IL-1 family member upregulated by UVB and implicated in immune suppression and skin tumour immune evasion (Byrne et al. 2011). Inflammatory doses of UVB, but not UVA led to a dramatic increase in the expression of IL-33 both in keratinocytes and CD45 negative dermal cells. IL-33-expressing dermal cells become surrounded by mast cells and neutrophils whose chemoattraction to and activation within UV-exposed skin is likely to have been mediated by IL-33 (Alves-Filho et al. 2010; Hueber et al. 2011; Enoksson et al. 2012). UV-induced platelet activating factor (PAF) is partly responsible for the upregulation of IL-33 whereas blocking IL-33 with neutralising antibodies prevents UV-immune suppression (Byrne et al. 2011). UV-induced skin tumours that evade immunological destruction (but not those destroyed by the anti-tumour immune response) also produce large amounts of IL-33. Together this provides compelling evidence that UV-induced IL-33 is a key player in UV-immune suppression and carcinogenesis. Whether targeting IL-33 is clinically beneficial requires the development of novel anti-IL-33 reagents.

Three other new IL-1 family members include IL-36, IL-1F7 (IL-37) and IL-1F10 (IL-38) (Garlanda et al. 2013). While IL-36 and IL-37 expression is altered in psoriatic skin (Keermann et al. 2015), it remains to be determined whether expression of these newly described IL-1 family members are affected by UV exposure.

A feature of the induction of biologically active IL-1 family members is the post-translational caspase-1-mediated cleavage and activation of the pro-forms of the cytokines. This often involves multiple signals leading to the formation of the NALP-3 inflammasome, which is crucial for generating active caspase-1 (Arend et al. 2008). UV does activate the inflammasome (Feldmeyer et al. 2007), which is consistent with an important role for biologically active IL-1, IL-18 and IL-33 in UV-induced inflammation and immune suppression. The molecular triggers for inflammasome formation are not entirely clear but may involve UV-induced uric acid (Leighton et al. 2013) and extracellular ATP (Park et al. 2010). These two extracellular compounds are already well known conspirators in NALP3 inflammasome activation (Iracheta-Vellve et al. 2015). Importantly, biological agents including Allopurinol (Table 10.1) and nicotinamide are already in clinical use and can interfere with uric acid formation and prevent ATP loss respectively. They provide us with novel therapeutic agents that could be used to reduce the detrimental affects of UV-induced IL-1 family members.

10.2.3 IL-6 Family Members

Members of the IL-6 cytokine family [IL-6, IL-11, IL-27, IL-31, IL-35 and Leukaemia Inhibitory Factor (LIF), amongst others (Garbers et al. 2012)] exert their diverse biological effects by binding to a common signal transducing receptor component called glycoprotein (gp)130 (Taniguchi and Karin 2014). IL-6 is rapidly upregulated in UV-exposed skin (within 6 h) (Scordi and Vincek 2000; Nishimura et al. 1999; Abeyama et al. 2000) and is now recognised as a powerful modulator of UV-induced inflammation (Nishimura et al. 1999) and UVA-mediated immune protection (Reeve et al. 2009). The molecular trigger for IL-6 production and release may involve IL-1β and/or hypoxia inducible factor (HIF)-1α (Cho et al. 2012). IL-11 is also upregulated by UV, albeit at slightly later time points (120 h post UV exposure) (Scordi and Vincek 2000). IL-11 reduces apoptosis in UVB-irradiated mouse skin (Scordi et al. 1999). In this way UV-induced IL-6 and IL-11 may act to restore homeostasis following exposure to an inflammatory dose of UVB.

LIF is constitutively expressed at cutaneous sites in humans (Paglia et al. 1996) and can be upregulated by UV in both mouse (Scordi and Vincek 2000) and human skin (McKenzie 2001). UV-upregulated LIF may contribute to skin carcinogenesis by promoting keratinocyte proliferation (Hu et al. 2000), suppressing adaptive immune responses (Akita et al. 2000) and/or enhancing the activity of dermal mast cells (Tanaka et al. 2001). Consistent with this hypothesis, expression of LIF mRNA was significantly elevated in squamous cell carcinomas compared with normal skin (Szepietowski et al. 2001).

10.2.4 Stem Cell Factor (SCF)

Stem Cell Factor (SCF; also known as mast cell growth factor and c-Kit ligand) is a growth factor that has since been shown to modulate the migration of cKIT+ cells. Indeed, SCF-mediated recruitment of cKIT+ mast cells drives inflammation and immune suppression in the tumour environment (Huang et al. 2008). Mice exposed to a relatively low dose [1 minimal erythemal dose (MED)] of UVB significantly upregulated the expression of SCF in the skin (Kligman and Murphy 1996). UVB also upregulates SCF in human skin (Hachiya et al. 2001; Baba et al. 2005). Being a potent mast cell growth factor (Grabbe et al. 1994) and chemoattractant (Meininger et al. 1992; Nilsson et al. 1994), this upregulation in SCF is thought to explain the increase in mast cell density observed in UV-exposed skin sites of mice (Kligman and Murphy 1996; Sarchio et al. 2014; Byrne et al. 2008) and humans (Grimbaldeston et al. 2003, 2006; Kim et al. 2008). SCF is also involved in activating c-Kit+ melanocytes to increase skin pigmentation (Hachiya et al. 2001). In this way UV-induced SCF may act not only as a chemoattractant for immune modulating, tumour-promoting mast cells, but also as a powerful driver of melanocyte growth and differentiation, as well as melanoma migration and metastasis.

10.2.5 C-C Motif Chemokine Family Members

The most abundantly expressed chemokine in skin is C-C motif ligand 27 (CCL27; previously known as Cutaneous T cell-Attracting ChemoKine or "CTACK") (Morales et al. 1999). Binding of CCL27 to its receptor CCR10 is a major way in which CCR10+ cells, particularly memory T cells, home to the skin. Epidermal CCL27 levels are, perhaps not surprisingly, abnormally elevated in patients with Mycosis fungoides, the most common form of cutaneous T-cell lymphoma (Fujita et al. 2006; Goteri et al. 2012). Paradoxically, successful treatment of Mycosis fungoides patients with interferon (IFN)-α and Psoralen+UVA (PUVA) upregulated CCL27 (Goteri et al. 2009) suggesting that alterations to CCL27 levels may not be efficaciously associated. In the skin of lupus erythematosus patients UVB induces the release and subsequent "leakage" of CCL27 from the basal epidermis into the papillary dermis (Meller et al. 2005). This UV-triggered CCL27 release in turn up-regulates the expression of the inflammatory chemokines CCL5, CCL20, CCL22, and CXCL8 (Meller et al. 2005). This may explain part of the mechanism by which exposure to UV elicits the cutaneous eruptions associated with lupus erythematosus. In contrast to these observations in human skin diseases, mouse models show that exposure to UV has minimal impact on cutaneous CCL27 levels (Merad et al. 2002). It should be noted these previous studies were performed using 254 nm UVC that is unlikely to be physiologically relevant.

UV-upregulation of CCL5 (previously known as **R**egulated upon **A**ctivation, **N**ormal **T** cell **E**xpressed and **S**ecreted or RANTES) was responsible for a rise in mast cell numbers within UV-exposed skin (Van Nguyen et al. 2011). This would be consistent with a more recent report showing that cutaneous CCL5 is partly responsible for the recruitment of mast cell progenitors into human papilloma virus infected-skin (Bergot et al. 2014). This is important as in addition to UV, HPV may be a risk factor for the development of non-melanoma skin cancer (Dubina and Goldenberg 2009). As previously mentioned, increased CCL5 is likely to explain not only the high numbers of mast cells found in UV-exposed and HPV-infected skin, but may be an important factor in immune suppression and carcinogenesis (Sarchio et al. 2012). Human melanoma expression of CCL5 is associated with enhanced tumour formation in nude mice (Mrowietz et al. 1999), which may explain, at least partially, the recruitment of Th17 to human tumours (Su et al. 2010). Antagonising any, or all of the receptors for CCL5 including CCR1, CCR3 and CCR5 (Zlotnik and Yoshie 2012) may therefore offer a unique approach to chemoprevent the immune modulating and carcinogenic effects of UV-induced CCL5. Indeed, a number of pharmacological strategies are being explored (Pease and Horuk 2009a, b) although many of the drugs developed to target specific chemokine receptors have met with limited success. There are two possible explanations for this. The first is that a large variety of different cells types, including dendritic cells, monocytes/macrophages, T and B cells, NK cells and mast cells express CCR1, CCR3 and/or CCR5 (Zabel et al. 2015). The second is that in addition to CCL5, these receptors are known to bind at least a dozen other chemokines (with varying affinity) (Zabel et al. 2015). Thus, antagonising chemokine receptors to chemoprevent skin cancer comes with a number of caveats including potential off-target effects and built-in redundancies. Maraviroc may be the exception (Table 10.1). Initially developed as a drug that blockes HIV entry and dissemination (Gulick et al. 2008), this highly specific CCR5 antagonist has also proven effective at blocking lymphocyte chemotaxis in graft versus host disease (Reshef et al. 2012). It remains to be determined whether Maraviroc could be deployed as a chemopreventative agent in patients at high risk of developing aggressive UV-induced skin cancers.

10.2.6 CXCL12/SDF-1α

C-X-C motif chemokine ligand 12 (CXCL12; previously stromal derived factor (SDF)-1α) is involved, either directly or indirectly, in the growth and metastasis of a number of different tumours including those of the breast (Müller et al. 2001; Yasuoka et al. 2008), esophagus, colon, ovaries (Sun et al. 2010) and skin (Müller et al. 2001; Murakami et al. 2002; Basile et al. 2008). Human melanomas that have metastasised to lymph nodes are also positive for the CXCL12 receptor, CXCR4 (Robledo et al. 2001). Indeed, for human metastatic melanoma (Scala et al. 2005) and aggressive non-melanoma skin cancers in particular (Basile et al. 2008), high levels of CXCR4 correlate with poor prognostic outcomes. Recently, primary cutaneous melanomas were shown to express both CXCR4 and CXCL12 (Mitchell et al. 2014) while human cutaneous squamous cell carcinomas (SCC), but not head and neck SCC (Clatot et al. 2015) also express the second CXCL12 receptor; CXCR7. This probably enables skin tumours to receive pro-survival signals from CXCL12 (Hu et al. 2014). Thus, human UV-induced skin cancers are positive for all three members of the CXCL12 chemokine family.

CXCR4-expressing cells migrate towards CXCL12 and UV alters this chemokine axis to direct the traffic of mast cells into and away from exposed skin (Byrne et al. 2008). Indeed, UV upregulates both CXCR4 and CXCL12 in murine (Sarchio et al. 2014) and human skin (Lee et al. 2013). Pharmacological interfering with UV-induced CXCL12 using the novel CXCR4-antagonist AMD3100 (brand names Mozobil and Plerixafor; Table 10.1) exposed the CXCL12 chemokine axis as a key mediator of UV-immunosuppression (Byrne et al. 2008) and skin carcinogenesis (Sarchio et al. 2014). AMD3100 is currently in clinical use as a stem cell mobilising agent (De Clercq 2009). There is significant potential therefore for this highly specific CXCR4 antagonist to be deployed as a novel photochemopreventative measure in human skin cancer patients.

10.2.7 Lipid Mediators

Most conventional cytokines/chemokines are proteins that require translation and transcription. Unless these cytokines are pre-made and stored in "ready-to-release" granules, as is the case for dermal mast cells, this production process can take many hours to manifest. UV can exert almost immediate biological effects by altering the production of a number of biologically active lipids (Kendall et al. 2015). Many of these lipid mediators of inflammation are produced in response to UV-induced reactive oxygen species and include platelet activating factor (PAF) receptor agonists (Travers et al. 2010), sphingosine 1 phosphate (S1P) (Uchida et al. 2010) and products of arachidonic acid metabolism such as prostaglandin (PG)-E_2 (Chen et al. 1996; Pentland and Mahoney 1990).

UV-induced PAF (and other PAF-receptor agonists) first came to the attention of skin tumour biologists when it was revealed to be a potent immune suppressant (Walterscheid et al. 2002). Mice treated with a PAF receptor antagonist were resistant to the carcinogenic effects of UV, thus confirming a role for PAF in UV-carcinogenesis (Sreevidya et al. 2008). More recently, PAF has been shown to contribute to UV-carcinogenesis by interfering with nucleotide excision repair (Sreevidya et al. 2010). UV-induced PAF plays a particularly important role in inducing both cell cycle arrest (Puebla-Osorio et al. 2015) and epigenetic modifications (Damiani et al. 2015) in mast cells. PAF is also responsible for upregulating the CXCR4 on dermal mast cells that facilitates their migration to skin-draining lymph nodes (Chacón-Salinas et al. 2014). Thus, drugs that antagonise PAF receptors in the skin will be particularly important pharmacological agents in any future chemopreventative strategies. A number of promising candidates exist (Table 10.1) that have even progressed to clinical trials in other inflammatory diseases including allergic rhinitis (Solans et al. 2008) and acquired cold urticaria (Metz et al. 2010). It remains to be determined whether such drugs display chemopreventative properties against skin cancer.

The hydrolytic conversion of pro-apoptotic ceramide to sphingosine in the skin allows for subsequent phosphorylation to S1P by sphingosine kinase 1. This is important because S1P was shown to protect keratinocytes from UVB-induced cell death (Uchida et al. 2010). UV-induced changes to S1P levels could also affect the maturation and migration of numerous cells including dendritic cells (Czeloth et al. 2005; Lamana et al. 2011), mast cells (Olivera and Rivera 2005) and T cells, especially those destined to be retained at cutaneous sites as resident memory T cells (Mackay et al. 2015). Pharmacologically targeting Cer-Sphingosine-S1P in skin is likely to be beneficial in skin cancer chemoprevention because sphingosine kinase 1 activators like K6PC-5 have been shown to reduce photo-damage in mice (Park et al. 2008) (Table 10.1).

UV irradiation of human skin explants also produces a dose-dependent increase in PGE_2 (Pentland et al. 1990), another major inflammatory product of arachidonic acid metabolism. PGE_2 is a potent immune suppressant that is upregulated, in part, by PAF (Walterscheid et al. 2002), MCP-1 and CCL5 (Conti and DiGioacchino 2001). UV-induced PGE_2 is a major inflammatory mediator of UV alterations to the bone marrow microenvironment (Ng et al. 2010), exerting its immune suppressive actions by signalling through the PGE_2-EP4 receptor (Soontrapa et al. 2011). While dendritic cells are a major immune cell target of UV-induced PGE_2 (Scandella et al. 2002; Luft et al. 2002; Legler et al. 2006), recruitment of regulatory T cells is also a possible explanation for why PGE_2 is immune suppressive (Karavitis et al. 2012).

Conversion of arachidonic acid to PGE_2 by the enzyme cyclo-oxygenase-2 (COX-2) is a key pathway leading to inflammation via the production of cytokines and chemokines (Liang et al. 2003a, b). It's perhaps not surprising therefore that a UV-induced increase in COX-2 is a major mechanism by which UV raises PGE_2 levels in the skin (Buckman et al. 1998).

10.2.8 Targeting PGE_2 by Modulating Cyclo-Oxygenase-2 (COX-2) Expression

Inhibitors of cyclo-oxygenase-2 (COX-2), including celecoxib, reduce photocarcinogenesis in mice (Fischer et al. 1999), clearly indicating the importance of UV-induced cytokines and chemokines in skin responses to UV (Halliday 2005). PGE_2 has affects additional to cytokine and chemokine induction that influence skin carcinogenesis, including immunosuppression and enhancement of tumour cell proliferation and invasion (Elmets et al. 2014). More than 90 % of human malignant melanomas expressed COX-2 with two-thirds expressing moderate to strong levels (Denkert et al. 2001). Moreover, production of PGE_2 by melanoma cells is important for their invasion in vitro (Denkert et al. 2001). Hence, therapeutic strategies that target COX-2 are likely to be beneficial in skin cancer chemopreventation. To that end, a double-blind placebo-controlled randomized trial compared oral celecoxib with placebo for 9 months of treatment in 240 subjects (Elmets et al. 2010). While celecoxib did not decrease the incidence of actinic keratosis at 9 months, at the end of the treatment period, the number of SCC and BCC was significantly reduced by celecoxib treatment and remained about 60 % lower at 2 months after completion of treatment.

Polyunsaturated fatty acids (PUFA) such as eicosapentaenoic acid (EPA) are essential fatty acids that can be provided from the diet, particularly marine animals such as oily fish. EPA competes with arachidonic acid for cyclooxygenases including COX-2 with EPA-derived products having less inflammatory effects and arachidonic acid-derived products. In this way polyunsaturated fatty acids such as EPA reduce COX-2 mediated inflammation and influence UV-induced cytokine production (Pilkington et al. 2011). EPA reduces UVB-induced IL-8 production by skin cells (Storey et al. 2005) and so is likely to inhibit the dermal recruitment of immune suppressive neutrophils. Supplementation of the diet of humans with omega-3 PUFAs including EPA significantly decreased lipopolysaccharide-induced production of the chemokines CCL5 and MCP-1 (Monocyte Chemotactic Protein-1) by peripheral blood mononuclear cells (Hung et al. 2015). This is important as both these chemokines have been shown to drive PGE_2 production (Conti and DiGioacchino 2001). In human clinical trials dietary EPA has been shown to alter the skin response to UV radiation with less pro-inflammatory products being produced (Pilkington et al. 2014). This results in protection from UV-induced immunosuppression in humans (Pilkington et al. 2013). Therefore modulation of COX-2 activity affects chemokine and cytokine production, affecting skin responses to UV radiation.

10.3 Promising New Photochemopreventative Agents

The major biological mechanisms that lead to skin cancer are UV-induced genetic damage, immunosuppression, and dysregulation of cell cycle control. Chemokines and cytokines are key regulators of these processes and are often targeted by or contribute to successful photchemopreventitive strategies. Strategies that enhance repair of damaged DNA, or prevent DNA damage from occurring, or prevent photoimmunosuppression, or enable cells to undergo cell cycle arrest to enhance the time available for DNA repair would all be expected to reduce the incidence of skin cancer.

10.3.1 Nicotinamide

Nicotinamide (NAM) is an amide form of vitamin B3 and there is a wealth of evidence that it is photochemoprotective. NAM and nicotinic acid, an alternate form of vitamin B3, reduces UV-induced immunosuppression and carcinogenesis in mice (Gensler 1997; Gensler et al. 1999). NAM (5 % cream) applied topically prior to or following solar-simulated UV, as well as NAM taken orally for 1 week prevented immunosuppression in humans. However the minimal erythemal dose (MED) was not changed by NAM. Therefore NAM protects from immunosuppression but not sunburn in humans. NAM's negligible absorbance, and protective capacity when applied after UV, indicates that it does not act as a sunscreen. Gene chip analysis indicated protection from UV downregulation of energy metabolism, complement and apoptosis pathways (Damian et al. 2008; Yiasemides et al. 2009). This was confirmed by Park et al. (2010) who showed that NAM protects from UV-induced blockade of glycolysis and ATP depletion but had no effect on reactive oxygen species (ROS) production in human keratinocytes. Thus NAM protects from the energy crisis that occurs in human keratinocytes following exposure to UV. This ability of NAM to normalise ATP production in UV irradiated skin is consistent with its known biochemical function as the primary precursor of nicotinamide adenine dinucleotide (NAD), which has a key function in ATP production. It is not clear how this normalisation of cellular energy pathways affects chemokine production but considering its ability to prevent UV immunosuppression it is likely that NAM would normalise UV-induced changes in cytokine and chemokine production.

Normalisation of ATP levels in UV exposed skin is likely to have many effects in chronically UV exposed skin, which is only beginning to be explored. DNA repair is increased by NAM in UV exposed human keratinocytes and melanocytes. The comet assay incorporating lesion specific excision enzymes was used to show that NAM increases repair of both cyclobutane pyrimidine dimers (CPDs) and 8-oxo-7,8-dihydro-2′-deoxyguanosine (8oxoG). Repair of both UV-induced CPDs and 8oxoG also occurred at a more efficient rate in ex vivo human skin treated with NAM as determined by immunostaining (Surjana et al. 2013; Thompson et al. 2014). Enhancement of the rate of repair of genetic damage would be expected to reduce the incidence of UV-induced mutations and therefore protect from UV-induced skin cancer. DNA repair is regulated by cytokines, with IL-12 having been shown to enhance DNA repair (Schwarz et al. 2002) but interactions between cytokine expression, ATP normalisation with NAM and DNA repair have not been adequately explored. NAM has been demonstrated to inhibit inflammatory cytokines (Ungerstedt et al. 2003). CD34(+) cells have increased migration to CXCL12 in the presence of NAM (Peled et al. 2012), and it also reduces expression of IL-6, IL-10, monocyte chemoattractant protein-1 and TNF mRNA in UV-irradiated keratinocytes (Monfrecola et al. 2013). It therefore appears that NAM plays a role in regulation of cytokine or chemokine expression, or their receptors, which could be involved in the photochemoprotective effects of this vitamin.

NAM reduces the incidence of skin cancer in humans. In two randomised double-blinded controlled phase II trials 500 mg NAM taken orally for 4 months once or twice per day significantly reduced the incidence of actinic keratosis (AK) by 29 and 35 % respectively (Surjana et al. 2012). These studies were relatively small with 41 patients in the once per day and 35 in the twice per day studies. AK are pre-malignant lesions that may progress into SCC and therefore this study indicated that NAM may be chemopreventive for skin cancer. This was directly investigated in a recent phase III, double-blind, randomized controlled trial where 386 participants who had a history of at least two NMSC received either 500 mg NAM or placebo twice per day in a 1:1 ratio for 12 months (Chen et al. 2015). In this study oral NAM significantly reduced the rate of new histologically confirmed NMSC by 23 % ($P = 0.02$). When the new NMSC were divided into BCC and SCC, the rates of reduction in the NAM group were similar but failed to achieve statistical significance due to the smaller number of skin cancer types. In these studies NAM was found to be safe with no side effects that could be attributed to this vitamin. It is also inexpensive, stable and readily available from stores selling vitamins. It therefore appears to be an effective and ideal chemopreventive agent.

10.3.2 Vitamin D

UV irradiation of 7-dehydrocholesterol results in production of the active vitamin D hormone, 1,25 dihydroxyvitamin D3 (1,25$(OH)_2$ D_3) in the skin (Bikle 2012). 1,25 $(OH)_2$ D_3 is important for bone and muscle health and is also an adaptive photo-protective response in the skin. 1,25$(OH)_2$ D_3 applied topically to mouse skin after each UV exposure reduced the number of mice in which tumours developed and the average number of tumours per mouse as well as increasing the time required for skin cancers to appear (Dixon et al. 2011). 1,25$(OH)_2$ D_3 reduces the level of CPDs in keratinocytes exposed to UV radiation in a dose and time-dependent dependent manner. UV-induced NO levels in keratinocytes were also reduced by 1,25$(OH)_2$ D_3 while p53 levels were increased. As a NO synthase inhibitor, like 1,25$(OH)_2$ D_3, reduced CPD levels, these events may be related and it is possible that 1,25$(OH)_2$ D_3 inhibition of NO levels could reduce oxidative damage to DNA repair enzymes, thus enhancing repair of UV-induced genetic damage (Gupta et al. 2007). Further evidence for this comes from studies showing that 1,25$(OH)_2$ D_3 additionally reduces UV-induced oxidative and nitrative DNA damage as well as CPDs and that treatment with nitric oxide donors results in the formation of all of these types of DNA damage in the absence of UV (Gordon-Thomson et al. 2012). Similar results were obtained using ex vivo human skin and in vivo in humans showing that the protective role of 1,25$(OH)_2$ D_3 occurred not only in isolated keratinocytes, but also in whole skin and in humans (Song et al. 2013; Damian et al. 2010). UV-induced NO can combine with ROS to produce peroxynitrite, which can cause oxidation and nitrosylation of not only DNA but also DNA repair enzymes. 1,25$(OH)_2$ D_3–

induced reduction in NO production could therefore enhance DNA repair, reducing the levels of DNA damage.

1,25$(OH)_2$ D_3 regulates pro-inflammatory cytokine and chemokine production in a variety of cell types (Svensson et al. 2015; Wang et al. 2015; Huang et al. 2015). NO can also regulate chemokine expression, depending on cell type and conditions (Kim et al. 2003; Tanese et al. 2012; Trifilieff et al. 2000). It is possible that 1,25 $(OH)_2$ D_3 may contribute to UV regulation of chemokines in a NO dependent manner however more work is required to clarify the roles of these molecules and whether this contributes to the photoprotective effects of 1,25$(OH)_2$ D_3.

10.3.3 Botanicals with Anti-inflammatory Activity

Agents found in botanical products have been shown to provide protection from the damaging effects of UV. The goji berry, *Lycium barbarum*, reduces UV-induced inflammatory oedema and immunosuppression in mice, possible due to its antioxidant activity (Reeve et al. 2010). Isoflavonoids, commonly found in plants, such as equol, protect from many of the damaging effects of UV, including inflammation, immunosuppression and photocarcinogenesis. In mice, protection by equol is inhibited by estrogen receptor antagonism suggesting that signaling through this receptor by equol is responsible for its photoprotective activity (Widyarini et al. 2006). Studies in knockout mice showed that this photoprotection is due to signaling via estrogen receptor-β which regulates UV control of production of a number of cytokines, including IFN-γ IL-12 and IL-10 (Cho et al. 2008). Antioxidant effects also contribute to the protective activity of equol (Widyarini et al. 2012). In humans a synthetic derivative of equol has been shown to protect the immune system from UV (Friedmann et al. 2004). The honeybee product propolis is another example of a photoprotective botanical that normalizes UV regulation of cytokines. Propolis corrects UV-induced overexpression of IL-10 and IL-6, and depletion of IL-12 (Cole et al. 2010).

Grape seed proanthocyanidins are another bioactive botanical that protects from UV-induced skin carcinogenesis. This is in part mediated by protecting the immune system and correcting UV induced changes in the cytokines IL-10 and IL-12 and increasing CD8+ T cell production of IFN-γ and IL-2 (Katiyar 2015). Silymarin, a plant flavonoid, protects from photocarcinogenesis and UV-induced immunosuppression. Injection of mice with neutralizing anti-IL-12 abrogated the protective effect of silymarin on immunosuppression indicating that it works at least in part by regulation of UV effects on cytokines (Meeran et al. 2006). Polyphenols from green tea significantly reduces skin carcinogenesis in UV irradiated wild type but not IL-12 knockout mice indicating that green tea polyphenols are photoprotective by a mechanism that includes regulation of IL-12. The proinflammatory cytokines TNF, IL-6 and IL-1β were also reduced in mice fed these polyphenols (Meeran et al. 2009). Green tea polyphenol supplementation of the diets of humans for 12 weeks has been shown to reduce the UV-induced sunburn response (Rhodes et al. 2013).

10.4 Summary and Conclusions

Decades of photobiological research into how chemokines and cytokines modulate UV damage have collided with the development of revolutionary biologics that serendipitously target these molecules. Successful photochemoprevention involves protection from UV induction of chemokines and cytokines, although other pathways are likely to also be involved. Photochemoprevention offers huge potential for skin cancer prevention and there has been considerable research to develop effective, safe and inexpensive photochemopreventive agents to be used in conjunction with strategies that shield from UV radiation such as sunscreens, sun avoidance and protective clothing. It is hoped that photochemoprevention *combined* with UV shielding will reduce the incidence of skin cancer further than what can be achieved by UV shielding alone. Adding at least some of these photochemopreventive approaches to our suite of established skin cancer preventive measures will be particularly important in individuals at high risk of developing aggressive UV-induced metastatic skin cancers.

References

Abeyama K, Eng W, Jester JV, Vink AA, Edelbaum D, Cockerell CJ et al (2000) A role for NF-kappaB-dependent gene transactivation in sunburn. J Clin Investig 105:1751–1759

Akita S, Ishihara H, Mohammad Abdur R, Fujii T (2000) Leukemia inhibitory factor gene improves skin allograft survival in the mouse model. Transplantation 70:1026–1031

Alard P, Niizeki H, Hanninen L, Streilein JW (1999) Local ultraviolet B irradiation impairs contact hypersensitivity induction by triggering release of tumor necrosis factor-alpha from mast cells. Involvement of mast cells and Langerhans cells in susceptibility to ultraviolet B. J Investig Dermatol 113:983–990

Allen MH, Skov L, Barber R, Trembath R, Simon J, Baadsgaard O, Barker J (1998) Ultraviolet B induced suppression of induction of contact sensitivity in human skin is not associated with tumour necrosis factor-alpha-308 or interleukin-10 genetic polymorphisms. Br J Dermatol 139:225–229

Alves-Filho JC, Sônego F, Souto FO, Freitas A, Verri WA, Auxiliadora-Martins M et al (2010) Interleukin-33 attenuates sepsis by enhancing neutrophil influx to the site of infection. Nat Med 16:708–712

Araneo BA, Dowell T, Moon HB, Daynes RA (1989) Regulation of murine lymphokine production in vivo. Ultraviolet radiation exposure depresses IL-2 and enhances IL-4 production by T cells through an IL-1-dependent mechanism. J Immunol 143:1737–1744

Arend WP, Palmer G, Gabay C (2008) IL-1, IL-18, and IL-33 families of cytokines. Immunol Rev 223:20–38

Baba H, Uchiwa H, Watanabe S (2005) UVB irradiation increases the release of SCF from human epidermal cells. J Invest Dermatol 124:1075–1077

Bachmann F, Buechner SA, Wernli M, Strebel S, Erb P (2001) Ultraviolet light downregulates CD95 ligand and TRAIL receptor expression facilitating actinic keratosis and squamous cell carcinoma formation. J Invest Dermatol 117:59–66

Bald T, Quast T, Landsberg J, Rogava M, Glodde N, Lopez-Ramos D et al (2014) Ultraviolet-radiation-induced inflammation promotes angiotropism and metastasis in melanoma. Nature 507:109–113

Basile J, Thiers B, Maize J, Lathers DM (2008) Chemokine receptor expression in non-melanoma skin cancer. J Cutan Pathol 35:623–629

Bergot A, Ford N, Leggatt GR, Wells JW, Frazer IH, Grimbaldeston MA (2014) HPV16-E7 expression in squamous epithelium creates a local immune suppressive environment via CCL2- and CCL5-mediated recruitment of mast cells. PLoS Pathog 10:e1004466

Bikle DD (2012) Vitamin D and the skin: physiology and pathophysiology. Rev Endocr Metab Disord 13:3–19

Buckman SY, Gresham A, Hale P, Hruza G, Anast J, Masferrer J, Pentland AP (1998) COX-2 expression is induced by UVB exposure in human skin: implications for the development of skin cancer. Carcinogenesis 19:723–729

Byrne SN, Halliday GM, Johnston LJ, King NJC (2001) Interleukin-1 beta but not tumor necrosis factor is involved in West Nile Virus-induced Langerhans cell migration from the skin in C57BL/6 mice. J Investig Dermatol 117:702–709

Byrne SN, Limon-Flores AY, Ullrich SE (2008) Mast cell migration from the skin to the draining lymph nodes upon UV-irradiation represents a key step in the induction of immune suppression. J Immunol 180:4648–4655

Byrne SN, Beaugie C, O'Sullivan C, Leighton S, Halliday GM (2011) the immune-modulating cytokine and endogenous alarmin interleukin-33 is upregulated in skin exposed to inflammatory UVB radiation. Am J Pathol 179:211–222

Cai H, Santiago FS, Prado-Lourenco L, Wang B, Patrikakis M, Davenport MP et al (2012) DNAzyme targeting c-jun suppresses skin cancer growth. Sci Transl Med 4:139ra82

Chacón-Salinas R, Chen L, Chávez-Blanco AD, Limón-Flores AY, Ma Y, Ullrich SE (2014) An essential role for platelet-activating factor in activating mast cell migration following ultraviolet irradiation. J Leukoc Biol 95:139–148

Chen X, Gresham A, Morrison A, Pentland AP (1996) Oxidative stress mediates synthesis of cytosolic phospholipase A2 after UVB injury. Biochim Biophys Acta 1299:23–33

Chen AC, Martin AJ, Choy B, Fernández-Peñas P, Dalziell RA, McKenzie CA et al (2015) A phase 3 randomized trial of nicotinamide for skin-cancer chemoprevention. N Engl J Med 373:1618–1626

Cho D, Seung Kang J, Hoon Park J, Kim YI, Hahm E, Lee J et al (2002) The enhanced IL-18 production by UVB irradiation requires ROI and AP-1 signaling in human keratinocyte cell line (HaCaT). Biochem Biophys Res Commun 298:289–295

Cho JL, Allanson M, Domanski D, Arun SJ, Reeve VE (2008) Estrogen receptor-beta signaling protects epidermal cytokine expression and immune function from UVB-induced impairment in mice. Photochem Photobiol Sci 7:120–125

Cho JL, Allanson M, Reeve VE (2012) Hypoxia inducible factor-1α contributes to UV radiation-induced inflammation, epidermal hyperplasia and immunosuppression in mice. Photochem Photobiol Sci 11:309–317

Cho EA, Moloney FJ, Cai H, Au-Yeung A, China C, Scolyer RA et al (2013) Safety and tolerability of an intratumorally injected DNAzyme, Dz13, in patients with nodular basal-cell carcinoma: a phase 1 first-in-human trial (DISCOVER). Lancet 381:1835–1843

Chung JH, Youn SH, Koh WS, Eun HC, Cho KH, Park KC, Youn JI (1996) Ultraviolet B irradiation-enhanced interleukin (IL)-6 production and mRNA expression are mediated by IL-1 alpha in cultured human keratinocytes. J Invest Dermatol 106:715–720

Clatot F, Cornic M, Berghian A, Marchand V, Choussy O, El Ouakif F et al (2015) CXCL12 and CXCR4, but not CXCR7, are primarily expressed by the stroma in head and neck squamous cell carcinoma. Pathology 47:45–50

Cole N, Sou PW, Ngo A, Tsang KH, Severino JA, Arun SJ et al (2010) Topical 'Sydney' propolis protects against UV-radiation-induced inflammation, lipid peroxidation and immune suppression in mouse skin. Int Arch Allergy Immunol 152:87–97

Conti P, DiGioacchino M (2001) MCP-1 and RANTES are mediators of acute and chronic inflammation. Allergy Asthma Proc 22:133–137

Czeloth N, Bernhardt G, Hofmann F, Genth H, Forster R (2005) Sphingosine-1-phosphate mediates migration of mature dendritic cells. J Immunol 175:2960–2967

Damian DL, Patterson CR, Stapelberg M, Park J, Barnetson RS, Halliday GM (2008) UV radiation-induced immunosuppression is greater in men and prevented by topical nicotinamide. J Invest Dermatol 128:447–454

Damian DL, Kim YJ, Dixon KM, Halliday GM, Javeri A, Mason RS (2010) Topical calcitriol protects from UV-induced genetic damage but suppresses cutaneous immunity in humans. Exp Dermatol 19:e23–e30

Damiani E, Puebla-Osorio N, Gorbea E, Ullrich SE (2015) Platelet-activating factor induces epigenetic modifications in human mast cells. J Invest Dermatol 135:3034–3040

De Clercq E (2009) The AMD3100 story: the path to the discovery of a stem cell mobilizer (Mozobil). Biochem Pharmacol 77:1655–1664

Denkert C, Köbel M, Berger S, Siegert A, Leclere A, Trefzer U, Hauptmann S (2001) Expression of cyclooxygenase 2 in human malignant melanoma. Cancer Res 61:303–308

Dixon KM, Norman AW, Sequeira VB, Mohan R, Rybchyn MS, Reeve VE et al (2011) 1α,25 $(OH)_2$-vitamin D and a nongenomic vitamin D analogue inhibit ultraviolet radiation-induced skin carcinogenesis. Cancer Prev Res (Phila) 4:1485–1494

Dubina M, Goldenberg G (2009) Viral-associated nonmelanoma skin cancers: a review. Am J Dermatopathol 31:561–573

Elmets CA, Viner JL, Pentland AP, Cantrell W, Lin HY, Bailey H et al (2010) Chemoprevention of nonmelanoma skin cancer with celecoxib: a randomized, double-blind, placebo-controlled trial. J Natl Cancer Inst 102:1835–1844

Elmets CA, Ledet JJ, Athar M (2014) Cyclooxygenases: mediators of UV-induced skin cancer and potential targets for prevention. J Invest Dermatol 134:2497–2502

Enoksson M, Möller-Westerberg C, Wicher G, Fallon PG, Forsberg-Nilsson K, Lunderius-Andersson C, Nilsson G (2012) Intraperitoneal influx of neutrophils in response to IL-33 is mast cell dependent. Blood 121:530–536

Fahmy RG, Waldman A, Zhang G, Mitchell A, Tedla N, Cai H et al (2006) Suppression of vascular permeability and inflammation by targeting of the transcription factor c-Jun. Nat Biotechnol 24:856–863

Feldmeyer L, Keller M, Niklaus G, Hohl D, Werner S, Beer HD (2007) The inflammasome mediates UVB-induced activation and secretion of interleukin-1beta by keratinocytes. Curr Biol 17:1140–1145

Fischer SM, Lo HH, Gordon GB, Seibert K, Kelloff G, Lubet RA, Conti CJ (1999) Chemopreventive activity of celecoxib, a specific cyclooxygenase-2 inhibitor, and indomethacin against ultraviolet light-induced skin carcinogenesis. Mol Carcinog 25:231–240

Friedmann AC, Halliday GM, Barnetson RS, Reeve VE, Walker C, Patterson CR, Damian DL (2004) The topical isoflavonoid NV-07alpha reduces solar-simulated UV-induced suppression of Mantoux reactions in humans. Photochem Photobiol 80:416–421

Fujita Y, Abe R, Sasaki M, Honda A, Furuichi M, Asano Y et al (2006) Presence of circulating CCR10+ T cells and elevated serum CTACK/CCL27 in the early stage of mycosis fungoides. Clin Cancer Res 12:2670–2675

Gahring L, Baltz M, Pepys MB, Daynes R (1984) Effect of ultraviolet radiation on production of epidermal cell thymocyte-activating factor/interleukin 1 in vivo and in vitro. Proc Natl Acad Sci U S A 81:1198–1202

Garbers C, Hermanns HM, Schaper F, Müller-Newen G, Grötzinger J, Rose-John S, Scheller J (2012) Plasticity and cross-talk of interleukin 6-type cytokines. Cytokine Growth Factor Rev 23:85–97

Garlanda C, Dinarello CA, Mantovani A (2013) The interleukin-1 family: back to the future. Immunity 39:1003–1018

Gensler HL (1997) Prevention of photoimmunosuppression and photocarcinogenesis by topical nicotinamide. Nutr Cancer 29:157–162

Gensler HL, Williams T, Huang AC, Jacobson EL (1999) Oral niacin prevents photocarcinogenesis and photoimmunosuppression in mice. Nutr Cancer 34:36–41

Golab J, Stoklosa T (2005) Technology evaluation: SB-485232, GlaxoSmithKline. Curr Opin Mol Ther 7:85–93

Gordon-Thomson C, Gupta R, Tongkao-on W, Ryan A, Halliday GM, Mason RS (2012) 1α,25 dihydroxyvitamin D3 enhances cellular defences against UV-induced oxidative and other forms of DNA damage in skin. Photochem Photobiol Sci 11:1837–1847

Goteri G, Rupoli S, Campanati A, Costagliola A, Sabato S, Stramazzotti D et al (2009) Lesional skin chemokine CTACK/CCL27 expression in mycosis fungoides and disease control by IFN-alpha and PUVA therapy. Am J Transl Res 1:203–210

Goteri G, Rupoli S, Campanati A, Zizzi A, Picardi P, Cardelli M et al (2012) Serum and tissue CTACK/CCL27 chemokine levels in early mycosis fungoides may be correlated with disease-free survival following treatment with interferon alfa and psoralen plus ultraviolet A therapy. Br J Dermatol 166:948–952

Grabbe J, Welker P, Dippel E, Czarnetzki BM (1994) Stem cell factor, a novel cutaneous growth factor for mast cells and melanocytes. Arch Dermatol Res 287:78–84

Grewe M, Gyufko K, Budnik A, Ruzicka T, Olaizola-Horn S, Berneburg M, Krutmann J (1996) Interleukin-1 receptors type I and type II are differentially regulated in human keratinocytes by ultraviolet B radiation. J Invest Dermatol 107:865–870

Griffith JW, Sokol CL, Luster AD (2014) Chemokines and chemokine receptors: positioning cells for host defense and immunity. Annu Rev Immunol 32:659–702

Grimbaldeston MA, Simpson A, Finlay-Jones JJ, Hart PH (2003) The effect of ultraviolet radiation exposure on the prevalence of mast cells in human skin. Brit J Dermatol 148:300–306

Grimbaldeston MA, Finlay-Jones JJ, Hart PH (2006) Mast cells in photodamaged skin: what is their role in skin cancer? Photochem Photobiol Sci 5:177–183

Gulick RM, Lalezari J, Goodrich J, Clumeck N, DeJesus E, Horban A et al (2008) Maraviroc for previously treated patients with R5 HIV-1 infection. N Engl J Med 359:1429–1441

Gupta R, Dixon KM, Deo SS, Holliday CJ, Slater M, Halliday GM et al (2007) Photoprotection by 1,25 dihydroxyvitamin D3 is associated with an increase in p53 and a decrease in nitric oxide products. J Invest Dermatol 127:707–715

Hachiya A, Kobayashi A, Ohuchi A, Takema Y, Imokawa G (2001) The paracrine role of stem cell factor/c-kit signaling in the activation of human melanocytes in ultraviolet-B-induced pigmentation. J Invest Dermatol 116:578–586

Hacker E, Muller K, Whiteman DC, Pavey S, Hayward N, Walker G (2008) Reduced expression of IL-18 is a marker of ultraviolet radiation-induced melanomas. Int J Cancer 123:227–231

Halliday GM (2005) Inflammation, gene mutation and photoimmunosuppression in response to UVR-induced oxidative damage contributes to photocarcinogenesis. Mutat Res 571:107–120

Hart PH, Grimbaldeston MA, Swift GJ, Sedgwick JD, Körner H, Finlay-Jones JJ (1998) TNF modulates susceptibility to UVB-induced systemic immunomodulation in mice by effects on dermal mast cell prevalence. Eur J Immunol 28:2893–2901

Hu J, Ono S, Katayama H, Imai T, Shimizu N, Nakagawa H (2000) Leukemia inhibitory factor induces epidermal hyperplasia in patients with amyotrophic lateral sclerosis. J Invest Dermatol 115:486–492

Hu SC, Yu HS, Yen FL, Chen GS, Lan CC (2014) CXCR7 expression correlates with tumor depth in cutaneous squamous cell carcinoma skin lesions and promotes tumor cell survival through ERK activation. Exp Dermatol 23:902–908

Huang B, Lei Z, Zhang GM, Li D, Song C, Li B et al (2008) SCF-mediated mast cell infiltration and activation exacerbate the inflammation and immunosuppression in tumor microenvironment. Blood 112:1269–1279

Huang YN, Ho YJ, Lai CC, Chiu CT, Wang JY (2015) 1,25-Dihydroxyvitamin D3 attenuates endotoxin-induced production of inflammatory mediators by inhibiting MAPK activation in primary cortical neuron-glia cultures. J Neuroinflammation 12:147

Hueber AJ, Alves-Filho JC, Asquith DL, Michels C, Millar NL, Reilly JH et al (2011) IL-33 induces skin inflammation with mast cell and neutrophil activation. Eur J Immunol 41:2229–2237

Hung AM, Booker C, Ellis CD, Siew ED, Graves AJ, Shintani A et al (2015) Omega-3 fatty acids inhibit the up-regulation of endothelial chemokines in maintenance hemodialysis patients. Nephrol Dial Transplant 30:266–274

Iracheta-Vellve A, Petrasek J, Satishchandran A, Gyongyosi B, Saha B, Kodys K et al (2015) Inhibition of sterile danger signals, uric acid and ATP, prevents inflammasome activation and protects from alcoholic steatohepatitis in mice. J Hepatol 63:1147–1155

Ito T, Seo N, Yagita H, Tsujimura K, Takigawa M, Tokura Y (2003) Alterations of immune functions in barrier disrupted skin by UVB irradiation. J Dermatol Sci 33:151–159

Karavitis J, Hix LM, Shi YH, Schultz RF, Khazaie K, Zhang M (2012) Regulation of COX2 expression in mouse mammary tumor cells controls bone metastasis and PGE2-induction of regulatory T cell migration. PLoS ONE 7:e46342

Katiyar SK (2015) Proanthocyanidins from grape seeds inhibit UV-radiation-induced immune suppression in mice: detection and analysis of molecular and cellular targets. Photochem Photobiol 91:156–162

Keermann M, Kõks S, Reimann E, Abram K, Erm T, Silm H, Kingo K (2015) Expression of IL-36 family cytokines and IL-37 but not IL-38 is altered in psoriatic skin. J Dermatol Sci 80:150

Kendall AC, Pilkington SM, Massey KA, Sassano G, Rhodes LE, Nicolaou A (2015) Distribution of bioactive lipid mediators in human skin. J Invest Dermatol 135:1510–1520

Kim JY, Kim D, Lee EM, Choi I, Park CG, Kim KS et al (2003) Inducible nitric oxide synthase inhibitors prolonged the survival of skin xenografts through selective down-regulation of pro-inflammatory cytokine and CC-chemokine expressions. Transpl Immunol 12:63–72

Kim MS, Kim YK, Lee DH, Seo JE, Cho KH, Eun HC, Chung JH (2008) Acute exposure of human skin to ultraviolet or infrared radiation or heat stimuli increases mast cell numbers and tryptase expression in human skin in vivo. Br J Dermatol 20:357–360

Kligman LH, Murphy GF (1996) Ultraviolet B radiation increases hairless mouse mast cells in a dose-dependent manner and alters distribution of UV-induced mast cell growth factor. Photochem Photobiol 63:123–127

Kock A, Schwarz T, Kirnbauer R, Urbanski A, Perry P, Ansel JC, Luger TA (1990) Human keratinocytes are a source for tumor necrosis factor alpha: evidence for synthesis and release upon stimulation with endotoxin or ultraviolet light. J Exp Med 172:1609–1614

Kondo S, Sauder DN, Kono T, Galley KA, McKenzie RC (1994) Differential modulation of interleukin-1 alpha (IL-1 alpha) and interleukin-1 beta (IL-1 beta) in human epidermal keratinocytes by UVB. Exp Dermatol 3:29–39

Konnikov N, Pincus SH, Dinarello CA (1989) Elevated plasma interleukin-1 levels in humans following ultraviolet light therapy for psoriasis. J Invest Dermatol 92:235–239

Kothny-Wilkes G, Kulms D, Luger TA, Kubin M, Schwarz T (1999) Interleukin-1 protects transformed keratinocytes from tumor necrosis factor-related apoptosis-inducing ligand- and CD95-induced apoptosis but not from ultraviolet radiation-induced apoptosis. J Biol Chem 274:28916–28921

Kupper TS, Chua AO, Flood P, McGuire J, Gubler U (1987) Interleukin 1 gene expression in cultured human keratinocytes is augmented by ultraviolet irradiation. J Clin Invest 80:430–436

Lamana A, Martin P, de la Fuente H, Martinez-Muñoz L, Cruz-Adalia A, Ramirez-Huesca M et al (2011) CD69 modulates sphingosine-1-phosphate-induced migration of skin dendritic cells. J Invest Dermatol 131:1503–1512

Lee E, Han J, Kim K, Choi H, Cho EG, Lee TR (2013) CXCR7 mediates SDF1-induced melanocyte migration. Pigment Cell Melanoma Res 26:58–66

Legler DF, Krause P, Scandella E, Singer E, Groettrup M (2006) Prostaglandin E2 is generally required for human dendritic cell migration and exerts its effect via EP2 and EP4 receptors. J Immunol 176:966–973

Leighton S, Kok LF, Halliday GM, Byrne SN (2013) Inhibition of UV-induced uric acid production using Allopurinol prevents suppression of the contact hypersensitivity response. Exp Dermatol 22:189–194

Lew W, Lee SH, Park YK (1995) Opposing effects of ultraviolet B irradiation on interleukin-1 receptor antagonist and interleukin-1 alpha messenger RNA expression in a human epidermoid carcinoma cell line. Photodermatol Photoimmunol Photomed 11:91–94

Liang L, Hu D, Liu W, Williams JP, Okunieff P, Ding I (2003a) Celecoxib reduces skin damage after radiation: selective reduction of chemokine and receptor mRNA expression in irradiated skin but not in irradiated mammary tumor. Am J Clin Oncol 26:S114–S121

Liang L, Hu DP, Liu WM, Williams JP, Okunieff P, Ding I (2003b) Celecoxib reduces *skin* damage after radiation. Am J Clin Oncol Cancer Clin Trials 26:S114–S121

Loser K, Mehling A, Loeser S, Apelt J, Kuhn A, Grabbe S et al (2006) Epidermal RANKL controls regulatory T-cell numbers via activation of dendritic cells. Nat Med 12:1372–1379

Luft T, Jefford M, Luetjens P, Toy T, Hochrein H, Masterman KA et al (2002) Functionally distinct dendritic cell (DC) populations induced by physiologic stimuli: prostaglandin E-2 regulates the migratory capacity of specific DC subsets. Blood 100:1362–1372

Mackay LK, Braun A, Macleod BL, Collins N, Tebartz C, Bedoui S et al (2015) Cutting edge: CD69 interference with sphingosine-1-phosphate receptor function regulates peripheral T cell retention. J Immunol 194:2059–2063

Maeda A, Beissert S, Schwarz T, Schwarz A (2008) Phenotypic and functional characterization of ultraviolet radiation-induced regulatory T cells. J Immunol 180:3065–3071

Malaviya R, Ikeda T, Ross E, Abraham SN (1996) Mast cell modulation of neutrophil influx and bacterial clearance at sites of infection through TNF-alpha. Nature 381:77–80

McKenzie RC (2001) Ultraviolet radiation B (UVB)-induction of leukaemia inhibitory factor (LIF) in human keratinocytes. Photodermatol Photoimmunol Photomed 17:284–285

Meeran SM, Katiyar S, Elmets CA, Katiyar SK (2006) Silymarin inhibits UV radiation-induced immunosuppression through augmentation of interleukin-12 in mice. Mol Cancer Ther 5:1660–1668

Meeran SM, Akhtar S, Katiyar SK (2009) Inhibition of UVB-induced skin tumor development by drinking green tea polyphenols is mediated through DNA repair and subsequent inhibition of inflammation. J Invest Dermatol 129:1258–1270

Meininger CJ, Yano H, Rottapel R, Bernstein A, Zsebo KM, Zetter BR (1992) The c-kit receptor ligand functions as a mast cell chemoattractant. Blood 79:958–963

Meller S, Winterberg F, Gilliet M, Müller A, Lauceviciute I, Rieker J et al (2005) Ultraviolet radiation-induced injury, chemokines, and leukocyte recruitment: an amplification cycle triggering cutaneous lupus erythematosus. Arthritis Rheum 52:1504–1516

Merad M, Manz MG, Karsunky H, Wagers A, Peters W, Charo I et al (2002) Langerhans cells renew in the skin throughout life under steady-state conditions. Nat Immunol 3:1135–1141

Metz M, Scholz E, Ferrán M, Izquierdo I, Giménez-Arnau A, Maurer M (2010) Rupatadine and its effects on symptom control, stimulation time, and temperature thresholds in patients with acquired cold urticaria. Ann Allergy Asthma Immunol 104:86–92

Mitchell B, Leone D, Feller K, Menon S, Bondzie P, Yang S et al (2014) Protein expression of the chemokine receptor CXCR4 and its ligand CXCL12 in primary cutaneous melanoma–biomarkers of potential utility? Hum Pathol 45:2094–2100

Monfrecola G, Gaudiello F, Cirillo T, Fabbrocini G, Balato A, Lembo S (2013) Nicotinamide downregulates gene expression of interleukin-6, interleukin-10, monocyte chemoattractant protein-1, and tumour necrosis factor-α gene expression in HaCaT keratinocytes after ultraviolet B irradiation. Clin Exp Dermatol 38:185–188

Moodycliffe AM, Kimber I, Norval M (1994) Role of tumour necrosis factor-alpha in ultraviolet B light-induced dendritic cell migration and suppression of contact hypersensitivity. Immunology 81:79–84

Morales J, Homey B, Vicari AP, Hudak S, Oldham E, Hedrick J et al (1999) CTACK, a skin-associated chemokine that preferentially attracts skin-homing memory T cells. Proc Natl Acad Sci U S A 96:14470–14475

Mrowietz U, Schwenk U, Maune S, Bartels J, Küpper M, Fichtner I et al (1999) The chemokine RANTES is secreted by human melanoma cells and is associated with enhanced tumour formation in nude mice. Br J Cancer 79:1025–1031

Müller A, Homey B, Soto H, Ge N, Catron D, Buchanan ME et al (2001) Involvement of chemokine receptors in breast cancer metastasis. Nature 410:50–56

Murakami T, Maki W, Cardones AR, Fang H, Tun Kyi A, Nestle FO, Hwang ST (2002) Expression of CXC chemokine receptor-4 enhances the pulmonary metastatic potential of murine B16 melanoma cells. Canc Res 62:7328–7334
Ng RLX, Bisley JL, Gorman S, Norval M, Hart PH (2010) Ultraviolet irradiation of mice reduces the competency of bone marrow-derived CD11c+ Cells via an indomethacin-inhibitable pathway. J Immunol 185:7207–7215
Nilsson G, Butterfield JH, Nilsson K, Siegbahn A (1994) Stem cell factor is a chemotactic factor for human mast cells. J Immunol 153:3717–3723
Nishimura N, Tohyama C, Satoh M, Nishimura H, Reeve VE (1999) Defective immune response and severe skin damage following UVB irradiation in interleukin-6-deficient mice. Immunology 97:77–83
Olivera A, Rivera J (2005) Sphingolipids and the balancing of immune cell function: lessons from the mast cell. J Immunol 174:1153–1158
Oxholm A, Oxholm P, Staberg B, Bendtzen K (1988) Immunohistological detection of interleukin I-like molecules and tumour necrosis factor in human epidermis before and after UVB-irradiation in vivo. Br J Dermatol 118:369–376
Paglia D, Kondo S, Ng KM, Sauder DN, McKenzie RC (1996) Leukaemia inhibitory factor is expressed by normal human keratinocytes in vitro and in vivo. Br J Dermatol 134:817–823
Park HY, Youm JK, Kwon MJ, Park BD, Lee SH, Choi EH (2008) K6PC-5, a novel sphingosine kinase activator, improves long-term ultraviolet light-exposed aged murine skin. Exp Dermatol 17:829–836
Park J, Halliday GM, Surjana D, Damian DL (2010) Nicotinamide prevents ultraviolet radiation-induced cellular energy loss. Photochem Photobiol 86:942–948
Pease JE, Horuk R (2009a) Chemokine receptor antagonists: part 1. Expert Opin Ther Pat 19:39–58
Pease JE, Horuk R (2009b) Chemokine receptor antagonists: part 2. Expert Opin Ther Pat 19:199–221
Peled T, Shoham H, Aschengrau D, Yackoubov D, Frei G, Rosenheimer GN et al (2012) Nicotinamide, a SIRT1 inhibitor, inhibits differentiation and facilitates expansion of hematopoietic progenitor cells with enhanced bone marrow homing and engraftment. Exp Hematol 40(342–55):e1
Pentland AP, Mahoney MG (1990) Keratinocyte prostaglandin synthesis is enhanced by IL-1. J Invest Dermatol 94:43–46
Pentland AP, Mahoney M, Jacobs SC, Holtzman MJ (1990) Enhanced prostaglandin synthesis after ultraviolet injury is mediated by endogenous histamine stimulation. A mechanism for irradiation erythema. J Clin Invest 86:566–574
Pilkington SM, Watson RE, Nicolaou A, Rhodes LE (2011) Omega-3 polyunsaturated fatty acids: photoprotective macronutrients. Exp Dermatol 20:537–543
Pilkington SM, Massey KA, Bennett SP, Al-Aasswad NM, Roshdy K, Gibbs NK et al (2013) Randomized controlled trial of oral omega-3 PUFA in solar-simulated radiation-induced suppression of human cutaneous immune responses. Am J Clin Nutr 97:646–652
Pilkington SM, Rhodes LE, Al-Aasswad NM, Massey KA, Nicolaou A (2014) Impact of EPA ingestion on COX- and LOX-mediated eicosanoid synthesis in skin with and without a pro-inflammatory UVR challenge—report of a randomised controlled study in humans. Mol Nutr Food Res 58:580–590
Puebla-Osorio N, Damiani E, Bover L, Ullrich SE (2015) Platelet-activating factor induces cell cycle arrest and disrupts the DNA damage response in mast cells. Cell Death Dis 6:e1745
Reeve VE, Tyrrell RM, Allanson M, Domanski D, Blyth L (2009) The role of interleukin-6 in UVA protection against UVB-induced immunosuppression. J Invest Dermatol 129:1539–1546
Reeve VE, Allanson M, Arun SJ, Domanski D, Painter N (2010) Mice drinking goji berry juice (Lycium barbarum) are protected from UV radiation-induced skin damage via antioxidant pathways. Photochem Photobiol Sci 9:601–607
Reshef R, Luger SM, Hexner EO, Loren AW, Frey NV, Nasta SD et al (2012) Blockade of lymphocyte chemotaxis in visceral graft-versus-host disease. N Engl J Med 367:135–145

Rhodes LE, Darby G, Massey KA, Clarke KA, Dew TP, Farrar MD et al (2013) Oral green tea catechin metabolites are incorporated into human skin and protect against UV radiation-induced cutaneous inflammation in association with reduced production of pro-inflammatory eicosanoid 12-hydroxyeicosatetraenoic acid. Br J Nutr 110:891–900

Ribeiro RA, Flores CA, Cunha FQ, Ferreira SH (1991) IL-8 causes in vivo neutrophil migration by a cell-dependent mechanism. Immunology 73:472–477

Rivas JM, Ullrich SE (1994) The role of IL-4, IL-10, and TNF-alpha in the immune suppression induced by ultraviolet radiation. J Leukoc Biol 56:769–775

Robledo MM, Bartolome RA, Longo N, Rodríguez-Frade JM, Mellado M, Longo I et al (2001) Expression of functional chemokine receptors CXCR3 and CXCR4 on human melanoma cells. J Biol Chem 276:45098–45105

Sarchio SN, Kok L-F, O'Sullivan C, Halliday GM, Byrne SN (2012) Dermal mast cells affect the development of sunlight-induced skin tumours. Exp Dermatol 21:241–248

Sarchio SNE, Scolyer RA, Beaugie C, McDonald D, Marsh-Wakefield F, Halliday GM, Byrne SN (2014) Pharmacologically antagonizing the CXCR4-CXCL12 chemokine pathway with AMD3100 inhibits sunlight-induced skin cancer. J Invest Dermatol 134:1091–1100

Scala S, Ottaiano A, Ascierto PA, Cavalli M, Simeone E, Giuliano P et al (2005) Expression of CXCR4 predicts poor prognosis in patients with malignant melanoma. Clin Cancer Res 11:1835–1841

Scandella E, Men Y, Gillessen S, Forster R, Groettrup M (2002) Prostaglandin E2 is a key factor for CCR7 surface expression and migration of monocyte-derived denctritic cells. Blood 100:1354–1361

Schwarz T, Urbanski A, Kirnbauer R, Köck A, Gschnait F, Luger TA (1988) Detection of a specific inhibitor of interleukin 1 in sera of UVB-treated mice. J Invest Dermatol 91:536–540

Schwarz A, Ständer S, Berneburg M, Böhm M, Kulms D, van Steeg H et al (2002) Interleukin-12 suppresses ultraviolet radiation-induced apoptosis by inducing DNA repair. Nat Cell Biol 4:26–31

Schwarz A, Maeda A, Stander S, van Steeg H, Schwarz T (2006) IL-18 reduces ultraviolet radiation-induced DNA damage and thereby affects photoimmunosuppression. J Immunol 176:2896–2901

Scordi IA, Vincek V (2000) Timecourse study of UVB-induced cytokine induction in whole mouse skin. Photodermatol Photoimmunol Photomed 16:67–73

Scordi IA, Nassiri M, Hanly AJ, Vincek V (1999) Interleukin 11 reduces apoptosis in UVB-irradiated mouse skin. Dermatology 199:296–301

Singh RK, Gutman M, Reich R, Bar-Eli M (1995) Ultraviolet B irradiation promotes tumorigenic and metastatic properties in primary cutaneous melanoma via induction of interleukin 8. Cancer Res 55:3669–3674

Solans A, Izquierdo I, Donado E, Antonijoan R, Peña J, Nadal T et al (2008) Pharmacokinetic and safety profile of rupatadine when coadministered with azithromycin at steady-state levels: a randomized, open-label, two-way, crossover, phase I study. Clin Ther 30:1639–1650

Song EJ, Gordon-Thomson C, Cole L, Stern H, Halliday GM, Damian DL, Reeve VE, Mason RS (2013) 1α,25-Dihydroxyvitamin D3 reduces several types of UV-induced DNA damage and contributes to photoprotection. J Steroid Biochem Mol Biol 136:131–138

Soontrapa K, Honda T, Sakata D, Yao C, Hirata T, Hori S et al (2011) Prostaglandin E2-prostoglandin E receptor subtype 4 (EP4) signaling mediates UV irradiation-induced systemic immunosuppression. Proc Natl Acad Sci U S A 108:6668–6673

Sreevidya CS, Khaskhely NM, Fukunaga A, Khaskina P, Ullrich SE (2008) Inhibition of photocarcinogenesis by platelet-activating factor or serotonin receptor antagonists. Cancer Res 68:3978–3984

Sreevidya CS, Fukunaga A, Khaskhely NM, Masaki T, Ono R, Nishigori C, Ullrich SE (2010) Agents that reverse UV-Induced immune suppression and photocarcinogenesis affect DNA repair. J Invest Dermatol 130:1428–1437

Ständer S, Schwarz T (2005) Tumor necrosis factor-related apoptosis-inducing ligand (TRAIL) is expressed in normal skin and cutaneous inflammatory diseases, but not in chronically UV-exposed skin and non-melanoma skin cancer. Am J Dermatopathol 27:116–121

Storey A, McArdle F, Friedmann PS, Jackson MJ, Rhodes LE (2005) Eicosapentaenoic acid and docosahexaenoic acid reduce UVB- and TNF-alpha-induced IL-8 secretion in keratinocytes and UVB-induced IL-8 in fibroblasts. J Invest Dermatol 124:248–255

Strickland I, Rhodes LE, Flanagan BF, Friedmann PS (1997) TNF-alpha and IL-8 are upregulated in the epidermis of normal human skin after UVB exposure: correlation with neutrophil accumulation and E-selectin expression. J Invest Dermatol 108:763–768

Su X, Ye J, Hsueh EC, Zhang Y, Hoft DF, Peng G (2010) Tumor microenvironments direct the recruitment and expansion of human Th17 cells. J Immunol 184:1630–1641

Sun X, Cheng G, Hao M, Zheng J, Zhou X, Zhang J et al (2010) CXCL12/ CXCR4/CXCR7 chemokine axis and cancer progression. Cancer Metastasis Rev 29:709–722

Surjana D, Halliday GM, Martin AJ, Moloney FJ, Damian DL (2012) Oral nicotinamide reduces actinic keratoses in phase II double-blinded randomized controlled trials. J Invest Dermatol 132:1497–1500

Surjana D, Halliday GM, Damian DL (2013) Nicotinamide enhances repair of ultraviolet radiation-induced DNA damage in human keratinocytes and ex vivo skin. Carcinogenesis 34:1144–1149

Svensson D, Nebel D, Nilsson BO (2015) Vitamin D3 modulates the innate immune response through regulation of the hCAP-18/LL-37 gene expression and cytokine production. Inflamm Res 65:25–32

Szepietowski JC, Walker C, McKenna DB, Hunter JA, McKenzie RC (2001) Leukaemia inhibitory factor and interleukin-8 expression in nonmelanoma skin cancers. Clin Exp Dermatol 26:72–78

Tanaka T, Morita E, Mihara S, Kanno M, Yamamoto S (2001) Identification of leukemia inhibitory factor as a potent mast cell growth-enhancing factor produced by mouse keratinocyte cell line, KCMH-1. Arch Dermatol Res 293:18–25

Tanese K, Grimm EA, Ekmekcioglu S (2012) The role of melanoma tumor-derived nitric oxide in the tumor inflammatory microenvironment: its impact on the chemokine expression profile, including suppression of CXCL10. Int J Cancer 131:891–901

Taniguchi K, Karin M (2014) IL-6 and related cytokines as the critical lynchpins between inflammation and cancer. Semin Immunol 26:54–74

Teunissen MB, Piskin G, di Nuzzo S, Sylva-Steenland RM, de Rie MA, Bos JD (2002) Ultraviolet B radiation induces a transient appearance of IL-4+ neutrophils, which support the development of Th2 responses. J Immunol 168:3732–3739

Thompson BC, Surjana D, Halliday GM, Damian DL (2014) Nicotinamide enhances repair of ultraviolet radiation-induced DNA damage in primary melanocytes. Exp Dermatol 23:509–511

Travers JB, Berry D, Yao Y, Yi Q, Konger RL, Travers JB (2010) Ultraviolet B radiation of human skin generates platelet-activating factor receptor agonists. Photochem Photobiol 86:949–954

Trifilieff A, Fujitani Y, Mentz F, Dugas B, Fuentes M, Bertrand C (2000) Inducible nitric oxide synthase inhibitors suppress airway inflammation in mice through down-regulation of chemokine expression. J Immunol 165:1526–1533

Uchida Y, Houben E, Park K, Douangpanya S, Lee YM, Wu BX et al (2010) Hydrolytic pathway protects against ceramide-induced apoptosis in keratinocytes exposed to UVB. J Invest Dermatol 130:2472–2480

Ungerstedt JS, Blömback M, Söderström T (2003) Nicotinamide is a potent inhibitor of proinflammatory cytokines. Clin Exp Immunol 131:48–52

Van Nguyen H, Di Girolamo N, Jackson N, Hampartzoumian T, Bullpitt P, Tedla N, Wakefield D (2011) Ultraviolet radiation-induced cytokines promote mast cell accumulation and matrix metalloproteinase production: potential role in cutaneous lupus erythematosus. Scand J Rheumatol 40:197–204

Vermeer M, Streilein JW (1990) Ultraviolet B light-induced alterations in epidermal Langerhans cells are mediated in part by tumor necrosis factor-alpha. Photodermatol Photoimmunol Photomed 7:258–265

Vincek V, Kurimoto I, Medema JP, Prieto E, Streilein JW (1993) Tumor necrosis factor alpha polymorphism correlates with deleterious effects of ultraviolet B light on cutaneous immunity. Cancer Res 53:728–732

Walterscheid JP, Ullrich SE, Nghiem DX (2002) Platelet-activating factor, a molecular sensor for cellular damage, activates systemic immune suppression. J Exp Med 195:171–179

Wang LF, Chien CY, Tai CF, Chiang FY, Chen JY (2015) Vitamin D decreases the secretion of eotaxin and RANTES in nasal polyp fibroblasts derived from Taiwanese patients with chronic rhinosinusitis with nasal polyps. Kaohsiung J Med Sci 31:63–69

Widyarini S, Domanski D, Painter N, Reeve VE (2006) Estrogen receptor signaling protects against immune suppression by UV radiation exposure. PNAS 103:12837–12842

Widyarini S, Domanski D, Painter N, Reeve VE (2012) Photoimmune protective effect of the phytoestrogenic isoflavonoid equol is partially due to its antioxidant activities. Photochem Photobiol Sci 11:1186–1192

Yasuoka H, Tsujimoto M, Yoshidome K, Nakahara M, Kodama R, Sanke T, Nakamura Y (2008) Cytoplasmic CXCR4 expression in breast cancer: induction by nitric oxide and correlation with lymph node metastasis and poor prognosis. BMC Cancer 8:340

Yiasemides E, Sivapirabu G, Halliday GM, Park J, Damian DL (2009) Oral nicotinamide protects against ultraviolet radiation-induced immunosuppression in humans. Carcinogenesis 30:101–105

Yoshikawa T, Kurimoto I, Streilein JW (1992) Tumour necrosis factor-alpha mediates ultraviolet light B-enhanced expression of contact hypersensitivity. Immunology 76:264–271

Yoshiki R, Kabashima K, Sakabe J, Sugita K, Bito T, Nakamura M et al (2010) The mandatory role of IL-10-producing and OX40 ligand-expressing mature Langerhans cells in local UVB-induced immunosuppression. J Immunol 184:5670–5677

Zabel BA, Rott A, Butcher EC (2015) Leukocyte chemoattractant receptors in human disease pathogenesis. Annu Rev Pathol 10:51–81

Zlotnik A (2006) Chemokines and cancer. Int J Cancer 119:2026–2029

Zlotnik A, Yoshie O (2012) The chemokine superfamily revisited. Immunity 36:705–716

Chapter 11
TLR3 and Inflammatory Skin Diseases: From Environmental Factors to Molecular Opportunities

Risa Tamagawa-Mineoka, Mayumi Ueta and Norito Katoh

Abstract Toll-like receptors (TLRs) are cellular sensors designed to recognize pathogens. TLR3 recognizes viral double-stranded RNA, which is a molecular pattern produced by most viruses. Interestingly, there is increasing recognition of the role of TLR3 in non-infectious inflammatory diseases as well as viral infections. In addition, TLR3 recognizes not only exogenous threats such as virus but also endogenous host molecules associated with tissue injury. TLR3 is expressed on various cell types including keratinocytes, Langerhans cells, mast cells, and fibroblasts in the skin. Recent findings show that upon stimulation of TLR3 with exogenous or endogenous ligands, these cells are closely involved in the pathogenesis of infectious or inflammatory skin diseases such as viral infections or allergic and irritant contact dermatitis. Furthermore, TLR3 signaling is associated with barrier repair after tissue injury and itching sensation in the skin. Therefore, TLR3 may serve as a new therapeutic target for inflammatory skin diseases.

Keywords Toll-like receptor 3 · Skin · Virus · Polyinosinic:polycytidylic acid · Barrier repair · Contact dermatitis · Stevens-Johnson syndrome · Toxic epidermal necrolysis · Itch

R. Tamagawa-Mineoka (✉) · N. Katoh
Department of Dermatology, Graduate School of Medical Science, Kyoto Prefectural University of Medicine, 465 Kajii-cho, Kawaramachi-hirokoji, Kamigyo-ku, Kyoto 602-8566, Japan
e-mail: risat@koto.kpu-m.ac.jp

M. Ueta
Frontier Medical Science and Technology for Ophthalmology, Graduate School of Medical Science, Kyoto Prefectural University of Medicine, Kyoto, Japan

G.T. Wondrak (ed.), *Skin Stress Response Pathways*,
DOI 10.1007/978-3-319-43157-4_11

11.1 Introduction

Toll-like receptors (TLRs) are pattern recognition receptors which play important roles in both innate and adaptive immune responses (Ishii and Akira 2008; Kawai and Akira 2011). At least 11 different TLRs have been identified and are expressed on both immune and non-immune cells. TLR signaling leads to the activation of nuclear factor κB, interferon-regulatory factor, and their target genes that induce the production of various antimicrobial and proinflammatory cytokines (Fig. 11.1).

Skin consists of a three-layer structure: the epidermis, dermis, and subcutaneous tissues. TLRs are expressed on various cell types in the skin (Fig. 11.2). The most important epidermal cells expressing TLRs include keratinocytes, which express TLRs 1-6, 9, and 10 (Baker et al. 2003; Ermertcan et al. 2011) and Langerhans

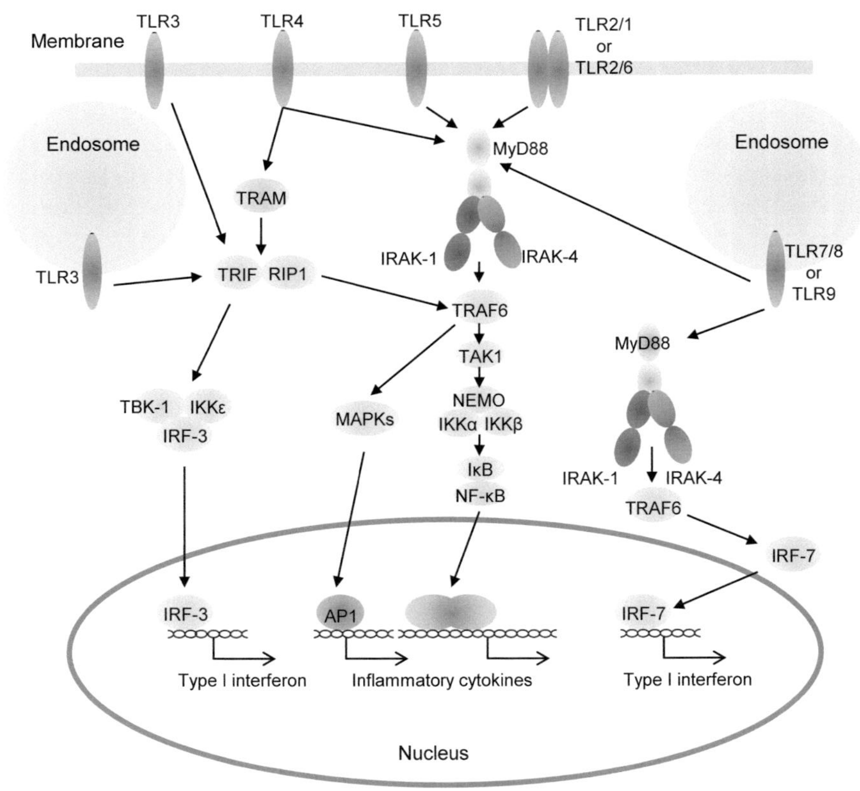

Fig. 11.1 TLR signaling pathway. Upon stimulation with ligands, TLR1, 2 and 4-9 recruit MyD88, IRAKs and TRAF6. And TLR signaling diverges at TRAF6 to two different pathways to produce inflammatory cytokines. TLR3 utilizes TRIF for the activation of the TRIF-dependent pathway to produce type I interferons and inflammatory cytokines

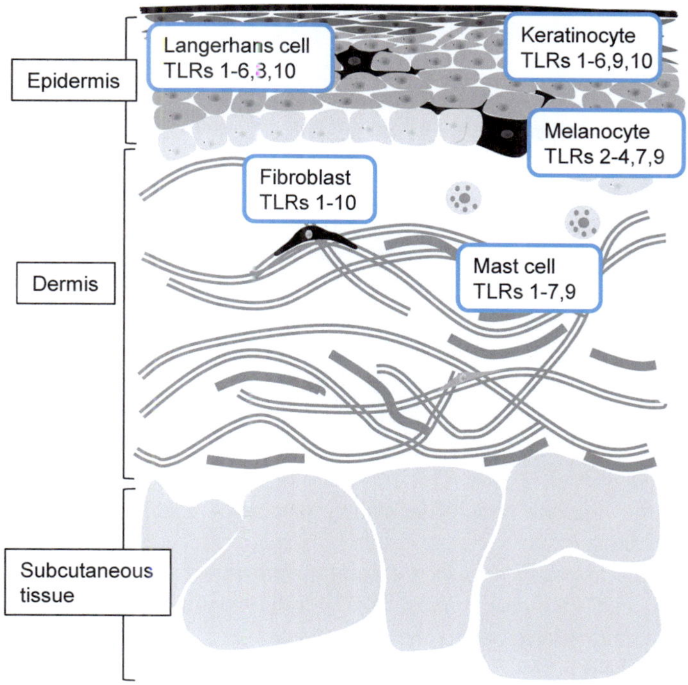

Fig. 11.2 TLR expression in the skin. Skin consists of a three-layer structure: the epidermis, dermis, and subcutaneous tissues. TLRs are expressed on several cell types including keratinocytes, Langerhans cells, melanocytes, mast cells, and fibroblasts in the skin

cells, which express TLRs 1-6, 8, and 10 (Renn et al. 2006; Ermertcan et al. 2011). In the dermis, resident cells such as mast cells and fibroblasts also express TLRs (Jang et al. 2012; Taves and Ji 2015).

TLR3 recognizes viral double-stranded RNA and polyinosinic:polycytidylic acid (Poly(I:C)), a mimic of viral double-stranded RNA, which is a molecular pattern produced by most viruses (Ishii and Akira 2008; Kawai and Akira 2011). It is reported that epithelial cells such as ocular surface (cornea and conjunctiva) epithelial cells (Ueta et al. 2005) and retinal pigment epithelial cells (Kleinman et al. 2008) expressed TLR3 on their cell surface and that among TLRs 1-10, TLR3 is the most intensely expressed TLR ocular surface epithelial cells (Ueta et al. 2005). Interestingly, there is increasing recognition of the role of TLR3 in non-infectious inflammatory skin diseases as well as viral infections. The aim of this chapter is to review the involvement of TLR3 signaling in the pathogenesis of skin infectious and inflammatory skin diseases.

11.2 Skin Infectious Diseases

The skin directly contacts with the outside environment, therefore, it has numerous opportunities to interact with various pathogens such as virus. TLR3 has an important role in immune responses to commonly encountered viral infections in various organs including the skin. Verruca vulgaris and molluscum contagiosum are common viral skin infectious diseases (Lowy and Androphy 2003a, b). Verruca is a benign proliferation of the skin that results from infection with human papilloma virus. A subset of human papilloma virus has been associated with the development of epithelial malignancies (Lowy and Androphy 2003a, b). On the other hand, molluscum contagiosum is a wart that forms as a result of infection by molluscum contagiosum virus (Lowy and Androphy 2003a, b). In the skin lesions of both diseases, epidermal TLR3 expression is greatly elevated with increased expression of interferon-β and tumor necrosis factor-α, compared with that of normal skin (Ku et al. 2008). This finding suggests that TLR3 signaling is associated with the immune and inflammatory responses against such common viral infections in the skin.

Herpes virus infection is also a common viral infection of the skin. In herpes simplex virus (HSV)-1 encephalitis, HSV-1 infects epithelial cells in the oral and nasal mucosa and progresses to the central nervous system via the trigeminal or olfactory nerves (Whitley 2006). It has been reported that patients deficient in TLR3 increase spreading of HSV-1 infection from keratinocytes to cranial nerves (Zhang et al. 2007; Mørk et al. 2015). In addition, there are mutations in the TLR3 signaling pathway including IRF3 and TRIF molecules in patients with herpes simplex encephalitis (Andersen et al. 2015; Mørk et al. 2015). These findings suggest that TLR3 signaling is closely related to suppression of expanding HSV infection.

11.3 Allergic and Irritant Contact Dermatitis

Allergic contact dermatitis (ACD) is a common allergic inflammatory skin disease characterized by pruritic eczematous lesions, and depends on the delay-type hypersensitivity reaction. The contact hypersensitivity response consists of two phases: sensitization and elicitation. In the sensitization phase of ACD, cutaneous dendritic cells ingest antigens that have penetrated into the skin, migrate to draining lymph nodes, and then present the antigens to naïve T cells. This process leads to the clonal expansion of antigen-specific T cells that can be recruited to the skin. It has been demonstrated that the sensitization process of the contact hypersensitivity response is not impaired in TLR3-deficient mice (Nakamura et al. 2015). Although dendritic cells and lymphocytes, which play a key role in the sensitization process, express TLR3 (Applequist et al. 2002), lack of TLR3 hardly affects the maturation, migration and antigen presentation of dendritic cells and proliferation of lymphocytes (Nakamura et al. 2015). These findings suggest that TLR3 signaling may not be closely related to the sensitization process of the contact hypersensitivity response.

The inflammatory responses in the elicitation phase of the contact hypersensitivity response depend on both antigen-dependent and -independent mechanisms (Grabbe and Schwarz 1998; Honda et al. 2013). Upon reexposure to haptens, antigen-specific T cells are stimulated by cutaneous antigen-presenting cells, secrete a variety of mediators, and induce activation of several cell types in the skin. On the other hand, keratinocytes are stimulated directly with haptens in an antigen-nonspecific manner, and then release numerous mediators such as cytokines and chemokines (Sebastiani et al. 2002; Honda et al. 2013). These reactions also affect each other, leading to increase of the inflammatory responses. It has been shown that the inflammatory responses in the elicitation phase of ACD are reduced in TLR3-deficient mice (Nakamura et al. 2015). In addition, this phenomenon is accompanied by decreased release of cytokines such as tumor necrosis factor-α, interleukin (IL)-1α and IL-1β and chemokines such as interferon-γ-inducible protein 10 (IP-10) and regulated on activation, normally T-cell expressed and secreted (RANTES) in the inflamed skin (Nakamura et al. 2015), that play a crucial role in the elicitation phase of ACD (Dufour et al. 2002; Watanabe et al. 2007; Canavese et al. 2010). Furthermore, the cytokines and chemokines including IP-10 and RANTES, which are important for inflammatory responses, are secreted from epithelial cells and fibroblasts by stimulation with a exogenous TLR3 ligand, poly (I:C) (Ueta et al. 2005, 2009, 2010; Kato et al. 2007; Farina et al. 2010). It has been demonstrated that no significant difference of the function of dendritic cells and lymphocytes between TLR3-deficient and wild-type mice (Nakamura et al. 2015). Taken together, these findings suggest that TLR3 signaling may be involved in the elicitation phase of ACD via release of cytokines and chemokines from keratinocytes and fibroblasts (Fig. 11.3).

In contrast to ACD, irritant contact dermatitis is caused by the direct action of chemical agents and shows non-antigen-specific cutaneous responses (Corsini and Galli 1998). The irritant contact dermatitis reaction following application of irritant agents is markedly decreased in TLR3-deficient mice, and is increased inTLR3-transgenic mice, compared with that in wild-type mice (Nakamura et al. 2015). These findings indicate that TLR3 signaling is related to non-antigen-specific cutaneous inflammation.

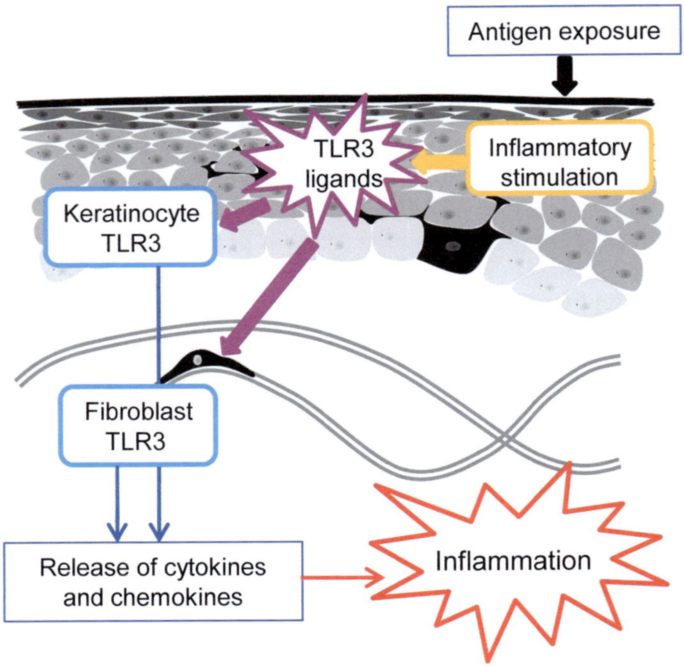

Fig. 11.3 Possible roles of TLR3 in skin inflammation. Skin resident cells such as keratinocytes release endogenous host molecules including RNA following inflammatory stimulation. Subsequently, activation of TLR3 via endogenous ligands induces release of cytokines and chemokines, leading to the development of skin inflammation

11.4 Endogenous TLR3 Ligands

TLRs recognize not only exogenous threats such as the bacteria and virus but also endogenous danger signals associated with cell necrosis and tissue damage (Table 11.1) (Seong and Matzinger 2004; Tsan and Gao 2004; Taves and Ji 2015). The skin suffers from outside hazards such as pathogenic microorganisms, mechanical insults, toxic chemicals, and ultraviolet irradiation, leading to tissue injury. In previous electron microscopic studies, necrosis of epidermal keratinocytes and Langerhans cells has been shown to be seen in inflammatory skin diseases such as allergic and irritant contact dermatitis (Willis et al. 1986, 1989). Therefore, endogenous host molecules may release from cells damaged during the inflammatory process in cutaneous diseases.

TLR3 could regulate allergic inflammation such as allergic conjunctivitis and allergic contact dermatitis in the absence of an exogenous viral infection or TLR3 ligand (Ueta et al. 2009; Nakamura et al. 2015). It is reported that in the absence of viral infection the TLR3 can amplify immune responses during acute inflammatory processes, which may involve stimulation of TLR3 by endogenous RNA from

Table 11.1 TLR ligands

TLR	Exogenous ligands	Endogenous ligands	References
TLR1/TLR2	Tri-acyl lipopeptides (bacteria)	Unknown	Takeuchi et al. (2002)
TLR2/TLR6	Lipoprotein/lipopeptides (various pathogens) Lipoteichoic acid (bacteria) Zymosan (fungi)	Heat shock proteins (HsP60, HsP70, Gp96) High mobility group box 1 protein (HMGB1)	Vabulas et al. (2001, (2002a, b), Asea et al. (2002), Park et al. (2004), Kawai and Akira (2011)
TLR3	Double-strand RNA (virus) Poly (I:C) (synthetic)	mRNA	Alexopoulou et al. (2001), Karikó et al. (2004)
TLR4	Lipopolysaccharide (gram-negative bacteria)	Heat shock proteins (HsP60, HsP70, Gp96) Fibrinogen Surfactant protein-A Fibronectin extra domain A HMGB1 Heparin sulfate Soluble hyaluronan β-defensin 2	Poltorak et al. (1998), Shimazu et al. (1999), Ohashi et al. (2000), Okamura et al. (2001), Smiley et al. (2001), Vabulas et al. (2001, 2002a, b), Asea et al. (2002), Biragyn et al. (2002), Bulut et al. (2002), Dybdahl et al. (2002), Guillot et al. (2002), Johnson et al. (2002), Termeer et al. (2002), Park et al. (2004), Kawai and Akira (2011)
TLR5	Flagellin (bacteria)	Unknown	Hayashi et al. (2001)
TLR7	Single-stranded RNA (virus) Imiquimod (synthetic) Resiquimod (R848) (synthetic) PolyURNA (synthetic)	Self-RNA MicroRNA	Diebold et al. (2004), Heil et al. (2004), Kawai and Akira (2011)
TLR8	Single-stranded RNA (virus) Resiquimod (R848) (Synthetic)	Self-RNA MicroRNA	Heil et al. (2004), Kawai and Akira (2011)
TLR9	CpG DNA (bacteria, virus) Hemozoin (plasmodium)	Self-DNA	Kawai and Akira (2011)
TLR10	Unknown	Unknown	
TLR11	Profilin-like protein (toxoplasma, bacteria)	Unknown	Yarovinsky et al. (2005)

necrotic cells (Cavassani et al. 2008). It is also possible that endogenous RNA from tissue or cells might stimulate TLR3 in allergic inflammation.

It has been shown that RNA released from necrotic cells such as damaged keratinocytes (Lai et al. 2009; Zhang et al. 2011; Bernard et al. 2012) and neutrophils (Cavassani et al. 2008) acts as a ligand for TLR3 in several cell types such as keratinocytes (Karikó et al. 2004; Cavassani et al. 2008; Lai et al. 2009; Zhang et al. 2011; Bernard et al. 2012). In addition, it has been demonstrated that ultraviolet-damaged self RNAs or ultraviolet-damaged keratinocytes are detected by TLR3 (Bernard et al. 2012). Furthermore, ultraviolet B irradiation increases cytokine production in the skin and affects the cutaneous inflammatory responses in a TLR3-dependent manner. These findings suggest that RNA released from cells damaged in inflammation can activate TLR3 on various cell types in the skin, leading to the development of non-infectious cutaneous inflammation.

11.5 Skin Barrier Repair

TLR3 signaling is involved in barrier repair after skin injury. Activation of TLR3 by endogenous ligands such as noncoding double-stranded RNA increases the expression of various key genes that are associated with permeability repair, including the ATP-binding cassette subfamily A, member 12 (ABCA12), glucocerebrosidase, acid sphingomyelinase, serine palmitoyltransferase, glucosylceramide synthase, and transglutaminase 1 (Borkowski et al. 2013). In addition, activation of TLR3 increases the number of lamellar bodies and keratohyalin granules in keratinocytes, which contain important molecules such as profilaggrin in the formation of skin barrier (Borkowski et al. 2013). It has been also demonstrated that the ability of mice to repair the skin barrier after ultraviolet B irradiation is delayed in TLR3-deficient mice (Borkowski et al. 2014). Furthermore, the products of ultraviolet B-damaged keratinocytes increase the expression of ABCA12, glucocerebrosidase, acid sphingomyelinase, and transglutaminase 1 (Borkowski et al. 2014). These findings suggest that TLR3 signaling via endogenous ligands such as double-stranded RNA is required for skin barrier repair after skin injury.

11.6 Itching

Itching is a sensation that provokes a desire to scratch, and is the main symptom of several skin inflammatory diseases, such as atopic dermatitis, contact dermatitis, and xerosis. Patients with these diseases often scratch their skin due to severe itching. Itch-scratch cycles result in further skin damage that exacerbates the symptoms. Itching signals are transmitted from the periphery to the brain via the dorsal horn by primary sensory neurons and spinothalamic tract neurons.

In the periphery, skin resident cells such as keratinocytes and mast cells can release numerous mediators including nerve growth factor (NGF), histamine, serotonin (5-hydroxytryptamine), and proteinase, which trigger itch sensation (Kuraishi 2013). Keratinocytes and mast cells are the main sources of NGF (Ikoma et al. 2006). In a dry skin-induced itch mouse model, the expression of NGF is elevated in the skin, followed by increased intradermal nerve fibers (Tominaga et al. 2007). Interestingly, lack of TLR3 inhibits the increase of NGF expression and scratching behaviors in dry skin (Liu et al. 2012). Epithelium-derived cytokine, thymic stromal lymphopoietin (TSLP), which is deeply involved in the development of inflammatory responses in atopic dermatitis (Kabashima 2013), act directly on a subset of primary sensory neurons and induce itch sensation (Wilson et al. 2013). Because activation of TLR3 induces the release of TSLP from epithelial cells (Ueta et al. 2009), TSLP secreted from keratinocytes may not only promotes inflammatory responses but also activates primary sensory neurons via TLR3 signaling in the lesions of atopic dermatitis. Taken together, these findings suggest that skin resident cells such as keratinocytes may release several mediators such as NGF and TSLP via TLR3 signaling and contribute to the itch signaling pathway in the periphery (Fig. 11.4).

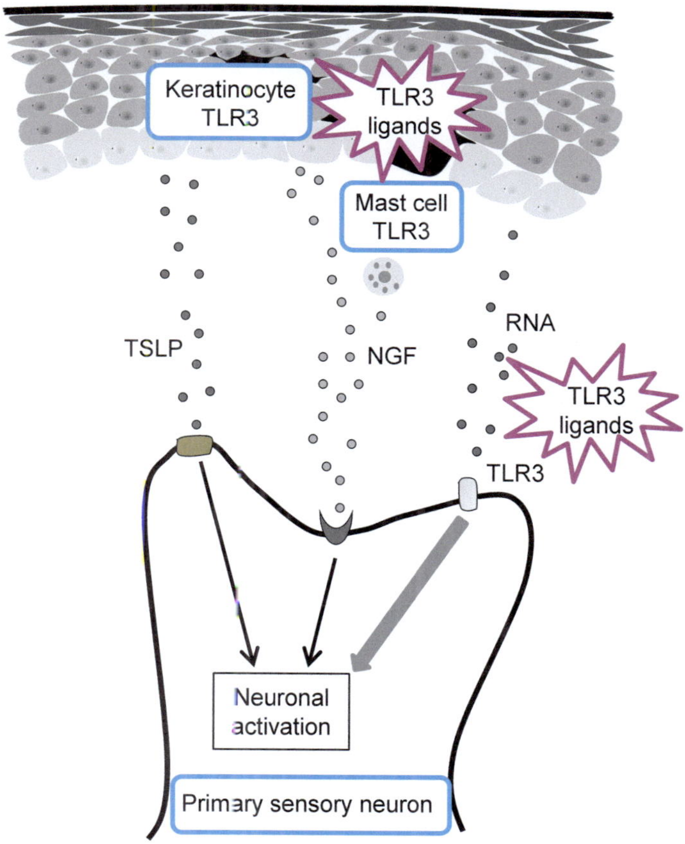

Fig. 11.4 Possible roles of TLR3 in itching signals. In the periphery, skin resident cells such as keratinocytes and mast cells secrete various mediators such as NGF and TSLP, which can trigger itch sensation, in a TLR3-dependent manner. In addition, activation of TLR3 in primary sensory neurons can affect itching signals

Itch signals in the dorsal horn are also important for pruritus. TLRs such as TLR3, TLR4, and TLR7 are expressed in sensory neurons in dorsal root and trigeminal ganglions (Wadachi and Hargreaves 2006; Diogenes et al. 2011; Liu et al. 2010, 2012). TLR3 is expressed mostly by small-sized primary sensory neurons in dorsal root ganglions that express transient receptor potential subtype V1 and gastrin-releasing peptide. It has been demonstrated that lack of TLR3 suppresses histamine-dependent itching induced by intradermal injection of compound 48/80, via histamine release from mast cells. In addition, administration of histamine-independent pruritogens also reduces scratching behaviors in TLR3-deficient mice (Liu et al. 2012). These findings suggest TLR3 in primary sensory neurons is involved in itching signals (Fig. 11.4). Therefore, TLR3 may serve as a new therapeutic target for pruritus.

11.7 Stevens-Johnson Syndrome (SJS)/Toxic Epidermal Necrolysis (TEN)

SJS and TEN are severe, acute multisystem inflammatory diseases of the skin and mucous membranes. These disorders are characterized by rapidly expanding, irregular macules and involvement of more than one mucosal site (oral, conjunctival, and anogenital), and are closely related, differing only in the extent of body surface area involved (Fritsch and Ruiz-Maldonado 2003). Both are closely related to infectious agents and/or drugs. Although the pathophysiological mechanisms of SJS/TEN is not fully established, previous findings have suggested that genetic and environmental factors including the human leukocyte antigen haplotype are associated with the onset of SJS/TEN (Fritsch and Ruiz-Maldonado 2003).

Interestingly, the association between the onset of SJS/TEN with severe ocular complications (SOC) and TLR3 signaling has been reported (Ueta et al. 2007, 2012). It is also reported that about 80 % of the Japanese SJS/TEN with SOC patients have developed SJS/TEN within several days after treatment for the common cold (Ueta et al. 2014) and that focusing on the cold medicine related (CM-) SJS/TEN with SOC, the significant association with TLR3 remains (Ueta et al. 2015). Interestingly, EP3, one of the receptors for PGE_2, SNPs also significantly associated with CM-SJS/TEN with SOC (Ueta et al. 2015) and PGE_2 acts at EP3 and negative regulates mucocutaneous inflammation induced by TLR3 (Ueta et al. 2012). Moreover, cold medicine such as NSAIDs (e.g., ibuprofen and loxoprofen) and cold medicine ingredients (e.g., acetaminophen) have the suppressive effect of the production of prostanoid, including PGE_2.

Therefore, the pathogenesis of CM-SJS/TEN with SOC may be possibly associated with the innate immune system including TLR3 signaling.

References

Alexopoulou L, Holt AC, Medzhitov R, Flavell RA (2001) Recognition of double-stranded RNA and activation of NF-kappaB by Toll-like receptor 3. Nature 413:732–738

Andersen LL, Mørk N, Reinert LS, Kofod-Olsen E, Narita R, Jørgensen SE, Skipper KA, Höning K, Gad HH, Østergaard L, Ørntoft TF, Hornung V, Paludan SR, Mikkelsen JG, Fujita T, Christiansen M, Hartmann R, Mogensen TH (2015) Functional IRF3 deficiency in a patient with herpes simplex encephalitis. J Exp Med 212:1371–1379

Applequist SE, Wallin RPA, Ljunggren HG (2002) Variable expression of toll-like receptor in murine innate and adaptive immune cell lines. Int Immunol 14:1065–1074

Asea A, Rehli M, Kabingu E, Boch JA, Bare O, Auron PE, Stevenson MA, Calderwood SK (2002) Novel signal transduction pathway utilized by extracellular hsp 70: role of toll-like receptor (TLR)2 and TLR4. J Biol Chem 277:15028–15034

Baker BS, Ovigne JM, Powles AV, Corcoran S, Fry L (2003) Normal keratinocytes express toll-like receptors (TLRs) 1, 2 and 5: modulation of TLR expression in chronic plaque psoriasis. Br J Dermatol 148:670–679

Bernard JJ, Cowing-Zitron C, Nakatsuji T, Muehleisen B, Muto J, Borkowski AW, Martinez L, Greidinger EL, Yu BD, Gallo RL (2012) Ultraviolet radiation damages self noncoding RNA and is detected by TLR3. Nat Med 18:1286–1290

Biragyn A, Ruffini PA, Leifer CA, Klyushnenkova E, Shakhov A, Chertov O, Shirakawa AK, Farber JM, Segal DM, Oppenheim JJ, Kwak LW (2002) Toll-like receptor 4-dependent activation of dendritic cells by β-defensin 2. Science 298:1025–1029

Borkowski AW, Park K, Ucida Y, Gallo RL (2013) Activation of TLR3 in keratinocytes increases expression of genes involved in formation of the epidermis, lipid accumulation, and epidermal organelles. J Invest Dermatol 133:2031–2040

Borkowski AW, Kuo IH, Bernard JJ, Yoshida T, Williams MR, Hung NJ, Yu BD, Beck LA, Gallo RL (2014) Toll-like receptor 3 activation is required for normal skin barrier repair following UV damage. J Invest Dermatol 135:569–578

Bulut Y, Faure E, Thomas L, Karahashi H, Michelsen KS, Equils O, Morrison SG, Morrison RP, Arditi M (2002) Chlamydial heat shock protein 60 activates macrophages and endothelial cells through toll-like receptor 4 and MD2 in a My D88-dependent pathway. J Immunol 162:3212–3219

Canavese M, Altruda F, Silengo L (2010) Therapeutic efficacy and immunological response of CCL5 antagonists in models of contact skin reaction. PLoS ONE 5:e8725

Cavassani KA, Ishii M, Wen H, Schaller MA, Lincoln PM, Lukacs NW, Hogaboam CM, Kunkel SL (2008) TLR3 is an endogenous sensor of tissue necrosis during acute inflammatory events. J Exp Med 205:2609–2621

Corsini E, Galli CL (1998) Cytokines and irritant contact dermatitis. Toxicol Lett 102–3:277–282

Diebold SS, Kaisho T, Hemmi H, Akira S, Reis e Sousa C (2004) Innate antiviral responses by means of TLR7-mediated recognition of single-stranded RNA. Science 303:1529–1531

Diogenes A, Ferraz CC, Akopian AN, Henry MA, Hargreaves KM (2011) LPS sensitizes TRPV1 via activation of TLR4 in trigeminal sensory neurons. J Dent Res 90(6):759–764

Dufour JH, Dziejman M, Liu MT, Leung JH, Lane TE, Luster AD (2002) IFN-gamma-inducible protein 10 (IP-10; CXCL10)-deficient mice reveal a role for IP-10 in effector T cell generation and trafficking. J Immunol 168:3195–3204

Dybdahl B, Wahba A, Lien E, Flo TH, Waage A, Qureshi N, Sellevold OF, Espevik T, Sundan A (2002) Inflammatory response after open heart surgery: release of heat-shock protein 70 and signaling through toll-like receptor-4. Circulation 105:685–690

Ermertcan AT, Öztürk F, Gündüz K (2011) Toll-like receptors and skin. J Eur Acad Dermatol Venereol 25:997–1006

Farina GA, York MR, Di Marzio M, Collins CA, Meller S, Homey B, Rifkin IR, Marshak-Rothstein A, Radstake TR, Lafyatis R (2010) Poly(I:C) drives type I IFN- and TGFβ-mediated inflammation and dermal fibrosis simulating altered gene expression in systemic sclerosis. J Invest Dermatol 130:2583–2593

Fritsch PO, Ruiz-Maldonado R (2003) Erythema multiforme, Stevens-Johnson syndrome, and toxic epidermal necrolysis. In: Freedberg IM, Eisen AZ, Wolff K, Austen KF, Goldsmith LA, Katz SI (eds) Fitzpatrick's dermatology in general medicine, 6th edn. McGraw-hill, New York, pp 543–557

Grabbe S, Schwart T (1998) Immunoregulatory mechanism involved in elicitation of allergic contact hypersensitivity. Immunol Today 19:37–44

Guillot L, Balloy V, McCormack FX, Golenbock DT, Chignard M, Si-Tahar M (2002) Cutting edge: the immunostimulatory activity of the lung surfactant protein-A involves toll-like receptor 4. J Immunol 168:5989–5992

Hayashi F, Smith KD, Ozinsky A, Hawn TR, Yi EC, Goodlett DR, Eng JK, Akira S, Underhill DM, Aderem A (2001) The innate immune response to bacterial flagellin is mediated by toll-like receptor 5. Nature 410:1099–1103

Heil F, Hemmi H, Hochrein H, Ampenberger F, Kirschning C, Akira S, Lipford G, Wagner H, Bauer S (2004) Species-specific recognition of single-stranded RNA via toll-like receptor 7 and 8. Science 303:1526–1529

Honda T, Egawa G, Grabbe S, Kabashima K (2013) Update of immune events in the murine contact hypersensitivity model: toward the understanding of allergic contact dermatitis. J Invest Dermatol 133:303–315

Ikoma A, Steinhoff M, Stander S, Yosipovitch G, Schmelz M (2006) The neurobiology of itch. Nat Rev Neurosci 7:535–547

Ishii KJ, Akira S (2008) Innate immunity. In: Rich RR, Fleisher TA, Shearer WT, Schroeder HW Jr, Frew AJ, Weyand CM (eds) Clinical immunology principles and practice, 3rd edn. Elsevier Ltd, Philadelphia, pp 39–51

Jang S, Park JS, Won YH, Yun SJ, Kim SJ (2012) The expression of toll-like receptors (TLRs) in cultured human skin fibroblast in modulated by histamine. Chonnam Med J 48:7–14

Johnson GB, Brunn GJ, Kodaira Y, Platt JL (2002) Receptor-mediated monitoring of tissue well-being via detection of soluble heparin sulfate by toll-like receptor 4. J Immunol 168:5233–5239

Kabashima K (2013) New concept of the pathogenesis of atopic dermatitis: interplay among the barrier, allergy and pruritus as a trinity. J Dermatol Sci 70:3–11

Karikó K, Ni H, Capodici J, Lamphier M, Weissman D (2004) mRNA is an endogenous ligand for toll-like receptor 3. J Biol Chem 279:12542–12550

Kato A, Favoreto S Jr, Avila PC, Schleimer RP (2007) TLR3- and Th2 cytokine-dependent production of thymic stromal lymphopoietin in human airway epithelial cells. J Immunol 179:1080–1087

Kawai T, Akira S (2011) Toll-like receptor and their crosstalk with other innate receptors in infection and immunity. Immunity 34:637–650

Kleinman ME, Yamada K, Takeda A, Chandrasekaran V, Nozaki M, Baffi JZ, Albuquerque RJC, Yamasaki S, Itaya M, Pan Y, Appukuttan B, Gibbs D, Yang Z, Karikó K, Ambati BK, Wilgus TA, DiPietro LA, Sakurai E, Zhang K, Smith JR, Taylor EW, Ambati J (2008) Sequence- and target-independent angiogenesis suppression by siRNA via TLR3. Nature 452:591–597

Ku JK, Kwon HJ, Kim MY, Kang H, Song PI, Armstrong CA, Ansel JC, Kim HO, Park YM (2008) Expression of Toll-like receptors in verruca and molluscum contagiosum. J Korean Med Sci 23(2):307–314

Kuraishi Y (2013) Potential new therapeutic targets for pathological pruritus. Biol Pharm Bull 36:1228–1234

Lai Y, Di Nardo A, Nakatsuji T, Leichtle A, Yang Y, Cogen AL, Wu ZR, Hooper LV, Schmidt RR, von Aulock S, Radek KA, Huang CM, Ryan AF, Gallo RL (2009) Commensal bacteria regulate Toll-like receptor 3-dependent inflammation after skin injury. Nat Med 15:1377–1382

Liu T, Xu ZZ, Park CK, Berta T, Ji RR (2010) Toll-like receptor 7 mediates pruritus. Nat Neurosci 13:1460–1462

Liu T, Berta T, Xu ZZ, Park CK, Zhang L, Lü N, Liu Q, Liu Y, Gao YJ, Liu YC, Ma Q, Dong X, Ji RR (2012) TLR3 deficiency impairs spinal cord synaptic transmission, central sensitization, and pruritus in mice. J Clin Invest 122:2195–2207

Lowy DR, Androphy EJ (2003a) Molluscum Contagiosum. In: Freedberg IM, Eisen AZ, Wolff K, Austen KF, Goldsmith LA, Katz SI (eds) Fitzpatrick's dermatology in general medicine, 6th edn. McGraw-hill, New York, pp 2114–2116

Lowy DR, Androphy EJ (2003b) Warts. In: Freedberg IM, Eisen AZ, Wolff K, Austen KF, Goldsmith LA, Katz SI (eds) Fitzpatrick's dermatology in general medicine, 6th edn. McGraw-hill, New York, pp 2119–2130

Mørk N, Kofod-Olsen E, Sørensen KB, Bach E, Ørntoft TF, Østergaard L, Paludan SR, Christiansen M, Mogensen TH (2015) Mutations in the TLR3 signaling pathway and beyond in adult patients with herpes simplex encephalitis. Genes Immun 16:552–566

Nakamura N, Tamagawa-Mineoka R, Ueta M, Kinoshita S, Katoh N (2015) Toll-like receptor 3 increases allergic and irritant contact dermatitis. J Invest Dermatol 135:411–418

Ohashi K, Burkart V, Flohé S, Kolb H (2000) Cutting edge: heat shock protein 60 is a putative endogenous ligand of the toll-like receptor-4 complex. J Immunol 164:558–561

Okamura Y, Watari M, Jerud ES, Young DW, Ishizaka S, Rose J, Chow JC, Strauss JF III (2001) The extra domain A of fibronectin activates toll-like receptor 4. J Biol Chem 276:10229–10233

Park JS, Svetkauskaite D, He Q, Kim JY, Strassheim D, Ishizaka A, Abraham E (2004) Involvement of toll-like receptors 2 and 4 in cellular activation by high mobility group box 1 protein. J Biol Chem 279:7370–7377

Poltorak A, He X, Smirnova I, Liu MY, Van Huffel C, Du X, Birdwell D, Alejos E, Silva M, Galanos C, Freudenberg M, Ricciardi-Castagnoli P, Layton B, Beutler B (1998) Defective LPS signaling in C3H/HeJ and C57BL/10ScCr mice: mutations in Tlr4 gene. Science 282:2085–2088

Renn CN, Sanchez DJ, Ochoa MT, Legaspi AJ, Oh CK, Liu PT, Krutzik SR, Sieling PA, Cheng G, Modlin RL (2006) TLR activation of Langerhans cell-like dendritic cells triggers an antiviral immune response. J Immunol 177:298–305

Sebastiani S, Albanesi C, De PO, Puddu P, Cavani A, Girolomoni G (2002) The role of chemokines in allergic contact dermatitis. Arch Dermatol Res 293:552–559

Seong SY, Matzinger P (2004) Hydrophobicity: an ancient damage-associated molecular pattern that initiates innate immune responses. Nat Rev Immunol 4:469–478

Shimazu R, Akashi S, Ogata H, Nagai Y, Fukudome K, Miyake K, Kimoto M (1999) MD-2, a molecule that confers lipopolysaccharide responsiveness on toll-like receptor 4. J Exp Med 189:1777–1782

Smiley ST, King JA, Hancock WW (2001) Fibrinogen stimulates macrophage chemokine secretion through toll-like receptor 4. J Immunol 167:2887–2894

Takeuchi O, Sato S, Horiuchi T, Hoshino K, Takeda K, Dong Z, Modlin RL, Akira S (2002) Cutting edge: role of toll-like receptor 1 in mediating immune response to microbial lipoproteins. J Immunol 169:10–14

Taves S, Ji RR (2015) Itch control by toll-like receptors. Handb Exp Pharmacol 226:135–150

Termeer C, Benedix F, Sleeman J, Fieber C, Voith U, Ahrens T, Miyake K, Freudenberg M, Galanos C, Simon JC (2002) Oligosaccharides of hyaluronan activate dendritic cells via toll-like receptor 4. J Exp Med 195:99–111

Tominaga M, Ozawa S, Tengara S, Ogawa H, Takamori K (2007) Intraepidermal nerve fibers increase in dry skin of acetone-treated mice. J Dermatol Sci 48(2):103–111

Tsan MF, Gao B (2004) Endogenous ligands of toll-like receptors. J Leukoc Biol 76:514–523

Ueta M, Hamuro J, Kiyono H, Kinoshita S (2005) Triggering of TLR3 by polyI: C in human corneal epithelial cells to induce inflammatory cytokines. Biochem Biophys Res Commun 331:285–294

Ueta M, Sotozono C, Inatomi T, Kojima K, Tashiro K, Hamuro J, Kinoshita S (2007) Toll-like receptor 3 gene polymorphisms in Japanese patients with Stevens-Johnson syndrome. Br J Ophthalmol 91:962–965

Ueta M, Uematsu S, Akira S, Kinoshita S (2009) Toll-like receptor 3 enhances late-phase reaction of experimental allergic conjunctivitis. J Allergy Clin Immunol 123:1187–1189

Ueta M, Mizushima K, Yokoi N, Naito Y, Kinoshita S (2010) Gene-expression analysis of polyI: C-stimulated primary human conjunctival epithelial cells. Br J Ophthalmol 94:1528–1532

Ueta M, Tamiya G, Tokunaga K, Sotozono C, Ueki M, Sawai H, Inatomi T, Matsuoka T, Akira S, Narumiya S, Tashiro K, Kinoshita S (2012) Epistatic interaction between toll-like recep-tor 3 (TLR3) and prostaglandin E receptor 3 (PTGER3) genes. J Allergy Clin Immunol 129:1413–1416

Ueta M, Kaniwa N, Sotozonol C, Tokunaga K, Saito Y, Sawai H, Miyadera H, Sugiyama E, Maekawa K, Nakamura R, Nagato M, Aihara M, Matsunaga K, Takahashi Y, Furuya H, Muramatsu M, Ikezawa Z, Kinoshital S (2014) Independent strong association of HLA-A*02:06 and HLA-B*44:03 with cold medicine-related Stevens-Johnson syndrome with severe mucosal involvement. Sci Rep 30:4862

Ueta M, Tokunaga K, Sotozono C, Sawai H, Yoon KC, Kim MK, Seo KY, Joo CK, Tashiro K (2015) Kinoshita S (2015) HLA-A*02:06 and PTGER3 polymorphism exert additive effects in cold medicine-related Stevens-Johnson syndrome with severe ocular complications. Hum Genome Var 2:15023

Vabulas RM, Ahmad-Nejad P, da Costa C, Miethke T, Kirschning CJ, Häcker H, Wagner H (2001) Endocytosed HSP60 s use toll-like receptor 2 (TLR2) and TLR4 to activate the toll/interleukin-1 receptor signaling pathway in innate immune cells. J Biol Chem 276:31332–31339

Vabulas RM, Ahmad- Nejad P, Ghose S, Kirschning CJ, Issels RD, Wagner H (2002a) Hsp70 as endogenous stimulus of the toll/interleukin-1 receptor signal pathway. J Biol Chem 277:15107–15112

Vabulas RM, Braedel S, Hilf N, Singh-Jasuja H, Herter S, Ahmad-Nejad P, Kirschning CJ, Da Costa C, Rammensee HG, Wagner H, Schild HA (2002b) The endoplasmic reticulum-resident heat shock protein Gp96 activates dendritic cells via the toll-like receptor 2/4 pathway. J Biol Chem 277:20847–20853

Wadachi R, Hargreaves KM (2006) Trigeminal nociceptors express TLR-4 and CD14: a mechanism for pain due to infection. J Dent Res 85(1):49–53

Watanabe H, Gaide O, Pétrilli V, Martinon F, Contassot E, Roques S, Kummer JA, Tschopp J, French LE (2007) Activation of IL-1β-processing inflammasome is involved in contact hypersensitivity. J Invest Dermatol 127:1956–1963

Whitley RJ (2006) Herpes simplex encephalitis: adolescents and adults. Antiviral Res 71:141–148

Willis CM, Young E, Brandon DR, Wilkinson JD (1986) Immunopathological and ultrastructural findings in human allergic and irritant contact dermatitis. Br J Dermatol 115:305–316

Willis CM, Stephens CJM, Wilkinson JD (1989) Epidermal damage induced by irritants in man. A light and electron microscopy study. J Invest Dermatol 93:695–700

Wilson SR, Thé L, Batia LM, Beattie K, Katibah GE, McClain SP, Pellegrino M, Estandian DM, Bautista DM (2013) The epithelial cell-derived atopic dermatitis cytokine TSLP activates neurons to induce itch. Cell 155:285–295

Yarovinsky F, Zhang D, Andersen JF, Bannenberg GL, Serhan CN, Hayden MS, Hieny S, Sutterwala FS, Flavell RA, Ghosh S, Sher A (2005) TLR11 activation of dendritic cells by a protozoan profilin-like protein. Science 308:1626–1629

Zhang S, Liu S, Yu N, Xiang L (2011) RNA released from necrotic keratinocytes upregulates intercellular adhesion molecule-1 expression in melanocytes. Arch Dermatol Res 303:771–776

Zhang SY, Jouanguy E, Ugolini S, Smahi A, Elain G, Romero P, Segal D, Sancho-Shimizu V, Lorenzo L, Puel A, Picard C, Chapgier A, Plancoulaine S, Titeux M, Cognet C, von Bernuth H, Ku CL, Casrouge A, Zhang XX, Barreiro L, Leonard J, Hamilton C, Lebon P, Héron B, Vallée L, Quintana-Murci L, Hovnanian A, Rozenberg F, Vivier E, Geissmann F, Tardieu M, Abel L, Casanova JL (2007) TLR3 deficiency in patients with herpes simplex encephalitis. Science 317(5844):1522–1527

Chapter 12
Sirtuins and Stress Response in Skin Cancer, Aging, and Barrier Function

Yu-Ying He

Abstract Sirtuins (SIRT1-7) are mammalian counterparts of the yeast silent information regulator 2 (Sir2) and are a family of NAD-dependent protein deacetylases and ADP ribosyltransferases. Sirtuins regulate numerous pathways in metabolism, aging and cancer. They are critical modulators in the cellular response to metabolic, oxidative, or genotoxic stress. Recent advances have demonstrated the pivotal role of sirtuin proteins in aging and a wide range of diseases including cancer in many organs. Skin is the essential barrier protecting organisms against environmental insults and minimizing water loss from the body. New evidence in mouse models and in vitro systems has illustrated that sirtuins have important roles in skin physiology, in the barrier function, aging, and diseases such as skin cancer. This review summarizes recent advances in understanding how sirtuins regulate the skin stress response in skin cancer, aging, and barrier integrity at the molecular, cellular, and organismal levels, and in how modulating sirtuins may help prevent or treat skin cancer, skin barrier defects, and other skin diseases.

Keywords Sirtuins · SIRT1 · SIRT2 · SIRT3 · SIRT6 skin cancer · Skin aging · Skin barrier · UV · DNA repair

12.1 Introduction and Overview on Sirtuins

Sirtuins (SIRT1-7) are NAD-dependent proteins with the enzymatic activity of deacetylases and ADP ribosyltransferases (Blander and Guarente 2004; Haigis and Guarente 2006; Haigis and Sinclair 2010; Michan and Sinclair 2007; Saunders and Verdin 2007). They are mammalian counterparts of the yeast silent information regulator 2 (Sir2). Since SIRT1 was first discovered about 15 years ago, there have been major breakthroughs in understanding the critical roles of sirtuins in

Y.-Y. He (✉)
Department of Medicine, Section of Dermatology, University of Chicago,
5841 S Maryland Ave, MC 5067, Chicago, IL 60637, USA
e-mail: yyhe@medicine.bsd.uchicago.edu

G.T. Wondrak (ed.), *Skin Stress Response Pathways*,
DOI 10.1007/978-3-319-43157-4_12

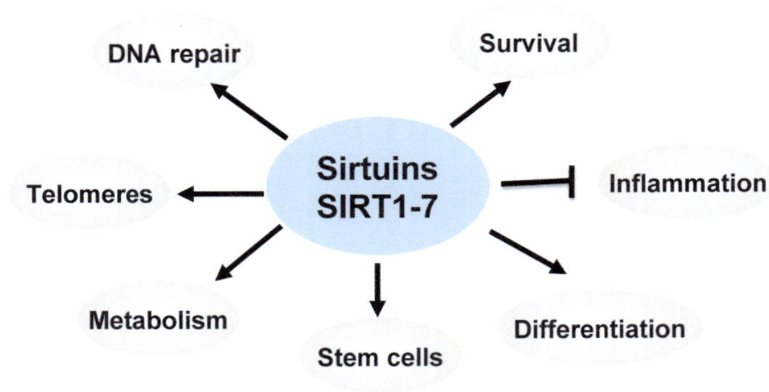

Fig. 12.1 Sirtuins regulates numerous cellular functions in stress response and homeostasis

physiology and pathology (Blander and Guarente 2004; Haigis and Guarente 2006; Haigis and Sinclair 2010; Michan and Sinclair 2007; Saunders and Verdin 2007). Sirtuins regulate a wide variety of proteins in the nucleus, cytosol and mitochondria. They are crucial regulators of tissue homeostasis and adaptation under metabolic, oxidative, or genotoxic stress. Using animal models, recent advances have demonstrated the illuminating roles of sirtuins in DNA repair, telomere integrity, metabolism, survival, inflammation, cell differentiation and stem cell biology in many human diseases including cancer and age-related diseases (Blander and Guarente 2004; Chalkiadaki and Guarente 2015; Haigis and Guarente 2006; Haigis and Sinclair 2010; Michan and Sinclair 2007; Saunders and Verdin 2007; Sebastian and Mostoslavsky 2015) (Fig. 12.1). Based on the molecular and cellular targets identified, sirtuins are considered to have important roles in skin cancer and age-related skin diseases (Serravallo et al. 2013). Indeed, using mouse models and in vitro systems, recent studies have illustrated critical roles of sirtuin proteins in the skin stress response, homeostasis, and skin diseases. This review focuses on recent advances in understanding the important roles of sirtuins at the molecular, cellular and organismal levels in the skin stress response and their function in skin cancer, aging, and barrier integrity.

12.2 Sirtuins in Skin Cancer

Skin cancer is the most common cancer in the US. In 2012, more than 5.4 million cases of nonmelanoma skin cancer were treated in over 3.3 million people (Rogers et al. 2015). The incidence of skin cancer continues to rise at an alarming rate. The average annual number of adults treated for skin cancer increased from 3.4 million in 2002–2006 to 4.9 million in 2007–2011 (Guy et al. 2015). Both genetic alterations and environmental risk factors play important roles in the pathogenesis of all three types of skin cancer—basal cell carcinoma, squamous cell carcinoma, and melanoma. In particular, important genetic alterations may be oncogenic or tumor suppressive; these may increase cell survival and proliferation, impair DNA repair and checkpoint activation, and induce inflammation in vivo (Bowden 2004; Cleaver 2005; Sundaresan et al. 2012). Targeting these molecular pathways has been demonstrated to hold promise for skin cancer prevention (Bowden 2004; Ratushny et al. 2012).

12.2.1 SIRT1 Has a Dual Role in Skin Cancer

Sirtuin 1 (SIRT1) is a proto member of the mammalian sirtuin family. It has been revealed that SIRT1 regulates various pathways in metabolism, aging, and cancer (Avivar-Valderas et al. 2011; Blander and Guarente 2004; Chalkiadaki and Guarente 2015; Haigis and Guarente 2006; Haigis and Sinclair 2010; Michan and Sinclair 2007; Saunders and Verdin 2007). Over the past decade, SIRT1 has attracted enormous attention due to its beneficial role in cell metabolism and survival in in vitro and in vivo animal studies (Avivar-Valderas et al. 2011; Blander and Guarente 2004; Chalkiadaki and Guarente 2015; Haigis and Guarente 2006; Haigis and Sinclair 2010; Michan and Sinclair 2007; Saunders and Verdin 2007). Both histone and non-histone targets of SIRT1 have been identified, including FOXO, p53, PGC-1α, NF-κB, and PPARγ (Blander and Guarente 2004; Brooks and Gu 2009; Michan and Sinclair 2007). Accumulating evidence suggests that the role of SIRT1 in cancer is complex. It remains under debate whether SIRT1 acts as a tumor suppressor or as an oncogene in many cancers (Brooks and Gu 2009; Deng 2009; Haigis and Sinclair 2010).

In skin cancer, ultraviolet radiation (UV) serves as the major risk factor by causing damage to the DNA and other molecules in the cells. By promoting deacetylation of xeroderma pigmentosum protein A (XPA) (Fan and Luo 2010) and promoting the expression of xeroderma pigmentosum C (XPC) (Ming et al. 2010), SIRT1 promotes nucleotide excision repair, which removes UV-induced DNA damage (Fig. 12.2). In addition, SIRT1 is down-regulated in UV-associated human skin cancers from Caucasian patients (who are at highest risk) (Ming et al. 2010), suggesting that in these cancers it is a tumor suppressor. In addition, UV radiation down-regulates SIRT1, and inhibiting SIRT1 increases p53 acetylation (Cao et al. 2009). The small molecule in grapes, a SIRT1 activator called resveratrol, reduces skin cancer development in mice treated with UVB radiation or chemical carcinogens (Aziz et al. 2005; Boily et al. 2009). Interestingly, the chemopreventive effect of resveratrol seems to depend on SIRT1 (Boily et al. 2009).

To elucidate the precise function of SIRT1 in cancer development in vivo, we have created mice with a keratinocyte-specific SIRT1 deletion and monitored tumor development following chronic UVB irradiation. Partial loss of SIRT1 increases UVB-induced tumorigenesis, while complete loss of SIRT1 decreases UV-induced

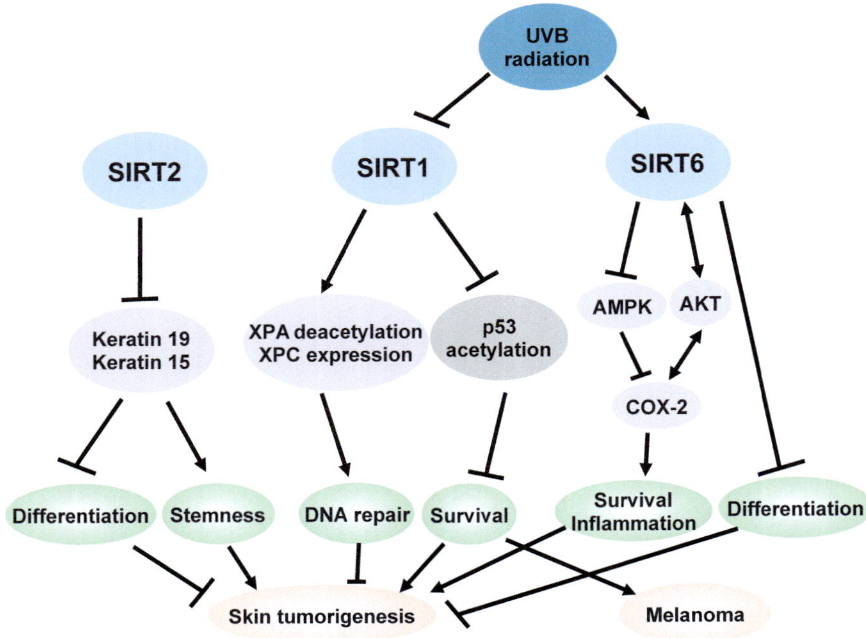

Fig. 12.2 SIRT1, SIRT2, and SIRT6 regulate DNA repair, survival, differentiation, and inflammation during tumorigenesis and each has distinct roles in skin tumorigenesis and cancer pathology

tumorigenesis, which is consistent with its role in promoting UVB-induced DNA damage repair and suppressing UVB-induced p53-mediated apoptosis (Ming et al. 2015a) (Fig. 12.2). These findings support a gene-dose-dependent role of SIRT1 in skin cancer in mice.

12.2.2 SIRT1 Is Oncogenic in Melanoma Cells

In addition to non-melanoma skin cancer, SIRT1 also plays an important role in melanoma. SIRT1 is found to be overexpressed in human melanoma and its small molecule inhibition imparts an anti-proliferative response via p53 activation (Wilking et al. 2014) (Fig. 12.2). SIRT1 regulates the level of many proteins, including p53 target genes (Singh et al. 2014; Wilking et al. 2014). In melanoma cells SIRT1 is regulated by the transcription factor MITF and promotes melanoma cell growth and survival (Ohanna et al. 2014). These studies indicate that SIRT1 has an oncogenic role, and inhibiting SIRT1 may improve anti-melanoma therapy.

12.2.3 SIRT2 Is a Tumor Suppressor in Skin

SIRT2 is a member of the mammalian sirtuin family. As compared with other sirtuins, SIRT2 is localized primarily in the cytoplasm. It regulates multiple physiological processes by deacetylating several proteins, including alpha-tubulin (North et al. 2003) and FOXO1 (Jing et al. 2007); it also deacetylates histone H4 at lysine 16 (Vaquero et al. 2006). In addition, SIRT2 modulates the mitotic deposition of H4K20 methylation and suppresses skin tumorigenesis (Serrano et al. 2013) (Fig. 12.2). SIRT2 also plays an important role in other cancers. In gliomas, melanomas, and gastric carcinomas, SIRT2 protein and RNA levels are decreased (de Oliveira et al. 2012). Using mice with SIRT2 ablation, we have shown that SIRT2 suppresses skin tumorigenesis, and suggest that SIRT2 promotes keratinocyte differentiation and suppresses tumor cell stemness in association with down-regulating keratin 19 (Ming et al. 2014b). Knockdown of SIRT2 increased the level of K19, but did not affect UVB-induced DNA damage repair and apoptosis. K19 has been considered to be a putative marker for epidermal stem cells in the hair follicle bulge (Michel et al. 1996). As loss of differentiation is known to promote tumorigenesis (Aymard et al. 2011; Kim et al. 2012), our data indicate that inhibition of SIRT2 may promote tumor growth in skin through inhibition of differentiation and increasing stemness (Ming et al. 2014b; Wang et al. 2014) (Fig. 12.2).

12.2.4 SIRT6 Is an Oncogene in Skin

SIRT6 is a member of the sirtuin family and an anti-aging protein important for many aspects of organismal health (Lombard et al. 2008; Sebastian et al. 2012a; Tennen and Chua 2011). At the molecular and cellular level, SIRT6 regulates multiple molecular pathways to modulate gene transcription, glucose homeostasis, DNA repair, and telomere integrity (Lombard et al. 2008; Sebastian et al. 2012a; Tennen and Chua 2011). As a positive regulator of genomic integrity, SIRT6 is predicted to act as a tumor suppressor. Indeed, it is found to suppress tumorigenesis in the intestine and liver in mice (Marquardt et al. 2013; Min et al. 2012; Sebastian et al. 2012b). However, a recent study showed that SIRT6 promotes transforming growth factor-β1 (TGF-β1)/H_2O_2/HOCl-mediated enhancement of hepatocellular carcinoma cell tumorigenicity by suppressing cellular senescence (Feng et al. 2015). TGF-β1/H_2O_2/HOCl up-regulates SIRT6 to inhibit cellular senescence (Feng et al. 2015). In addition, SIRT6 has been implicated as an oncogene in skin cancer (Lefort et al. 2013) and prostate cancer (Liu et al. 2013). It seems that its function may be tissue- and context-dependent.

Using mice with skin-specific SIRT6 ablation, we found that skin-specific SIRT6 deletion inhibits skin tumorigenesis. SIRT6 promotes the expression of the pro-inflammatory and pro-survival protein COX-2 through suppressing AMPK signaling, an energy-sensing pathway, and increases cell survival and proliferation (Ming et al. 2014a) (Fig. 12.2). UVB induces SIRT6 expression through activating the AKT pathway. SIRT6 is up-regulated in human squamous cell carcinoma (Ming et al. 2014a). SIRT6 also inhibits keratinocyte differentiation and is suppressed by microRNA-34a, which can also promote skin tumorigenesis (Lefort et al. 2013) (Fig. 12.2). These findings demonstrate that SIRT6 is an oncogene in skin.

12.3 Sirtuins in Skin Aging

Sirtuins have been shown to reduce the aging process in a broad range of organisms including mammals (Guarente 2013). Sirtuin activation can inhibit the progression of aging diseases, including neurodegeneration, diabetes, cardiovascular diseases and many types of cancer (Guarente 2013; Haigis and Sinclair 2010).

12.3.1 SIRT1 in Skin Aging

Using transgenic mice moderately overexpressing SIRT1 under its own regulatory elements (Sirt1-tg), a recent study showed that old Sirt1-tg mice present lower levels of DNA damage, decreased expression of the ageing-associated gene $p16^{Ink4a}$, better general health, and fewer spontaneous carcinomas and sarcomas. Sirt1-tg mice show improved wound healing, providing direct proof of the anti-aging activity of SIRT1 in mammalian skin and other tissues (Herranz et al. 2010) (Fig. 12.3). Loss of SIRT1 accelerates retinoic acid-induced embryonic stem cell differentiation by increasing CRABPII acetylation and thus cellular retinoic acid signaling (Tang et al. 2014). It is possible that SIRT1 is critical for adult stem cell maintenance in the skin as well. SIRT1 is down-regulated in later passage fibroblasts (Kim et al. 2015). In dermal fibroblasts, SIRT1 suppresses the expression of matrix metalloproteinases 1 and 3 (MMP1 and MMP3) under basal conditions or exposure to interleukin 1beta (Ohguchi et al. 2010) (Fig. 12.3), suggesting that SIRT1 inhibits the aging process in the dermis at the basal level and under inflammation conditions and that agents targeting SIRT1 may reduce the production of MMPs and thereby slow down the skin aging process.

12.3.2 SIRT6 Has a Potential Role in Skin Aging

SIRT6 regulates various molecular pathways in genomic stability, metabolism, and aging. SIRT6 knockout mice have displayed genomic instability and several phenotypes of accelerated premature aging (Mostoslavsky et al. 2006). Overexpressing SIRT6 extends lifespans in male mice but not in female mice (Kanfi et al. 2012).

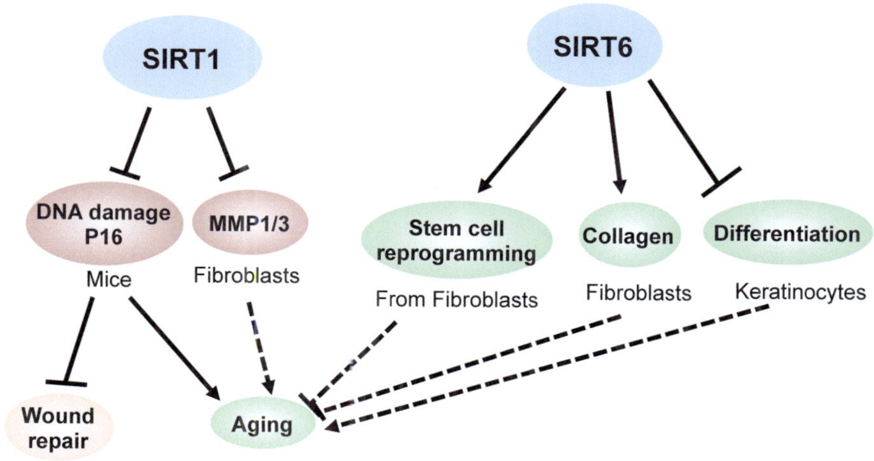

Fig. 12.3 SIRT1 and SIRT6 regulate keratinocyte and fibroblast functions in response to stress and homeostasis

Ablation of neural SIRT6 causes obesity in mice (Schwer et al. 2010). SIRT6 is a protein deacetylase that deacetylates Histone H3 lysine 9 (H3K9), required for telomere maintenance (Michishita et al. 2008; Tennen and Chua 2011). It suppresses NF-kB by interacting with the NF-kB RELA subunit and deacetylating H3K9 to delay the signs of aging (Kawahara et al. 2009), and it blocks IGF-AKT signaling to protect against development of cardiac hypertrophy (Sundaresan et al. 2012). It regulates glucose homeostasis (Kim et al. 2010; Xiao et al. 2010), repressing HIF1a (Zhong et al 2010) and activating acetyltransferase GCN5 (Dominy et al. 2012). In addition, SIRT6 regulates double strand break (DSB) repair through recruiting SNF2H to DNA strand breaks, (Toiber et al. 2013), deacetylating the DSB resection protein CtIP (Kaidi et al. 2010), activating PARP1 under oxidative stress (Mao et al. 2011), and stabilizing DNA-dependent protein kinase (McCord et al. 2009). SIRT6 reverses the decline of homologous recombination repair during replicative senescence (Mao et al. 2012).

SIRT6 may have a role in skin aging as well. SIRT6 promotes reprogramming of induced pluripotent stem cells from human dermal fibroblasts (Sharma et al. 2013), and also regulates skin aging by modulating collagen metabolism in dermal fibroblasts (Baohua and Li 2012) (Fig. 12.3). SIRT6 is down-regulated in later passage fibroblasts (Kim et al. 2015). In addition, in keratinocytes SIRT6 loss accelerates keratinocyte differentiation and senescence (Kawahara et al. 2009; Lefort et al. 2013) (Fig. 12.3).

12.4 Sirtuins in Keratinocyte Differentiation, Stress Response, and Skin Barrier Function

Skin is the essential barrier protecting organisms against environmental insults including infectious pathogens, chemicals and UV radiation, and minimizing water loss from the body. As the most abundant cells forming the epidermis, keratinocytes proliferate and differentiate to form an impermeable barrier. Defects in the skin barrier have an active role in the pathogenesis of several chronic inflammatory skin diseases, including atopic dermatitis (Elias 2008; Elias and Schmuth 2009; Elias and Wakefield 2011; Jin et al. 2009).

12.4.1 SIRT1 Loss Disrupts Skin Barrier Function

Previously SIRT1 has been shown to promote differentiation of normal human keratinocytes in vitro (Blander et al. 2009), suggesting a possible role in barrier function and thus the development of atopic dermatitis (AD). Using mice with epidermis-specific SIRT1 deletion, we showed that SIRT1 is critical for skin barrier integrity (Ming et al. 2015b). Epidermis-specific SIRT1 ablation causes AD-like skin lesions in mice, and mice with the epidermal SIRT1 deletion are sensitive to percutaneous challenge by the protein allergen ovalbumin. In normal human keratinocytes and mouse skin, SIRT1 knockdown or genetic deletion down-regulates the barrier molecule filaggrin, and regulation of filaggrin expression by SIRT1 requires the deacetylase activity of SIRT1. SIRT1 also promotes the activation of the aryl hydrocarbon receptor (AhR), and the AhR ligand benzo[*a*]pyrene (BaP) restores filaggrin expression in SIRT1-inhibited cells (Fig. 12.4). As compared with normal human skin, SIRT1 is down-regulated in the lesions of atopic dermatitis as well as non-atopic dermatitis (Ming et al. 2015b). Interestingly, loss of filaggrin in flaky-tail mice reduced SIRT1 expression (Nakai et al. 2012) (Fig. 12.4), suggesting that SIRT1 and filaggrin form a positive feedback loop in maintaining the availability of both proteins and thus skin barrier function. These findings demonstrate a critical role of SIRT1 in the skin barrier function, which may open up new opportunities to use SIRT1 as a pharmacological target for AD prevention and therapy.

12.4.2 SIRT3 in Keratinocyte Differentiation and Stress Response

Dysregulation in the balance of reactive oxygen species homeostasis may play a role in keratinocyte differentiation. SIRT3 is a mitochondrial sirtuin deacetylase and found to be a tumor suppressor (Chalkiadaki and Guarente 2015). A recent report

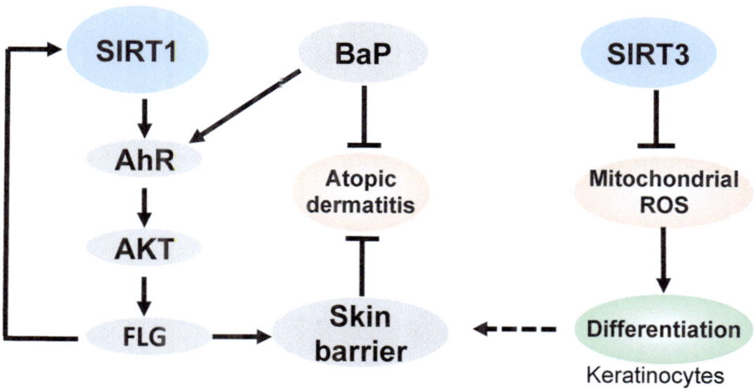

Fig. 12.4 SIRT1 and SIRT3 regulate keratinocyte differentiation and stress response and SIRT1 is required for skin barrier integrity

has shown that SIRT3 suppresses the generation of mitochondrial reactive oxygen species during keratinocyte differentiation (Bause et al. 2013) (Fig. 12.4). SIRT3 expression is down-regulated during keratinocyte differentiation, in parallel with an increase in mitochondrial superoxide levels. Loss of SIRT3 in keratinocytes increased superoxide levels and promoted the expression of differentiation markers, whereas overexpression decreased superoxide levels and reduced the expression of differentiation markers (Bause et al. 2013). In human cells with mitochondrial dysfunction caused by a pathogenic mtDNA mutation, increased intracellular ROS levels might modulate the expression of Sirt3, which deacetylates and activates the mitochondrial enzyme F(o)F(1)ATPase (Wu et al. 2013). Therefore targeting SIRT3 may help treat mitochondrial disorders. Ozone also decreases the levels of SIRT3 (McCarthy et al. 2013). Ozone is an environmental pollutant that has detrimental effects on human health. Understanding the role of SIRT3 in the epidermal response to ozone can help prevent or treat skin diseases associated with ozone exposure (Syed and Mukhtar 2013).

12.5 Conclusion and Future Perspectives

As summarized, in a wide range of experimental models, recent overwhelming evidence has connected the role of sirtuins in stress response in associating with skin cancer, aging, and skin barrier dysfunction. The sirtuin members have different roles in response to genotoxic UV stress, oxidative stress, and metabolic stress at the molecular, cellular and organismal levels. In the past decade multiple small molecular modulators targeting SIRT1 have been discovered and tested in metabolism stress response and cancer. There is growing interest in applying those small molecule sirtuin modulators in skin diseases. However, specific small molecular modulators for most of the sirtuin enzyme are still lacking or limited. Targeting specific sirtuins is necessary to achieve the desired preventative or therapeutic needs for a particular pathological condition. It is also critical to identify new regulatory and functional roles of sirtuins in the skin and to expand our knowledge of the functions of sirtuins in skin cancer, aging and barrier function. This may provide a wealth of new preventive and therapeutic opportunities for skin cancer and age-related or barrier-related diseases.

Acknowledgments We apologize to those investigators whose work could not be directly referenced owing to space limitations. Work in the authors' laboratory was supported by NIH/NIEHS grants ES016936 and ES024373 (YYH), the American Cancer Society (ACS) grant RSG-13-078-01 (YYH), the University of Chicago Cancer Research Center (P30 CA014599), the CTSA (UL1 TR000430), and the University of Chicago Friends of Dermatology Endowment Fund. I thank Dr. Ann Motten for a critical reading of the manuscript.

References

Avivar-Valderas A, Salas E, Bobrovnikova-Marjon E, Diehl JA, Nagi C, Debnath J, Aguirre-Ghiso JA (2011) PERK integrates autophagy and oxidative stress responses to promote survival during extracellular matrix detachment. Mol Cell Biol 31:3616–3629

Aymard E, Barruche V, Naves T, Bordes S, Closs B, Verdier M, Ratinaud MH (2011) Autophagy in human keratinocytes: an early step of the differentiation? Exp Dermatol 20:263–268

Aziz MH, Reagan-Shaw S, Wu J, Longley BJ, Ahmad N (2005) Chemoprevention of skin cancer by grape constituent resveratrol: relevance to human disease? FASEB J 19:1193–1195

Baohua Y, Li L (2012) Effects of SIRT6 silencing on collagen metabolism in human dermal fibroblasts. Cell Biol Int 36:105–108

Bause AS, Matsui MS, Haigis MC (2013) The protein deacetylase SIRT3 prevents oxidative stress-induced keratinocyte differentiation. J Biol Chem 288:36484–36491

Blander G, Guarente L (2004) The Sir2 family of protein deacetylases. Annu Rev Biochem 73:417–435

Blander G, Bhimavarapu A, Mammone T, Maes D, Elliston K, Reich C, Matsui MS, Guarente L, Loureiro JJ (2009) SIRT1 promotes differentiation of normal human keratinocytes. J Invest Dermatol 129:41–49

Boily G, He XH, Pearce B, Jardine K, McBurney MW (2009) SirT1-null mice develop tumors at normal rates but are poorly protected by resveratrol. Oncogene 28:2882–2893

Bowden GT (2004) Prevention of non-melanoma skin cancer by targeting ultraviolet-B-light signalling. Nat Rev Cancer 4:23–35

Brooks CL, Gu W (2009) How does SIRT1 affect metabolism, senescence and cancer? Nat Rev Cancer 9:123–128

Cao C, Lu S, Kivlin R, Wallin B, Card E, Bagdasarian A, Tamakloe T, Wang WJ, Song X, Chu WM et al (2009) SIRT1 confers protection against UVB- and H2O2-induced cell death via modulation of p53 and JNK in cultured skin keratinocytes. J Cell Mol Med 13:3632–3643

Chalkiadaki A, Guarente L (2015) The multifaceted functions of sirtuins in cancer. Nat Rev Cancer 15:608–624

Cleaver JE (2005) Cancer in xeroderma pigmentosum and related disorders of DNA repair. Nat Rev Cancer 5:564–573

de Oliveira RM, Sarkander J, Kazantsev AG, Outeiro TF (2012) SIRT2 as a Therapeutic Target for Age-Related Disorders. Front Pharmacol 3:82

Deng CX (2009) SIRT1, is it a tumor promoter or tumor suppressor? Int J Biol Sci 5:147–152

Dominy JE Jr, Lee Y, Jedrychowski MP, Chim H, Jurczak MJ, Camporez JP, Ruan HB, Feldman J, Pierce K, Mostoslavsky R et al (2012) The deacetylase Sirt6 activates the acetyltransferase GCN5 and suppresses hepatic gluconeogenesis. Mol Cell 48:900–913
Elias PM (2008) Skin barrier function. Curr Allergy Asthma Rep 8:299–305
Elias PM, Schmuth M (2009) Abnormal skin barrier in the etiopathogenesis of atopic dermatitis. Curr Opin Allergy Clin Immunol 9:437–446
Elias PM, Wakefield JS (2011) Therapeutic implications of a barrier-based pathogenesis of atopic dermatitis. Clin Rev Allergy Immunol 41:282–295
Fan W, Luo J (2010) SIRT1 regulates UV-induced DNA repair through deacetylating XPA. Mol Cell 39:247–258
Feng XX, Luo J, Liu M, Yan W, Zhou ZZ, Xia YJ, Tu W, Li PY, Feng ZH, Tian DA (2015) Sirtuin 6 promotes transforming growth factor-beta1/H2O2/HOCl-mediated enhancement of hepatocellular carcinoma cell tumorigenicity by suppressing cellular senescence. Cancer Sci 106:559–566
Guarente L (2013) Calorie restriction and sirtuins revisited. Genes Dev 27:2072–2085
Guy GP Jr, Machlin SR, Ekwueme DU, Yabroff KR (2015) Prevalence and costs of skin cancer treatment in the U.S., 2002–2006 and 2007–2011. Am J Prev Med 48:183–187
Haigis MC, Guarente LP (2006) Mammalian sirtuins–emerging roles in physiology, aging, and calorie restriction. Genes Dev 20:2913–2921
Haigis MC, Sinclair DA (2010) Mammalian sirtuins: biological insights and disease relevance. Annu Rev Pathol 5:253–295
Herranz D, Munoz-Martin M, Canamero M, Mulero F, Martinez-Pastor B, Fernandez-Capetillo O, Serrano M (2010) Sirt1 improves healthy ageing and protects from metabolic syndrome-associated cancer. Nat Commun 1:3
Jin H, He R, Oyoshi M, Geha RS (2009) Animal models of atopic dermatitis. J Invest Dermatol 129:31–40
Jing E, Gesta S, Kahn CR (2007) SIRT2 regulates adipocyte differentiation through FoxO1 acetylation/deacetylation. Cell Metab 6:105–114
Kaidi A, Weinert BT, Choudhary C, Jackson SP (2010) Human SIRT6 promotes DNA end resection through CtIP deacetylation. Science 329:1348–1353
Kanfi Y, Naiman S, Amir G, Peshti V, Zinman G, Nahum L, Bar-Joseph Z, Cohen HY (2012) The sirtuin SIRT6 regulates lifespan in male mice. Nature 483:218–221
Kawahara TL, Michishita E, Adler AS, Damian M, Berber E, Lin M, McCord RA, Ongaigui KC, Boxer LD, Chang HY et al (2009) SIRT6 links histone H3 lysine 9 deacetylation to NF-kappaB-dependent gene expression and organismal life span. Cell 136:62–74
Kim HS, Xiao C, Wang RH, Lahusen T, Xu X, Vassilopoulos A, Vazquez-Ortiz G, Jeong WI, Park O, Ki SH et al (2010) Hepatic-specific disruption of SIRT6 in mice results in fatty liver formation due to enhanced glycolysis and triglyceride synthesis. Cell Metab 12:224–236
Kim M, Cho KH, Lee JH, Chang MS, Cho S (2012) Intratumoral mast cell number is negatively correlated with tumor size and mitosis in dermatofibrosarcoma protuberans. Exp Dermatol 21:559–561
Kim KS, Park HK, Lee JW, Kim YI, Shin MK (2015) Investigate correlation between mechanical property and aging biomarker in passaged human dermal fibroblasts. Microsc Res Tech 78:277–282
Lefort K, Brooks Y, Ostano P, Cario-Andre M, Calpini V, Guinea-Viniegra J, Albinger-Hegyi A, Hoetzenecker W, Kolfschoten I, Wagner EF et al (2013) A miR-34a-SIRT6 axis in the squamous cell differentiation network. EMBO J 32:2248–2263
Liu Y, Xie QR, Wang B, Shao J, Zhang T, Liu T, Huang G, Xia W (2013). Inhibition of SIRT6 in prostate cancer reduces cell viability and increases sensitivity to chemotherapeutics. Protein Cell 4(9):702–710
Lombard DB, Schwer B, Alt FW, Mostoslavsky R (2008) SIRT6 in DNA repair, metabolism and ageing. J Intern Med 263:128–141
Mao Z, Hine C, Tian X, Van Meter M, Au M, Vaidya A, Seluanov A, Gorbunova V (2011) SIRT6 promotes DNA repair under stress by activating PARP1. Science 332:1443–1446

Mao Z, Tian X, Van Meter M, Ke Z, Gorbunova V, Seluanov A (2012) Sirtuin 6 (SIRT6) rescues the decline of homologous recombination repair during replicative senescence. Proc Natl Acad Sci USA 109:11800–11805

Marquardt JU, Fischer K, Baus K, Kashyap A, Ma S, Krupp M, Linke M, Teufel A, Zechner U, Strand D et al (2013) Sirtuin-6-dependent genetic and epigenetic alterations are associated with poor clinical outcome in hepatocellular carcinoma patients. Hepatology 58:1054–1064

McCarthy JT, Pelle E, Dong K, Brahmbhatt K, Yarosh D, Pernodet N (2013) Effects of ozone in normal human epidermal keratinocytes. Exp Dermatol 22:360–361

McCord RA, Michishita E, Hong T, Berber E, Boxer LD, Kusumoto R, Guan S, Shi X, Gozani O, Burlingame AL et al (2009) SIRT6 stabilizes DNA-dependent protein kinase at chromatin for DNA double-strand break repair. Aging (Albany NY) 1:109–121

Michan S, Sinclair D (2007) Sirtuins in mammals: insights into their biological function. Biochem J 404:1–13

Michel M, Torok N, Godbout MJ, Lussier M, Gaudreau P, Royal A, Germain L (1996) Keratin 19 as a biochemical marker of skin stem cells in vivo and in vitro: keratin 19 expressing cells are differentially localized in function of anatomic sites, and their number varies with donor age and culture stage. J Cell Sci 109(Pt 5):1017–1028

Michishita E, McCord RA, Berber E, Kioi M, Padilla-Nash H, Damian M, Cheung P, Kusumoto R, Kawahara TL, Barrett JC et al (2008) SIRT6 is a histone H3 lysine 9 deacetylase that modulates telomeric chromatin. Nature 452:492–496

Min L, Ji Y, Bakiri L, Qiu Z, Cen J, Chen X, Chen L, Scheuch H, Zheng H, Qin L et al (2012) Liver cancer initiation is controlled by AP-1 through SIRT6-dependent inhibition of survivin. Nat Cell Biol 14:1203–1211

Ming M, Shea CR, Guo X, Li X, Soltani K, Han W, He YY (2010) Regulation of global genome nucleotide excision repair by SIRT1 through xeroderma pigmentosum C. Proc Natl Acad Sci USA 107:22623–22628

Ming M, Han W, Zhao B, Sundaresan NR, Deng CX, Gupta MP, He YY (2014a) SIRT6 promotes COX-2 expression and acts as an oncogene in skin cancer. Cancer Res. In press

Ming M, Qiang L, Zhao B, He YY (2014b) Mammalian SIRT2 inhibits keratin 19 expression and is a tumor suppressor in skin. Exp Dermatol 23:207–209

Ming M, Soltani K, Shea CR, Li X, He YY (2015a) Dual role of SIRT1 in UVB-induced skin tumorigenesis. Oncogene 34:357–363

Ming M, Zhao B, Shea CR, Shah P, Qiang L, White SR, Sims DM, He YY (2015b) Loss of sirtuin 1 (SIRT1) disrupts skin barrier integrity and sensitizes mice to epicutaneous allergen challenge. J Allergy Clin Immunol 135(936–945):e934

Mostoslavsky R, Chua KF, Lombard DB, Pang WW, Fischer MR, Gellon L, Liu P, Mostoslavsky G, Franco S, Murphy MM et al (2006) Genomic instability and aging-like phenotype in the absence of mammalian SIRT6. Cell 124:315–329

Nakai K, Yoneda K, Hosokawa Y, Moriue T, Presland RB, Fallon PG, Kabashima K, Kosaka H, Kubota Y (2012) Reduced expression of epidermal growth factor receptor, E-cadherin, and occludin in the skin of flaky tail mice is due to filaggrin and loricrin deficiencies. Am J Pathol 181:969–977

North BJ, Marshall BL, Borra MT, Denu JM, Verdin E (2003) The human Sir2 ortholog, SIRT2, is an NAD + -dependent tubulin deacetylase. Mol Cell 11:437–444

Ohanna M, Bonet C, Bille K, Allegra M, Davidson I, Bahadoran P, Lacour JP, Ballotti R, Bertolotto C (2014) SIRT1 promotes proliferation and inhibits the senescence-like phenotype in human melanoma cells. Oncotarget 5:2085–2095

Ohguchi K, Itoh T, Akao Y, Inoue H, Nozawa Y, Ito M (2010) SIRT1 modulates expression of matrix metalloproteinases in human dermal fibroblasts. Br J Dermatol 163:689–694

Ratushny V, Gober MD, Hick R, Ridky TW, Seykora JT (2012) From keratinocyte to cancer: the pathogenesis and modeling of cutaneous squamous cell carcinoma. J Clin Invest 122:464–472

Rogers HW, Weinstock MA, Feldman SR, Coldiron BM (2015) Incidence Estimate of Nonmelanoma Skin Cancer (Keratinocyte Carcinomas) in the US Population, 2012. JAMA Dermatol 151:1081–1086

Saunders LR, Verdin E (2007) Sirtuins: critical regulators at the crossroads between cancer and aging. Oncogene 26:5489–5504

Schwer B, Schumacher B, Lombard DB, Xiao C, Kurtev MV, Gao J, Schneider JI, Chai H, Bronson RT, Tsai LH et al (2010) Neural sirtuin 6 (Sirt6) ablation attenuates somatic growth and causes obesity. Proc Natl Acad Sci U S A 107:21790–21794

Sebastian C, Mostoslavsky R (2015) The role of mammalian sirtuins in cancer metabolism. Semin Cell Dev Biol 43:33–42

Sebastian C, Satterstrom FK, Haigis MC, Mostoslavsky R (2012a) From sirtuin biology to human diseases: an update. J Biol Chem 287:42444–42452

Sebastian C, Zwaans BM, Silberman DM, Gymrek M, Goren A, Zhong L, Ram O, Truelove J, Guimaraes AR, Toiber D et al (2012b) The histone deacetylase SIRT6 is a tumor suppressor that controls cancer metabolism. Cell 151:1185–1199

Serrano L, Martinez-Redondo P, Marazuela-Duque A, Vazquez BN, Dooley SJ, Voigt P, Beck DB, Kane-Goldsmith N, Tong Q, Rabanal RM et al (2013) The tumor suppressor SirT2 regulates cell cycle progression and genome stability by modulating the mitotic deposition of H4K20 methylation. Genes Dev 27:639–653

Serravallo M, Jagdeo J, Glick SA, Siegel DM, Brody NI (2013) Sirtuins in dermatology: applications for future research and therapeutics. Arch Dermatol Res 305:269–282

Sharma A, Diecke S, Zhang WY, Lan F, He C, Mordwinkin NM, Chua KF, Wu JC (2013) The role of SIRT6 protein in aging and reprogramming of human induced pluripotent stem cells. J Biol Chem 288:18439–18447

Singh CK, George J, Nihal M, Sabat G, Kumar R, Ahmad N (2014) Novel downstream molecular targets of SIRT1 in melanoma: a quantitative proteomics approach. Oncotarget 5:1987–1999

Sundaresan NR, Vasudevan P, Zhong L, Kim G, Samant S, Parekh V, Pillai VB, Ravindra PV, Gupta M, Jeevanandam V et al (2012) The sirtuin SIRT6 blocks IGF-Akt signaling and development of cardiac hypertrophy by targeting c-Jun. Nat Med 18:1643–1650

Syed DN, Mukhtar H (2013) Ozone and SIRT3: an unexplored paradigm. Exp Dermatol 22:396

Tang S, Huang G, Fan W, Chen Y, Ward JM, Xu X, Xu Q, Kang A, McBurney MW, Fargo DC et al (2014) SIRT1-mediated deacetylation of CRABPII regulates cellular retinoic acid signaling and modulates embryonic stem cell differentiation. Mol Cell 55:843–855

Tennen RI, Chua KF (2011) Chromatin regulation and genome maintenance by mammalian SIRT6. Trends Biochem Sci 36:39–46

Toiber D, Erdel F, Bouazoune K, Silberman DM, Zhong L, Mulligan P, Sebastian C, Cosentino C, Martinez-Pastor B, Giacosa S et al (2013) SIRT6 recruits SNF2H to DNA break sites, preventing genomic instability through chromatin remodeling. Mol Cell 51:454–468

Vaquero A, Scher MB, Lee DH, Sutton A, Cheng HL, Alt FW, Serrano L, Sternglanz R, Reinberg D (2006) SirT2 is a histone deacetylase with preference for histone H4 Lys 16 during mitosis. Genes Dev 20:1256–1261

Wang M, Yue Z, Paus R, Ramot Y (2014) SIRT2 as a new player in epigenetic programming of keratinocyte differentiation and a candidate tumor suppressor. Exp Dermatol 23:636–638

Wilking MJ, Singh C, Nihal M, Zhong W, Ahmad N (2014) SIRT1 deacetylase is overexpressed in human melanoma and its small molecule inhibition imparts anti-proliferative response via p53 activation. Arch Biochem Biophys 563:94–100

Wu YT, Lee HC, Liao CC, Wei YH (2013) Regulation of mitochondrial F(o)F(1)ATPase activity by Sirt3-catalyzed deacetylation and its deficiency in human cells harboring 4977 bp deletion of mitochondrial DNA. Biochim Biophys Acta 1832:216–227

Xiao C, Kim HS, Lahusen T, Wang RH, Xu X, Gavrilova O, Jou W, Gius D, Deng CX (2010) SIRT6 deficiency results in severe hypoglycemia by enhancing both basal and insulin-stimulated glucose uptake in mice. J Biol Chem 285:36776–36784

Zhong L, D'Urso A, Toiber D, Sebastian C, Henry RE, Vadysirisack DD, Guimaraes A, Marinelli B, Wikstrom JD, Nir T et al (2010) The histone deacetylase Sirt6 regulates glucose homeostasis via Hif1alpha. Cell 140:280–293

Chapter 13
Cutaneous Opioid Receptors and Stress Responses: Molecular Interactions and Opportunities for Therapeutic Intervention

Hanane Chajra

Abstract Opioid receptors (μ opioid receptor, δ opioid receptor, κ opioid receptor, orphan opioid-like nociceptin receptor and opioid growth factor receptor) and their endogenous ligands (β-endorphins, enkephalins, and dynorphins) are not only expressed in central and peripheral nervous systems but also in others tissues and especially in the skin. Indeed, recent studies on the complex cutaneous opioid system involving several receptors and ligands (—endogenous or exogenous such as morphine or naltrexone—) have shown that it is not only in charge of pain and itching control sensations but also in wound healing phases (inflammation, proliferation and maturation), skin homeostasis, and skin ageing. In this chapter, published findings on the cutaneous opioid system concerning the treatment of skin pain, itching, wound healing, homeostasis, and ageing will be discussed. Based on the current knowledge of the cutaneous opioid system open opportunities for medical and cosmetic applications will be suggested.

Keywords Skin · Opioid receptors · Delta opioid receptor · Kappa opioid receptor · Mu opioid receptor · Zeta opioid receptor · Wound healing · Itching · Ageing · Homeostasis

13.1 Introduction

The human skin is a complex and large organ covering the whole body. Skin is a multi-layered tissue composed of a stratified and non-vascularized epithelium called epidermis. The dermis, a vascularized connective tissue, is tucked away

H. Chajra (✉)
Givaudan Active Beauty, Libragen, 3 rue des satellites, 31400 Toulouse, France
e-mail: hanane.chajra@givaudan.com

G.T. Wondrak (ed.), *Skin Stress Response Pathways*,
DOI 10.1007/978-3-319-43157-4_13

between the epidermis and the hypodermis. The skin contains also appendages including hair follicles, sebaceous glands, and finally sweat glands penetrating deeply into the hypodermis. Skin functions are critical for human being survival (Roosterman et al. 2006). The skin is able to maintain local and systemic homeostasis in an autonomous manner by reacting to environmental changes induced by biological, chemical, and physical factors. Skin, by a close communication with central nervous system and its own organized and independent neuro-immuno-endocrine system, ensures body homeostasis (Roosterman et al. 2006; Arck et al. 2006). This organized neuro-immuno-endocrine system is composed first of resident and circulating cells of the epidermis and dermis, hypodermis and adnexal structures expressing receptors. Second, it is composed by circulating molecules in stress and unstress situations such as neuro-transmitters, neuro-hormones, hormones, and cytokines. Skin cells also produce hormones, and neuropeptides (Slominski et al. 1998; Skobowiat et al. 2011; Slominski 2003). These molecules are able to activate cutaneous sensory nerve endings that then alert the brain in stress situation. In this chapter, it will be focused only on cutaneous opioids receptors. In skin, five classes of opioid receptor (OR) have been identified: mu (μ, MOR) (Bigliardi et al. 1998), delta (δ, DOR) (Salemi et al. 2005), kappa (κ, KOR) (Salemi et al. 2005), orphan opioid-like nociceptin receptor (NOP) and opioid growth factor receptor also called zeta receptor (ζ, OGFR) (Zagon et al. 2009). MOR, DOR and KOR receptors belong to the G protein- coupled receptor family (GPCR) and are located on the cell membrane. ζ receptor (zeta) is located on the nuclear membrane. The orphan receptor is less studied than others opioid receptors. All opioid receptors have been found in keratinocytes (Neumann et al. 2015), fibroblasts, melanocytes, sebocytes, immune cells and cutaneous sensory nerve ending (Tachibana and Nawa 2005). They are all capable of mediating the effects of endogenous opioids. Endogenous opioids are peptides resulting from the conversion of three prohormones called proenkephalins (pro-Leu-enkephalin and pro-Met-enkephalin) (Nissen and Kragballe 1997; Hughes et al. 1997), prodynorphin and pro-opiomelanocortin. Proenkephalins (PENK) and proenkephalin derived peptides (Met- and Leu-enkephalin) (Slominski et al. 2011) and their receptors are expressed predominantly in the suprabasal layer of the epidermis (Neumann et al. 2015; Chajra et al. 2015).

Exogenous opioids such as morphine are also known to interact with these opioid receptors. Because signalling involving opioid receptors in skin can also affect cell differentiation, cell proliferation (Immonen et al. 2014) and cell migration process (Slominski 2003), it is rightful to assume that opioid receptors are involved in the regulation of skin homeostasis in response to stresses (trauma, irradiation, chemical irritation, insects bites, viral and bacterial insults). In this chapter, the last findings related to opioid receptors in medical (wound healing, itching, pain relief, inflammation) and cosmetic fields (skin ageing) will be discussed in detail.

13.2 Opioid Receptors and Skin Sensations

13.2.1 *Pain (Algesia)*

Somatosensory neurons are involved in pain transduction and itch (or pruritus) sensations facilitating our detection of threats coming from external insults (insects, toxic plants or chemical irritants) or perturbation of skin homeostasis resulting of physiological abnormalities. Acute pain sensation and limited itching act as danger signals, providing a protection to the body (Luo et al. 2015).

Unfortunately, a persistent pain followed or not by itching sensation is often debilitating. First-line therapies for chronic pain include prescriptions for common μ opioid receptor agonists such as morphine and its various derivatives (tramadol, oxymorphone, tapentadol, oxycodone, hydrocodone, fentanyl, buprenorphine) (Trescot et al. 2008). Most of these treatments are provided orally to the patient with the exception of fentanyl and buprenorphine), delivered via transdermal route. Fentanyl is an effective and well-tolerated μ opioid agonist drug (Duragesic^{TM}) administrated by transdermal route for the treatment of chronic pain caused by malignant and non-malignant diseases in children and in adult (Kornick et al. 2003). Transdermal fentanyl is a useful drug for cancer patients who are unable to swallow or have gastrointestinal issues. Transdermal fentanyl is indicated only for patients who require continuous opioid administration for the treatment of chronic pain that cannot be managed with other medications. Buprenorphine is a lipid-soluble drug also used in the management of chronic pain in cancer and non-cancer suffering patients. It is a partial agonist to μ-opioid receptors, an antagonist to κ-opioid receptors, an agonist to δ-opioid receptors and a partial agonist at ORL-1 (nociceptin) receptors. Several side effects associated with buprenorphine use include headache, dizziness, somnolence, constipation, dry mouth, nausea, vomiting, pruritus and erythema (Kitzmiller et al. 2015). Transdermal buprenorphine as transdermal fentanyl has significant potential for managing chronic pain. In addition to increased convenience and efficacy advantages, they decrease tolerance. Compared with oral opioids, the advantages of transdermal fentanyl include a lower incidence and impact of adverse effects (constipation, nausea and vomiting), a higher degree of patient satisfaction, an improved quality of life, an improved convenience and compliance resulting from administration every 72 h, and finally a decreased use of rescue medication (Muijsers and Wagstaff 2001). It has been shown that morphine topically applied at low dose on two children suffering of epidermolysis bullosa (Watterson et al. 2004) induced a decrease in pain sensation without the adverse effects provided by oral administration. As described above, current treatment of chronic pain relies on the activation of μ opioid receptors associated with side effects such as itching and scratching. Though δ opioid agonists are described in scientific literature to be also potent analgesics without induction of scratching (Trescot et al. 2008), there is no drug approved on the market specifically covering this specific delta opioid receptor. Some researchers are working on the combination of molecules having double

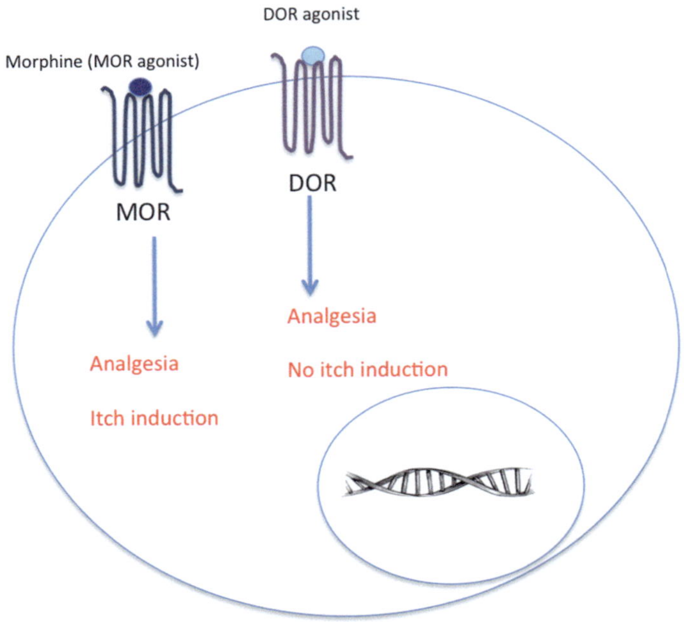

Fig. 13.1 Schematic representation of analgesia coupled or not with itching sensation after activation of MOR (μ opioid receptor) or DOR (δ opioid receptor) by their respective agonists. MOR agonist such as morphine induces analgesia with itch induction, whereas DOR agonist is known to induce analgesia without itch induction

activation μ and δ opioid receptors for pain control with less side-effect (Podolsky et al. 2013). The anti-nociception molecular mechanism of opioids receptors involved in analgesia is well described in literature (Jordan and Devi 1998). Figure 13.1 is a summary of action of DOR and MOR agonists in pain control.

Interestingly, in contrast to animal studies, in human application, any tolerance to opioids topically applied was recorded. These studies open the way to the application of such therapeutic to other diseases involving pain such as burns, or post-operative wounds (Stein and Kuchler 2013).

13.2.2 Itching

Persistent itching associated with scratching is frequently encountered in a variety of inflammatory skin pathologies. Antihistamines and specifically histamine H_1-receptor blockers are commonly used as treatment for all types of persistent itching resulting from renal and liver diseases, as well as from serious skin diseases such as atopic dermatitis. Nevertheless, these antihistamines often lack efficacy in such situations due to the fact that other receptors are involved in the itching process such as opioid receptors, or thermoreceptors (Tominaga and Takamori 2014).

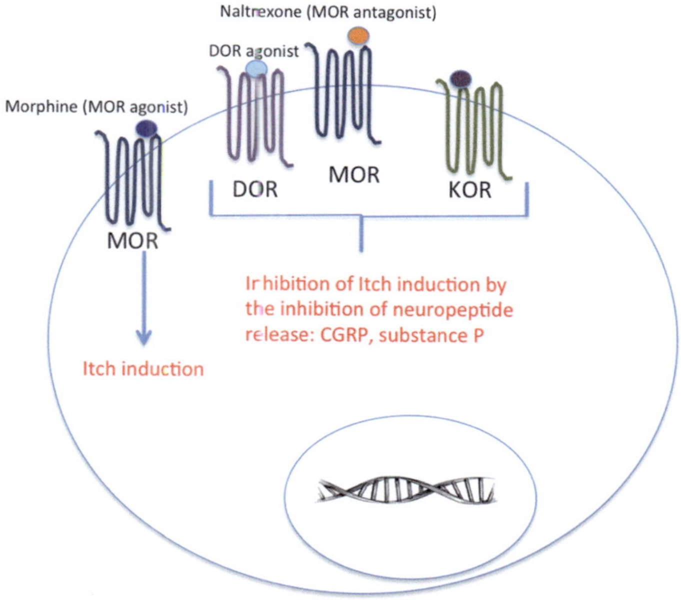

Fig. 13.2 Schematic representation of itching induction or inhibition by opioid receptors (MOR, DOR and KOR). MOR agonist induces itching sensation whereas MOR antagonist, DOR agonist and KOR agonist inhibit itching sensation. The mechanism of itching inhibition is due to a decrease in the release of neuropeptides such as CGRP and substance P

In this review, we will focus only on opioid receptors and itching. Indeed, itching is only mediated by μ opioid receptors (Ganesh and Maxwell 2007; Stander et al. 2002). In contrast to μ opioid agonists, κ opioid agonists and δ opioid agonists inhibit scratching. Nalfurafine (κ opioid agonist) has been shown to inhibit scratching in animal models (Schmelz 2009; Phan et al. 2012; Ko and Husbands 2009) and in patients suffering from uraemic pruritus. Nalfurafine is approved for the treatment of chronic pruritus in Japan. Opioids act by the inhibition of the release of inflammatory neuropeptides involved in itching such as substance P (SP) and calcitonine gene related peptide (CGRP) (Stander et al. 2002). This specificity is interesting as it has been shown that δ opioid receptors are not involved in itching sensations and that κ opioid receptor is a target for limiting itching, allowing their use in wound healing treatment or cosmetic indications such as anti-ageing or pigmentation control. In fact, ageing and pigmentation are two processes modulated by inflammation. Figure 13.2 is a summary of the mechanism of action of opioid receptors in itching mediation or repression.

13.2.3 Inflammation

Cutaneous inflammation is a consequence of trauma, metabolic dysfunction (diabetes), genetic disease (psoriasis) or infection. Because classical (steroids and nonsteroidal anti-inflammatory drugs) and non-classical (inhibitors of janus kinases or tumor necrosis factor) anti-inflammatory treatments currently used are either associated with side effects (cushing syndrome, intestinal ulcers, cardiac disease or potential tumor induction) or too expensive, the use of molecules interacting with opioid receptors could be considered as a relevant alternative. Indeed, it has been demonstrated that immune cells involving macrophages, lymphocytes and monocytes express opioid peptides (pro-opiomelanocortin POMC and beta endorphin) under inflammatory conditions (Busch-Dienstfertig and Stein 2010; Stein and Kuchler 2012; Sharp 2006). Consequently, the use of opioids or inhibitor of opioids degradation (Tominaga and Takamori 2014; Ganesh and Maxwell 2007) as potential anti-inflammatory molecules could be promising alternatives in anti-inflammatory drug discovery field (Stein and Kuchler 2013). Nevertheless, human studies confirming that opioid peptides and receptors have powerful effects in anti-inflammatory processes are lacking (Farley 2011; LeBon et al. 2009). Moreover, chronic inflammation is often associated with pathologies and ageing (Tabas and Glass 2013). As a consequence, targeting inflammation via opioid receptor activation could be very interesting as these receptors are also modulated with ageing.

13.3 Opioid Receptors and Cutaneous Tissue Wound Healing

Usually, tissue injury is followed by the acute inflammatory phase, the proliferation phase also called reepithelialisation phase, and the maturation phase. These 3 phases encompass wound-healing process. It has been demonstrated in several animals' studies that opioids topically applied on full thickness wound are able to help the healing process at different steps. Table 13.1 summarises, the observed effects of opioids topically applied on full thickness wound either in a normal or in a pathological wound-healing situation. Opioid molecules most used in wound healing animal studies were morphine and naltrexone (an exogenous antagonist ligand to μ and ζ opioid receptor). Recently, Bigliardi et al. have tested an antagonist molecule of the δ opioid receptor in normal and pathological wound mice model, naltrindole. They conclude that topically applied naltrindole stimulates wound healing, with a minimization of scarring. Likewise, the McLaughlin team has shown in non-diabetic and diabetic rats an improvement of wound closure after topical application of naltrexone. They confirmed an acceleration of re-epithelialization with less contracture (McLaughlin et al. 2011).

Interestingly, topical application of opioids improved only two phases in the wound healing process, the proliferative and maturation phases. In contrast, the initiation phase of wound healing seems to be delayed by the use of opioids suggesting that there is a specific time for their use in healing process. Chronic wounds observed in psoriatic, or atopic dermatitis, or diabetic patents characterized by a chronic impairment in wound healing process over express β endorphin,

Table 13.1 Summary of the roles described in literature for two opioid molecules (morphine and naltrexone) in the 3 phases of the wound healing process

Wound healing phases studied in animal models or in vitro	Biological phenomenon	Action of opioids	References
Inflammatory phase	Inflammatory cells infiltration: neutrophils, monocytes, eosinophils.	Morphine dose-dependently reduces the infiltration of neutrophils and morphine decreases local cytokines expression.	Clark et al. (2007)
	Pro-inflammatory neuropeptides secretion (substance P, tachykinin, neurokinin A release) and modulation of neurokinin receptor.	Morphine inhibits the peripheral release of neuropeptides. Morphine alters neurokinin receptor expression.	Rook and McCarson (2007, 2008, 2009)
Proliferative phase/reepithelialisation/granulation tissue formation	Keratinocyte migration and proliferation	Morphine stimulates keratinocytes migration and epithelialization. Dalargin (Opioid peptide) increases epithelialization.	Bigliardi-Qi and Bigliardi (2015) Shekhter et al. (1988) Kuchler et al. (2010)
	Collagen synthesis	Morphine enhances collagen synthesis. Naltrexone enhances collagen formation and maturation.	Immonen et al. (2013) Chang et al. (2010) Shekhter et al. (1988)
	Angiogenesis	Naltrexone stimulates angiogenesis.	Shekter et al. (1988)
	Fibroblasts migration, proliferation	Naltrexone stimulates fibroblasts migration.	Immonen et al. (2014)

(continued)

Table 13.1 (continued)

Wound healing phases studied in animal models or in vitro	Biological phenomenon	Action of opioids	References
		Naltrindole stimulates fibroblast migration in vitro	Bigliardi-Qi and Bigliardi (2015) Shekhter et al. (1988)
	FGF-2 and FGF-7	Naltrexone increases expression of FGF-2.	McLaughlin et al. (2013)
Maturation	Fibroblasts/Myofibroblasts	Naltrexone increases myofibroblats cells.	Rook et al. (2008) McLaughlin et al. (2013)

met-enkephalin and under-express μ opioid receptors (Bigliardi et al. 2003, 2009; Bigliardi-Qi et al. 2006). These observations are complementary to those describing an impairment of wound closure process observed in knock out mice model for δ and κ opioid receptors (Bigliardi-Qi et al. 2006; Neuman et al. 2015). Stimulation of keratinocytes migration by opioids from endogenous (Bigliardi et al. 2002, 2009; Bigliardi-Qi and Bigliardi 2015) or exogenous origins (Wolf et al. 2009; Charbaji et al. 2012) was reported in several studies, confirming this healing property. Moreover, it has been shown on fibroblasts cultured in vitro using wound scratching assay, a faster migration in presence of the DOR antagonist (naltrindole), and no effect with the agonist SNC80 (Bigliardi-Qi and Bigliardi 2015). These data suggest that there is an interaction between antagonist and agonist in the regulation of opioid receptors activities. These results suggest that selective antagonists of these receptors are promising targets to help wound healing process (Fig. 13.3).

The ζ opioid receptor is also an interesting target in wound healing strategies. Indeed, this receptor is directly connected to cell growth control by the regulation of p16 and p21 genes expression. The activation of this pathway stops the cell cycle by an active negative feedback (Fig. 13.4) and an up regulation of this receptor delays the wound healing process (McLaughlin et al. 2012). Naltrexone is an antagonist for ζ opioid receptor: inhibits the activation of opioid growth factor

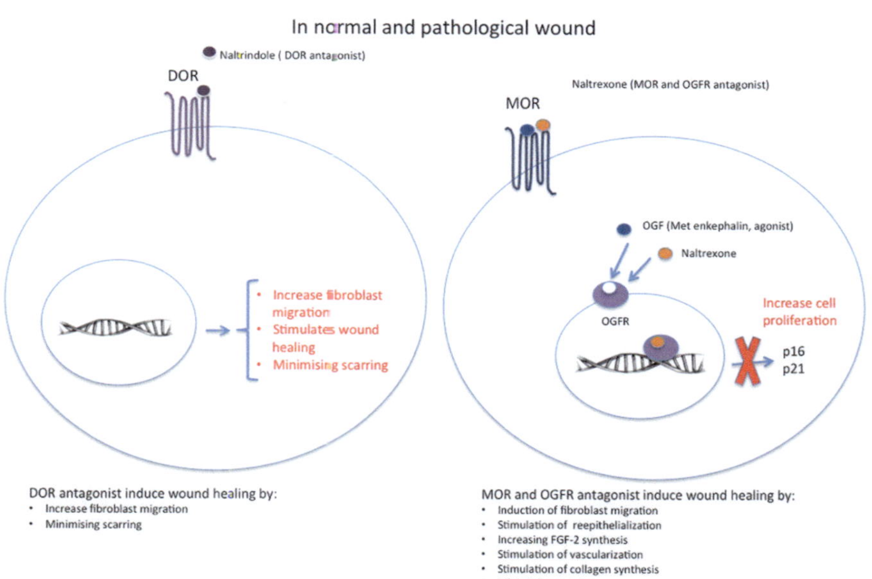

Fig. 13.3 Mechanism of action of antagonist molecules to opioid receptors in normal and pathological wound healing process. DOR antagonists help the wound healing process by increasing fibroblast migration, and no other effect has been demonstrated to date. MOR and OGFR antagonists induce fibroblast migration, epidermis re-epithelialization, promote vascularization and collagen synthesis. It is important to underline, when thinking about skin care, that all antagonists improve the aesthetic quality of the wound with fewer scars

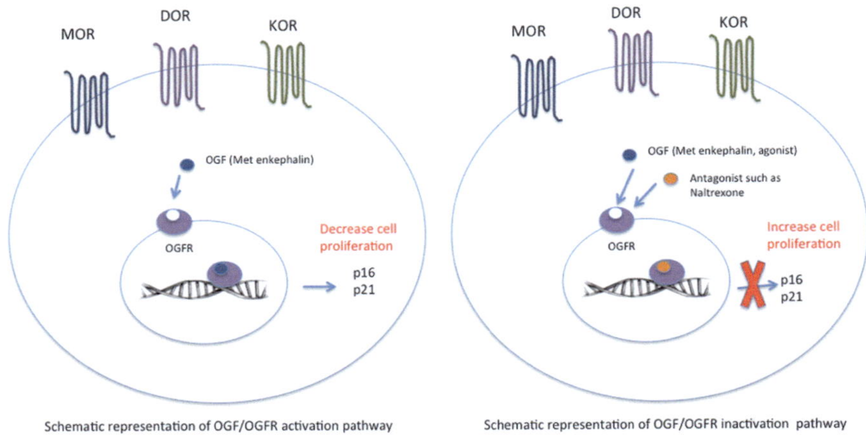

Fig. 13.4 Schematic representation of OGF/OGFR pathway: Once OGFR activated by its agonist OGF or [Met^5] enkephalin, the cell proliferation is decrease due to expression of p16 and p21 factors. In contrast, OGFR antagonist such as naltrexone competes with OGF molecule blocking this activation pathway, allowing cell proliferation

(OGF)-OGF receptor (OGFR) pathway (McLaughlin et al. 2011; McLaughlin and Zagon 2015), thus allowing the cell proliferation needed to repair the tissue.

All these data confirm the involvement of μ, κ, δ delta and ζ opioid receptors and their specific ligands in normal and abnormal wound healing process at different steps, revealing their promising use in wound healing therapies. In contrast, in hypertrophic scars, the over-expression of all opioid receptors was noticed (Cheng et al. 2008, 2011).

13.4 Opioid Receptors and Skin Homeostasis

The epidermis is a biological and physical barrier involved in the maintenance of skin homeostasis (Feingold and Elias 2014). Epidermis reacts to various external or internal insults such as ultraviolet irradiation, pollution, chemicals, infection, inflammation by more and more described system involving opioid receptors and their specific endogenous ligands (Slominski and Wortsman 2000; Slominski et al. 2012). The control of epidermis thickness by opioids receptors was demonstrated on knock-out animal models for μ, κ and δ opioid receptors (Bigliardi-Qi et al. 2007). We have published results showing for the first time, on inflammatory human reconstructed epidermises, a down regulation of δ opioid receptors, associated with epidermis barrier function deficiencies (Chajra et al. 2015). Interestingly the level of κ opioid receptor and its ligand dynorphin A were decreased in psoriatic epidermis in comparison to healthy skin (Taneda et al. 2011). Psoriatic skin is an inflammatory skin with known barrier function deficiencies. Under inflammatory conditions, beta-endorphin expression (endogenous ligand to μ opioid receptor,

Glinski et al. 1994) was increased leading to down regulation of μ opioid receptor associated with an increase of cytokeratin 16 expression a marker of psoriatic differentiation (Bigliardi-Qi et al. 2000). The down regulation of μ opioid receptor seen in this work is probably also due to oct-1 expression (Wei and Loh 2011). Beta-endorphin is produced in epidermis but also in dermis after a stress such as UVB irradiation (Skobowiat et al. 2013). Proenkephalin (PENK, endogenous ligand of δ opioid receptor) was also stimulated under UV irradiation (Slominski et al. 2011). Proenkephalin is required, for apoptosis induction, in response to activation or over-expression of p53 and nuclear factor κ B (NF-κB). The apoptosis is a necessary mechanism for the maintenance of epidermis homeostasis and to trigger an anti-tumor response (McTavish et al. 2007). Morphine gets also a potent cyto-protective effects for oral epithelial cells against irradiation. So it could be possible to extend this property to other opioids ligands. Our findings demonstrate also that Rubixyl™ (δ opioid agonist) topically applied on inflammatory epidermis maintains the expression of δ opioid receptor (or blocks its internalization) (Chajra et al. 2015). They also show that it restores barrier function by the stimulation of epidermis differentiation markers. Expression of δ opioid receptor is up-regulated either by an agonist such as Rubixyl™ or SNC-80 or by antagonist such as naltrindole (Bigliardi team's patent). McLaughlin and Zagon (2012) introduced the principle of a local axis of opioid growth factor OGF receptor (Fig. 13.4), acting also as a homeostatic regulator of the epidermis. Proliferation and differentiation of keratinocytes required in maintenance of epidermis homeostasis are tightly regulated by cellular transcription factors, including activator protein-1 (AP-1), nuclear factor-κB proteins and POU (Pit-Oct-Unc) transcription factors. Three POU transcription factors (Oct-1, Oct-6, and Skn-1a) are expressed in the epidermis. Wei and Loh (2002, 2011) demonstrated that opioid receptors are transcriptionally regulated by proliferation and differentiation factors. For example, oct-1 down- regulates MOR expression and AP-1 induces DOR expression, confirming its major role in cell differentiation. c-Myc (a transcription factor coded by Myc gene) induces KOR expression, whereas nuclear factor-κB induces MOR and DOR expression (Wei and Loh 2011). Interestingly, it has been demonstrated that an agonist of δ opioid receptor down regulates also skn-1a expression (Skn-1a also known as POU2F3), helping the differentiation process as confirmed by keratin 10 expression. δ opioid receptors modulate also keratinocyte proliferation and differentiation (Neumann et al. 2015) via the activation of mitogen-activated protein kinase (MAPK) pathway. It was found that Skn-1a was over-expressed in psoriasis skin in comparison to normal skin, justifying the undifferentiated and proliferative phenotypes observed in psoriatic keratinocytes (Takemoto et al. 2010). In cell such as macrophages, monocytes, fibroblasts, keratinocytes, opioid receptors involved also MAPK pathway ERK1/2 (Neumann et al. 2015; Jordan et al. 2000) or Phospholipase C pathways (Moore et al. 2007; Zollner and Stein 2007). Once activated MAPK pathway ERK1/2 in turn activates several proteins such as c-fos, c-jun, c-myc, or stat3. ERK1/2 is able to modulate cell proliferation or differentiation (Sharp 2006).

In conclusion, μ, δ, and κ opioids receptors expression is modulated by transcription factors expressed in normal or in pathologic conditions (such as AP-1, nuclear factor-κB, c-Myc). Finally, all opioids receptors (μ, δ, κ and ζ) are crucial in the control of skin homeostasis in normal or pathological conditions because they are either directly regulated by major transcription factors or because they regulate also major cell signalling pathways.

13.5 Opioid Receptors and Skin Ageing

Opioid receptors and especially δ opioid receptors could be beneficial targets in anti-ageing strategies for skin cosmetic purposes. Indeed, it has been demonstrated that a negative correlation exists between signs of aging (aged spots, wrinkles) and DOR expression, with in particular DOR mRNA expression being decreased in intrinsic ageing. It has been shown in vitro that melanocytes are impacted by DOR modulation. Furthermore, an agonist of δ opioid receptor, naltrindole, upregulates mRNA DOR expression. The interest of δ opioid ligand in skin anti-ageing cosmetic field was confirmed by our research (Chajra et al. 2015) done in a double blind clinical study performed on human volunteers showing clinical signs of ageing (periocular and perilabial wrinkles). It is concluded that Rubixyl™ induces a significant decrease in wrinkle depth. It must nevertheless be underlined that Rubixyl™ is an agonist, whereas naltrindole is an antagonist for δ opioid receptors. Both ligands have positive effects in anti-ageing strategies but the mechanism underlying their efficacy is not clear. Rubixyl™ probably acts by inhibiting the internalization of DOR whereas naltrindole acts by increasing DOR expression.

13.6 Conclusion

This chapter demonstrates that all cutaneous opioid receptors (δ, κ, μ and ζ) are involved in many biological situations such as skin sensations (pain, itching, and inflammation), wound healing, skin homeostasis and skin ageing. This review shows that opioid receptors ligands are very promising molecules for cosmetic or medical applications. Nevertheless, the ideal molecule doesn't exist and probably the need of a combination of opioid receptors ligands (agonist and antagonists) could be the best solution. The future development of efficient cosmetic or medical treatment should be based on the understanding of the molecular mechanism of action of each opioid receptor associated either with its agonist or antagonist ligand, and triggering fewer drawbacks such as scratching.

References

Arck PC, Slominski A, Theoharides TC, Peters EM, Paus R (2006) Neuroimmunology of stress: skin takes center stage. J Invest Dermatol 126(8):1697–1704

Bigliardi PL, Bigliardi-Qi M, Buechner S, Rufli T (1998) Expression of mu-opiate receptor in human epidermis and keratinocytes. J Invest Dermatol 111(2):297–301

Bigliardi PL, Buchner S, Rufli T, Bigliardi-Qi M (2002) Specific stimulation of migration of human keratinocytes by mu-opiate receptor agonists. J Recept Signal Transduction Res 22 (1–4):191–199

Bigliardi PL, Sumanovski LT, Buchner S, Rufli T, Bigliardi-Qi M (2003) Different expression of mu-opiate receptor in chronic and acute wounds and the effect of beta-endorphin on transforming growth factor beta type II receptor and cytokeratin 16 expression. J Invest Dermatol 120(1):145–152

Bigliardi PL, Tobin DJ, Gaveriaux-Ruff C, Bigliardi-Qi M (2009) Opioids and the skin—where do we stand? Exp Dermatol 18(5):424–430

Bigliardi-Qi M, Bigliardi PL (2015) The role of opioid receptors in migration and wound recovery in vitro in cultured human keratinocytes and fibroblasts. Methods Mol Biol 1230:273–277

Bigliardi-Qi M, Bigliardi PL, Eberle AN, Buchner S, Rufli T (2000) beta-endorphin stimulates cytokeratin 16 expression and downregulates mu-opiate receptor expression in human epidermis. J Invest Dermatol 114(3):527–532

Bigliardi-Qi M, Gaveriaux-Ruff C, Zhou H et al (2006) Deletion of delta-opioid receptor in mice alters skin differentiation and delays wound healing. Differ Res Biol Diversity 74(4):174–185

Bigliardi-Qi M, Gaveriaux-Ruff C, Pfaltz K et al (2007) Deletion of mu- and kappa-opioid receptors in mice changes epidermal hypertrophy, density of peripheral nerve endings, and itch behavior. J Invest Dermatol 127(6):1479–1488

Busch-Dienstfertig M, Stein C (2010) Opioid receptors and opioid peptide-producing leukocytes in inflammatory pain–basic and therapeutic aspects. Brain Behav Immun 24(5):683–694

Chajra H, Amstutz B, Schweikert K, Auriol D, Redziniak G, Lefevre F (2015) Opioid receptor delta as a global modulator of skin differentiation and barrier function repair. Int J Cosmet Sci 37:386–394

Chang PJ, Chen MY, Huang YS et al (2010) Morphine enhances tissue content of collagen and increases wound tensile strength. J Anesth 24(2):240–246

Charbaji N, Schafer-Korting M, Kuchler S (2012) Morphine stimulates cell migration of oral epithelial cells by delta-opioid receptor activation. PLoS ONE 7(8):e42616

Cheng B, Liu HW, Fu XB, Sheng ZY, Li JF (2008) Coexistence and upregulation of three types of opioid receptors, mu, delta and kappa, in human hypertrophic scars. Br J Dermatol 158(4): 713–720

Cheng B, Liu HW, Fu XB (2011) Update on pruritic mechanisms of hypertrophic scars in postburn patients: the potential role of opioids and their receptors. J Burn Care Res: Official Publ Am Burn Assoc 32(4):e118–e125

Clark JD, Shi X, Li X et al (2007) Morphine reduces local cytokine expression and neutrophil infiltration after incision. Mol Pain 3:28

Farley P (2011) Should topical opioid analgesics be regarded as effective and safe when applied to chronic cutaneous lesions? J Pharm Pharmacol 63(6):747–756

Feingold K, Elias P (2014) The important role of lipids in the epidermis and their role in the formation and maintenance of the cutaneous barrier. Biochim Biophys Acta 1841(3):279

Ganesh A, Maxwell LG (2007) Pathophysiology and management of opioid-induced pruritus. Drugs 67(16):2323–2333

Glinski W, Brodecka H, Glinska-Ferenz M, Kowalski D (1994) Increased concentration of beta-endorphin in sera of patients with psoriasis and other inflammatory dermatoses. Br J Dermatol 131(2):260–264

Hughes J, Kosterlitz HW, Smith TW (1997) The distribution of methionine-enkephalin and leucine-enkephalin in the brain and peripheral tissues. Br J Pharmacol 120(4 Suppl):428–436 (discussion 426–427)
Immonen JA, Zagon IS, Lewis GS, McLaughlin PJ (2013) Topical treatment with the opioid antagonist naltrexone accelerates the remodeling phase of full-thickness wound healing in type 1 diabetic rats. Exp Biol Med 238(10):1127–1135
Immonen JA, Zagon IS, McLaughlin PJ (2014) Selective blockade of the OGF-OGFr pathway by naltrexone accelerates fibroblast proliferation and wound healing. Exp Biol Med 239(10): 1300–1309
Jordan B, Devi LA (1998) Molecular mechanisms of opioid receptor signal transduction. Br J Anaesth 81(1):12–19
Jordan BA, Cvejic S, Devi LA (2000) Kappa opioid receptor endocytosis by dynorphin peptides. DNA Cell Biol 19(1):19–27
Kitzmiller JP, Barnett CJ, Steiner NS et al (2015) Buprenorphine: revisiting the efficacy of transdermal delivery system. Ther Deliv 6(4):419–422
Ko MC, Husbands SM (2009) Effects of atypical kappa-opioid receptor agonists on intrathecal morphine-induced itch and analgesia in primates. J Pharmacol Exp Ther 328(1):193–200
Kornick CA, Santiago-Palma J, Moryl N, Payne R, Obbens EA (2003) Benefit-risk assessment of transdermal fentanyl for the treatment of chronic pain. Drug Saf 26(13):951–973
Kuchler S, Wolf NB, Heilmann S et al (2010) 3D-wound healing model: influence of morphine and solid lipid nanoparticles. J Biotechnol 148(1):24–30
LeBon B, Zeppetella G, Higginson IJ (2009) Effectiveness of topical administration of opioids in palliative care: a systematic review. J Pain Symptom Manage 37(5):913–917
Luo J, Feng J, Liu S, Walters ET, Hu H (2015) Molecular and cellular mechanisms that initiate pain and itch. Cell Mol Life Sci CMLS 72(17):3201–3223
McLaughlin PJ, Zagon IS (2012) The opioid growth factor-opioid growth factor receptor axis: homeostatic regulator of cell proliferation and its implications for health and disease. Biochem Pharmacol 84(6):746–755
McLaughlin PJ, Zagon IS (2015) Duration of opioid receptor blockade determines biotherapeutic response. Biochem Pharmacol 97(3):236–246
McLaughlin PJ, Pothering CA, Immonen JA, Zagon IS (2011) Topical treatment with the opioid antagonist naltrexone facilitates closure of full-thickness wounds in diabetic rats. Exp Biol Med 236(10):1122–1132
McLaughlin PJ, Keiper CL, Verderame MF, Zagon IS (2012) Targeted overexpression of OGFr in epithelium of transgenic mice suppresses cell proliferation and impairs full-thickness wound closure. Am J Physiol Regul Integr Comp Physiol 302(9):R1084–R1090
McLaughlin PJ, Immonen JA, Zagon IS (2013) Topical naltrexone accelerates full-thickness wound closure in type 1 diabetic rats by stimulating angiogenesis. Exp Biol Med 238(7): 733–743
McTavish N, Copeland LA, Saville MK, Perkins ND, Spruce BA (2007) Proenkephalin assists stress-activated apoptosis through transcriptional repression of NF-kappaB- and p53-regulated gene targets. Cell Death Differ 14(9):1700–1710
Moore CA, Milano SK, Benovic JL (2007) Regulation of receptor trafficking by GRKs and arrestins. Annu Rev Physiol 69:451–482
Muijsers RB, Wagstaff AJ (2001) Transdermal fentanyl: an updated review of its pharmacological properties and therapeutic efficacy in chronic cancer pain control. Drugs 61(15):2289–2307
Neumann C, Bigliardi-Qi M, Widmann C, Bigliardi PL (2015) The delta-opioid receptor affects epidermal homeostasis via ERK-dependent inhibition of transcription factor POU2F3. J Invest Dermatol 135(2):471–480
Nissen JB, Kragballe K (1997) Enkephalins modulate differentiation of normal human keratinocytes in vitro. Exp Dermatol 6(5):222–229
Phan NQ, Lotts T, Antal A, Bernhard JD, Stander S (2012) Systemic kappa opioid receptor agonists in the treatment of chronic pruritus: a literature review. Acta Derm-Venereol 92(5):555–560

Podolsky AT, Sandweiss A, Hu J et al (2013) Novel fentanyl-based dual mu/delta-opioid agonists for the treatment of acute and chronic pain. Life Sci 93(25–26):1010–1016
Rook JM, McCarson KE (2007) Delay of cutaneous wound closure by morphine via local blockade of peripheral tachykinin release. Biochem Pharmacol 74(5):752–757
Rook JM, Hasan W, McCarson KE (2008) Temporal effects of topical morphine application on cutaneous wound healing. Anesthesiology 109(1):130–136
Rook JM, Hasan W, McCarson KE (2009) Morphine-induced early delays in wound closure: involvement of sensory neuropeptides and modification of neurokinin receptor expression. Biochem Pharmacol 77(11):1747–1755
Roosterman D, Goerge T, Schneider SW, Bunnett NW, Steinhoff M (2006) Neuronal control of skin function: the skin as a neuroimmunoendocrine organ. Physiol Rev 86(4):1309–1379
Salemi S, Aeschlimann A, Reisch N et al (2005) Detection of kappa and delta opioid receptors in skin–outside the nervous system. Biochem Biophys Res Commun. 338(2):1012–1017
Schmelz M (2009) Opioid-induced pruritus. Mechanisms and treatment regimens. Der Anaesthesist 58(1):61–65
Sharp BM (2006) Multiple opioid receptors on immune cells modulate intracellular signaling. Brain Behav Immun 20(1):9–14
Shekhter AB, Solov'eva AI, Spevak SE, Titov MI (1988) Effects of opioid peptide dalargin on reparative processes in wound healing. Biulleten' eksperimental'noi biologii i meditsiny 106(10):487–490
Skobowiat C, Dowdy JC, Sayre RM, Tuckey RC, Slominski A (2011) Cutaneous hypothalamic-pituitary-adrenal axis homolog: regulation by ultraviolet radiation. Am J Physiol Endocrinol Metab 301(3):E484–E493
Skobowiat C, Nejati R, Lu L, Williams RW, Slominski AT (2013) Genetic variation of the cutaneous HPA axis: an analysis of UVB-induced differential responses. Gene 530(1):1–7
Slominski AT (2013) Beta-endorphin/mu-opiate receptor system in the skin. J Invest Dermatol 120(6):xii–xiii
Slominski AT, Wortsman J (2000) Neuroendocrinology of the skin. Endocr Rev 21(5):457–487
Slominski AT, Mazurkiewicz J, Baker J, Wortsman J (1998) Characterization of corticotropin-releasing hormone (CRH) in human skin. J Clin Endocrinol Metab 83(3):1020–1024
Slominski AT, Zmijewski MA, Zbytek B et al (2011) Regulated proenkephalin expression in human skin and cultured skin cells. J Invest Dermatol 131(3):613–622
Slominski AT, Zmijewski MA, Skobowiat C, Zbytek B, Slominski RM, Steketee JD (2012) Sensing the environment: regulation of local and global homeostasis by the skin's neuroendocrine system. Adv Anat Embryol Cell Biol 212:v, vii, 1–115
Stander S, Gunzer M, Metze D, Luger T, Steinhoff M (2002) Localization of mu-opioid receptor 1A on sensory nerve fibers in human skin. Regul Pept 110(1):75–83
Stein C, Kuchler S (2012) Non-analgesic effects of opioids: peripheral opioid effects on inflammation and wound healing. Curr Pharm Des 18(37):6053–6069
Stein C, Kuchler S (2013) Targeting inflammation and wound healing by opioids. Trends Pharmacol Sci 34(6):303–312
Tabas I, Glass CK (2013) Anti-inflammatory therapy in chronic disease: challenges and opportunities. Science 339(6116):166–172
Tachibana T, Nawa T (2005) Immunohistochemical reactions of receptors to met-enkephalin, VIP, substance P, and CGRP located on Merkel cells in the rat sinus hair follicle. Arch Histol Cytol 68(5):383–391
Takemoto H, Tamai K, Akasaka E et al (2010) Relation between the expression levels of the POU transcription factors Skn-1a and Skn-1n and keratinocyte differentiation. J Dermatol Sci 60 (3):203–205
Taneda K, Tominaga M, Negi O et al (2011) Evaluation of epidermal nerve density and opioid receptor levels in psoriatic itch. Br J Dermatol 165(2):277–284
Tominaga M, Takamori K (2014) Sensitization of itch signaling: itch sensitization-nerve growth factor, semaphorins itch: mechanisms and treatment. Taylor & Francis Group, LLC., Boca Raton

Trescot AM, Datta S, Lee M, Hansen H (2008) Opioid pharmacology. Pain Phys 11(2 Suppl): S133–S153
Watterson G, Howard R, Goldman A (2004) Peripheral opioids in inflammatory pain. Arch Dis Child 89(7):679–681
Wei LN, Loh HH (2002) Regulation of opioid receptor expression. Curr Opin Pharmacol 2(1): 69–75
Wei LN, Loh HH (2011) Transcriptional and epigenetic regulation of opioid receptor genes: present and future. Annu Rev Pharmacol Toxicol 51:75–97
Wolf NB, Kuchler S, Radowski MR et al (2009) Influences of opioids and nanoparticles on in vitro wound healing models. Eur J Pharm Biopharm: Official J Arbeitsgemeinschaft fur Pharmazeutische Verfahrenstechnik e.V. 73(1):34–42
Zagon IS, Donahue RN, McLaughlin PJ (2009) Opioid growth factor-opioid growth factor receptor axis is a physiological determinant of cell proliferation in diverse human cancers. Am J Physiol Regul Integr Comp Physiol 297(4):R1154–R1161
Zollner C, Stein C (2007) Opioids. Handb Exp Pharmacol 177:31–63

Chapter 14
Regulation of Cutaneous Stress Response Pathways by the Circadian Clock: From Molecular Pathways to Therapeutic Opportunities

Elyse van Spyk, Milton Greenberg, Faraj Mourad and Bogi Andersen

Abstract The skin is a protective barrier that defends against harmful environmental stressors such as solar radiation, chemical toxins, and pathogenic microbes. Our environment is highly dynamic, with robust time-of-day dependent fluctuations in temperature, solar radiation, and probability of injury and infections. In addition, oxidative metabolism and cell-cycle progression in epidermal stem cells show prominent diurnal rhythms. Accumulating evidence suggests that the skin's circadian clock optimizes its physiology to meet the demands of this changing environment. The responsiveness of the skin to external stressors such as UVB radiation from the sun, and toxic pollutants, is regulated in a circadian manner on multiple levels. Furthermore, the robustness of inflammatory responses following injury, infections, exposure to allergens, pollutants, and drugs is dependent on the time of day in which exposure occurs. The diurnal variation in the responsiveness to external stressors may be important for skin integrity and organismal health. We speculate that such circadian gating may be important as constitutively high activation of stress response pathways could be deleterious for health; for example constant high activity of the immune system could contribute to the development of autoimmune diseases.

Keywords Circadian clock · Skin · Stem cells · Stress response · UV exposure · Reactive oxygen species · DNA damage · Antioxidants · Immunity · Aging · Cell cycle · Autoimmune disease

E. van Spyk · B. Andersen (✉)
Department of Biological Chemistry, University of California, Irvine 92697, CA, USA
e-mail: bogi@uci.edu

M. Greenberg
Schmid College of Science and Technology, Chapman University, Orange 92866, CA, USA

F. Mourad · B. Andersen
Department of Medicine, Division of Endocrinology, School of Medicine,
University of California, Irvine, CA 92697, USA

G.T. Wondrak (ed.), *Skin Stress Response Pathways*,
DOI 10.1007/978-3-319-43157-4_14

14.1 The Circadian Clock and the Skin Stress Response

As a forefront barrier between us and the environment, the skin is exposed to externally-derived insults, including ultraviolet B (UVB) radiation, toxic chemicals, and pathogenic microbes. Within epidermal stem and progenitor cells, desynchronization of oxidative/reductive metabolism and cellular division may facilitate genomic damage, apoptosis and proteolysis, resulting in skin ageing and/or cancer (Sancar et al. 2015; Plikus et al. 2015; Wilking et al. 2013; Stringari et al. 2015; Pluquet et al. 2014). These external insults and perturbations in homeostasis activate the skin's stress response pathways, triggering diverse activities such as DNA damage repair, reactive oxygen species (ROS) extermination, and immune modulation (Valacchi et al. 2012).

The body-autonomous circadian clock harmonizes an organism's physiology with the daily light/dark cycle caused by the earth's rotation. Numerous physiological processes, including organismal metabolism and the sleep-wake cycle, are directly or indirectly regulated by an organism's circadian rhythm. The clock is an evolutionarily conserved mechanism—all phyla possess an internal clock with a period of approximately 24 h—indicating that the clock optimizes fitness and survival. While earlier studies assumed that the circadian clock was a property of the suprachiasmatic nucleus (SCN) only, work in the 1990s showed that most, if not all, cells of the body have active clocks (reviewed in Mohawk et al. 2012; Dibner et al. 2010). Consistent with this idea, more recent work has demonstrated the existence of a skin circadian clock (Lin et al. 2009; Tanioka et al. 2009) with important roles in skin biology (reviewed in Plikus et al. 2015). In addition to functional experiments in genetically modified mice, epidemiological research has illustrated the importance of the circadian clock in promoting human fitness. Disturbed circadian rhythms caused by abnormal lighting schedules, sleep deprivation, and aberrant feeding times are thought to promote maladaptation and pathologies ranging from cancer to metabolic diseases, as well as early ageing (Sancar et al. 2015; Pluquet et al. 2014; Wilking et al. 2013; Kondratov et al. 2006; Sigurdardottir et al. 2012; Armstrong et al. 2013; Lengyel et al. 2013; Libert et al. 2012).

Exposure to many external insults, including solar radiation and endogenous cellular stresses, is highly diurnal. Therefore, it is reasonable to propose a stress response role for the circadian clock, an ancient system that has evolved to better adapt to environmental changes over the day. In this chapter we will highlight studies supporting this notion. While there is strong evidence supporting the role of the circadian clock in modulating certain stress response pathways in the skin, the clock's involvement in other stress-activated pathways is more speculative. In addition to outlining this evidence, we also discuss therapeutic implications of the skin circadian clock, and how dysregulation of clock mechanisms through altered sleep, eating and/or light exposure may impair the skin's capacity to cope with external stressors.

14.2 Structure of the Skin

In the skin, several different cell types cooperate to maintain homeostasis in the face of an ever-changing environment and external stressors. The epidermis, the surface epithelium of the skin, is separated from the underlying dermis by a basement membrane (Fig. 14.1). At the base of the epidermis, epidermal progenitor/stem cells divide and give rise to post-mitotic keratinocytes which migrate upwards as they differentiate and start expressing structural proteins, adhesion molecules, and lipid-producing enzymes, all required for the formation of an effective epidermal barrier. At the top of the epidermis, these cells lose their nucleus, forming the outermost layer of the epidermis, the stratum corneum, a layer of cells with heavily crosslinked protein/lipid structure sealed with lipids. The epidermis also contains melanocytes that transfer melanin to keratinocytes, an important mechanism countering UVB-induced DNA damage.

Below the epidermis resides the dermis, composed mainly of fibroblasts, adipocytes, and leukocytes. Fibroblasts secrete extracellular matrix components that support the tensile strength of the skin, while adipocytes store energy and leukocytes contribute to pathogen clearance; leukocytes will be discussed later in the chapter. The dermis is divided into two layers, the papillary layer abutting the epidermis, and the reticular layer residing deeper under the papillary layer. Epidermal appendages extending into the dermis include hair follicles, sebaceous glands, and sweat glands. In addition, the dermis is richly innervated and vascularized.

The skin contains numerous hematopoietic cell types that contribute to inflammatory responses and the barrier role of the skin (Pasparakis et al. 2014). Under homeostasis, Langerhans cells (LC) in the epidermis sample pathogens in the environment through dendritic projections, and epidermal T cells help maintain epithelial integrity, and protect against the development of cutaneous malignancies (Girardi et al. 2001; Sumaria et al. 2011). Upon skin infection or damage, both LCs and dermal dendritic cells (DDCs) phagocytose and present antigens to T cells, enabling adaptive immune responses. In addition, the skin's microbiome composition is highly complex and dynamic. Changes in signals from the skin commensal microorganisms remodel the skin immune landscape with potential implications for skin immunity and pathologies (Naik et al. 2015). While the microbiome composition is known to vary in a circadian manner in the gut epithelium (Zarrinpar et al. 2014), diurnal variations in microbial populations in the skin and their effects on host defense, homeostasis, and chronic disease have not been extensively explored.

14.3 The Circadian Clock

14.3.1 The Circadian Clock at an Organismal Level

The circadian clock, a cell-intrinsic transcriptional network that is present in most, if not all, cells of the body, coordinates the organism's physiology with the

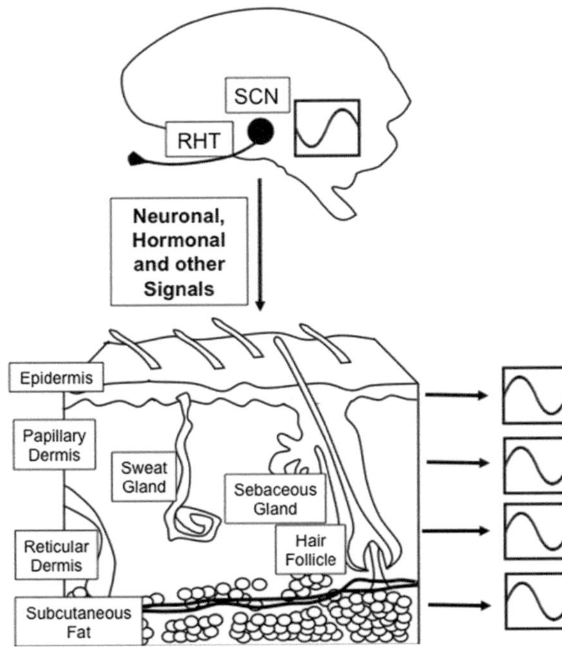

Fig. 14.1 Organization of the skin circadian clock. Light input is received in the ganglion neurons in the retina, and signals are sent to the suprachiasmatic nucleus (SCN) in the hypothalamus via the retinohypothalamic tract (RHT). The SCN then transmits signals through neuronal efferents and hormonal pathways to other organ of the body, including the skin. These SCN-derived signals coordinate the circadian phase of different cell types in the skin

day-night cycle. In vertebrates, the central circadian clock is located in the SCN of the hypothalamus. While this clock is highly autonomous, its phase is primarily set by light input that activates ganglionic cells in the retina, which in turn send signals through the retinohypothalamic tract (RHT) to the SCN. The SCN, composed of 15–20,000 neurons, acts as the central pacemaker by synchronizing the clocks in peripheral organs, presumably through neuronal and hormonal pathways (Reppert and Weaver 2002) (Fig. 14.1). Light input signaling to the SCN is not the only stimulus that can entrain the peripheral clocks as physical activity, timing of food intake, and the metabolic state have been shown to affect the rhythm of the circadian clock in the peripheral organs independent of the rhythm produced by the SCN (Brown et al. 2002; Dibner et al. 2010). Work in recent years has established a role for peripheral clocks in most organs where about 10–20 % of the genome exhibits diurnal change in expression. The diurnal transcriptome in each organ is relatively unique and often composed of genes that confer functions prototypical for each organ (Mohawk et al. 2012; Geyfman et al. 2012).

14.3.2 Molecular Mechanism of the Clock

The molecular clock is driven by the rhythmic transcriptional activity of two transcription factors, Circadian Locomotor Output Cycles Kaput (CLOCK) and Brain and Muscle Arylhydrocarbon Receptor Nuclear Translocator-Like 1 (BMAL1). CLOCK

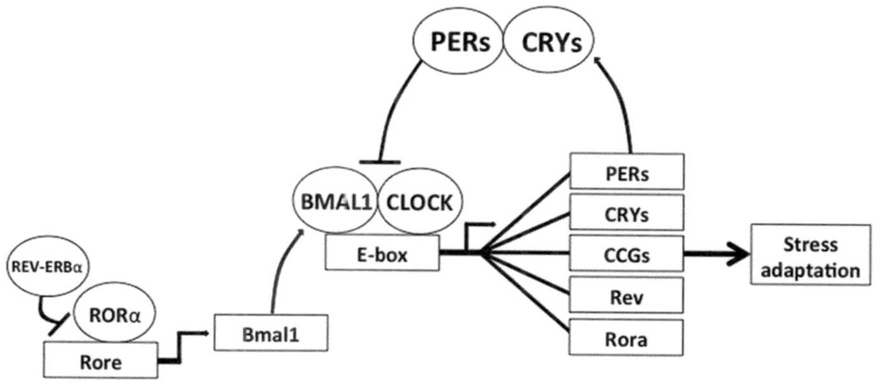

Fig. 14.2 The molecular mechanism of the clock. CLOCK and BMAL1 form a heterodimer that initiates transcription of multiple genes through binding to E-box sequences in target gene promoters. An autoregulatory feedback loop is created, as BMAL1 and CLOCK promote the transcription of their own inhibitors (Per1/2/3 and Cry1/2). Furthermore, CLOCK:BMAL1 promotes the transcription of RORα and REV-ERBα which induce and repress, respectively, BMAL1 expression. Other CLOCK:BMAL1 target genes encode for critical functions in peripheral organs, including genes regulating the response to stressors. CCGs, Clock-controlled genes

and BMAL1 form a heterodimer via their respective PAS domains and bind to E-box sequences in gene promoters, activating the expression of clock-controlled genes (CCGs) (reviewed in Buhr and Takahashi 2013; Mohawk et al. 2012). Among the CCGs, are genes encoding repressors of the CLOCK:BMAL1 complex, including *Period 1, Period 2, Period 3* (*PER1/2/3*), *Cryptochrome 1* and *Cryptochrome 2* (*CRY1/2*). PER1/2/3 and CRY1/2 accumulate in the cytoplasm and then return to the nucleus to form heterodimers that inhibit the activity of CLOCK:BMAL1 on E boxes in the promoters of target genes, thus inhibiting their own expression. The duration of this loop of CLOCK:BMAL1-mediated transcriptional activation followed by inhibition by PER1/2/3:CRY1/2 heterodimers is approximately 24 h, resulting in the rhythmic expression of CCGs. This rhythmicity is further sustained by an auxiliary loop whereby CCGs RORα/ß/γ and REV-ERBα activate and inhibit, respectively, *Bmal1* gene expression (Preitner et al. 2002) (Fig. 14.2). In addition, post-transcriptional mechanisms controlling the stability of clock proteins play important roles in the circadian clock; for a more thorough review, see (Mohawk et al. 2012).

14.3.3 The Circadian Clock in the Skin

Like other peripheral organs, the skin possesses an intrinsic circadian clock that is entrained by signals originating from the core clock in the SCN (Lin et al. 2009; Tanioka et al. 2009; Geyfman et al. 2012; Plikus et al. 2013). Based on studies in other organs, it has been assumed that the skin clock in mice develops rhythmicity within the first month of life (Sladek et al. 2004; Ansari et al. 2009). While the skin clock maintains rhythmicity in the absence of light input, the rhythms depend on an intact SCN (Tanioka et al. 2009). How the SCN transmits its signals to the skin clock has not been established although it is assumed that both hormonal and neuronal signals are important. The circadian clock seems to be active throughout the skin, but particularly robust clock output has been noted in quiescent bulge stem cells, the hair matrix, the dermal papillae, the interfollicular epidermis, and the secondary hair germ (Lin et al. 2009; Plikus et al. 2013; Janich et al. 2011). The circadian clock in the skin is important for skin physiology; *Bmal1*-deleted (*Bmal1*$^{-/-}$) mice have many skin-related pathologies including delayed wound healing (Kowalska et al. 2013), cellular senescence (Kondratov et al. 2006; Khapre et al. 2011), and delayed hair regrowth (Kondratov et al. 2006).

14.4 Role of the Circadian Clock in the Skin's Response to Endogenous and External Stressors

14.4.1 Circadian Regulation of Cellular Metabolism and the Cell Cycle

Skin, similar to gastrointestinal epithelium and bone marrow, requires high levels of progenitor cell proliferation for its maintenance. In mice, the fraction of epidermal progenitors in S-phase is higher during the night than during the day; this is opposite to the phase in human skin, which exhibits peak S-phase during the day (Brown 1991; Clausen et al. 1979; Geyfman et al. 2012; reviewed in Bjarnason and Jordan 2002). The rhythmic cell proliferation is controlled by the circadian clock as circadian knockout mice have a constant fraction of epidermal progenitor cells in S-phase over the day (Geyfman et al. 2012; Plikus et al. 2013; Gaddameedhi et al. 2011). While the function of the prominent diurnal variation in cellular proliferation remains unknown, it is proposed that the circadian clock may have evolved to coordinate the phases of different cellular processes (Jouffe et al. 2013; Geyfman et al. 2012; Panda et al. 2002; Gillette and Sejnowski 2005). For epidermal stem cells, the clock's function may be to synchronize the cell cycle with intermediary metabolism, thus minimizing cellular damage from ROS created through oxidative phosphorylation (Stringari et al. 2015). This idea is supported by a recent study in which diurnal metabolic oscillations in the ratio of bound to free NADH (indicative of the balance between oxidative phosphorylation and glycolysis) in stem cells of the interfollicular epidermis were measured by fluorescence lifetime imaging (Stringari et al. 2015). It was found that oxidative phosphorylation was anti-phasic to the rhythm of S-phase, and that diurnal metabolic oscillations and rhythms of proliferation in skin progenitors were abolished, becoming constitutively upregulated in the absence of the clock. These findings are corroborated by previous studies in *Bmal1*$^{-/-}$ mice showing that they have elevated levels of ROS (Stringari et al. 2015; Geyfman et al. 2012). High ROS levels present during S-phase might contribute to the deleterious phenotypes seen in circadian knockout mice including reduced lifespans (Libert et al. 2012) and various symptoms of premature aging (Kowalska et al. 2013; Kondratov et al. 2006; Khapre et al. 2011). The involvement of elevated ROS in the premature aging phenotypes of *Bmal1*$^{-/-}$ mice is supported by a study showing that antioxidants could assuage the age-dependent weight loss and development of cataracts typically seen in *Bmal1*$^{-/-}$ mice (Kondratov et al. 2009). Interestingly, some of the aging phenotypes in *Bmal1*$^{-/-}$ mice, including the hair regrowth defect, require *Bmal1* to be ablated early in development before the clock machinery has matured, suggesting a potential non-circadian role of BMAL1 during development (Yang et al. 2016).

Apart from its detrimental effects, ROS also function as signaling molecules that regulate biological activities (Finkel 2011). ROS are implicated in regulating normal homeostatic maintenance in other stem cell niches (Le Belle et al. 2011). The question as to whether these signaling functions of ROS are regulated by the clock in epidermal progenitor cells remains unanswered.

14.4.2 Circadian Clock Control of the Unfolded Protein Response

In response to stressful conditions such as wounding, infections, UV exposure, hypoxia, nutrient deprivation and ROS accumulation, cells upregulate proteins that help prevent the accumulation of misfolded proteins in the endoplasmic reticulum; this response is called the Unfolded Protein Response (UPR). For example, the UPR is activated in proliferating fibroblasts during wound healing (Matsuzaki et al. 2015). Although the UPR is most commonly thought of as a response to perturbation, it is activated in differentiating keratinocytes of the skin in the most differentiated layers of the epidermis (Sugiura 2013). Interestingly, in mouse skin, several mRNAs encoding UPR-associated proteins oscillate diurnally, with most of them exhibiting peak expression in the late night/early morning (Fig. 14.3a). One of these genes, *HERPUD1* is affected in *Bmal1*$^{-/-}$ mice. Although no studies to date have investigated the functional significance of the diurnal expression of components of the UPR in the skin, studies in the liver have shown that circadian UPR activation is coordinated with the timing of maximum protein secretion in mouse liver (Cretenet et al. 2010; Mauvoisin et al. 2014). Moreover, *Cry1*$^{-/-}$; *Cry2*$^{-/-}$ mice exhibit dysregulation of endoplasmic reticulum-resident enzymes and perturbed lipid metabolism (Cretenet et al. 2010), suggesting a direct clock role in modulating the UPR in the liver. The potential role of the circadian clock in modulating the UPR in the skin is unknown and merits further investigation.

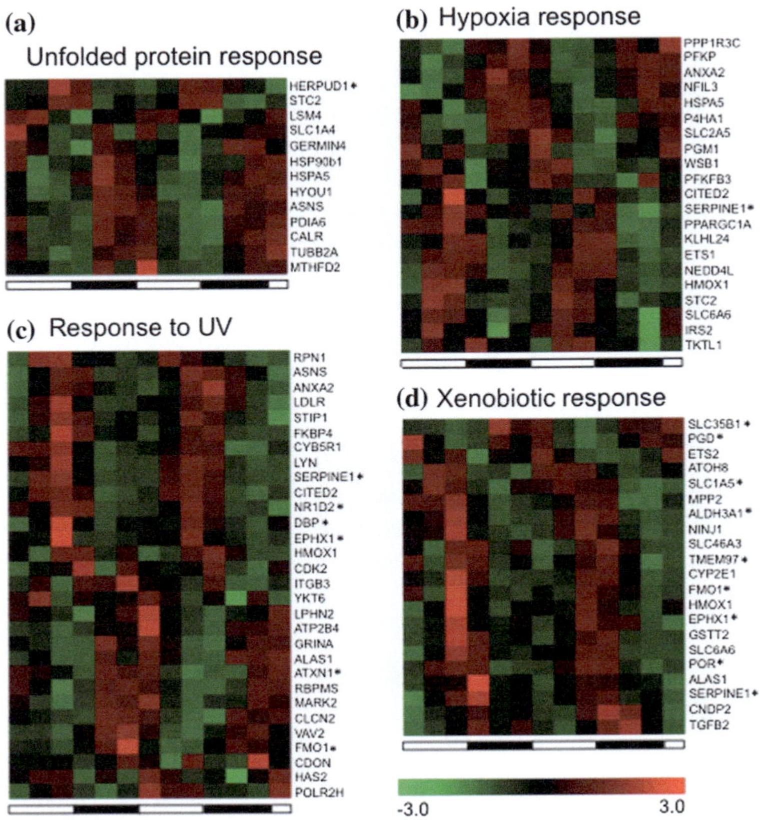

Fig. 14.3 Circadian expression of stress response pathways in the skin. Heat maps showing the expression of genes in the skin over 2 days based on previously published whole skin microarrays performed in mice (Geyfman et al. 2012). The MSigDB database was used to identify significantly enriched stress response pathways. Shown are diurnal genes associated with unfolded protein response (**a**), hypoxia response (**b**), UV response (**c**), and xenobiotic response (**d**). Asterisks indicate genes whose expression is significantly different in the skin of *Bmal1*$^{-/-}$ versus wildtype mice (Geyfman et al. 2012), suggesting the possibility of direct clock regulation

14.4.3 Response to Wounding

The skin has evolved highly effective regenerative mechanisms to close wound defects. The review of wound healing is beyond the scope of this chapter but suffice to say, complicated signaling networks that are activated in response to wounding promote closure of the wound through enhanced migration and proliferation of fibroblasts and keratinocytes. In addition, polarizing immune cells are recruited to the wound to clear up debris and kill off intruding microbes. Studies suggest that the clock facilitates proper wound healing as evidenced by less epithelial coverage and decreased fibroblast proliferation after wounding in *Bmal1*$^{-/-}$ mice (Kowalska et al.

2013). It is possible that healing defects observed in *Bmal1*$^{-/-}$ mice are at least partially related to the dampened ability of *Bmal1*$^{-/-}$ keratinocytes to respond to pro-proliferative signals in older mice (Janich et al. 2011).

The microenvironment of wounded tissues is hypoxic and has impaired nutrient supply due to vascular perturbation and high oxygen utilization by cells at the wound edge (Pai and Hunt 1972). Hypoxia induces the expression of heat shock proteins, which facilitate epithelial cell migration, thus contributing to re-epithelialization. The mRNA levels for heat shock proteins (Hsp90 and Hsp70), as well as several other proteins involved in the response to hypoxia, exhibit diurnal expression rhythms in mouse skin under homeostasis (Fig. 14.3b).

14.4.4 UVB- and γ-Irradiation-Induced DNA Damage

Intricately linked to the cell cycle, the susceptibility to UVB-induced DNA damage in mouse skin exhibits a diurnal rhythm. UVB-induced DNA damage in the form of (6-4) photoproducts and cyclobutane pyrimidine dimers is greater when UVB is applied at night compared to the day. This effect may be explained at least in part by the diurnal expression of a rate-limiting protein essential for the nucleotide excision repair pathway, Xeroderma pigmentosum complementation group A (XPA) (Cleaver 1968), which is lowly expressed in mouse skin during the night compared to day. The stage of the cell cycle may also contribute to this effect, as DNA is most vulnerable to damage during the S-phase of the cell cycle (Pantazis 1980), which also peaks during the night in epidermal progenitors (Geyfman et al. 2012). Recently, other physiological aspects of the mouse skins' response to UVB-induced damage, including sunburn apoptosis, inflammatory cytokine production, and erythema were found to be time-of-day dependent, with maximal response induced by UVB exposure at night (Gaddameedhi et al. 2015). Most strikingly, the same group found that UVB-induced squamous cell carcinomas accrue more rapidly in mice exposed to UVB at night (Gaddameedhi et al. 2011). Notably, in mouse skin under homeostasis, multiple mRNAs encoding proteins in the "response to UV" gene set exhibit diurnal oscillations, suggesting the possibility that other genes play a role in the diurnal UVB response (Fig. 14.3c). These findings are all in nocturnal mice, which have opposite phase of the circadian clock compared to diurnal humans where the maximum sensitivity to UVB-induced DNA epidermal damage may be during the day, the time of maximum solar exposure (Geyfman et al. 2012; Gaddameedhi et al. 2011).

Studies have shown that cells in the M phase are most susceptible to γ-irradiation-induced DNA damage (Sinclair and Morton 1965; Terasima and Tolmach 1961). Consistent with this fact, γ-irradiation causes more extensive hair loss when applied to skin during the early morning versus in the afternoon (Plikus et al. 2013). *Cry1*$^{-/-}$; *Cry2*$^{-/-}$ mice, which are arrhythmic, exhibit similar and enhanced levels of hair loss in response to γ-irradiation regardless of time of day, implicating a role for the circadian clock in this process (Plikus et al. 2013).

Together, these studies support a role for the circadian clock in modulating the epidermal response to exogenous stressors in the form of UVB- and γ-irradiation radiation.

14.4.5 Antioxidant Defense

The skin possesses an intricate network of antioxidant mechanisms poised to assuage oxidant stress caused by exposure to solar radiation, chemicals, inflammation, and endogenous metabolic processes. Antioxidant systems in the skin include proteins that protect against ROS, such as catalase (CAT), glutathione peroxidase (GPx), and superoxide dismutase (SOD), as well as antioxidants like vitamins A, C, and E, melatonin, and glutathione (GSH). Many of these components exhibit diurnal rhythmicity throughout the body. For example, Melatonin, most well known for its role as a primary circadian effector hormone, is also a potent ROS- and NOS-scavenger. The structure of melatonin allows it to neutralize many forms of radicals such as H_2O_2, $^{\cdot}OH$, singlet oxygen ($^1O_2$), superoxide anion ($^{\cdot}O_2^-$), peroxynitrite anion ($ONOO^-$) and peroxyl radical ($LOO^{\cdot}$) (Tan et al. 2002). The neutralization of these oxidizing molecules is especially important for skin health due to the epidermis' high rate of cell proliferation, which correlates with its propensity to become cancerous (Tomasetti and Vogelstein 2015). Apart from its direct actions, melatonin also works in the skin by inhibiting the depletion of antioxidant enzymes including CAT, GPx, and SODs after UV radiation-mediated photodamage (Fischer et al. 2013).

Another mechanism by which the skin and other organs fight the accumulation of harmful free radicals is through the action of SODs, which catalyze the dismutation of O_2^- into O_2 and H_2O_2. SODs are integral to skin homeostasis, as heterozygous deletion of SOD2 results in an "immune-ageing" phenotype, with enhanced T cell-mediated contact hypersensitivity (Scheurmann et al. 2014) as well as nuclear DNA damage, and cellular senescence in the mouse epidermis (Velarde et al. 2012). SODs are expressed in a diurnal manner in many tissues including rat intestine, lung, and cerebellum (Martin et al. 2003). *Per2* mutant mice show dampened SOD expression levels in the liver, while *Per1/2* double knockout mice have a shift in phase of SOD gene expression (Jang et al. 2011), suggesting that this mechanism is modulated by the circadian clock.

GSH is a critical antioxidant that neutralizes ROS in a process catalyzed by GPx proteins, in which GSH becomes oxidized to form glutathione disulfide (GSSG). GSH and GSSG, as well as other components of the GSH pathway, such as GPx, GR, and GST, are robustly diurnal in multiple tissues (Baydas et al. 2002a; Lapenna et al. 1992; Maurice et al. 1991) with a peak expression of GSH during the light phase in mice and during the night in humans (Atkinson and Babbitt 2009). A few Glutathione *S*-transferases, including GSTT1 and GSTA3, exhibit diurnal rhythmicity in their mRNA expression in the skin and are altered in *Bmal1*$^{-/-}$ mice (Geyfman et al. 2012). Although there are no studies to date investigating the physiological significance of the circadian rhythmicity of these GSH-associated genes in the skin, higher oxidized GSH levels are often seen in lesional and non-lesional skin from patients with chronic irritant dermatitis, suggesting this pathway is integral for maintaining skin homeostasis (Kaur et al. 2001).

14.4.6 Xenobiotic Detoxification

The skin protects against the effects of man-made genotoxic drugs and cytotoxic compounds found in nature. The Aryl hydrocarbon receptor (AhR) is a ligand-dependent transcription factor that plays a critical role in metabolism of small molecules, including dioxins, polycyclic aromatic hydrocarbons, plant polyphenols, and tryptophan photoproducts (Rannug and Fritsche 2006). Upon ligand binding, AhR translocates to the nucleus and dimerizes with ARNT, inducing transcription of xenobiotic-metabolizing enzymes, including cytochrome P450 (CYP) 1A1 and CYP1A2/B1. The CYP proteins then degrade chemical toxins and, as a by-product, produce ROS. AhR also activates the expression of nuclear factor-erythroid 2-related factor-2 (Nrf2), which regulates the expression of myriad of antioxidant proteins including NAD(P)H dehydrogenase [quinone] 1 (Nqo1) and Heme oxygenase 1 (HO-1) that protect against genotoxicity due to elevated ROS (Cho et al. 2002). In the mouse lung epithelium, circadian Nrf2 levels control the pulmonary response to oxidative injury in a lung fibrosis model, with greater fibrosis accruing during the early evening, corresponding to lowest Nrf2 levels (Pekovic-Vaughan et al. 2014). Moreover, reduced Nrf2 and GSH expression in the lungs of *Clock*$^{\Delta 19}$ mice is linked to increased oxidative damage of proteins and spontaneous development of fibrosis in the airways (Perovic-Vaughan et al. 2014). In the mouse skin, the expression of Nrf2, Nqo1, and HO-1 is diurnal with a peak in expression a few hours prior to the onset of night; in addition, Nqo1 and Nrf2 mRNA expression is altered in *Bmal1*$^{-/-}$ mice (Geyfman et al. 2012), suggesting these genes are controlled by the CLOCK:BMAL1 complex.

The AhR pathway and the circadian clock exhibit a dynamic, reciprocal interaction. On the one hand, AhR expression and DNA binding activity have a 24-h rhythmicity; core clock proteins regulate AhR-mediated enzyme expression and detoxification activity in the rat pituitary and liver (Huang et al. 2002; Tanimura et al. 2011). On the other hand, activation of the AhR pathway by dioxins impacts the expression of core clock genes in mouse liver and hematopoietic stem cells (Xu et al. 2010). It is currently unknown whether this disruption occurs in epidermal and follicular progenitor cells. However, if it does, this would suggest yet another pathway by which dioxins (acting through AhR activation) exert their damaging effects on the skin.

AhR is expressed in the upper part of the hair follicle including the infundibulum (Ikuta et al. 2009). Although the mRNA expression of AhR itself is not circadian in mouse skin, transcripts for genes associated with the xenobiotic response such as CYP2E1 and epoxide hydrolase 1 exhibit diurnal rhythmicity, peaking around the onset of night in mouse skin under homeostasis (Geyfman et al. 2012) (Fig. 14.3d). The functional significance of the circadian regulation of xenobiotic metabolism within the skin may be to prepare for and/or respond to chemical toxins encountered during the night, when mice are most active.

14.5 Circadian Regulation of Skin Immunity

14.5.1 Circadian Rhythm in Skin Innate Immunity

In addition to the barrier mechanisms described above, a diverse army of inflammatory cells in the skin deals with environmental insults by reacting, attacking, and relaying danger signals to the rest of the body. Epidermal keratinocytes, which compose the bulk of cells in the skin, secrete antimicrobial defensin peptides to resist pathogenic microbial colonization. Defensin β23 mRNA exhibits a striking circadian rhythmicity in mouse skin under homeostasis (Geyfman et al. 2012). Skin immunity also relies on evolutionarily conserved pattern recognition receptors (PRRs), including TLR 1, 2, 3, 5, 9 and 10, which enable innate inflammatory responses to a variety of immunogenic stimuli including bacterial, fungal, viral, and apoptotic molecules (Miller et al. 2005; Köllisch et al. 2005; Lebre et al. 2007). Skin-resident leukocytes derived from the hematopoietic system contribute to barrier defense, expressing a diverse array of PRRs, including TLRs 1-10 (Renn et al. 2006) and C-type lectin receptors. In healthy mouse whole skin, TLR 4, 7, 8, and 9 expression oscillates diurnally (Geyfman et al. 2012). PRR engagement induces nuclear translocation of inflammatory transcription factors, including nuclear factor κB (NF-κB), enabling pro-inflammatory gene expression. The circadian clock regulates the magnitude of these inflammatory responses following PRR engagement. The most profound example of the circadian regulation of PRR sensitivity is exhibited by the increased mortality following systemic lipopolysaccharide (LPS) administration immediately preceding or during the evening in mice; this effect is clock-dependent as *Per2* mutant mice are resistant to LPS-induced endotoxic shock (Liu et al. 2006). LPS is a microbial component of gram-negative bacteria which induces inflammatory cytokine secretion through activation of TLR4, and systemic administration results in endotoxic shock and sepsis. Results in mouse LPS models are recapitulated in human sepsis, in which greater mortality is observed during the night (Smolensky et al. 1972).

Immune cell sensitivity to pathogenic challenges is regulated by the circadian clock in numerous epithelial barriers. Lung epithelium responds diurnally to challenge by LPS or *S. pneumoniae*, where inflammatory chemokine release and neutrophil recruitment peaks during the early day in mice (Gibbs et al. 2014). This diurnal variation in reactivity to exogenous particulates in the lung epithelium may contribute to the potent early morning symptoms of wheezing in asthma patients (Barnes 1985) and decreased lung function in COPD patients (Calverley and Walker 2003). In addition, the ability of the gut epithelium to respond to, and defend against, ingested microbes is dependent on the circadian expression of defensins (Froy et al. 2005) and PPRs in intestinal epithelial cells that both peak at the intersection between late night and early day (Mukherji et al. 2013). The physiological outcome of the circadian regulation of these proteins was revealed in experiments where investigators fed mice with *Salmonella,* and found that mice infected during the day showed increased colonization levels and pathology scores compared to nighttime-infected mice (Bellet et al. 2013). These findings support the idea that the circadian clock in epithelia promotes immunity during night, when mice are active and feeding, and thus most likely to encounter pathogenic microorganisms.

14.5.2 Circadian Rhythm in Skin Adaptive Immunity

In addition to innate PRR-mediated immunity, the skin epithelium is home to a complex network of leukocytes which also permit adaptive humoral and cell-mediated immunity (Pasparakis et al. 2014). Allergic contact dermatitis occurs in the skin following exposure to environmental chemicals, e.g. poison ivy, resulting in delayed type hypersensitivity (DTH). DTH is a cell-mediated response, requiring leukocyte migration to the lymph nodes and antigen presentation by skin-resident macrophages and dendritic cells to T cells. DTH has become a favorite animal model for human chronic inflammatory disease as the inflammatory pathology that occurs in skin DTH mirrors numerous cellular processes which also occur in chronic autoimmune disease in multiple organs. Prendergast et al. (2013) found that circadian trafficking of antigen presenting $CD11c^+$ dendritic cells in response to DTH became arrhythmic after a disruptive phase shift (DPS) procedure.

Psoriasis, a common chronic human autoimmune disease affecting 2 % of the population, is characterized by increased epidermal proliferation, epidermal thickening, altered epidermal differentiation, and organized lymphoid infiltrates in the reticular dermis. Psoriasis pathology is thought to be initiated by immuno-triggering environmental exposures and infections in patients with susceptibility to immune de-regulation due to genetic risk factors (reviewed in Harden et al. 2015). Innate immune cells such as dendritic cells expressing PRRs become activated to migrate to lymph nodes where they stimulate the differentiation of T cells into inflammatory subsets which become competent to enter the skin. T cell cytokine and growth factor secretion in the skin alters the transcriptional profile of keratinocytes and endothelial cells, resulting in a hyperproliferative state and self-perpetuating chronic inflammatory responses. The diurnal rhythmicity of psoriasis immunopathology was first published in the 1980s where Pigatto et al. (1985) found a substantial diurnal rhythmicity in neutrophil recruitment to the psoriatic lesions.

Work with psoriasis animal models suggests a circadian regulation of skin immunopathology. The psoriasiform lesion-inducing drug Imiquimod (IMQ) functions as a pathogen-associated molecular pattern (PAMP) and activates TLR7 signaling in skin-resident dendritic cells, resulting in the influx of inflammatory cells, proinflammatory cytokine secretion, and epidermal alterations (acanthosis, parakeratosis) similar to human psoriasis. These symptoms are more pronounced when mice are treated with IMQ at night than during the day (Ando et al. 2015). Knockout studies and circadian disruption studies support the modulatory role of the circadian clock in maintaining proper immune responsiveness to external PAMPs and antigens. Mice with mutated *Clock* genes have damped psoriatic lesion formation in response to IMQ, while *Per2* knockout mice have exacerbated pathogenesis (Ando et al. 2015). In other studies, mice subjected to disrupted lighting cycles and treated with the psoriatic-inducing agent human neutrophil elastase developed exacerbated psoriatic histopathology and pro-inflammatory cytokine production compared to mice housed under normal 12L:12D conditions (Hirotsu et al. 2012).

Nocturnal pruritus, or increased itchiness at night, has been well described in patients with various dermatological disorders, including psoriasis (Yosipovitch et al. 2000), atopic dermatitis (Yosipovitch and Tang 2002), lichen simplex chronicus (Koca et al. 2006), and scabies (Chouela et al. 2002). There are many factors that may contribute to this effect, one of them being histamine release by mast cells, which is modulated by the circadian clock (Baumann et al. 2013). Time-of-day–dependent variations in a mouse model of IgE/mast cell–mediated allergic reaction (passive cutaneous anaphylactic (PCA) reaction) peaked during at night. Furthermore, these rhythms in reactivity were reliant on a functional clock protein, *Per2* (Nakamura et al. 2011). Together, these studies illustrate the powerful modulatory role of the circadian clock on immune responses in the skin.

14.6 Conclusions and Opportunities for Chronotherapy

Our skin maintains a dynamic barrier, protecting us from harmful external stimuli like fluctuating temperatures, humidity levels, UV rays, pollution, and infections. Work on the role of the circadian clock in skin suggests that it has evolved to coordinate the skins' protective function with changes in the external environment, allowing for optimal response to external insults. The clock also functions to temporally gate internal cellular processes such as oxidative phosphorylation, cell division, and antioxidant pathways within the skin, perhaps helping to keep ROS-induced DNA damage at bay (Fig. 14.4). Most of the experimental work on the skin role of the circadian clock has been performed in mice, which are nocturnal, while humans are diurnal. Therefore, a number of circadian clock-modulated processes described in this review may exhibit antiphasic patterns in humans. It will be important to take this fact into consideration when thinking about the implications of these findings in the realm of human physiology and disease.

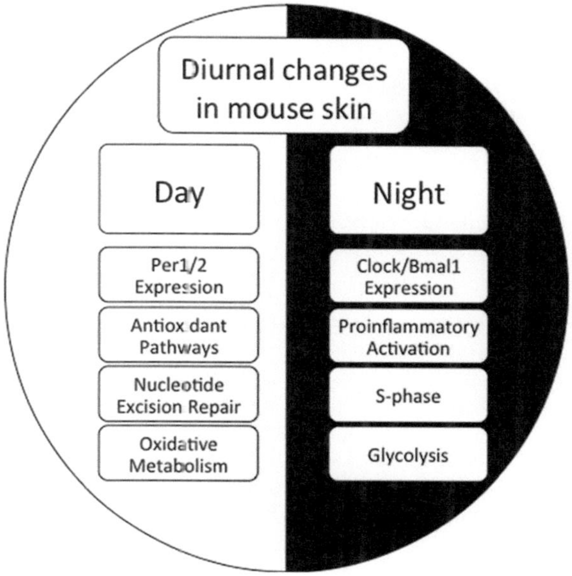

Fig. 14.4 Diurnal activities of circadian stress response pathways in the skin. In mouse skin, circadian clock proteins, BMAL1 and CLOCK, exhibit peak expression during the night when most epidermal progenitor cells are in S-phase and glycolysis is the predominant metabolic pathway in these cells. The propensity for immune activation also peaks at night, which may help defend against invading pathogens encountered during the active phase. Conversely, oxidative metabolism and ROS production is higher during the day, coinciding with antioxidant pathway activity. DNA damage repair also peaks during the day in mice

This chapter highlights the importance of the circadian clock in gating skin's stress response. In part, this notion is well supported by experimental data, but, in part, the evidence is more speculative, pointing to the importance of further work in this field. Circadian disruption, a common phenomenon in today's society, may impair the skin's ability to handle stressors and infections.

Understanding the mechanisms by which the clock gates the skin's responsiveness to external stimuli, as well as the physiological outcomes of this regulation, is of paramount importance for the development of chronotherapy. Chronotherapy aims to administer drugs at specific times of the day to maximize the beneficial effects of the treatment and/or to minimize side effects. For example, 5-fluorouricil treatment of tumor bearing mice wielded more potent anti-tumor effects when dosed in the early morning compared to other times of the day (Kojima et al. 1999). The pro-inflammatory effects of another anti-tumor/anti-viral drug, the TLR7 agonist IMQ, have recently been shown to be diurnal with peak activity induced after nighttime treatment in mice (Ando et al. 2015). Studies on skin active drugs should consider time of day as a potentially important variable, modulating effectiveness and side effects.

References

Ando N, Nakamura Y, Aoki R, Ishimaru K, Ogawa H, Okumura K, Shibata S, Shimada S, Nakao A (2015) Circadian gene clock regulates psoriasis-like skin inflammation in mice. J Invest Dermatol 135(12):3001–3008

Ansari N, Agathagelidis M, Lee C, Korf HW, von Gall C (2009) Differential maturation of circadian rhythms in clock gene proteins in the suprachiasmatic nucleus and the pars tuberalis during mouse ontogeny. Eur J Neurosci 29(3):477–489

Armstrong AW, Harskamp CT, Armstrong EJ (2013) Psoriasis and metabolic syndrome: a systematic review and meta-analysis of observational studies. J Am Acad Dermatol 68:654–662

Atkinson HJ, Babbitt PC (2009) Glutathione transferases are structural and functional outliers in the thioredoxin fold. Biochemistry 48(46):11108–11116

Barnes PJ (1985) Circadian variation in airway function. Am J Med 79(6A):5–9

Baumann A, Gönnenwein S, Bischoff SC, Sherman H, Chapnik N, Froy O, Lorentz A (2013) The circadian clock is functional in eosinophils and mast cells. Immunology 140(4):465–474

Baydas G, Gursu MF, Yilmaz S, Canpolat S, Yasar A, Cikim G, Canatan H (2002a) Daily rhythm of glutathione peroxidase activity, lipid peroxidation and glutathione levels in tissues of pinealectomized rats. Neurosci Lett 323(3):195–198

Bellet MM, Deriu E, Liu JZ, Grimaldi B, Blaschitz C, Zeller M, Edwards RA, Sahar S, Dandekar S, Baldi P, George MD, Raffatellu M, Sassone-Corsi P (2013) Circadian clock regulates the host response to Salmonella. Proc Natl Acad Sci USA 110(24):9897–9902

Bjarnason GA, Jordan R (2002) Rhythms in human gastrointestinal mucosa and skin. Chronobiol Int 19(1):129–140

Brown WR (1991) A review and mathematical analysis of circadian rhythms in cell proliferation in mouse, rat, and human epidermis. J Invest Dermatol 97(2):273–280

Brown SA, Zumbrunn G, Fleury-Olela F, Preitner N, Schibler U (2002) Rhythms of mammalian body temperature can sustain peripheral circadian clocks. Curr Biol 12(18):1574–1583

Buhr ED, Takahashi JS (2013) Molecular components of the Mammalian circadian clock. Handb Exp Pharmacol 217:3–27

Calverley PM, Walker P (2003) Chronic obstructive pulmonary disease. Lancet 362(9389): 1053–1061

Cho HY, Jedlicka AE, Reddy SP, Kensler TW, Yamamoto M, Zhang LY, Kleeberger SR (2002) Role of NRF2 in protection against hyperoxic lung injury in mice. Am J Respir Cell Mol Biol 26(2):175–182

Chouela E, Abeldaño A, Pellerano G, Hernández MI (2002) Diagnosis and treatment of scabies: a practical guide. Am J Clin Dermatol 3(1):9–18

Clausen OP, Thorud E, Bjerknes R, Elgjo K (1979) Circadian rhythms in mouse epidermal basal cell proliferation: variations in compartment size, flux and phase duration. Cell Tissue Kinet 12:319–337

Cleaver JE (1968) Defective repair replication of DNA in xeroderma pigmentosum. Nature 218 (5142):652–656

Cretenet G, Le Clech M, Gachon F (2010) Circadian clock-coordinated 12 Hr period rhythmic activation of the IRE1alpha pathway controls lipid metabolism in mouse liver. Cell Metab 11 (1):47–57

Dibner C, Schibler U, Albrecht U (2010) The mammalian circadian timing system: organization and coordination of central and peripheral clocks. Annu Rev Physiol 72:517–549

Finkel T (2011) Signal transduction by reactive oxygen species. J Cell Biol 194(1):7–15

Fischer TW, Kleszczyński K, Hardkop LH, Kruse N, Zillikens D (2013) Melatonin enhances antioxidative enzyme gene expression (CAT, GPx, SOD), prevents their UVR-induced depletion, and protects against the formation of DNA damage (8-hydroxy-2′-deoxyguanosine) in ex vivo human skin. J Pineal Res 54(3):303–312

Froy O, Chapnik N, Miskin R (2005) Mouse intestinal cryptdins exhibit circadian oscillation. FASEB J. 19:1920–1922
Gaddameedhi S, Selby CP, Kaufmann WK, Smart RC, Sancar A (2011) Control of skin cancer by the circadian rhythm. Proc Natl Acad Sci USA 108(46):18790–18795
Gaddameedhi S, Selby CP, Kemp MG, Ye R, Sancar A (2015) The circadian clock controls sunburn apoptosis and erythema in mouse skin. J Invest Dermatol 135(4):1119–1127
Geyfman M, Kumar V, Liu Q, Ruiz R, Gordon W, Espitia F, Cam E, Millar SE, Smyth P, Ihler A, Takahashi JS, Andersen B (2012) Brain and muscle Arnt-like protein-1 (BMAL1) controls circadian cell proliferation and susceptibility to UVB-induced DNA damage in the epidermis. Proc Natl Acad Sci 109(29):11758–11763
Gibbs J, Ince L, Matthews L, Mei J, Bell T, Yang N, Saer B, Begley N, Poolman T, Pariollaud M, Farrow S, Demayo F, Hussel T, Worthen GS, Ray D, Loudon A (2014) An epithelial circadian clock controls pulmonary inflammation and glucocorticoid action. Nat Med 20(8):919–926
Gillette MU, Sejnowski TJ (2005) Physiology. Biological clocks coordinately keep life on time. Science 309(5738):1196–1198
Girardi M, Oppenheim DE, Steele CR, Lewis JM, Glusac E, Filler R, Hobby P, Sutton B, Tigelaar RE, Hayday AC (2001) Regulation of cutaneous malignancy by gammadelta T cells. Science 294(5542):605–609
Harden JL, Krueger JG, Bowcock AM (2015) The immunogenetics of psoriasis: a comprehensive review. J Autoimmun 64:66–73
Hirotsu C, Rydlewski M, Araújo MS, Tufik S, Andersen ML (2012) Sleep loss and cytokines levels in an experimental model of psoriasis. PLoS ONE 7(11):e51183
Huang P, Ceccatelli S, Håkansson H, Grandison L, Rannug A (2002) Constitutive and TCDD-induced expression of Ah receptor-responsive genes in the pituitary. Neurotoxicology 23(6):783–793
Ikuta T, Namiki T, Fujii-Kuriyama Y, Kawajiri K (2009) AhR protein trafficking and function in the skin. Biochem Pharmacol 77(4):588–596
Jang YS, Lee MH, Lee SH, Bae K (2011) Cu/Zn superoxide dismutase is differentially regulated in period gene-mutant mice. Biochem Biophys Res Commun 409:22–27
Janich P, Pascual G, Merlos-Suárez A, Batlle E, Ripperger J, Albrecht U, Cheng HY, Obrietan K, Di Croce L, Benitah SA (2011) The circadian molecular clock creates epidermal stem cell heterogeneity. Nature 480(7376):209–214
Jouffe C, Cretenet G, Symul L, Martin E, Atger F, Naef F, Gachon F (2013) The circadian clock coordinates ribosome biogenesis. PLoS Biol 11(1):e1001455
Kaur S, Zilmer M, Eisen M, Kullisaar T, Rehema A, Vihalemm T (2001) Patients with allergic and irritant contact dermatitis are characterized by striking change of iron and oxidized glutathione status in nonlesional area of the skin. J Invest Dermatol 116(6):886–890
Khapre RV, Kondratova AA, Susova O, Kondratov RV (2011) Circadian clock protein BMAL1 regulates cellular senescence in vivo. Cell Cycle 10(23):4162–4169
Koca R, Altin R, Konuk N, Altinyazar HC, Kart L (2006) Sleep disturbance in patients with lichen simplex chronicus and its relationship to nocturnal scratching: A case control study. South Med J 99(5):482–485
Kojima H, Sakamoto J, Yasue (1999) Circadian rhythm-modulated chemotherapy with high dose 5-fluorouracil against gastrointestinal cancers: evaluation and case report. Nagoya J Med Sci 62:29–38
Köllisch G, Kalali BN, Voelcker V, Wallich R, Behrendt H, Ring J, Bauer S, Jakob T, Mempel M, Ollert M (2005) Various members of the toll-like receptor family contribute to the innate immune response of human epidermal keratinocytes. Immunology 114(4):531–541
Kondratov RV, Kondratova AA, Gorbacheva VY, Vykhovanets OV, Antoch MP (2006) Early aging and age-related pathologies in mice deficient in BMAL1, the core component of the circadian clock. Genes Dev 20(14):1868–1873
Kondratov RV, Vykhovanets O, Kondratova AA, Antoch MP (2009) Antioxidant N-acetyl-L-cysteine ameliorates symptoms of premature aging associated with the deficiency of the circadian protein BMAL1. Aging 1:979–987

Kowalska E, Ripperger JA, Hoegger DC, Bruegger P, Buch T, Birchler T, Mueller A, Albrecht U, Contaldo C, Brown SA (2013) NONO couples the circadian clock to the cell cycle. Proc Natl Acad Sci USA 110(5):1592–1599

Lapenna D, de Gioia S, Ciofani G, Mezzetti A, Ucchino S, Calafiore AM, Napolitano AM, Di Ilio C, Cuccurullo F (1992) Circadian variations in antioxidant defences and lipid peroxidation in the rat heart. Free Radic Res Commun 17(3):187–194

Le Belle JE, Orozco NM, Paucar AA, Saxe JP, Mottahedeh J, Pyle AD, Wu H, Kornblum HI (2011) Proliferative neural stem cells have high endogenous ROS levels that regulate self-renewal and neurogenesis in a PI3 K/Akt-dependant manner. Cell Stem Cell 8(1):59–71

Lebre MC, van der Aar AM, van Baarsen L, van Capel TM, Schuitemaker JH, Kapsenberg ML, de Jong EC (2007) Human keratinocytes express functional toll-like receptor 3, 4, 5, and 9. J Invest Dermatol 127(2):331–341

Lengyel Z, Battyani Z, Szekeres G, Csernus V, Nagy AD (2013) Circadian clocks and tumor biology: what is to learn from human skin biopsies? Gen Comp Endocrinol 188:67–74

Libert S, Bonkowski MS, Pointer K, Pletcher SD, Guarente L (2012) Deviation of innate circadian period from 24 h reduces longevity in mice. Aging Cell 11(5):794–800

Lin KK, Kumar V, Geyfman M, Chudova D, Ihler AT, Smyth P, Paus R, Takahashi JS, Andersen B (2009) Circadian clock genes contribute to the regulation of hair follicle cycling. PLoS Genet 5(7):e1000573

Liu J, Malkani G, Mankani G, Shi X, Meyer M, Cunningham-Runddles S, Ma X, Sun ZS (2006) The circadian clock period 2 gene regulates gamma interferon production of NK cells in host response to lipopolysaccharide-induced endotoxic shock. Infect Immun 74(8):4750–4756

Martín V, Sainz RM, Mayo JC, Antolín I, Herrera F, Rodríguez C (2003) Daily rhythm of gene expression in rat superoxide dismutases. Endocr Res 29(1):83–95

Matsuzaki S, Hiratsuka T, Taniguchi M, Shingaki K, Kubo T, Kiya K, Fujiwara T, Kanazawa S, Kanematsu R, Maeda T, Takamura H, Yamada K, Miyoshi K, Hosokawa K, Tohyama M, Katayama T (2015) Physiological ER stress mediates the differentiation of fibroblasts. PLoS One 10(4):e0123578

Maurice DV, Lightsey SF, Hsu KT, Rhoades JF (1991) Comparison of glutathione S-transferase activity in the rat and birds: tissue distribution and rhythmicity in chicken (*Gallus domesticus*) liver. Comp Biochem Physiol B 100(3):471–474

Mauvoisin D, Wang J, Jouffe C, Martin E, Atger F, Waridel P, Quadroni M, Gachon F, Naef F (2014) Circadian clock-dependent and -independent rhythmic proteomes implement distinct diurnal functions in mouse liver. Proc Natl Acad Sci USA 111(1):167–172

Miller LS, Sørensen OE, Liu PT, Jalian HR, Eshtiaghpour D, Behmanesh BE, Chung W, Starner TD, Kim J, Sieling PA, Ganz T, Modlin RL (2005) TGF-alpha regulates TLR expression and function on epidermal keratinocytes. J Immunol 174(10):6137–6143

Mohawk JA, Green CB, Takahashi JS (2012) Central and peripheral circadian clocks in mammals. Annu Rev Neurosci 35:445–462

Mukherji A, Kobiita A, Ye T, Chambon P (2013) Homeostasis in the intestinal epithelium is orchestrated by the circadian clock and microbiota cues transduced by TLRs. Cell 153(4):812–827

Naik S, Bouladoux N, Linehan JL, Han SJ, Harrison OJ, Wilhelm C, Conlan S, Himmelfarb S, Byrd AL, Deming C, Quinones M, Brenchley JM, Kong HH, Tussiwand R, Murphy KM (2015) Commensal-dendritic-cell interaction specifies a unique protective skin immune signature. 520(7545):104–108

Nakamura Y, Harama D, Shimokawa N, Hara M, Suzuki R, Tahara Y, Ishimaru K, Katoh R, Okumura K, Ogawa H, Shibata S, Nakao A (2011) Circadian clock gene Period2 regulates a time-of-day-dependent variation in cutaneous anaphylactic reaction. J Allergy Clin Immunol 127 (4):1038–1045.e1031-1033

Pai MP, Hunt TK (1972) Effect of varying oxygen tensions on healing of open wounds. Surg Gynecol Obstet 135(5):756–758

Panda S, Antoch MP, Miller BH, Su AI, Schook AB, Straume M, Schultz PG, Kay SA, Takahashi JS, Hogenesch JB (2002) Coordinated transcription of key pathways in the mouse by the circadian clock. Cell 109(3):307–320

Pantazis P (1980) Sensitivity of DNA synthetic phase to near-ultraviolet radiation: chromatid damage at early and late replication periods. Cancer Lett 10(3):253–259

Pasparakis M, Haase I, Nestle FO (2014) Mechanisms regulating skin immunity and inflammation. Nat Rev Immunol 14(5):289–301

Pekovic-Vaughan V, Gibbs J, Yoshitane H, Yang N, Pathiranage D, Guo B, Sagami A, Taguchi K, Bechtold D, Loudon A, Yamamoto M, Chan J, van der Horst GT, Fukada Y, Meng QJ (2014) The circadian clock regulates rhythmic activation of the NRF2/glutathione-mediated antioxidant defense pathway to modulate pulmonary fibrosis. Genes Dev 28(6):548–560

Pigatto PD, Radaelli A, Tadini G, Polenghi MM, Brambilla L, Altomare G, Carandente F (1985) Circadian rhythm of the in vivo migration of neutrophils in psoriatic patients. Arch Dermatol Res 277:185–189

Plikus MV, Van Spyk EN, Pham K, Geyfman M, Kumar V, Takahashi JS, Andersen B (2015) The circadian clock in skin: Implications for adult stem cells, tissue regeneration, cancer, aging, and immunity. J Biol Rhythms 30(3):163–182

Plikus MV, Vollmers C, de la Cruz D, Chaix A, Ramos R, Panda S, Chuong CM (2013) Local circadian clock gates cell cycle progression of transient amplifying cells during regenerative hair cycling. Proc Natl Acad Sci 110(23):E2106–E2115

Pluquet O, Dejeans N, Chevet E (2014) Watching the clock: endoplasmic reticulum-mediated control of circadian rhythms in cancer. Ann Med 46(4):233–243

Preitner N, Damiola F, Lopez-Molina L, Zakany J, Duboule D, Albrecht U, Schibler U (2002) The orphan nuclear receptor REV-ERBalpha controls circadian transcription within the positive limb of the mammalian circadian oscillator. Cell 110(2):251–260

Prendergast BJ, Cable EJ, Patel PN, Pyter LM, Onishi KG, Stevenson TJ, Ruby NF, Bradley SP (2013) Impaired leukocyte trafficking and skin inflammatory responses in hamsters lacking a functional circadian system. Brain Behav Immun 32:94–104

Rannug A, Fritsche E (2006) The aryl hydrocarbon receptor and light. Biol Chem 387(9): 1149–1157

Renn CN, Sanchez DJ, Ochoa MT, Legaspi AJ, Oh CK, Liu PT, Krutzik SR, Sieling PA, Cheng G, Modlin RL (2006) TLR activation of langerhans cell-like dendritic cells triggers an antiviral immune response. J Immunol 177(1):298–305

Reppert SM, Weaver DR (2002) Coordination of circadian timing in mammals. Nature 418 (6901):935–941

Sancar A, Lindsey-Boltz LA, Gaddameedhi S, Selby CP, Ye R, Chiou YY, Kemp MG, Hu J, Lee JH, Ozturk N (2015) Circadian clock, cancer, and chemotherapy. Biochemistry 54(2): 110–123

Scheurmann J, Treiber N, Weber C, Renkl AC, Frenzel D, Trenz-Buback F, Ruess A, Schulz G, Scharffetter-Kochanek K, Weiss JM (2014) Mice with heterozygous deficiency of manganese superoxide dismutase (SOD2) have a skin immune system with features of "inflamm-aging". Arch Dermatol Res 306(2):143–155

Sigurdardottir LG, Valdimarsdottir UA, Fall K, Rider JR, Lockley SW, Schernhammer E, Mucci LA (2012) Circadian disruption, sleep loss, and prostate cancer risk: a systematic review of epidemiologic studies. Cancer Epidemiol Biomarkers Prev 21:1002–1011

Sinclair WK, Morton RA (1965) X-ray and ultraviolet sensitivity of synchronized Chinese hamster cells at various stages of the cell cycle. Biophys J 5:1–25

Sladek M, Sumova A, Kovacikova Z, Bendova Z, Laurinova K, et al. (2004) Insight into molecular core clock mechanism of embryonic and early postnatal rat suprachiasmatic nucleus. PNAS 292(3):R1224–9

Smolensky M, Halberg F, Sargent F (1972) Chronobiology of the life sequence. In: Ito S, Ogata K, Yohimura H (eds) Advances in climatic physiology. Igaku Shoin, Tokyo, pp 281–318

Stringari C, Wang H, Geyfman M, Crosignani V, Kumar V, Takahashi JS, Andersen B, Gratton E (2015) In vivo single-cell detection of metabolic oscillations in stem cells. Cell Rep 10(1):1–7

Sugiura K (2013) Unfolded protein response in keratinocytes: impact on normal and abnormal keratinization. J Dermatol Sci 69(3):181–186

Sumaria N, Roediger B, Ng LG, Qin J, Pinto R, Cavanagh LL, Shklovskaya E, de St Fazekas, Groth B, Triccas JA, Weninger W (2011) Cutaneous immunosurveillance by self-renewing dermal gammadelta T cells. J Exp Med 208(3):505–518

Tan DX, Reiter RJ, Manchester LC, Yan MT, El-Sawi M, Sainz RM, Mayo JC, Kohen R, Allegra M, Hardeland R (2002) Chemical and physical properties and potential mechanisms: melatonin as a broad spectrum antioxidant and free radical scavenger. Curr Top Med Chem 2 (2):181–197

Tanimura N, Kusunose N, Matsunaga N, Koyanagi S, Ohdo S (2011) Aryl hydrocarbon receptor-mediated Cyp1a1 expression is modulated in a CLOCK-dependent circadian manner. Toxicology 290(2–3):203–207

Tanioka M, Yamada H, Doi M, Bando H, Yamaguchi Y (2009). Molecular clocks in mouse skin. J Invest Dermatol 129:1225–1231

Terasima T, Tolmach LJ (1961) Changes in x-ray sensitivity of HeLa cells during the division cycle. Nature 190:1210–1211

Tomasetti C, Vogelstein B (2015) Cancer etiology. Variation in cancer risk among tissues can be explained by the number of stem cell divisions. Science 347(6217):78–81

Valacchi G, Sticozzi C, Pecorelli A, Cervellati F, Cervellati C, Maioli E (2012) Cutaneous responses to environmental stressors. Ann NY Acad Sci 1271:75–81

Velarde MC, Flynn JM, Day NU, Melov S, Campisi J (2012) Mitochondrial oxidative stress caused by Sod2 deficiency promotes cellular senescence and aging phenotypes in the skin. Aging (Albany NY) 4(1):3–12

Wilking M, Ndiaye M, Mukhtar H, Ahmad N (2013) Circadian rhythm connections to oxidative stress: implications for human health. Antioxid Redox Signal 19(2):192–208

Xu CX, Krager SL, Liao DF, Tischkau SA (2010) Disruption of CLOCK-BMAL1 transcriptional activity is responsible for aryl hydrocarbon receptor-mediated regulation of Period1 gene. Toxicol Sci 115(1):98–108

Yang G, Chen L, Grant GR, Paschos G, Song W, Musiek ES, Lee V, McLoughlin SC, Grosser T, Cotsarelis G, FitzGerald GA (2016) Timing of expression of the core clock gene *Bmal1* influences its effects on aging and survival. Sci Trans Med 8 (324):324ra16

Yosipovitch G, Tang MB (2002) Practical management of psoriasis in the elderly: epidemiology, clinical aspects, quality of life, patient education and treatment options. Drugs Aging 19 (11):847–863

Yosipovitch G, Goon A, Wee J, Chan YH, Goh CL (2000) The prevalence and clinical characteristics of pruritus among patients with extensive psoriasis. Br J Dermatol 143(5):969–973

Zarrinpar A, Chaix A, Yooseph S, Panda S (2014) Diet and feeding pattern affect the diurnal dynamics of the gut microbiome. Cell Metab 20(6):1006–1017

Chapter 15
Endocannabinoids and Skin Barrier Function: Molecular Pathways and Therapeutic Opportunities

Sergio Oddi and Mauro Maccarrone

Abstract As an interface between the organism and its environment, skin is continuously subjected to a myriad of insults that could impair its structural and functional integrity, ultimately leading to clinical manifestations. Skin reacts to external stresses through a vast array of cellular and molecular components, which form a highly sophisticated and well-organized signaling network. Our knowledge of the molecular pathways underlying this complex interplay and accounting for skin homeostasis, both under normal and pathological conditions, is still in its infancy. Among these pathways, the endocannabinoid system has emerged as a key actor in skin biology, by controlling epidermal barrier formation and maintenance, modulating growth and terminal differentiation of cutaneous cells, and regulating skin inflammatory responses via pleiotropic mechanisms. This chapter summarizes our current knowledge of the manifold effects of endocannabinoids in skin, in order to put in a better perspective their potential as next-generation therapeutics against disorders of this organ, particularly those involving dysregulation of immune system and epidermal barrier, such as allergic and atopic dermatitis, localized scleroderma and psoriasis.

Keywords Endocannabinoids · Endocannabinoid system · Skin biology · Homeostasis · Psoriasis · Atopic dermatitis · Allergic contact dermatitis · Localized scleroderma · Skin barrier · Immunomodulation

---

S. Oddi (✉)
Faculty of Veterinary Medicine, University of Teramo, Via Renato Balzarini 1, 64100 Teramo, Italy
e-mail: soddi@unite.it

S. Oddi · M. Maccarrone
European Center for Brain Research (CERC)/Santa Lucia Foundation IRCCS, Via del Fosso di Fiorano 64, 00143 Rome, Italy
e-mail: m.maccarrone@unicampus.it

M. Maccarrone
Department of Medicine, Campus Bio-Medico University of Rome, Via Alvaro del Portillo 21, 00128 Rome, Italy

G.T. Wondrak (ed.), *Skin Stress Response Pathways*,
DOI 10.1007/978-3-319-43157-4_15

15.1 Introduction

Skin, or cutis, is the outermost and largest organ in the body and serves as primary barrier against physical, chemical and biological insults. The physical barrier of the skin is almost exclusively provided by the stratum corneum, the outer part of the epidermis, consisting of corneocytes, i.e., keratinocytes terminally differentiated in horny lamellae, made of specialized proteins and lipids. In addition to provide a passive physical barrier, the skin also contains elements of innate and adaptive immune systems, such as macrophages, dendritic cells and lymphocytes, which allow an active fight against infections (Bos 2005).

To support its specialized functions, the skin possesses a highly dynamic structure with remarkable self-renewing properties, which allow cutaneous barrier to continuously regenerate and to repair upon damage. Skin homeostasis is tightly regulated by multiple molecular and cellular mechanisms, such as the release of pro-inflammatory or anti-inflammatory cytokines, proliferation and differentiation of keratinocytes and melanocytes, as well as the recruitment and activation of immune cells. Each of these activities is controlled and integrated by a number of distinct cellular signal transduction systems, which allow skin cells to appropriately cope with a variety of stresses.

In the last few years, the endocannabinoid (eCB) system has emerged as a prominent lipid signaling system widely expressed in the body and involved in multiple adaptive responses to stressful internal and/or environmental insults (Maccarrone et al. 2015). By virtue of its capability of modulating cell functions, generally in a pro-homeostatic manner, the eCB signaling is currently regarded as a promising target for multimodal drug approaches for the treatment of an equally wide variety of pathological conditions, including neurodegenerative, cardiovascular and metabolic disorders (Di Marzo 2008).

In this chapter, we highlight the relevance of eCB signaling in skin physiology, and its therapeutic potential in maintaining/restoring the cutaneous barrier function in a vast range of skin diseases. We begin with a brief overview of the eCB system, giving a summary of its key components as well as of the main signaling pathways that it can elicit. Then, we focus on the possible role of eCBs in skin homeostasis, describing how these bioactive lipids may regulate the biological processes involved in the structural and functional integrity of the skin, such as keratinization, melanogenesis, sebogenesis, dermal fibrogenesis and immune response. Finally, we also describe current evidence supporting that targeted manipulation of eCB signaling by eCB-oriented medicines may represent a valuable strategy for a broad variety of dermatoses.

15.2 The Endocannabinoid System

Fifty years ago (1964) the psychoactive ingredient of cannabis (*Cannabis sativa*), Δ^9-tetrahydrocannabinol (THC), was isolated, and approximately 30 years later the endogenous counterparts of THC, collectively termed eCBs, were discovered: *N*-arachidonoylethanolamine (AEA), also known as anandamide, in 1992, and 2-arachidonoylglycerol (2-AG) in 1995 (Mechoulam and Parker 2013). Since then, many research efforts have shed light on the impact of eCBs on human health and disease, identifying an ensemble of proteins that bind, synthesize and degrade them, and that altogether form the eCB system (Di Patrizio and Piomelli 2012; Galve-Roperh et al. 2013; Maccarrone et al. 2014). The eCBs control basic biological processes, including cell-choice between survival and death, immune response, neuronal development, neurotransmission, energy homeostasis and reproduction, just to mention a few. Unsurprisingly, in the last two decades they have been recognized as key mediators of several aspects of human pathophysiology, and thus have emerged among the most versatile signaling molecules discovered at the end of the past millennium. On this basis, a better understanding of the key-factors that drive at the right time one eCB to the right target among many available candidates in the same cell, holds potential to decipher basic molecular details of energy homeostasis and drug dependence, as well as to develop more effective therapeutics against a variety of human diseases, stress conditions and pain (Di Marzo 2008).

The regulation of eCB levels by biosynthetic and hydrolyzing enzymes, and their mode of action, are being uncovered and appear characterized by an increasing degree of redundancy of pathways and promiscuity of molecular targets. The main elements of this "eCB system" are summarized in Table 15.1.

15.2.1 Metabolism

The eCBs are produced from membrane lipid precursors by multiple biosynthetic pathways "on demand", namely when and where needed upon (patho)physiological stimuli (Mechoulam and Parker 2013).

AEA is produced from the hydrolysis of the corresponding *N*-acyl-phosphatidylethanolamine (NArPE). This can occur in one step, when catalyzed by the NAPE-selective phospholipase D (NAPE-PLD) enzyme, or in two or three steps through alternative routes. 2-AG is produced in one step from the hydrolysis of diacylglycerols (DAGs) by either of two *sn*-1-diacylglycerol lipases (DAGLs), namely DAGLα and DAGLβ (Fezza et al. 2014).

The signaling action of eCBs is terminated by cellular uptake and intracellular degradation by specific hydrolases. The mechanism by which cells take up these bioactive lipids has not been fully understood yet, but it is likely to involve membrane transporters, intracellular carriers and endocytosis (Maccarrone et al. 2010;

Table 15.1 The main elements of the eCB system

Member	Description	Function
AEA	*N*-Arachidonoylethanolamine	Bioactive lipid
2-AG	2-Arachidonoylglycerol	Bioactive lipid
CB_1	Type-1 Cannabinoid receptor	G protein coupled receptor, associated with Gi/o, Gs and Gq/11
CB_2	Type-2 Cannabinoid receptor	G protein coupled receptor, associated with Gi/o, Gs and Gq/11
TRPV1	Type-1 Transient receptor potential vanilloid channel	Non-selective cation channel with a preference for Ca^{2+}
PPARs	Peroxisome proliferator-activated receptors	Ligand-activated transcription factors
NAPE-PLD	NArPE-selective phospholipase D	Ca^{2+}-dependent hydrolase responsible for AEA synthesis
DAGL	Diacylglycerol lipase	Ca^{2+}-dependent hydrolase responsible for 2-AG synthesis
FAAH	Fatty acid amide hydrolase	Hydrolase responsible for AEA degradation
MAGL	Monoacylglycerol lipase	Hydrolase responsible for 2-AG degradation

Nicolussi and Gertsch 2015). The most relevant AEA-catabolizing enzyme is the serine hydrolase fatty acid amide hydrolase (FAAH), an endo-membrane-bound enzyme that hydrolyzes AEA to release arachidonic acid and ethanolamine (Cravatt and Lichtman 2002). 2-AG is mainly hydrolyzed by a monoacylglycerol lipase (MAGL) by other emerging lipases, like αβ-hydrolases 6 (ABH6) and 12 (ABH12), and FAAH (Ueda et al. 2011). Additionally, both AEA and 2-AG are also oxidized by the cyclooxygenase 2 (COX2), lipoxygenases 12 (12-LOX) and 15 (15-LOX), and cytochrome P450 to a series of hydroperoxy, hydroxy and epoxy derivatives with distinct biological properties compared to the parent compounds (Kozak et al. 2002; Snider et al. 2010; Kuc et al. 2012; Urquhart et al. 2015). The metabolism of AEA and 2-AG is schematically depicted in Fig. 15.1.

15.2.2 Molecular Targets

AEA and 2-AG bind with different affinity and potency type-1 (CB_1) and type-2 (CB_2) cannabinoid receptors (Pertwee et al. 2010), two well-characterized 7-transmembrane G protein-coupled receptors (GPCRs). In addition, eCBs are described to interact with several non-cannabinoid receptors. Some of them have an intracellular binding site, like the transient receptor potential vanilloid type-1 (TRPV1) ion channel (Di Marzo and De Petrocellis 2010). Others are localized in the nucleus, like the peroxisome proliferator-activated receptors (PPAR) α and γ (Pistis and Melis 2010).

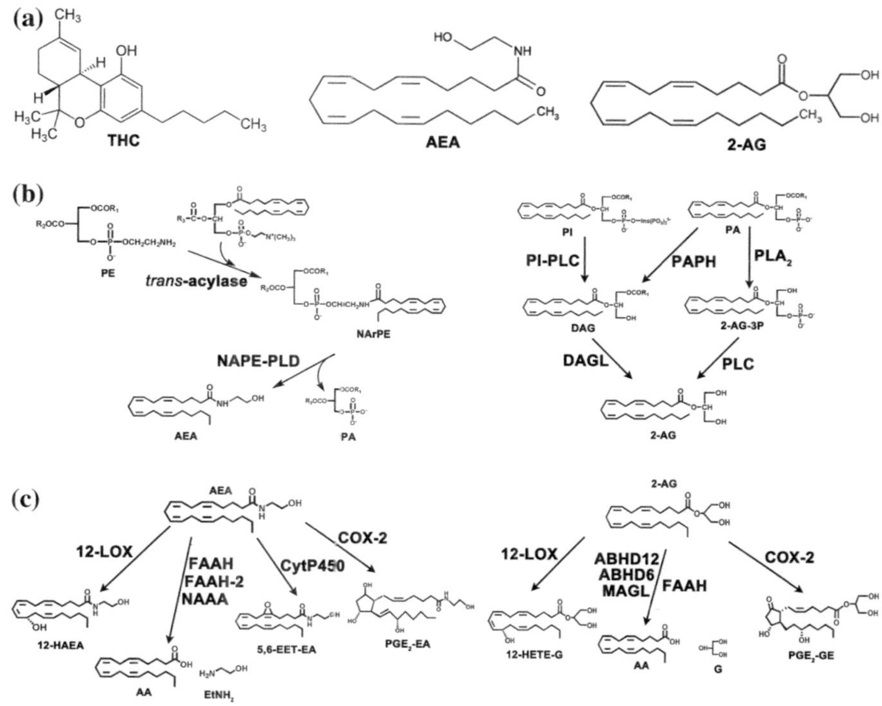

Fig. 15.1 Endocannabinoid metabolism. Chemical structures of THC and two prominent eCBs (**a**). Alternative biosynthetic and degradative pathways of AEA (**b**) and 2-AG (**c**). Abbreviations: *2-AG-3P* 2-arachidonoylglycerol-3-phosphate; *12-HAEA* 12-hydroxyanandamide; *12-LOX* 12-lipoxygenase; *5,5-EET-EA* 5,5-epoxyeicosatrienoyl ethanolamide; *12-HETE-G* 12-hydroxyarachidonoyl-glycerol; *AA* arachidonic acid; *ABHD6/12* α/β-hydrolase domain 6/12; *Cyt P450* cytochrome P450; *COX-2* cyclooxygenase-2; *DAG* diacylglycerol; *DAGL* diacylglycerol lipase; *EtNH*$_2$ ethanolamine; *FAAH* fatty acid amide hydrolase; *FAAH-2* fatty acid amide hydrolase-2; *G* glycerol; *MAGL* monoacylglycerol lipase; *NAAA* *N*-acylethanolamine-hydrolyzing acid amidase; *NArPE* *N*-arachidonoyl-phosphatidylethanolamine; *NAPE-PLD* *N*-acyl-phosphatidyl-ethanolamines-hydrolyzing phospholipase D; *PA* phosphatidic acid; *PAPH* phosphatidic acid phosphohydrolase; *PI* phosphatidylinositol; *PE* phosphatidylethanolamine; *PGE*$_2$*-G* prostaglandin glycerol E$_2$; *PLA*$_2$ phospholipase A$_2$; *PLC* phospholipase C

15.2.2.1 Cannabinoid Receptors

CB$_1$ and CB$_2$ receptors are members of the rhodopsin-like family of heptahelical transmembrane-spanning GPCRs. They are encoded for by different genes, and exhibit 44 % amino acid identity throughout the whole protein, and 68 % within the transmembrane domains. These receptors show a quite broad, and sometimes overlapping, distribution (Pertwee et al. 2010).

CB$_1$ receptors are predominantly found in the central nervous system, where they are highly expressed in brain areas associated with cognition, memory, emotionality, motor function, and pain, including cortex, limbic system, hippocampus, cerebellum and several nuclei of the basal ganglia. CB_1 receptors are also expressed in non-neuronal cells, including immune cells (Chiurchiù et al. 2015).

CB_2 receptors are mainly expressed in the immune system, including the marginal zone of the spleen and macrophages, generally mediating anti-inflammatory and immunosuppressive effects. There is also evidence that CB_2 receptors are also expressed in central and peripheral neurons, both under physiological conditions and upon stress (Van Sickle et al. 2005; Viscomi et al. 2009; Onaivi et al. 2012).

Cannabinoid receptors can couple to multiple heterotrimeric G-proteins to elicit specific signaling pathways, often in a cell-type-specific, agonist-specific or dose-dependent manner (Howlett 2005). Typically, their stimulation has been shown to lead to: inhibition or, less often, stimulation of adenylyl cyclase (AC), via Gi/o or Gs proteins, with subsequent inhibition, or stimulation, of protein kinase A (PKA), respectively; (ii) activation of different members of the mitogen-activated protein kinase (MAPK) family, such as extracellular signal-regulated kinase (ERK) (Bouaboula et al. 1995), c-Jun N-terminal kinase (JNK) and p38 MAPK (Liu et al. 2000), via Gi/o proteins; (iii) activation of phospholipase C (PLC) via either Gq/11 or βγ subunits of Gi/o proteins (Howlett 2005). Finally, CB_1 receptors can cause Gi/o-mediated inhibition of voltage-gated Ca^{2+} channels (L, N, and P/Q-type) and activation of A-type and inwardly rectifying K^+ channels (Howlett 2005). CB_2 receptors share with CB_1 receptors similar signal transduction mechanisms in terms of their actions on adenylyl cyclase and MAPKs, but they seem to be unable to regulate ion channels as do CB_1 receptors. However, it has been demonstrated that CB_2 receptors are coupled, via inositol trisphosphate receptor, to Ca^{2+}-activated Cl^- channels in pyramidal neurons of the rodent medial prefrontal cortex, suggesting that also these receptors may regulate ion homeostasis and cell excitability (den Boon et al. 2012).

15.2.2.2 Transient Receptor Potential Vanilloid Type-1 Channel

The best-established non-cannabinoid receptor for eCBs is the TRPV1 channel, previously discovered as the receptor for capsaicin, the pungent agent in hot-chilli peppers (Caterina et al. 1997). TRPV1 is a non-selective cation channel with a preference for Ca^{2+}, that is involved in the transmission and modulation of pain (nociception), as well as in the integration of diverse painful and inflammatory stimuli. Therefore, it senses, directly or indirectly, a wide range of cellular and environmental signals, including noxious temperature, mild acidification, and local mediators of inflammation, such as histamine, bradykinin, nerve-growth factor, eicosanoids, ADP and ATP (Szallasi et al. 2007). TRPV1 is primarily expressed in primary sensory neurons, but it is also widely expressed in the body, including the central nervous system (Szallasi et al. 2007).

15.2.2.3 Peroxisome Proliferator-Activated Receptors

Endogenous, synthetic, and natural cannabinoids are also reported to activate PPARs, ligand-activated transcription factors that are primarily involved in the regulation of metabolism and energy homeostasis, cell differentiation, and immune function (Kersten et al. 2000). Three different PPAR isoforms are known (α, γ and δ), that are ubiquitously expressed, even though with a different tissue distribution. PPARα is mainly expressed in liver and brown adipose tissue, and to a lesser extent in kidney, heart and skeletal muscle; PPARγ is expressed in adipose tissue and colon, immune system and retina; PPARδ is widely expressed in the body, with the highest expression in heart, gut and kidney (Kersten et al. 2000).

Once activated by ligand binding, PPARs heterodimerize with the receptor of 9-*cis*-retinoic acid, and bind to specific peroxisome proliferator response elements to regulate the transcription of target genes. Endogenous ligands for PPARs are eicosanoids, fatty acids and fatty acid derivatives, including eCBs (Pistis and Melis 2010).

It has been described that AEA and 2-AG, at micromolar concentrations, directly bind to and activate both PPARα and PPARγ. In particular, AEA induces expression of several PPARγ-sensitive genes in 3T3-L1 fibroblasts (Bouaboula et al. 2005), and causes inhibition of interleukin (IL)-2 expression by activating PPARγ in primary splenocytes (Rockwell and Kaminski 2004). Finally, AEA controls adipocyte differentiation by activating PPARγ (Gasperi et al. 2007) and induces vasorelaxant responses on the ophthalmic artery through activation of PPARα (Romano and Lograno 2012).

15.3 The Cutaneous Endocannabinoid System

15.3.1 *Expression*

As in other parts of the body, the eCB system is ubiquitously expressed by all cellular components of the skin (Oddi and Maccarrone 2014). The eCBs are produced and released by different skin cell populations, including keratinocytes (Maccarrone et al. 2003; Toth et al. 2011; Magina et al. 2011), sebocytes (Dobrosi et al. 2008), melanocytes (Pucci et al. 2012), sweat gland epithelial cells (Czifra et al. 2012), and macrophages (Jiang et al. 2009), under basal and stimulated conditions. The levels of AEA and 2-AG have been measured in rodent paw skin (Felder et al. 1996; Khasabova et al. 2012), reaching pmol/g and nmol/g concentrations, respectively, similar to those found in the brain.

The presence in the skin of diacylglycerol lipase, DAGL, and monoacylglycerol lipase, MAGL, the main enzymes involved in 2-AG biosynthesis and catabolism, respectively, has been assessed in cultured keratinocytes (Berdyshev et al. 2000; Maccarrone et al. 2003; Oddi et al. 2005), melanocytes (Hamtiaux et al. 2012; Pucci et al. 2012), sebocytes (Dobrosi et al. 2008), and fibroblasts (McPartland 2008). Also AEA-metabolizing enzymes, namely FAAH and NAPE-PLD, have been documented in rodent skin (Karsak et al. 2007; Petrosino et al. 2010; Khasabova et al. 2012).

Immunohistological investigations of the precise localization of CB_1 and CB_2 receptors in sections of human and rodent skin revealed that both receptors are expressed in virtually all skin cell populations. In particular, both receptors are present in keratinocytes, cutaneous nerve fibers, dermal cells, and specialized cells with adnexal structures (Casanova et al. 2003; Ibrahim et al. 2005; Stander et al. 2005). Notably, in one of these immunohistochemical studies on human skin, CB_1 and CB_2 have been found to be distributed in a complementary fashion in epidermis, hair follicle, and sebaceous gland, with CB_1 and CB_2 being predominantly expressed in differentiated and undifferentiated cells, respectively. Therefore, it can be suggested that these two receptors play nonredundant roles during differentiation of keratinocytes and sebocytes. In the skin, CB_2 is expressed beyond the basal layer, but fairly uniformly distributed throughout the epidermis (Ibrahim et al. 2005). In the dermis, CB_1 and CB_2 are both expressed in the myoepithelial cells of the secretory portion of eccrine sweat glands, but not in secretory cells (Stander et al. 2005). Positive immunoreactivity for CB_1 and CB_2 has been also documented in mast cells and in most (but not all) CD68-positive macrophages (Stander et al. 2005; Sugawara et al. 2012). In mouse skin, CB_2 is present in myofibroblasts and vascular smooth muscle cells (Zheng et al. 2012). Concerning their localization in human primary sensory nerves, CB_1 and CB_2 are expressed in large (myelinated) and thin (unmyelinated) calcitonin gene-related peptide positive nerve fibers (Stander et al. 2005). Finally, both receptors are functionally expressed in cultured melanocytes (Magina et al. 2011; Pucci et al. 2012), fibroblasts (McPartland 2008), sebocytes (Dobrosi et al. 2008) and sweat gland epithelial cells (Czifra et al. 2012).

A wide expression in both neuronal and non-neuronal cells of the skin has also documented for TRPV1 and all the isotypes of PPARs, in several cases with an overlapping expression CB_1 and CB_2 receptors. TRPV1 is located in a neurochemically heterogeneous population of small-diameter primary afferent fibers and with small-diameter nerve fibers in the skin of rodents and humans (Guo et al. 1999; Stander et al. 2004; Bodo et al. 2004). Moreover, TRPV1 ion channels have been described in numerous non-neuronal cell types, including keratinocytes, mast cells and dendritic cells (Stander et al. 2004; Bodo et al. 2004). PPARδ is present throughout all epidermal layers, whereas PPARα and PPARγ are mainly located in suprabasal compartments (Di-Poi et al. 2004).

15.3.2 *Endocannabinoids and Skin Barrier Function*

15.3.2.1 Activity in Epidermal Barrier Formation

Growing evidence supports a functional role of eCB signaling in regulating key biological processes of keratinocytes, such as proliferation, differentiation and apoptosis, which are essential for formation and maintenance of epidermal barrier structure and function.

For example, AEA inhibits the formation of cornified envelope in differentiating keratinocyte, through a CB_1-dependent reduction of transglutaminase and protein kinase C activities (Maccarrone et al. 2003), suggesting an important role of eCB signaling in epidermal differentiation. This anti-differentiative activity of AEA has been found to be associated with the silencing of genes involved in keratinocyte differentiation (i.e., keratin 1, keratin 10, involucrin, and transglutaminase 5) by p38-MAPK-mediated DNA methylation of their promoters (Paradisi et al. 2008). On the other hand, in hair follicles it has been demonstrated that CB_1 activation by AEA inhibits hair shaft elongation and the proliferation of hair matrix keratinocytes, and also induces intraepithelial apoptosis and premature hair follicle regression (Telek et al. 2007). Interestingly, these cells failed to respond to 2-AG stimulation, highlighting the nonredundancy of these two prototypic eCBs (Telek et al. 2007). Consistent with an inhibitory role of AEA in keratinocyte growth, CB_1 activation by AEA has been found to markedly suppress proliferation and induce cell death in both human cultured keratinocytes and skin organ-culture models (Toth et al. 2011), possibly by elevating intracellular Ca^{2+} concentration through activation of TRPV1.

Histological phenotyping of CB_1 and CB_2 deficient mice revealed that these two receptors operate in an opposite manner to regulate epidermal barrier homeostasis and epidermal differentiation (Roelandt et al. 2012). In particular, the loss of CB_1 receptor enhances proliferation and reduces differentiation of keratinocytes, causing the formation of a thicker epidermis with altered lipid bilayer structures. Conversely, the targeted disruption of CB_2 leads to the formation of a thinner epidermis with reduced proliferative rates of keratinocytes, paralleled by a strong expression of the main epidermal differentiation markers: involucrin, loricrin, filaggrin and caspase 14 activation (Roelandt et al. 2012). Moreover, functional data from these mouse models demonstrated that the recovery of the permeability barrier function of the epidermis following acute removal of corneocytes from the stratum corneum is impaired in $CB_1^{-/-}$, whilst it was enhanced in $CB_2^{-/-}$ mice. These findings strongly suggest that CB_1 signaling is a positive regulator, whereas CB_2 signaling is a negative regulator, of epidermal permeability barrier and stratum corneum structure (Roelandt et al. 2012).

Since it is well-established that an increase of intracellular 3′,5′-cyclic adenosine monophosphate (cAMP) in epidermal keratinocytes delays barrier recovery, that instead is accelerated by cAMP antagonists (Denda et al. 2004), it is tempting to speculate that the opposite effects exerted by cannabinoid receptors on epidermal homeostasis could be due to their different regulation of adenylyl cyclase activity. Furthermore, it should also be kept in mind that Ca^{2+} is a central regulator of keratinocyte differentiation (Elsholz et al. 2014) and that the eCBs can strongly influence cytosolic Ca^{2+} levels via cannabinoid receptors and TRPV1, which are co-expressed in keratinocytes. However, additional studies are needed to better clarify the physiological relevance of eCB signaling in keratinocyte differentiation, as well as in epidermal barrier homeostasis.

15.3.2.2 Activity in Non-keratinocyte Skin Cells

Beyond the pivotal role played by keratinocytes, structure and function of the skin barrier are both strongly influenced by the activity of many other specialized cells, such as sebocytes, melanocytes and sweat gland cells, that regulate the content of sebum, melanin pigmentation and hydration of the skin, respectively. Moreover, dermis, the collagen-rich connective tissue of the skin, is produced, organized and maintained by the activity of fibroblasts, the main resident cells of the dermis.

On these cells, most likely because of the variety of their targets and of their underlying signaling pathways, eCBs and their synthetic counterparts evoke complex, and even biphasic, actions. In particular, it has been documented that human sebocytes express CB_2 but not CB_1 receptors, and that AEA stimulates lipid production at low concentrations, but induces apoptosis at higher levels, in a CB_2-mediated manner (Dobrosi et al. 2008). Similarly, in melanocytes AEA produces melanogenic, mitogenic, and dendritogenic effects at low doses (via CB_1) and proapoptotic effects at higher doses (via TRPV1) (Pucci et al. 2012). Additionally, activation of CB_1 inhibits basal and ultraviolet B-induced melanogenesis in a human melanoma cell line (Magina et al. 2011). In human eccrine sweat gland epithelial cells both AEA and 2-AG are able to (i) suppress proliferation, (ii) induce apoptosis, (iii) alter expression of various structural proteins (i.e., involucrin, filaggrin, loricrin, and keratins), and (iv) upregulate lipid synthesis; remarkably, all these effects have been found to be exerted in a CB_1–, CB_2–, and TRPV1-independent manner (Czifra et al. 2012). In dermal fibroblasts, it has been reported that synthetic cannabinoid agonists, acting via non-CB receptors, limit extracellular matrix (ECM) production by disrupting the transforming growth factor β (TGFβ) cascade, and downregulating proliferation and activation (Servettaz et al. 2010; Balistreri et al. 2011). On the same cells, it has been demonstrated that AjA, a synthetic THC analogue, inhibits collagen synthesis through activation of PPARγ in skin fibroblasts (Garcia-Gonzalez et al. 2012).

15.3.2.3 Activity in Skin Immunity

In addition to being a physical barrier, the skin is an immunological barrier, consisting in a combination of specialized cell types with distinct roles in innate and adaptive immunity, including macrophages, mast cells, dendritic cells, Langerhans cells, keratinocytes, fibroblasts, as well as B and T lymphocytes.

It is well-established that CB_2, and to a lesser extent CB_1, receptors are expressed in several cell lineages of the immune system (Chiurchiù et al. 2015). It is also widely recognized that their stimulation by exogenous and/or endogenous cannabinoids generally suppresses acute and chronic inflammatory conditions. Although the precise mechanisms of (e)CB-induced immunomodulation have not been fully elucidated yet, it is likely that they depend on the ability of the eCB system to manipulate those signaling cascades (such as cAMP, Ca^{2+} and MAPK cascades), that are essential for maturation and function of immune cells (Chiurchiù et al. 2015).

One major mechanism of immunosuppression by (e)CBs is the induction of apoptosis in immune cell populations. For example, activation of cannabinoid receptors (mainly CB_2) by THC and other cannabinoid ligands induces cell death in macrophages, dendritic cells, T- and B-lymphocytes (Klein 2005). Similarly, low doses of AEA cause significant inhibition of proliferation of lymphocytes and dendritic cells, inducing cell death by apoptosis, while 2-AG has been shown to exhibit biological activity in mouse splenocytes, by producing strong immunomodulatory activity on mitogen-induced lymphocyte proliferation (Schwarz et al. 1994; Lee et al. 1995; Do et al. 2004).

Another relevant immunomodulatory action mediated by the eCB system is the regulation of inflammatory cytokine production by immune cells. In particular, THC and eCBs have been shown to cause blockade of pro-inflammatory Th1 cytokines, such as interferon-γ and interleukin (IL)-2, and increase the expression of anti-inflammatory Th2 cytokines, such as IL-4 and IL-10, which are important for humoral immunity, and TGF-α which has immunosuppressive properties (Pacifici et al. 2003). Regarding skin cells, it has been recently shown that CB_1 activation in keratinocytes leads to a reduced secretion of proinflammatory chemokines C–C motif ligand 8 (CCL8) and C–X–C motif ligand 10 (CXCL10) in a mouse model of allergic contact dermatitis. Both substances regulate T cell-dependent inflammation, and attenuate thymic stromal lymphopoietin- (TSLP-) and CCL8-dependent Th2-type allergic inflammatory responses (Gaffal et al. 2013, 2014). Moreover, AEA has been reported to reduce tumor necrosis factor (TNF)-α-induced IL-8 and CCL2 release from keratinocytes, acting in an anti-inflammatory manner (Leonti et al. 2010). Finally, in a very recent study we found that AEA reduces production and release of IL-12 and IL-23 (Th1- and Th17-inducing cytokines, respectively) from inflamed keratinocytes in a CB_1-dependent manner, suggesting that CB_1 could negatively drive the polarization of CD4 naive T cells into Th1 and Th17 (unpublished results).

Regarding the influence of the eCB system on phagocytosis, which is a crucial step in the induction of innate and acquired immunity, it has been shown that 2-AG augments the phagocytosis of HL-60 cells differentiated to a macrophage-like phenotype, via CB_2-mediated signaling, possibly involving Akt and ERK cascades (Gokoh et al. 2007). In contrast, a more recent study reported that CB_1, but not

CB_2, enhances phagocytic activity of human macrophages, through Gαi/o-dependent RhoA/ROCK pathways (Mai et al. 2015).

Finally, another cannabinoid-mediated mechanism of immunomodulation involves the ability of cannabinoids to perturb the recruitment of leukocytes at sites of inflammation, by regulating their adhesion to endothelium, extravasation and migration in the tissue (Klein 2005). In particular, there is a large body of data that supports a functional relevance of (e)CBs in inhibiting migratory activities of a diverse array of immune cell types, primarily through CB_2-mediated pathways (Joseph et al. 2004; Kurihara et al. 2006). However, there are also some discrepancies regarding the impact of 2-AG in mediating the trafficking of immune cells. In particular, in peripheral blood eosinophils the activation of CB_2 by 2-AG, but not by AEA, induces cell migration, suggesting that 2-AG acts as a chemotactic agent and may be involved in allergic responses by promoting eosinophil infiltration (Oka et al. 2004). The active involvement of 2-AG into cell migration has been also found in myeloid and normal splenocytes (Jorda et al. 2002), and in other different lymphoid lineages, such as macrophage-like cells HL-60, U937, THP-1, as well as and human peripheral blood monocytes (Kishimoto et al. 2003). This effect of 2-AG appears to occur via CB_2-mediated signaling, that seems to involve Rho kinase and MAPK cascades.

15.4 Therapeutic Opportunities

15.4.1 Atopic Dermatitis

Atopic dermatitis, also known as atopic eczema, is a multifactorial inflammatory skin disorder characterized by intense itching and recurrent eczematous lesions, that are prone to microbial infections. An altered lipid composition of the stratum corneum is responsible for the xerotic aspect of the skin, and may determine a higher permeability to allergens and pathogens. Atopic dermatitis skin is associated with a type I hypersensitivity reaction characterized by a pro-inflammatory cytokine milieu made by excessive infiltration of immune cells, including eosinophils, mast cells and T-cells, particularly Th2 cells, Th22 cells, and, to a lesser degree, Th1 and Th17 cells (Bos 2005).

Oral or topical administration of cannabinoid-based drugs has been shown to be effective in the treatment of atopic dermatitis-like skin lesions. Indeed, several studies reported beneficial effects of manipulating the eCB system in animal models of this disorder. For example, in an oxazolone-induced dermatitis, topical application of CB_1-specific agonist significantly accelerates the recovery of epidermal permeability barrier function and exerts marked anti-inflammatory activity (Kim et al. 2015). Similarly, mice lacking CB_1 receptors globally, or specifically in keratinocytes, show enhanced Th2-type contact hypersensitivity responses to fluorescein isothiocyanate (FITC), and a delayed epidermal barrier repair when compared with wild-type mice (Gaffal et al. 2014). In particular, mRNA levels for IL-4, TSLP and CCL8, proinflammatory mediators that drive Th2-type skin inflammation in atopic dermatitis, as well as eosinophil activity, are significantly increased in inflamed ear tissue of FITC-challenged $CB_1^{-/-}$ mice, confirming the involvement of CB_1 both in maintaining epidermal barrier homoeostasis and in attenuating Th2-type allergic inflammatory responses (Gaffal et al. 2014).

The eCB system has emerged as a key regulator of mast cells, which are key effector cell type in IgE-mediated immediate hypersensitivity and allergic responses in atopic dermatitis (Kawakami et al. 2009). Indeed, natural and synthetic cannabinoids and eCBs exert suppressive activity on mast cell functions, leading to protective effects both in acute and chronic inflammatory pathologies sustained by excessive accumulation and degranulation of these immunocompetent cells (Chiurchiù et al. 2015). More specifically, both the nonpsychotropic CB_2 agonists HU-308 and HU-320 strongly reduce edema in two different murine models of allergic inflammation (Hanus et al. 1999; Sumariwalla et al. 2004). Furthermore, AEA has been shown to inhibit mast cell degranulation, via CB_1-dependent mechanisms, both in vitro and in vivo (Maccarrone et al. 2002; Sugawara et al. 2012).

As compounds that interfere with the pathophysiology of pruritus, cannabinoids could be successfully applied in the management of pruritus commonly occurring in atopic dermatitis. Systemic activation of CB_1 receptor, via either directly-acting receptor agonists (i.e., THC) or inhibitors of AEA degradation, (i.e., by pharmacological blockade or genetic deletion of FAAH) reduces scratching in a murine model of pruritus (Schlosburg et al. 2009). Another study reported that CB_1 activation by HU210 effectively suppresses histamine-induced pruritus in humans (Dvorak et al. 2003). Moreover, oral administration of JTE-907, a selective CB_2 antagonist, significantly inhibits spontaneous scratching behavior in a mouse model of atopic dermatitis (Maekawa et al. 2006), suggesting a yet-to-be-clarified CB_2 involvement in allergic itch. Finally, PAC-14028, a TRPV1 antagonist, suppresses scratching behaviors in two different models of atopic dermatitis (Yun et al. 2011). Interestingly, in a T-cell mediated model of atopic dermatitis, histamine-independent itch induced by IL-31 is significantly reduced in $TRPV1^{-/-}$ mice compared to controls (Cevikbas et al. 2014). These findings suggest that eCB signaling is crucially involved in the neuronal/nonneuronal cellular network of pruritogenic stimuli in the skin, and that its manipulation can represent another therapeutic approach for the management of itching associated to atopic dermatitis, as well as to other inflammatory conditions.

15.4.2 Allergic Contact Dermatitis

Allergic contact dermatitis is a T-cell-mediated inflammatory reaction occurring at the site of challenge with a contact allergen in sensitized individuals. It is characterized by redness, papules, and vesicles, followed by scaling and dry skin.

Immunologically, contact dermatitis is a form of delayed type IV hypersensitivity consisting of two phases: sensitisation and elicitation. In the sensitisation phase, occurring at the first contact of the skin with the hapten, the resident antigen-presenting cells, i.e., Langerhans cells and dermal dendritic cells, pick up and process the antigen. Then, hapten-bearing dendritic cells migrate to the draining lymph nodes, where the allergen is exposed to naive T lymphocytes that differentiate into antigen-specific memory T cells. During the elicitation phase, after a new contact with the same antigen, memory T cells are activated and exert direct and indirect cytotoxic effects towards cells of the skin, causing edema, erythema and induration at the site of contact in sensitized humans or animals (Bos 2005).

Numerous preclinical studies have explored the role of the eCB system in contact dermatitis. Significant alterations in the components of the eCB system have been found in different mice models of this dermatosis. In particular, in an experimental allergy contact dermatitis induced by 2,4-dinitrofluorobenzene (DNFB), tissue levels of AEA and 2-AG were found to be increased, along with a downregulation of CB_1 receptors and an upregulation of NAPE-PLD, TRPV1 and CB_2 receptors (Karsak et al. 2007; Petrosino et al. 2010). An increase of 2-AG, but not of AEA, was also observed in another model of contact dermatitis induced by oxazolone (Oka et al. 2006).

Agonists and antagonists of cannabinoid receptors can produce both anti-allergic- and pro-allergic effects. Studies with animals genetically devoid of CB_1 and CB_2 receptors have generated contradictory findings about the effective contribution of these receptors, particularly of CB_2, to allergic dermatitis. On the one hand, single and double CB_1/CB_2 receptor knockout mice have been found to display exacerbated inflammation following treatment with DNFB, suggesting that both receptors exert a protective role in allergic reaction (Karsak et al. 2007). In particular, it has been reported that $CB_2^{-/-}$ mice experience pronounced chronic inflammation that is alleviated or exacerbated by CB_2 agonists or antagonists, respectively (Karsak et al. 2007). On the other hand, $CB_2^{-/-}$ mice have been found to exhibit a significant suppression of DNFB-induced edema and acanthosis (i.e., diffuse epidermal hyperplasia), and consistently a CB_2-selective antagonist has been found to alleviate chronic inflammation induced by DNFB in wild-type mice (Ueda et al. 2005; Mimura et al. 2012). Moreover, a CB_2-selective agonist induces ear swelling in wild-type mice (Ueda et al. 2007), suggesting that the CB_2 receptor plays a stimulatory role in the sensitization and exacerbation of allergic inflammation. Furthermore, in other contact dermatitis models, where ovalbumin or oxazolone were repeatedly applied, there was a significant decrease in ear swelling and acanthosis in $CB_2^{-/-}$ mice compared with wild-type animals, strongly supporting the notion that CB_2 and its endogenous ligand 2-AG enhance dermal reactions to allergens (Mimura et al. 2012). A possible explanation for these conflicting results could reside in the different doses of inflammatory stimuli used to induce a dermal reaction and, most likely, with the pleiotropic actions that CB_2 exerts on immune cells, including regulation in cell proliferation, activation and migration.

Less controversial seems to be the role of CB_1 receptors in allergic contact dermatitis. Indeed, mice lacking CB_1 in keratinocytes show enhanced and prolonged allergic responses following DNFB challenge (Gaffal et al. 2013). Interestingly, CB_1-deficient keratinocytes produced increased amounts of CXCL10 and CCL8 in response to IFN-γ (Gaffal et al. 2013), suggesting that peripheral CB_1 expressed on these cells helps to limit the secretion of proinflammatory chemokines that regulate T cell-dependent inflammation in the elicitation phase of allergic contact dermatitis.

15.4.3 Localized Scleroderma

Localized scleroderma is a rare disease of unknown etiology, characterized by inflammation and thickening of the skin from excessive collagen deposition. Available data suggest that the mechanism of pathogenesis of scleroderma is complex. Vessels, immune system and extracellular matrix are affected and may contribute to the development of the disease. Early stages of scleroderma are characterized by an infiltration of affected skin by inflammatory cells, mostly macrophages and activated T cells. Later stages of the disease are characterized by an excessive collagen synthesis and deposition by fibroblasts, resulting in pathologic dermal fibrosis (Bielsa 2013).

Activation of the eCB system can exerts both pro-fibrotic and anti-fibrotic-effects, by acting through CB_1 and CB_2 receptors, respectively. Indeed, $CB_1^{-/-}$ mice, or controls treated with CB_1 antagonists, are protected from bleomycin-induced skin fibrosis, exhibiting a reduced dermal thickening, associated with a decreased number of myofibroblasts, infiltrating T cells and macrophages. In marked contrast, $CB_2^{-/-}$ mice, or controls treated with CB_2 antagonists, are more susceptible to the same model of scleroderma, with clinical symptoms markedly worsened (Akhmetshina et al. 2009). Similarly, $CB_2^{-/-}$ mice develop a more exacerbated hypochlorite-induced fibrosis compared with wild-type animals (Servettaz et al. 2010). Experiments involving bone marrow transplantation revealed that these two receptors indirectly regulate the activation of fibroblasts by orchestrating the infiltration of leukocytes into lesional skin (Servettaz et al. 2010; Marquart et al. 2010). Finally, increased levels of AEA induced by inactivation of FAAH exacerbate experimental fibrosis primarily via activation of CB_1 fibrosis, suggesting that CB_1 is the predominant receptor for eCBs in skin fibrosis, and that AEA exerts fibrogenic activity (Palumbo-Zerr et al. 2012).

From these preclinical data it is arguable that selective antagonism and agonism of CB_1 and CB_2 receptors, respectively, may have therapeutic potential for the treatment of early inflammatory stages of skin scleroderma.

15.4.4 Psoriasis

Psoriasis is a chronic inflammatory skin disease characterized by sharply demarcated erythematous plaques appearing on the surface of the epidermis. These lesions result from intense skin inflammation with infiltration of inflammatory cells into the dermis and epidermis and keratinocyte hyperproliferation. Although the mechanism underlying psoriasis remains elusive, there is growing evidence that T-cell-mediated immune mechanisms, particularly those mediated by Th1 and Th17 cells, play a major role in the pathology of this disease (Bos 2005).

Although direct studies using (e)CBs on preclinical models of psoriasis have not yet been conducted, the above-mentioned biological effects of these compounds on keratinocytes, and their potential in regulating the activation and balance of Th1/Th2 cells, suggest that the eCB system could be a potential target for the development of new pharmacological approaches against this skin disease.

15.5 Concluding Remarks

There is a huge need for the development of new treatments for managing chronic skin disorders, such as psoriasis, atopic dermatitis, allergic contact dermatitis and localized scleroderma. The increased knowledge of the pathogenesis of these dermatoses has highlighted several molecular and cellular mechanisms, on which it would be advisable to intervene with higher selectivity and efficacy through novel pharmacological approaches. There are many good reasons to believe that (e)CBs could be a new valuable generation of dermatological drugs. In the first place, they modulate the activity of a signaling pathway, the so-called eCB system, which is involved in skin homeostasis by orchestrating anti-proliferative, anti-fibrotic and immunomodulatory actions. In the second place, these substances, by acting as direct or indirect agonists and antagonists of cannabinoid receptors, produce beneficial effects on relevant animal models of different skin disorders, also providing proof of concept that the eCB system has a pleiotropic homeostatic function in the skin (Table 15.2). In the third place, (e)CBs have favorable drug-safety profiles, being generally well-tolerated and showing low toxicity and moderate adverse effects. Finally, as lipophilic compounds, (e)CB-based drugs can be easily administered topically, for example in the form of cream, lotion or ointment. On the basis of accumulated evidence summarized in this chapter, there is certainly a hope that in the next future at least some of (e)CB-related compounds could contribute to expand the therapeutic arsenal of clinical dermatology.

Table 15.2 Preclinical evidence for a possible therapeutic role of the eCB system in skin diseases

Disorder	Preclinical model	Role of the eCB system	Receptors involved	Reference
Atopic dermatitis	Fluorescein isothiocyanate-induced atopic dermatitis	Edema is strongly exacerbated in $CB_1^{-/-}$ mice	CB_1	Gaffal et al. (2014)
Allergic contact dermatitis	2,4-Dinitrofluorobenzene-induced contact dermatitis	Edema is slightly exacerbated in $CB_1^{-/-}$, $CB_2^{-/-}$ and double $CB_1^{-/-}$ $CB_2^{-/-}$ mice THC decreases ear swelling and granulocyte infiltration	CB_1, CB_2	Karsak et al. (2007)
	Oxazolone-induced contact dermatitis Ovalbumin-induced contact dermatitis	Edema is suppressed in $CB_2^{-/-}$ mice CB_2 and 2-AG play important stimulative roles in the sensitization, elicitation, and exacerbation of allergic inflammation	CB_2	Mimura et al. (2012), Oka et al. (2006)
Scleroderma	Bleomycin-induced fibrosis Hypochlorite-induced fibrosis	Skin fibrosis is reduced in $CB_1^{-/-}$ mice and slightly exacerbated in $CB_2^{-/-}$ mice CB_1 and AEA play important stimulative roles in skin fibrogenesis	CB_1, CB_2	Akhmetshina et al. (2009), Servettaz et al. (2010), Marquart et al. (2010), Palumbo-Zerr et al. (2012)

References

Akhmetshina A, Dees C, Busch N, Beer J, Sarter K, Zwerina J, Zimmer A, Distler O, Schett G, Distler JHW (2009) The cannabinoid receptor CB2 exerts antifibrotic effects in experimental dermal fibrosis. Arthritis Rheum 60:1129–1136

Balistreri E, Garcia-Gonzalez E, Selvi E, Akhmetshina A, Palumbo K, Lorenzini S, Maggio R, Lucattelli M, Galeazzi M, Distler JWH (2011) The cannabinoid WIN55, 212-2 abrogates dermal fibrosis in scleroderma bleomycin model. Ann Rheum Dis 70:695–699

Berdyshev EV, Schmid PC, Dong Z, Schmid HH (2000) Stress-induced generation of N-acylethanolamines in mouse epidermal JB6 P+ cells. Biochem J 346(Pt 2):369–374
Bielsa IB (2013) Update on the classification and treatment of localized scleroderma. Actas Dermo-Sifiliográficas 104:654–666
Bodo E, Kovács I, Telek A, Varga A, Paus R, Kovács L, Biro T (2004) Vanilloid receptor-1 (VR1) is widely expressed on various epithelial and mesenchymal cell types of human skin. J Invest Dermatol 123:410–413
Bos JD (ed) (2005) Skin immune system: cutaneous immunology and clinical immunodermatology, 3rd edn. CRC Press, Boca Raton
Bouaboula M, Hilairet S, Marchand J, Fajas L, Le Fur G, Casellas P (2005) Anandamide induced PPARgamma transcriptional activation and 3T3-L1 preadipocyte differentiation. Eur J Pharmacol 517:174–181
Bouaboula M, Poinot-Chazel C, Bourrié B, Canat X, Calandra B, Rinaldi-Carmona M, Le Fur G, Casellas P (1995) Activation of mitogen-activated protein kinases by stimulation of the central cannabinoid receptor CB1. Biochem J 312(Pt 2):637–641
Casanova ML, Blázquez C, Martínez-Palacio J, Villanueva C, Fernández-Aceñero MJ, Huffman JW, Jorcano JL, Guzmán M (2003) Inhibition of skin tumor growth and angiogenesis in vivo by activation of cannabinoid receptors. J Clin Invest 111:43–50
Caterina MJ, Schumacher MA, Tominaga M, Rosen TA, Levine JD, Julius D (1997) The capsaicin receptor: a heat-activated ion channel in the pain pathway. Nature 389:816–824
Cevikbas F, Wang X, Akiyama T, Kempkes C, Savinko T, Antal A, Kukova G, Buhl T, Ikoma A, Buddenkotte J et al (2014) A sensory neuron—expressed IL-31 receptor mediates T helper cell—dependent itch: involvement of TRPV1 and TRPA1. J Allergy Clin Immunol 133:448–460
Chiurchiù V, Battistini L, Maccarrone M (2015) Endocannabinoid signalling in innate and adaptive immunity. Immunology 144:352–364
Cravatt BF, Lichtman AH (2002) The enzymatic inactivation of the fatty acid amide class of signaling lipids. Chem Phys Lipids 121:135–148
Czifra G, Szollosi AG, Toth BI, Demaude J, Bouez C, Breton L, Biro T (2012) Endocannabinoids regulate growth and survival of human eccrine sweat gland-derived epithelial cells. J Invest Dermatol 132:1967–1976
den Boon FS, Chameau P, Schaafsma-Zhao Q, van Aken W, Bari M, Oddi S, Kruse CG, Maccarrone M, Wadman WJ, Werkman TR (2012) Excitability of prefrontal cortical pyramidal neurons is modulated by activation of intracellular type-2 cannabinoid receptors. Proc Natl Acad Sci USA 109:3534–3539
Denda M, Fuziwara S, Inoue K (2004) Association of cyclic adenosine monophosphate with permeability barrier homeostasis of murine skin. J Invest Dermatol 122:140–146
Di Marzo V (2008) Targeting the endocannabinoid system: to enhance or reduce? Nat Rev Drug Discov 7:438–455
Di Marzo V, De Petrocellis L (2010) Endocannabinoids as regulators of transient receptor potential (TRP) channels: a further opportunity to develop new endocannabinoid-based therapeutic drugs. Curr Med Chem 17:1430–1449
Di Patrizio NV, Piomelli D (2012) The thrifty lipids: endocannabinoids and the neural control of energy conservation. Trends Neurosci 35:403–411
Di-Poi N, Michalik L, Desvergne B, Wahli W (2004) Functions of peroxisome proliferator-activated receptors (PPAR) in skin homeostasis. Lipids 39:1093–1099
Dobrosi N, Toth BI, Nagy G, Dozsa A, Geczy T, Nagy L, Zouboulis CC, Paus R, Kovacs L, Biro T (2008) Endocannabinoids enhance lipid synthesis and apoptosis of human sebocytes via cannabinoid receptor-2-mediated signaling. FASEB J 22:3685–3695
Do Y, McKallip RJ, Nagarkatti M (1950) Nagarkatti PS (2004) activation through cannabinoid receptors 1 and 2 on dendritic cells triggers NF-kappaB-dependent apoptosis: novel role for endogenous and exogenous cannabinoids in immunoregulation. J Immunol Baltim Md 173:2373–2382

Dvorak M, Watkinson A, McGlone F, Rukwied R (2003) Histamine induced responses are attenuated by a cannabinoid receptor agonist in human skin. Inflamm Res Off J Eur Histamine Res Soc Al 52:238–245

Elsholz F, Harteneck C, Muller W, Friedland K (2014) Calcium—a central regulator of keratinocyte differentiation in health and disease. Eur J Dermatol EJD 24:650–661

Felder CC, Nielsen A, Briley EM, Palkovits M, Priller J, Axelrod J, Nguyen DN, Richardson JM, Riggin RM, Koppel GA et al (1996) Isolation and measurement of the endogenous cannabinoid receptor agonist, anandamide, in brain and peripheral tissues of human and rat. FEBS Lett 393:231–235

Fezza F, Bari M, Florio R, Talamonti E, Feole M, Maccarrone M (2014) Endocannabinoids, related compounds and their metabolic routes. Mol Basel Switz 19:17078–17106

Gaffal E, Cron M, Glodde N, Bald T, Kuner R, Zimmer A, Lutz B, Tüting T (2013) Cannabinoid 1 receptors in keratinocytes modulate proinflammatory chemokine secretion and attenuate contact allergic inflammation. J Immunol 190:4929–4936

Gaffal E, Glodde N, Jakobs M, Bald T, Tüting T (2014) Cannabinoid 1 receptors in keratinocytes attenuate fluorescein isothiocyanate-induced mouse atopic-like dermatitis. Exp Dermatol 23:401–406

Galve-Roperh I, Chiurchiù V, Díaz-Alonso J, Bari M, Guzmán M, Maccarrone M (2013) Cannabinoid receptor signaling in progenitor/stem cell proliferation and differentiation. Prog Lipid Res 52:633–650

Garcia-Gonzalez E, Selvi E, Balistreri E, Akhmetshina A, Palumbo K, Lorenzini S, Lazzerini PE, Montilli C, Capecchi PL, Lucattelli M et al (2012) Synthetic cannabinoid ajulemic acid exerts potent antifibrotic effects in experimental models of systemic sclerosis. Ann Rheum Dis 71:1545–1551

Gasperi V, Fezza F, Pasquariello N, Bari M, Oddi S, Agrò AF, Maccarrone M (2007) Endocannabinoids in adipocytes during differentiation and their role in glucose uptake. Cell Mol Life Sci CMLS 64:219–229

Gokoh M, Kishimoto S, Oka S, Sugiura T (2007) 2-Arachidonoylglycerol enhances the phagocytosis of opsonized zymosan by HL-60 cells differentiated into macrophage-like cells. Biol Pharm Bull 30:1199–1205

Guo A, Vulchanova L, Wang J, Li X, Elde R (1999) Immunocytochemical localization of the vanilloid receptor 1 (VR1): relationship to neuropeptides, the P2X3 purinoceptor and IB4 binding sites. Eur J Neurosci 11:946–958

Hamtiaux L, Masquelier J, Muccioli GG, Bouzin C, Feron O, Gallez B, Lambert DM (2012) The association of N-palmitoylethanolamine with the FAAH inhibitor URB597 impairs melanoma growth through a supra-additive action. BMC Cancer 12:92

Hanus L, Breuer A, Tchilibon S, Shiloah S, Goldenberg D, Horowitz M, Pertwee RG, Ross RA, Mechoulam R, Fride E (1999) HU-308: a specific agonist for CB(2), a peripheral cannabinoid receptor. Proc Natl Acad Sci USA 96:14228–14233

Howlett AC (2005) Cannabinoid receptor signaling. Handb Exp Pharmacol 53–79

Ibrahim MM, Porreca F, Lai J, Albrecht PJ, Rice FL, Khodorova A, Davar G, Makriyannis A, Vanderah TW, Mata HP et al (2005) CB2 cannabinoid receptor activation produces antinociception by stimulating peripheral release of endogenous opioids. Proc Natl Acad Sci USA 102:3093–3098

Jiang L, Pu J, Han Z, Hu L, He B (2009) Role of activated endocannabinoid system in regulation of cellular cholesterol metabolism in macrophages. Cardiovasc Res 81:805–813

Jorda MA, Verbakel SE, Valk PJM, Vankan-Berkhoudt YV, Maccarrone M, Finazzi-Agrò A, Löwenberg B, Delwel R (2002) Hematopoietic cells expressing the peripheral cannabinoid receptor migrate in response to the endocannabinoid 2-arachidonoylglycerol. Blood 99:2786–2793

Joseph J, Niggemann B, Zaenker KS, Entschladen F (2004) Anandamide is an endogenous inhibitor for the migration of tumor cells and T lymphocytes. Cancer Immunol Immunother CII 53:723–728

Karsak M, Gaffal E, Date R, Wang-Eckhardt L, Rehnelt J, Petrosino S, Starowicz K, Steuder R, Schlicker E, Cravatt B et al (2007) Attenuation of allergic contact dermatitis through the endocannabinoid system. Science 316:1494–1497

Kawakami T, Ando T, Kimura M, Wilson BS, Kawakami Y (2009) Mast cells in atopic dermatitis. Curr Opin Immunol 21:666–678

Kersten S, Desvergne B, Wahli W (2000) Roles of PPARs in health and disease. Nature 405:421–424

Khasabova IA, Khasabov S, Paz J, Harding-Rose C, Simone DA, Seybold VS (2012) Cannabinoid type-1 receptor reduces pain and neurotoxicity produced by chemotherapy. J Neurosci 32:7091–7101

Kim HJ, Kim B, Park BM, Jeon JE, Lee SH, Mann S, Ahn SK, Hong S-P, Jeong SK (2015) Topical cannabinoid receptor 1 agonist attenuates the cutaneous inflammatory responses in oxazolone-induced atopic dermatitis model. Int J Dermatol 54:e401–e408

Kishimoto S, Gokoh M, Oka S, Muramatsu M, Kajiwara T, Waku K, Sugiura T (2003) 2-arachidonoylglycerol induces the migration of HL-60 cells differentiated into macrophage-like cells and human peripheral blood monocytes through the cannabinoid CB2 receptor-dependent mechanism. J Biol Chem 278:24469–24475

Klein TW (2005) Cannabinoid-based drugs as anti-inflammatory therapeutics. Nat Rev Immunol 5:400–411

Kozak KR, Crews BC, Morrow JD, Wang L-H, Ma YH, Weinander R, Jakobsson P-J, Marnett LJ (2002) Metabolism of the endocannabinoids, 2-arachidonylglycerol and anandamide, into prostaglandin, thromboxane, and prostacyclin glycerol esters and ethanolamides. J Biol Chem 277:44877–44885

Kuc C, Jenkins A, Van Dross RT (2012) Arachidonoyl ethanolamide (AEA)-induced apoptosis is mediated by J-series prostaglandins and is enhanced by fatty acid amide hydrolase (FAAH) blockade. Mol Carcinog 51:139–149

Kurihara R, Tohyama Y, Matsusaka S, Naruse H, Kinoshita E, Tsujioka T, Katsumata Y, Yamamura H (2006) Effects of peripheral cannabinoid receptor ligands on motility and polarization in neutrophil-like HL60 cells and human neutrophils. J Biol Chem 281:12908–12918

Lee M, Yang KH, Kaminski NE (1995) Effects of putative cannabinoid receptor ligands, anandamide and 2-arachidonyl-glycerol, on immune function in B6C3F1 mouse splenocytes. J Pharmacol Exp Ther 275:529–536

Leonti M, Casu L, Raduner S, Cottiglia F, Floris C, Altmann K-H, Gertsch J (2010) Falcarinol is a covalent cannabinoid CB1 receptor antagonist and induces pro-allergic effects in skin. Biochem Pharmacol 79:1815–1826

Liu J, Gao B, Mirshahi F, Sanyal AJ, Khanolkar AD, Makriyannis A, Kunos G (2000) Functional CB1 cannabinoid receptors in human vascular endothelial cells. Biochem J 346(Pt 3):835–840

Maccarrone M, Bari M, Battista N, Finazzi-Agrò A (2002) Endocannabinoid degradation, endotoxic shock and inflammation. Curr Drug Targets Inflamm Allergy 1:53–63

Maccarrone M, Di Rienzo M, Battista N, Gasperi V, Guerrieri P, Rossi A, Finazzi-Agrò A (2003) The endocannabinoid system in human keratinocytes. Evidence that anandamide inhibits epidermal differentiation through CB1 receptor-dependent inhibition of protein kinase C, activation protein-1, and transglutaminase. J Biol Chem 278:33896–33903

Maccarrone M, Dainese E, Oddi S (2010) Intracellular trafficking of anandamide: new concepts for signaling. Trends Biochem Sci 35:601–608

Maccarrone M, Guzmán M, Mackie K, Doherty P, Harkany T (2014) Programming of neural cells by (endo)cannabinoids: from physiological rules to emerging therapies. Nat Rev Neurosci 15:786–801

Maccarrone M, Bab I, Biro T, Cabral GA, Dey SK, Di Marzo V, Konje JC, Kunos G, Mechoulam R, Pacher P et al (2015) Endocannabinoid signaling at the periphery: 50 years after THC. Trends Pharmacol Sci 36:277–296

Maekawa T, Nojima H, Kuraishi Y, Aisaka K (2006) The cannabinoid CB2 receptor inverse agonist JTE-907 suppresses spontaneous itch-associated responses of NC mice, a model of atopic dermatitis. Eur J Pharmacol 542:179–183

Magina S, Esteves-Pinto C, Moura E, Serrão MP, Moura D, Petrosino S, Di Marzo V, Vieira-Coelho MA (2011) Inhibition of basal and ultraviolet B-induced melanogenesis by cannabinoid CB(1) receptors: a keratinocyte-dependent effect. Arch Dermatol Res 303:201–210

Mai P, Tian L, Yang L, Wang L, Yang L, Li L (2015) Cannabinoid receptor 1 but not 2 mediates macrophage phagocytosis by $G_{(\alpha)i/o}$/RhoA/ROCK signaling pathway. J Cell Physiol 230:1640–1650

Marquart S, Zerr P, Akhmetshina A, Palumbo K, Reich N, Tomcik M, Horn A, Dees C, Engel M, Zwerina J et al (2010) Inactivation of the cannabinoid receptor CB1 prevents leukocyte infiltration and experimental fibrosis. Arthritis Rheum 62:3467–3476

McPartland JM (2008) Expression of the endocannabinoid system in fibroblasts and myofascial tissues. J Bodyw Mov Ther 12:169–182

Mechoulam R, Parker LA (2013) The endocannabinoid system and the brain. Annu Rev Psychol 64:21–47

Mimura T, Ueda Y, Watanabe Y, Sugiura T (2012) The cannabinoid receptor-2 is involved in allergic inflammation. Life Sci 90:862–866

Nicolussi S, Gertsch J (2015) Endocannabinoid transport revisited. Vitam Horm 98:441–485

Oddi S, Maccarrone M (2014) Phytocannabinoids and skin disorders. In: Pertwee R (ed) Handbook of cannabis. Oxford University Press, pp 582–600

Oddi S, Bari M, Battista N, Barsacchi D, Cozzani I, Maccarrone M (2005) Confocal microscopy and biochemical analysis reveal spatial and functional separation between anandamide uptake and hydrolysis in human keratinocytes. Cell Mol Life Sci CMLS 62:386–395

Oka S, Ikeda S, Kishimoto S, Gokoh M, Yanagimoto S, Waku K, Sugiura T (2004) 2-arachidonoylglycerol, an endogenous cannabinoid receptor ligand, induces the migration of EoL-1 human eosinophilic leukemia cells and human peripheral blood eosinophils. J Leukoc Biol 76:1002–1009

Oka S, Wakui J, Ikeda S, Yanagimoto S, Kishimoto S, Gokoh M, Nasui M, Sugiura T (2006) Involvement of the cannabinoid CB2 receptor and its endogenous ligand 2-arachidonoylglycerol in oxazolone-induced contact dermatitis in mice. J Immunol 177:8796–8805

Onaivi ES, Ishiguro H, Gu S, Liu Q-R (2012) CNS effects of CB2 cannabinoid receptors: beyond neuro-immuno-cannabinoid activity. J Psychopharmacol Oxf Engl 26:92–103

Pacifici R, Zuccaro P, Pichini S, Roset PN, Poudevida S, Farré M, Segura J, De la Torre R (2003) Modulation of the immune system in cannabis users. JAMA 289:1929–1931

Palumbo-Zerr K, Horn A, Distler A, Zerr P, Dees C, Beyer C, Selvi E, Cravatt BF, Distler O, Schett G et al (2012) Inactivation of fatty acid amide hydrolase exacerbates experimental fibrosis by enhanced endocannabinoid-mediated activation of CB1. Ann Rheum Dis 71:2051–2054

Paradisi A, Pasquariello N, Barcaroli D, Maccarrone M (2008) Anandamide regulates keratinocyte differentiation by inducing DNA Methylation in a CB1 receptor-dependent manner. J Biol Chem 283:6005–6012

Pertwee RG, Howlett AC, Abood ME, Alexander SPH, Di Marzo V, Elphick MR, Greasley PJ, Hansen HS, Kunos G, Mackie K et al (2010) International union of basic and clinical pharmacology. LXXIX. Cannabinoid receptors and their ligands: beyond CB_1 and CB_2. Pharmacol Rev 62:588–631

Petrosino S, Cristino L, Karsak M, Gaffal E, Ueda N, Tüting T, Bisogno T, De Filippis D, D'Amico A, Saturnino C et al (2010) Protective role of palmitoylethanolamide in contact allergic dermatitis. Allergy 65 698–711

Pistis M, Melis M (2010) From surface to nuclear receptors: the endocannabinoid family extends its assets. Curr Med Chem 17:1450–1467

Pucci M, Pasquariello N, Battista N, Di Tommaso M, Rapino C, Fezza F, Zuccolo M, Jourdain R, Finazzi Agrò A, Breton L et al (2012) Endocannabinoids stimulate human melanogenesis via type-1 cannabinoid receptor. J Biol Chem 287:15466–15478

Rockwell CE, Kaminski NE (2004) A cyclooxygenase metabolite of anandamide causes inhibition of interleukin-2 secretion in murine splenocytes. J Pharmacol Exp Ther 311:683–690

Roelandt T, Heughebaert C, Bredif S, Giddelo C, Baudouin C, Msika P, Roseeuw D, Uchida Y, Elias PM, Hachem J-P (2012) Cannabinoid receptors 1 and 2 oppositely regulate epidermal permeability barrier status and differentiation. Exp Dermatol 21:688–693

Romano MR, Lograno MD (2012) Involvement of the peroxisome proliferator-activated receptor (PPAR) alpha in vascular response of endocannabinoids in the bovine ophthalmic artery. Eur J Pharmacol 683:197–203

Schlosburg JE, Boger DL, Cravatt BF, Lichtman AH (2009) Endocannabinoid modulation of scratching response in an acute allergenic model: a new prospective neural therapeutic target for pruritus. J Pharmacol Exp Ther 329:314–323

Schwarz H, Blanco FJ, Lotz M (1994) Anadamide, an endogenous cannabinoid receptor agonist inhibits lymphocyte proliferation and induces apoptosis. J Neuroimmunol 55:107–115

Servettaz A, Kavian N, Nicco C, Deveaux V, Chereau C, Wang A, Zimmer A, Lotersztajn S, Weill B, Batteux F (2010) Targeting the cannabinoid pathway limits the development of fibrosis and autoimmunity in a mouse model of systemic sclerosis. Am J Pathol 177:187–196

Snider NT, Walker VJ, Hollenberg PF (2010) Oxidation of the endogenous cannabinoid arachidonoyl ethanolamide by the cytochrome P450 monooxygenases: physiological and pharmacological implications. Pharmacol Rev 62:136–154

Stander S, Moormann C, Schumacher M, Buddenkotte J, Artuc M, Shpacovitch V, Brzoska T, Lippert U, Henz BM, Luger TA et al (2004) Expression of vanilloid receptor subtype 1 in cutaneous sensory nerve fibers, mast cells, and epithelial cells of appendage structures. Exp Dermatol 13:129–139

Stander S, Schmelz M, Metze D, Luger T, Rukwied R (2005) Distribution of cannabinoid receptor 1 (CB1) and 2 (CB2) on sensory nerve fibers and adnexal structures in human skin. J Dermatol Sci 38:177–188

Sugawara K, Biro T, Tsuruta D, Toth BI, Kromminga A, Zakany N, Zimmer A, Funk W, Gibbs BF, Zimmer A et al (2012) Endocannabinoids limit excessive mast cell maturation and activation in human skin. J Allergy Clin Immunol 129(726–738):e8

Sumariwalla PF, Gallily R, Tchilibon S, Fride E, Mechoulam R, Feldmann M (2004) A novel synthetic, nonpsychoactive cannabinoid acid (HU-320) with antiinflammatory properties in murine collagen-induced arthritis. Arthritis Rheum 50:985–998

Szallasi A, Cortright DN, Blum CA, Eid SR (2007) The vanilloid receptor TRPV1: 10 years from channel cloning to antagonist proof-of-concept. Nat Rev Drug Discov 6:357–372

Telek A, Biro T, Bodo E, Toth BI, Borbiro I, Kunos G, Paus R (2007) Inhibition of human hair follicle growth by endo- and exocannabinoids. FASEB J 21:3534–3541

Toth BI, Dobrosi N, Dajnoki A, Czifra G, Olah A, Szollosi AG, Juhasz I, Sugawara K, Paus R, Biro T (2011) Endocannabinoids modulate human epidermal keratinocyte proliferation and survival via the sequential engagement of cannabinoid receptor-1 and transient receptor potential vanilloid-1. J Invest Dermatol 131:1095–1104

Ueda Y, Miyagawa N, Matsui T, Kaya T, Iwamura H (2005) Involvement of cannabinoid CB(2) receptor-mediated response and efficacy of cannabinoid CB(2) receptor inverse agonist, JTE-907, in cutaneous inflammation in mice. Eur J Pharmacol 520:164–171

Ueda Y, Miyagawa N, Wakitani K (2007) Involvement of cannabinoid CB2 receptors in the IgE-mediated triphasic cutaneous reaction in mice. Life Sci 80:414–419

Ueda N, Tsuboi K, Uyama T, Ohnishi T (2011) Biosynthesis and degradation of the endocannabinoid 2-arachidonoylglycerol. BioFactors Oxf Engl 37:1–7

Urquhart P, Nicolaou A, Woodward DF (2015) Endocannabinoids and their oxygenation by cyclo-oxygenases, lipoxygenases and other oxygenases. Biochim Biophys Acta 1851:366–376

Van Sickle MD, Duncan M, Kingsley PJ, Mouihate A, Urbani P, Mackie K, Stella N, Makriyannis A, Piomelli D, Davison JS et al (2005) Identification and functional characterization of brainstem cannabinoid CB2 receptors. Science 310:329–332

Viscomi MT, Oddi S, Latini L, Pasquariello N, Florenzano F, Bernardi G, Molinari M, Maccarrone M (2009) Selective CB2 receptor agonism protects central neurons from remote axotomy-induced apoptosis through the PI3K/Akt pathway. J Neurosci Off J Soc Neurosci 29:4564–4570

Yun JW, Seo JA, Jang WH, Koh HJ, Bae IH, Park YH, Lim KM (2011) Antipruritic effects of TRPV1 antagonist in murine atopic dermatitis and itching models. J Invest Dermatol 131:1576–1579

Zheng JL, Yu TS, Li XN, Fan YY, Ma WX, Du Y, Zhao R, Guan DW (2012) Cannabinoid receptor type 2 is time-dependently expressed during skin wound healing in mice. Int J Legal Med 126:807–814

Chapter 16
The Aryl Hydrocarbon Receptor (AhR) as an Environmental Stress Sensor and Regulator of Skin Barrier Function: Molecular Mechanisms and Therapeutic Opportunities

Rebecca Justiniano and Georg T. Wondrak

Abstract The aryl hydrocarbon receptor (AhR) is a transcription factor responsive to both xenobiotic and endogenous ligands involved in skin barrier adaptations in response to environmental and endogenous stressors. Due to the fundamental role that AhR-controlled signaling plays in skin barrier formation, homeostasis, resilience to environmental stressors, and damage repair, AhR-directed pharmacological strategies that aim at AhR-orchestrated signaling for anti-inflammatory, immune-modulatory, cancer chemopreventive, and barrier enhancing intervention show great therapeutic promise, delivering unique patient-directed benefit by targeting specific skin pathologies (including psoriasis, atopic dermatitis, seborrheic dermatitis, and solar radiation-induced skin photodamage) that have remained elusive and difficult to treat. The ever expanding and accessible range of chemically diverse physiological and synthetic AhR-modulators that differ with regard to pharmacokinetic and pharmacodynamic profile, AhR-directed potency, metabolic stability, and off-target effects through engagement of other signaling pathways provides a versatile and accessible compound platform of prototype agents and therapeutic leads for experimental intervention through AhR engagement, potentially representing breakthrough therapeutics that can quickly be optimized, developed, and formulated into novel AhR-directed cutaneous therapeutic entities.

Keywords Aryl hydrocarbon receptor · TCDD · CYP1A1 · Tryptophan · FICZ · Kynurenine · ITE · Cinnabarinic acid · Malassezin · Ketoconazole · Seborrheic dermatitis · Psoriasis · Atopic dermatitis · Vitiligo · Melanoma · Photocarcinogenesis · Nrf2 · UVA · UVB · LINE-1

R. Justiniano · G.T. Wondrak (✉)
Department of Pharmacology and Toxicology, College of Pharmacy and the University of Arizona Cancer Center, University of Arizona, 1515 N. Campbell Ave., Tucson, AZ 85724, USA
e-mail: wondrak@pharmacy.arizona.edu

G.T. Wondrak (ed.), *Skin Stress Response Pathways*,
DOI 10.1007/978-3-319-43157-4_16

16.1 The Aryl Hydrocarbon Receptor: An Environmental Stress Sensor in Skin

The aryl hydrocarbon receptor (AhR) is an ubiquitous ligand-dependent cytosolic transcription factor involved in environmental stress response signaling, xenobiotic metabolism, immune function, developmental and redox regulation, and—potentially—circadian rhythmicity (Denison and Nagy 2003; Esser and Rannug 2015; Haarmann-Stemmann et al. 2015).

AhR belongs to the evolutionarily old basic helix-loop-helix Per-Arnt-Sim (bHLH-PAS) protein superfamily, recognized as sensors of environmental and developmental signals. The AhR consists of two PAS domains, PAS-A and PAS-B, which allow for ligand binding (PAS-B) and homo-/hetero-dimerization (PAS-A/PAS-B) to other PAS proteins (Wu et al. 2013) (Fig. 16.1). Furthermore, the N-terminal basic helix-loop-helix motif mediates DNA and protein binding (Gu et al. 2000). Within the N-terminal bHLH region resides the nuclear localization signal (NLS) and a nuclear export signal (NES), which mediate nuclear transportation

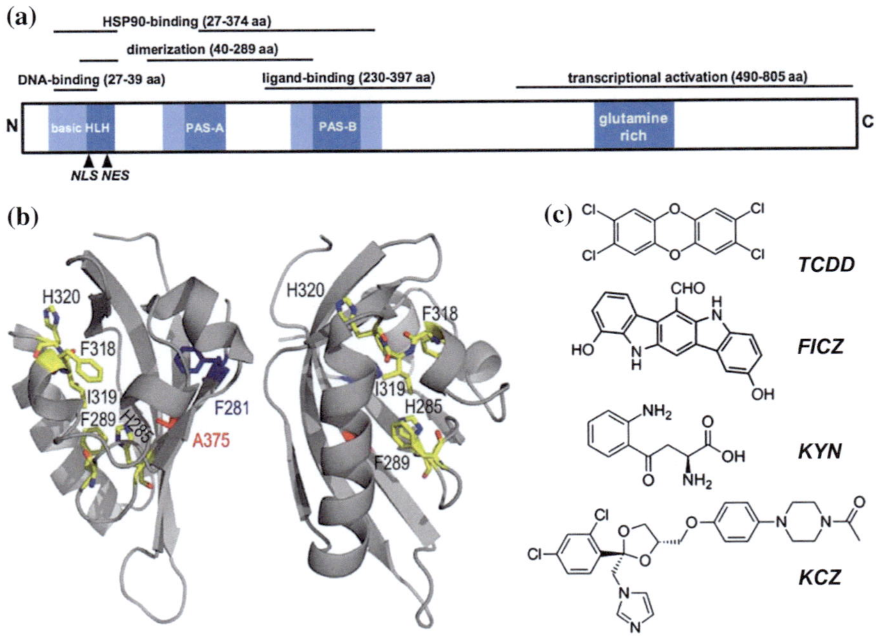

Fig. 16.1 **a** Primary AhR sequence (from N- to C-terminus) and domain coverage; *NLS* nuclear localization sequence; *NES* nuclear export signal. **b** Mouse AhR (mAhR) PASB domain; structural model; *yellow* residues involved in ligand-specific AhR activation. The residue involved in Hsp90 binding (Phe281) is indicated in *blue*, and ligand (TCDD) binding (Ala375) is indicated in *red* [reprinted with permission from: American Society for Microbiology (Soshilov and Denison 2014)]. **c** Prototype AhR modulators (from *top* to *bottom*): TCDD (dioxin); FICZ (6-formylindolo-[3,2-b]-carbazole); KYN (kynurenine); KCZ (ketoconazole)

following ligand-dependent AhR activation. Additionally, the C-terminal glutamine-rich transactivation domain (TAD) cooperates with co-activator proteins for enhanced transcriptional gene expression (Rowlands et al. 1996).

In the unliganded state, AhR is retained in the cytoplasm as an inactive protein complex consisting of an Hsp90 dimer, the chaperone prostaglandin E synthase 3 (PTGES3, p23), the immunophilin-like protein hepatitis B virus X-associated protein 2 (XAP2/ARA9/AIP), and other factors including the tyrosine kinase pp60src (Kazlauskas et al. 1999, 2001; Barouki et al. 2007). Hsp90 and p23 protect AhR from ubiquitin-dependent proteolysis maintaining an AhR conformation that is receptive to ligand binding. Consistent with AhR function as an Hsp90 client protein, Hsp90 inhibitors suppress AhR-mediated activation of AhR target gene *expression* causing pronounced down-regulation of AhR protein levels (Davis et al. 2015). After AhR ligands (such as dioxin, polycyclic aromatic hydrocarbons, and endogenous tryptophan-derivatives) engage the receptor, a conformational change exposes the NLS region critical for nuclear translocation. Nuclear AhR then hetero-dimerizes with AhR nuclear translocator protein (Arnt; also termed HIF-1β) via the PAS-A and PAS-B domains, and the AhR/Arnt heterodimer binds to DNA via the xenobiotic response element (XRE) promoter sequence (-also termed DRE, dioxin-response element; core DNA sequence: 5′-GCGTG-3′) located in the regulatory region of AhR-target genes.

The AhR ligand-binding domain exhibits a remarkable degree of promiscuity concerning ligand binding, and the structure activity relationship underlying small molecule AhR ligand activity remains poorly understood even though recent progress has been achieved based on in silico modeling and systematic site-directed mutagenesis. Specifically, homology modeling of the mouse, rat, and human AhR-ligand binding (LBD/PAS) domain was performed using the published NMR-based PAS domain structure of human hypoxia-inducible factor 2α (HIF2α), enabling virtual ligand docking (e.g. TCDD, FICZ, ITE) and screening of new AhR ligands (such as the flavonoid pinocembrin), characterized further in cellular assays measuring XRE-luciferase reporter transcriptional activation, AhR nuclear translocation, and AhR target gene expression (Bisson et al. 2009). Recently, the remarkable species (e.g. human versus murine)-specificity of some AhR agonists (including the microbiome-derived indole-type AhR agonists indole, 3-methylindole, and the indole-dimer-derived indirubin) has been attributed to the bimolecular (2:1) stoichiometry between ligand and AhR-LBD, a finding that has been interpreted as a molecular adaptation of the human AhR to sense microbiota-derived indoles as a prerequisite of maintaining intestinal and cutaneous commensal homeostasis and barrier function (Hubbard et al. 2015). In addition, comprehensive site-directed AhR-LBD mutagenesis has identified specific amino acid residues within the AhR-LBD, dictating selectivity of ligand binding, agonistic/antagonistic receptor interaction, and Hsp90 engagement (Soshilov and Denison 2014) (Fig. 16.1).

16.2 AhR Target Genes

The AhR gene battery comprises numerous genes involved in broad cellular biological functions. Nevertheless, AhR-mediated transcriptional changes are highly ligand, cell and species specific (Flaveny et al. 2010; Dere et al. 2011). The classical AhR target genes include the major phase one metabolizing cytochrome P450 monooxygenases (CYP1A1, CYP1A2, CYP2B1), aldehyde dehydrogenase-3 (ALDH3A1), and phase two enzymes including UDP-glucuronosyltransferase (UGT1A1, UGT1A6), NADPH quinone oxidoreductase (NQO1), and glutathione-S-transferase (GST). In addition, AhR is an important physiological regulator of cellular homeostasis by controlling the expression of genes involved in proliferation, differentiation, adhesion and matrix remodeling, as well as inflammation and immune responses as discussed below. Such genes include epidermal barrier proteins (e.g. keratin 10, loricrin, pro-filaggrin), cell growth regulators (e.g. transforming growth factors including TGF-α and TGF-β), and nuclear transcription factors (e.g. c-fos, c-jun) (van den Bogaard et al. 2013, 2015).

Activation of AhR is rapidly terminated by molecular pathways that negatively regulate AhR. First, AhR is subject to feedback inhibition by mediating transcription of the gene encoding the AhR repressor (AhRR), which competes with AhR for Arnt (Tsuchiya et al. 2003; Evans et al. 2008). Second, AhR undergoes nuclear export engaging the NES, followed by ubiquitination and 26S proteosomal-mediated degradation. Third, termination of AhR signaling is also achieved through rapid ligand metabolism by CYP1A1-dependent turnover, a mechanism effective for some ligands (FICZ) that are efficient CYP1A1 substrates but not for others (e.g. TCDD) that are metabolically inert, potentially representing the molecular basis of physiological versus pathological AhR engagement.

16.3 Exogenous and Endogenous AhR Ligands

Apart from 2,3,7,8-tetrachlorodibenzo-*p*-dioxin (TCDD), the prototypical AhR ligand, numerous other planar hydrocarbons including halogenated aromatic hydrocarbons (HAHs), polycyclic aromatic hydrocarbons (PAHs), and PAH-like compounds display high AhR affinity upstream of AhR-dependent cellular signaling. Importantly, metabolically stable dioxin-like HAH ligands (including TCDD, 2,3,7,8-tetrachlorodibenzofuran, and 3,3′,4,4′,5-pentachlorobiphenyl) cause dramatic AhR-mediated toxic effects that seem to originate from supra-physiological, dysregulated, and persistent stimulation of AhR signaling. In contrast, metabolically susceptible high affinity AhR ligands [such as the carcinogenic PAH 3-methylcholanthrene, the phytochemical β-naphthoflavone, and the endogenous ligand 6-formylindolo[3,2-b]carbazole (FICZ)] initiate transient AhR-dependent signaling and beneficial (or adverse) biological effects in the absence of specific toxicity resulting from sustained AhR activation due to rapid metabolic inactivation that attenuates pathological AhR signaling (Berghard et al. 1992; Kim et al. 2012).

16.3.1 Exogenous AhR Ligands

Exogenous ligands are synthetic ('anthropogenic') and natural compounds that are not generated within or on the surface of the human body. This category includes environmental pollutants (HAHs, PAHs and related compounds) (Safe 1990; Denison et al. 1998; Poland and Knutson 1982). Members of the planar hydrophobic HAH family are high-affinity AhR ligands including dibenzofurans, polyhalogenated dibenzo-p-dioxins, and biphenyls (Denison et al. 1998; Denison and Heath-Pagliuso 1998). The prototypical and most potent HAH is TCDD (Poland and Knutson 1982). In humans, TCDD has a half-life of 5-10 years due to its high lipophilicity and resistance to metabolic degradation resulting in the sustained induction of CYP1A1 (Aylward et al. 2005). Many studies have shown that TCDD exposure can cause a diverse array of tissue-specific biological and toxicological actions, most of which are mediated by AhR (Safe 1990, 1995; Devito 1994). The members of the PAH include compounds such as benzo[a]pyrene (BaP), benzoflavones, 3-methylcholanthrene and benzanthracenes (Denison and Heath-Pagliuso 1998; Devito 1994; Poland and Knutson 1982). The PAHs are more metabolically labile and have relatively lower binding affinity than HAHs towards AhR (Fraschini et al. 1996). The AhR binding affinity of the PAH 3-methylcholanthrene is almost equal to TCDD but rapid metabolic conversion results in only a transient induction of CYP1A1 expression. Other classes of exogenous AhR agonists include plant-derived phenolics including flavonoids (Ashida 2000; Ciolino et al. 1999) and curcumin (Ciolino et al. 1998), carotenoids (Gradelet et al. 1997), and indol-3-carbinol (I3C; Bjeldanes et al. 1991) that can reach skin by either topical application or dietary intake. Interestingly, flavonoids and other related polyphenols have been shown to have agonist/antagonist effects and may actually competitively block AhR activation by dioxin-like contaminants. Additionally, pharmacological agents have been reported to display AhR activity including the azole antifungal ketoconazole and the proton pump inhibitor omeprazole (Tsuji et al. 2012; Jin et al. 2014). Other AhR-directed FDA-approved drugs currently used for distinct therapeutic indications include flutamide, leflunomide, nimodipine, mexiletine, and tranilast (Hu et al. 2007; Jin et al. 2014).

16.3.2 Endogenous AhR Ligands

The cutaneous presence of endogenous AhR ligands supports a physiological role of AhR in skin barrier structure and function. In skin, tryptophan is available in free form and also as a constituent of cellular protein, serving as the major precursor of endogenous indolic AhR ligands. Key enzymes involved in the catabolism of free tryptophan such as indoleamine 2,3-dioxygenase 1/2 (IDO1/2), tryptophan 2,3-dioxygenase (TDO) and tryptophan hydroxylase are expressed in human skin cells engaged in the formation of tryptophan metabolites including kynurenine, 3-hydroxyanthranilic acid (HA), picolinic acid, and quinolinic acid (Moffett and Namboodiri 2003; Sheipouri et al. 2015). Tryptophan metabolites serve as precursors for the biosynthesis of niacin and nicotinamide adenine dinucleotide, kynurenine, melatonin, and serotonin (Thomas and Stocker 1999; Sheipouri et al. 2012, 2015). IDO depletes tryptophan, a crucial factor in T-cell proliferation, and AhR-KO mice display impaired IDO expression (Nguyen et al. 2010). The IDO-encoding gene is under transcriptional control of AhR, and IDO expression is impaired in murine AhR-deficient versus AhR-wt Langerhans cells (Jux et al. 2009). Kynurenines are known AhR agonists involved in the induction AhR-dependent regulatory T cells (Tregs) from naïve T cells, suggesting an immunosuppressive role that could potentially confer tolerance and may also play a role in tumor immune evasion (DiNatale et al. 2010; Mezrich et al. 2010; Nguyen et al. 2010; Opitz et al. 2011). In addition, the endogenous AhR ligand cinnabarinic acid, another kynurenine pathway metabolite derived from tryptophan, produced by the oxidation of 3-hydroxyanthranilic via non-enzymatic or enzymatic (such as laccase- or ceruloplasmin-dependent) oxidation, has been demonstrated to stimulate the differentiation of human and mouse T cells producing the Th17-associated cytokine IL-22 (Lowe et al. 2014). Initially linked to IL-17 as a pro-inflammatory cytokine, recent evidence suggests that IL-22 plays an independent immunoregulatory role in the context of non-hematopoietic cells, maintaining epithelial cell homeostasis in mucosal tissues and serving a specific role in tissue repair following inflammation. Other endogenous tryptophan metabolites with AhR-directed activity are tryptamine, 5-hydroxy-tryptophan (Bittinger et al. 2003), and indigo and indirubin (Spink et al. 2003; Adachi et al. 2001; Heath-Pagliuso et al. 1998); however, indigo and indirubin are detectable in human urine only at picomolar concentrations, well below the concentrations that would activate AhR-driven gene expression (Adachi et al. 2001; Guengerich et al. 2004). Only a few other tryptophan-derived endogenous AhR ligands have been identified such as 2-(1′H-indole-3′-carbonyl)-thiazole-4-carboxylic acid methyl ester (ITE), a novel nontoxic (i.e., non-chloracnegenic) AhR ligand, that efficiently suppresses T cell-immunity in an experimental model of autoimmune uveitis, but the potential physiological role of ITE in the context of skin barrier function remains largely undefined (Song et al. 2002; Nugent et al. 2013; Forrester et al. 2014).

It is well known that tryptophan photolysis generates photoproducts that can cause the AhR-dependent upregulation of Cyp expression in skin. These photoproducts are formed from tryptophan in response to UV and visible radiation through non-enzymatic photooxidative mechanisms (including hydroxylation, oxidative deamination, oxidative ring opening, condensation, and oxidative coupling) generating a range of potent AhR agonists including kynurenine, indole-3-acetic acid (IAA), tryptamine, 1-(1H-indol-3-yl)-9H-pyrido[3,4-b]indole,

6-formylindolo-[3,2-b]-carbazole (FICZ), indolo[3,2-b]carbazole (ICZ), 6,12-di-formylindolo[3,2-b]carbazole (dFICZ), and the FICZ oxidation product indolo [3,2-b]carbazole-6-carboxylic acid (CICZ) (Rannug et al. 1987; Helferich and Denison 1991; Wei et al. 2000; Denison and Nagy 2003; Oberg et al. 2005; Fritsche et al. 2007; Diani-Moore et al. 2011; Smirnova et al. 2016). Among these tryptophan-derived photolytic products, FICZ displays extraordinary activity as an AhR ligand with almost ten times higher AhR binding affinity than TCDD, suggesting a causative role of FICZ-induced AhR activity in the mediation of UV-driven effects on skin (Rannug et al. 1987, 1995; Wincent et al. 2012) (Fig. 16.2). More detailed biochemical analysis revealed that FICZ serves as an exceptionally efficient substrate for CYP1A1, CYP1A2, and CYP1B1, and its hydroxylated metabolites are substrates for the sulfotransferases SULT1A1, SULT1A2, SULT1B1, and SULT1E1; sulfoconjugates of phenolic FICZ

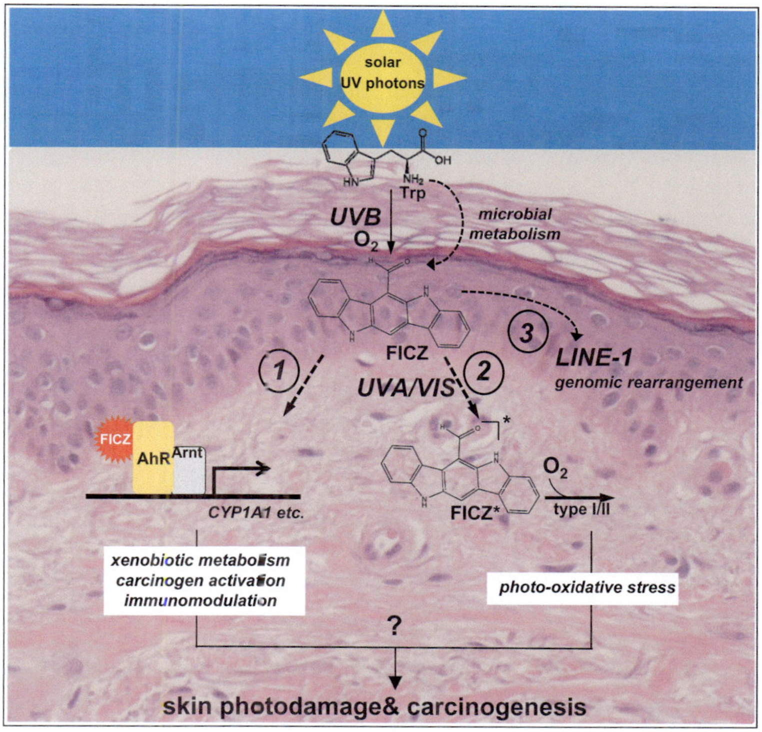

Fig. 16.2 Molecular pathways mediating FICZ-dependent effects in human skin downstream of its formation as a cutaneous microbial metabolite or solar UVB-induced tryptophan photooxidation product; *pathway 1*: FICZ as an AhR-ligand causing AhR/Arnt-dependent upregulation of target gene expression including *CYP1A1*; *pathway 2*: UVA-induced formation of FICZ photoexcited states (FICZ*) followed by generation of reactive oxygen species (ROS) through type I and II photosensitization reactions causing cutaneous photo-oxidative stress; *suggested pathway 3*: FICZ-induced AhR-independent genomic reorganization through stimulation of LINE-1 retrotransposition

metabolites are present in human urine (Wincent et al. 2009). LC/MS/MS analysis confirmed UVB-driven FICZ formation, followed by AhR nuclear translocation and upregulation of CYP1A1 mRNA levels as demonstrated in HaCaT keratinocytes (Fritsche et al. 2007), and inhibition of cytochrome P450-dependent clearance of FICZ has been suggested as a physiological mechanism for AhR activation and FICZ potentiation (Wei et al. 2000; Wincent et al. 2012). Indeed, elevated levels of unmetabolized FICZ are observable as a result of pharmacological AhR (using 3′-methoxy-4′-nitroflavone) or CYP inhibition (Bergander et al. 2004; Wincent et al. 2012). Remarkably, FICZ is also a fungal metabolite in cutaneous patient samples, detectable in seborrheic dermatitis and pityriasis versicolor skin specimens (Magiatis et al. 2013; Wincent et al. 2009).

Recently, in addition to light-dependent photooxidative or microbial biosynthetic formation of cutaneous FICZ, three light-independent oxidative pathways of FICZ formation with potential physiological relevance have been identified dependent on the intermediate formation of indole-3-acetaldehyde, the key chemical precursor of all pathways leading from tryptophan to FICZ: (i) nonenzymatic tryptophan oxidation by the endogenous oxidant H_2O_2, (ii) nonenzymatic oxidative conversion of indole-3-pyruvate formed enzymatically from tryptophan through L-amino acid oxidase, (iii) enzymatic oxidative deamination of tryptamine via mitochondrial monoamine oxidase. Due to the non-enzymatic nature of the reaction, formation of FICZ from tryptophan has the potential to produce a complex mixture of indole derivatives, some of which are CYP1A1 inhibitors (including tryptamine and melatonin), thereby potentially enhancing FICZ bioavailability through blockade of oxidative metabolism (Heath-Pagliuso et al. 1998; Chang et al. 2010; Smirnova et al. 2016).

16.4 The Skin Microbiome as a Source of Cutaneous AhR Agonists

Recent research indicates that the commensal cutaneous microbiome is a rich source of AhR-directed small molecules. Indeed, various species of human skin yeasts (e.g. *Malassezia)* generate tryptophan metabolites displaying AhR activity including indirubin, tryptanthrin, malassezin, FICZ, and ICZ (indole [3,2-b]-carbazole) (Fig. 16.2). Although the biochemical mechanism underlying the biosynthesis of theses compounds currently remains undetermined, it is evident that these AhR ligands have cutaneous functions influencing immunoregulation and barrier quality. For example, the fungus-derived metabolite malassezin induces AhR mediated apoptosis in melanocytes consistent with the molecular scenario relevant to long lasting depigmented plaques, a characteristic of pityriasis versicolor (Kramer et al. 2005), and absence of sunburn in pityriasis versicolor macules has been attributed to the indole pityriacitrin, which acts as a potent UV filter (Larangeira de Almeida and Mayser 2006). Other microbial indoles display various biological functions including the ultrapotent AhR ligand FICZ, whose AhR-dependent functions include pro- and anti-inflammatory effects and skin barrier modulation (Quintana et al. 2008; Wincent et al. 2009; Luecke et al. 2010; Prochazkova et al. 2011; Wincent et al. 2012; Gaitanis et al. 2012; Mexia et al. 2015). The potential immune-suppressive capacity of cutaneous microbiome-derived AhR ligands has been substantiated by experimental evidence indicating that these ligands impede Toll-like receptor-induced dendritic cell (DC) maturation and DC-induction of T-cell proliferation, representing an AhR-controlled mechanism of suppressed surveillance of microbial infections that might facilitate tolerance towards cutaneous microbial colonization (Vlachos et al. 2012).

Malassezia yeasts comprise the majority of the microbial flora of healthy skin, and these commensal fungi have also been implicated in the pathogenesis of skin diseases including seborrheic dermatitis, pityriasis versicolor, atopic dermatitis and psoriasis (Nakabayashi et al. 2000; Sugita et al. 2002; Gao et al. 2010; Gaitanis et al. 2012; Jagielski et al. 2014). Indeed, skin extracts from seborrheic dermatitis and pityriasis versicolor patient lesions indicate high quantities of *Malassezia furfur*-derived indoles (Gaitanis et al. 2008, 2012; Magiatis et al. 2013; Mexia et al. 2015), and it seems reasonable to postulate that the increased presence of these AhR-directed indoles alters local immune function relevant to pityriasis versicolor lesions and chronic inflammation, as seen in atopic dermatitis and seborrheic dermatitis (Gupta et al. 2004; Kuo et al. 2013).

Importantly, beyond the established fungal origin, AhR-directed tryptophan-derived and other metabolites can also originate from bacteria residing in human skin. Indeed, AhR has been identified as an intracellular pattern recognition receptor for virulent factors including phenazine (originating from *Pseudomonas aeruginosa*) and the naphthoquinone phthiocol (originating from *Mycobacterium tuberculosis*), indicating a role for AhR in immune modulation downstream of primary bacterial infections (Moura-Alves et al. 2014). Likewise, *Lactobacilli* convert tryptophan into indole-3-aldehyde (3-IAld) which has anti-inflammatory effects thought to originate from AhR-mediated induction of IDO1 (Zelante et al. 2013).

16.5 FICZ Functions that Occur Independent of AhR Ligand Activity

Recent research indicates that FICZ assumes additional biological functions that might impact skin barrier function in response to environmental stressors without involvement of AhR signaling (Fig. 16.2).

16.5.1 FICZ: A Nanomolar Endogenous UVA-Photosensitizer

Our own research has demonstrated that FICZ acts as a nanomolar photosensitizer potentiating UVA-induced oxidative stress in skin cells, human epidermal skin models, and murine skin, irrespective of AhR ligand activity (Park et al. 2015; Syed and Mukhtar 2015). Photosensitization, a phototoxic mechanism downstream of photon absorption by chromophores present in the human skin is a key mechanism of UV-induced oxidative stress (Wondrak et al. 2006). In human HaCaT and primary epidermal keratinocytes, photodynamic induction of apoptosis was elicited by the combined action of solar-simulated UVA [or visible (blue light)] photons and FICZ, whereas exposure to the isolated action of light (UVA/visible) or FICZ did not impair viability. In a human epidermal tissue reconstruct, FICZ/UVA co-treatment caused pronounced phototoxicity inducing keratinocyte cell death, and FICZ photodynamic activity was also substantiated in a murine skin exposure model. Array analysis revealed pronounced potentiation of cellular heat shock, endoplasmic reticulum stress, and oxidative stress response gene expression observed only upon FICZ/UVA co-treatment. FICZ photosensitization caused intracellular oxidative stress, and comet analysis revealed introduction of formamidopyrimidine-DNA glycosylase (Fpg)-sensitive oxidative DNA lesions suppressible by antioxidant cotreatment. Interestingly, FICZ but not its deformylated analogue ICZ, a potent agonist of equal AhR affinity as FICZ, displayed photosensitizer activity, consistent with the carbonyl group-associated triplet state being the ultimate structural determinant of FICZ-associated UVA- and blue light-induced phototoxicity.

Taken together, these data provide evidence that the endogenous AhR ligand FICZ displays nanomolar photodynamic activity representing a molecular mechanism of UVA-induced photooxidative stress potentially operative in human skin. It may be hypothesized that FICZ serves as an endogenous photosensitizer, a role similar to that attributed before to other endogenous chromophores such as riboflavin (vitamin B_2) and protoporphyrin IX, but the precise mechanism and photobiological relevance of FICZ-induced photo-oxidative stress operative in solar UV-exposed human skin remains to be elucidated. It also remains to be seen if FICZ-induced photo-oxidative stress may facilitate its generation from tryptophan, representing an autocatalytic mechanism that would be consistent with recent observations on FICZ excited state chemistry and non-enzymatic, non-photochemical FICZ formation originating from hydrogen peroxide-induced oxidation of tryptophan (Park et al. 2015; Smirnova et al. 2016).

16.5.2 FICZ: An Endogenous Activator of LINE-1 retrotransposition

Recent experimental evidence indicates that FICZ may cause genomic reorganization through stimulation of retrotransposition, a remarkable activity that impacts genomic integrity without AhR involvement. FICZ-induced retrotransposition of the long interspersed nucleotide element-1 (LINE-1) can be observed at picomolar concentrations in human HuH-7 and HeLa cells. LINE-1 is a genetic non-LTR retrotransposon comprising about 17 % of the human genome, of which 80–100 copies are competent as mobile elements. LINE-1 contains an internal polymerase II promoter and ORF1 (encoding a 40-kDa basic RNA-binding protein with RNA chaperone activity) and ORF2 (encoding a 150-kDa protein with endonuclease and reverse transcriptase activities), involved in L1 cDNA genomic integration. LINE-1 retrotransposition depends on AhR nuclear translocator-1 (Arnt1), and FICZ is thought to stimulate the interaction of the LINE-1-encoded ORF1 and Arnt1, recruiting ORF1 to chromatin downstream of activation of mitogen-activated protein kinase. Prior research has demonstrated the activation of human LINE-1 retrotransposition by benzo(a)pyrene, an ubiquitous environmental carcinogen, requiring DNA adduction after cytochrome P450-catalyzed oxidation of the parent hydrocarbon (Stribinskis and Ramos 2006), and a causative involvement of LINE-1 reverse transcriptase (encoded by ORF-2) has been substantiated in UV-induced transformation of cutaneous keratinocytes (Banerjee et al. 2005). However, the molecular mechanism underlying FICZ-induced LINE-1 retrotransposition and its potential role in the modulation of genomic adaptations to UV and other environmental stressors remain to be elucidated in more detail. In the context of genomic rearrangement as a result of LINE-1 retrotransposition in response to DNA damage, it is interesting that LINE-1 retrotransposition can be induced by oxidative DNA damage in human neuroblastoma cells exposed to hydrogen peroxide, and LINE-1 hypomethylation induced by ROS is mediated via depletion of S-adenosylmethionine, suggesting a mechanistic link between oxidative stress and LINE-1 driven insertional mutagenesis and genomic instability that may also be operative in human skin cells under environmental oxidative stress (Giorgi et al. 2011; Carreira et al. 2014; Kloypan et al. 2015). Based on the recent emergence of FICZ as a potent sensitizer of photo-oxidative stress via ROS formation upstream of oxidative (8-oxo-dG-mediated) genomic damage (Park et al. 2015), it is tempting to speculate that FICZ-driven AhR-independent LINE-1 transposition may also be impacted by FICZ-induced photo-oxidative stress, a hypothesis to be tested by future experimentation.

16.6 AhR: Cutaneous Functions and Therapeutic Opportunities

AhR is highly expressed in barrier organs such as skin, lung, and gut consistent with its role as a critical environmental stress sensor and orchestrator of environmental and endogenous stress responses (Esser and Rannug 2015; Haarmann-Stemmann et al. 2015).

16.6.1 AhR and Epidermal Barrier Function

Recent reports have demonstrated a critical role of AhR in epidermal differentiation, skin barrier formation and homeostasis (Sutter et al. 2011; van den Bogaard et al. 2013, 2015). Earlier studies have reported that AhR deficient mice display abnormalities in keratinocyte terminal differentiation suggesting a physiological role of AhR in skin morphogenesis (Loertscher et al. 2002). Using murine and human skin models it has recently been shown that AhR activation is required for normal keratinocyte differentiation as evidenced by impaired epidermal stratification resulting from AhR inactivation during human skin equivalent development (van den Bogaard EH et al. 2015). Comparative transcriptomic analysis between $AhR^{(-/-)}$ and $AhR^{(+/+)}$ murine keratinocytes indicated a significant enrichment of differentially expressed genes linked to epidermal differentiation, and $AhR^{(-/-)}$ keratinocytes showed a significant reduction in terminal differentiation gene and protein expression, an observation mimicked by pharmacological AhR antagonism using drug-like small molecule modulators (including GNF351, CH223191, SGA360). Likewise, monolayer cultured primary human keratinocytes subjected to pharmacological AhR antagonism also display an impaired terminal differentiation program. Based on these observations, pharmacological AhR activation employing synthetic or endogenous AhR ligands has now emerged as a novel therapeutic strategy targeting disturbed epidermal differentiation, a key clinical feature associated with numerous skin pathologies.

16.6.2 Lessons from TCDD-Induced Chloracne

Dysregulated expression of epidermal barrier proteins is thought to contribute to various cutaneous pathologies, and TCDD-induced overexpression of these genes may therefore cause detrimental effects including impairment of skin barrier function. Indeed, toxicity studies have reported that long-term exposure to TCDD causes chloracne, a severe acne-like condition characterized by aberrant epidermal hyperproliferation and hyperkeratinization involving the interfollicular squamous epithelium and hair follicles, as well as a metaplastic response of sebaceous glands

(Loertscher et al. 2001; Sutter et al. 2009, 2011). Chloracne is clinically characterized by widespread dissemination of epidermal and dermal cysts with severe atrophy of the sebaceous glands, and TCDD-induced transcriptional repression of genes involved in sebum lipid metabolism may underlie sebaceous gland-directed adverse effects (Saurat and Sorg 2010). Consequences of TCDD exposure are exacerbated by the toxicant's lipophilicity and metabolic inertness attributed to polyhalogenation, preventing (or at least attenuating) enzymatic oxidative bioconversion and deactivation, resulting in a prolonged biological half-life of TCDD in humans that exceeds one year. However, patho-mechanistic aspects of AhR engagement underlying the chloracne phenotype remain poorly understood. It has recently been shown that induction of a chloracne phenotype achieved in an epidermal equivalent model by TCDD depends on AhR activation and is not reproduced by AhR knockdown (Forrester et al. 2014). Indeed, when human epidermal equivalents were treated with TCDD or two AhR-directed non-chloracnegens [β-naphthoflavone (β-NF) and ITE], ligand-induced CYP1A1 and AhR degradation did not correlate with their chloracnegenic potential, and only TCDD induced a chloracne-like phenotype, whereas β-NF or ITE did not.

In a politically motivated assassination attempt using TCDD as a single toxicant in 2004, the victim, former Ukrainian president Viktor Yushchenko, was hospitalized displaying TCDD serum levels 50,000-fold above average levels in the general population (Sorg et al. 2009), a singular incident of TCDD-specific exposure different from mass exposure scenarios where victims of Agent Orange (Vietnam war; Poland et al. 1976), industrial accidents (Seveso, Italy; Reggiani 1978), and environmental disasters (Yusho, Japan; Kuratsune et al. 1971) were exposed to a mixture of chemicals including polychlorinated dibenzo-p-dioxins (PCDDs), polychlorinated dibenzofurans (PCDFs), and polychlorinated biphenyls (PCBs). Interestingly, two TCDD metabolites (2,3,7-trichloro-8-hydroxydibenzo-p-dioxin and 1,3,7,8-tetrachloro-2-hydroxydibenzo-p-dioxin) were identified in the patient's feces, blood serum, and urine. Biopsies of cutaneous lesions revealed high concentrations of TCDD that surpassed serum levels tenfold at eleven months post poisoning, accompanied by highly altered AhR-regulated gene expression indicative of sustained AhR signaling in skin (Saurat et al. 2012).

Importantly, it is now firmly established that the epidermal barrier is a functional target of the TCDD-activated AhR (Sutter et al. 2011). TCDD controls the expression of genes in the human epidermal differentiation complex (EDC) locus, a chromosomal region and gene complex spanning 1.9 Mbp (1q21) comprising over fifty genes encoding proteins involved in the terminal differentiation and cornification of epidermal keratinocytes underlying epidermal barrier function (Mischke et al. 1996). EDC gene expression is controlled by various transcription factors such as KLF4, GATA3, GRHL3, Nrf2, and AhR/Arnt (Kypriotou et al. 2012). The proteins encoded by EDC genes are functionally interrelated, representing members of three evolutionarily distinct gene families: (i) the cornified envelope precursor family [e.g. involucrin (*IVL*), loricrin (*LOR*), and various small proline-rich (*SPRR*s) and late cornified envelope proteins (*LCE*s)], (ii) the S100 protein family [e.g. psoriasin (*S100A7*), calgranulin A (*S100A8*), and calgranulin B (*S100A9*), some of which are serving as antimicrobial peptides], and (iii) the S100 fused type protein (SFTP) family [e.g. filaggrin (*FLG*), filaggrin-2 (*FLG2*), trichohyalin (*TCHH*), trichohyalin-like 1 protein (*TCHHL1*), hornerin (*HRNR*), repetin (*RPTN*), and cornulin (*CRNN*)].

The functional importance of the EDC is exemplified by the molecular pathogenesis of human diseases involving dramatic skin manifestations: For example, *FLG* (filaggrin) mutations have been established as strong risk factors for atopic dermatitis (AD) and AD-associated asthma. Expression of the EDC gene *FLG* encoding the epidermal barrier protein profilaggrin (i.e. 'filament aggregating protein'), part of the SFTP family within the EDC, is under AhR transcriptional regulation via XRE-promoter control. Interestingly, filaggrin aggregates keratin filaments important for creating the lipid-protein cornified envelope of differentiating keratinocytes, and proteolytic degradation of the histidine-rich filaggrin releases free hygroscopic amino acids serving as precursors of pyrrolidone carboxylic acid and trans-urocanic acid, important components of the natural moisturizing factor (NMF), produced in the cornified layer of skin involved in water retention and osmoprotection, pH control, UV signaling, and photoimmunosuppression (Pouillot et al. 2008). Gene expression analysis beyond AhR-dependent *FLG* modulation indicated that exposure of confluent human keratinocytes to TCDD (10 nM, 24 h) additionally upregulated mRNA levels including *RPTN*, *HRNR*, *FLG2*, *LCE3A*, *LCE3E*, *SPRR1A*, *SPRR2A*, *SPRR2B*, *S100A7*, *S100A9*, and *S100A12*, a finding consistent with XRE-identification in the respective gene promoter sequences (Bruhs et al. 2015; Furue et al. 2015). TCDD also increases the expression of genes required for de novo ceramide biosynthesis. Consistent with these gene expression changes, TCDD treatment of organotypic skin cultures resulted in accelerated keratinocyte terminal differentiation causing an augmented and irregular spatial distribution of several differentiation-specific proteins (filaggrin, involucrin, transglutaminase) (Loertscher et al. 2001). Other studies assessed the effects of in utero TCDD treatment on fetal C57BL/J6 murine skin morphogenesis detecting enhanced premature expression of filaggrin and alterations of late stage keratinocyte differentiation. TCDD-induced acceleration of in utero epidermal barrier formation was shown to be associated with increased expression of isoforms of late cornified envelope, isoforms of S100 calcium-binding protein, hornerin, and involucrin (Ray and Swanson 2003; Sutter et al. 2011).

16.6.3 AhR as an Environmental Stress Sensor: Ozone and Human Skin

A significant fraction of environmental oxidative damage targeting skin originates from the air pollutant ozone (trioxygen, O_3; Baudouin et al. 2002). Ground-level ozone, a major component of photochemical smog, is created near the Earth's surface by the action of solar UV on precursors pollutants, such as methane and those emitted during the combustion of fossil fuels. Ground level ozone impairs the respiratory system and lung function, and exposure to ozone increases the incidence of asthma, bronchitis, cardiovascular insult, and other cardiopulmonary problems. In skin, ozone is recognized as a powerful environmental oxidant that impairs cutaneous structure and function. Recently, AhR has been recognized as an ozone sensor in human skin (Afaq et al. 2009). In normal human epidermal keratinocytes (NHEKs) exposure to ozone (0.3 ppm) resulted in an increase in protein and mRNA expression of *CYP1A1*, *CYP1A2*, and *CYP1B1*, an effect that was blocked by AhR silencing (siRNA) validating AhR as an ozone sensitive target. NHEK exposure to ozone also resulted in nuclear AhR translocation and EGFR phosphorylation (Afaq et al. 2009).

16.6.4 Harnessing AhR-Nrf2 Crosstalk for Cutaneous Resilience Against Environmental Stressors and Maintenance of Barrier Function

In addition to AhR as a prototype environmental stress sensor pathway in skin, the redox-sensitive and environmental stress-activated CNC (*cap'n'collar*) basic leucine zipper transcription factor Nrf2 (nuclear factor-E2-related factor 2) orchestrates major cellular defense mechanisms including phase-II detoxification, inflammatory signaling, DNA repair, and antioxidant response relevant to skin barrier function. Nrf2 is a master regulator of keratinocyte redox signaling and has now been recognized as a promising molecular target for the pharmacological control of skin pathologies associated with oxidative stress and inflammatory dysregulation resulting from exposure to environmental electrophilic toxicants including ionizing radiation, solar UV photons (UVA and UVB) , reactive oxygen and nitrogen species (ROS/RNS), PAHs (and their epoxidized metabolites), reactive carbonyl compounds and lipid peroxidation products (e.g., acrolein and 4-hydroxynonenal), heavy metals (e.g. cadmium, zinc), and metalloids (arsenic) (McMahon et al. 2010; Schäfer and Werner 2015). Consequently, extensive mechanistic crosstalk between these two stress response pathways exists, determining skin adaptational responses and barrier function, and the AhR-Nrf2 pathway as operative in keratinocytes has recently been highlighted as a major molecular target for skin cancer chemoprevention (Haarmann-Stemmann et al. 2012).

Nrf2 transcriptional activity orchestrates major cellular antioxidant and phase-II detoxification and anti-inflammatory pathways that protect tissue against electrophilic insult. Numerous dietary chemopreventive factors activate Nrf2 through covalent adduction and/or oxidation of redox-sensitive thiol residues in Keap1 (Kelch-like ECH-associated protein 1), the negative regulator of Nrf2, and Nrf2 has emerged as an attractive target for potential cutaneous photo-chemopreventive intervention (Zhang and Hannink 2003; Saw et al. 2011; Knatko et al. 2015; Tao et al. 2015). Inhibition of Keap1-dependent ubiquitination and subsequent proteasomal degradation of Nrf2 allows nuclear translocation, a process followed by Nrf2-dependent transcriptional activation of target genes containing an antioxidant response element (ARE) regulatory sequence. Upregulation of target genes encoding cytoprotective enzymes such as γ-glutamylcysteinyl-synthetase, glutathione S-transferases, thioredoxin, peroxiredoxins, NAD(P)H quinone oxidoreductase 1 (NQO1), and heme oxygenase 1 is thought to underlie Nrf2-dependent protection against oxidative environmental insult (Tao et al. 2015). Nrf2 orchestrates and binds to antioxidant responsive element (ARE) sequences of target gene promoters involved in type 2 xenobiotic detoxification and oxidative stress. Upregulation of epidermal suprabasal Nrf2 activity leads to expression of ROS detoxifying enzymes and proteins involved in glutathione transport and biosynthesis establishing a trans-epidermal glutathione gradient, thought to underlie Nrf2-dependent protection of the suprabasal epidermis against UV irradiation and ROS-induced apoptosis enabling the preferential elimination of UVB-damaged basal keratinocytes (Schäfer et al. 2010).

Nrf2 control of epidermal barrier structure and function has recently been recognized (Schäfer and Werner 2015). Keap1 deficiency resulting in supra-physiological constitutive Nrf2 activation causes epidermal hyperkeratosis (with upregulation of loricrin, repetin and keratin 6 together with attenuation of involucrin synthesis), and Keap1-null mice are not viable postnatally due to severe gastrointestinal hyperkeratosis. Transgenic mice displaying pathologically enhanced Nrf2 activity in keratinocytes are characterized by epidermal upregulation of secretory leukocyte peptidase inhibitor (Slpi) and small proline-rich protein (Sprr2d), associated with inflammatory hyperkeratosis and epidermal thickening reminiscent of ichthyosis and chloracne/metabolizing acquired dioxin-induced skin hamartomas (MADISH) (Schäfer et al. 2012, 2014).

A role of pharmacological Nrf2 activation for skin protection against oxidative and inflammatory insult has recently been substantiated, and the therapeutic acceleration of diabetic wound healing by topical and systemic Nrf2-activators has been reported (Long et al. 2016). Moreover, recent studies strongly suggest a protective role of Nrf2-mediated gene expression in the suppression of cutaneous photodamage induced by solar UV radiation (Knatko et al. 2015). Nrf2 activation has been shown to protect cutaneous keratinocytes and fibroblasts against the cytotoxic effects of UVA and UVB (Wondrak et al. 2008; Tao et al. 2013; Schäfer and Werner 2015), and recent research performed in SKH-1 mice documents that constitutive genetic Nrf2 activation with retention of Keap1 negative control protects mice against acute photodamage and photocarcinogenesis (Saw et al. 2011; Knatko et al. 2015). Therefore, pharmacological modulation of Nrf2 has now attracted considerable attention as a novel approach to molecular skin photoprotection working synergistically with sunscreen-based strategies (Wondrak 2014). Indeed, protection of primary human keratinocytes from UVB-induced cell death by novel drug-like Nrf2 activators has been reported, a photoprotective effect attributed in part to Nrf2-dependent elevation of cellular glutathione levels (Lieder et al. 2012). Topical application of Nrf2 inducers, e.g. the synthetic Nrf2-activator TBE-31, has shown pronounced photoprotective and photochemopreventive activity in murine skin, and suppression of solar UV-induced human skin erythema was achieved by topical application of a standardized broccoli extract delivering the Nrf2 inducer sulforaphane (Knatko et al. 2015). Recently, we have been able to demonstrate that Nrf2-dependent skin photoprotection against sunburn and oxidative insult can be achieved by systemic administration of bixin, a water soluble apocarotenoid derived from the fruit of the achiote tree, used as a dietary additive all over tropical America since pre-Columbian times and now employed worldwide as an FDA-approved food colorant with established systemic availability and safety profile upon oral administration (Tao et al. 2015).

Mechanistic crosstalk between Nrf2 and AhR occurs at the gene expression level as supported by the co-occurrence of ARE- and XRE-sequences in the promoter region of several AhR-controlled genes (including NQO1 and GST) (Miao et al. 2005). Likewise, immunoprecipitation analysis confirmed direct AhR binding to XREs located in the Nrf2 promoter region, a finding in support of transcriptional crosstalk enabling AhR agonists including TCDD to induce mRNA and protein expression of Nrf2 (Miao et al. 2005). Moreover, Nrf2 seems to be essential to TCCD induction of classical AhR target genes (NQO1, UGTs, GST) based on the observation that in murine in vivo experiments TCDD treated Nrf2 deficient (−/−) mice expressed lower levels of these genes than TCDD-treated Nrf2 wild type (+/+) mice (Yeager et al. 2009). It is tempting to speculate that the AhR-Nrf2 interplay may represent a synergistic defense system blocking oxidative stress and environmental tissue injury that may also be induced by electrophilic AhR-ligand metabolites. Indeed, it has been observed that enhanced CYP1A1 enzymatic activity generates ROS that modulates oxidative stress responsive JNK, NFκB, and Nrf2 pathways, suggesting that AhR indirectly modulates cellular regulatory factors in other signaling pathways through CYP1A1-mediated oxidative stress as substantiated by prior studies on TCDD-induced CYP1A1-dependent oxidative stress (Park et al. 1996; Diry et al. 2006; Kopf et al. 2010).

Recently, the synthetic imidazole antifungal ketoconazole (KCZ) has been shown to display activity as an AhR-Nrf2 activator in cultured human keratinocytes representing the basis of its anti-inflammatory effect (Tsuji et al. 2012). In cultured human keratinocytes KCZ induces AhR nuclear translocation, resulting in the upregulation of CYP1A1 mRNA and protein expression. Furthermore, KCZ actively switched on Nrf2 nuclear translocation and NQO1 expression, and TNFα- and BaP-induced ROS and IL-8 production as well as BaP-induced 8-hydroxy-2-deoxyguanosine were effectively inhibited by KCZ treatment. Importantly, knockdown of either AhR or Nrf2 abolished the inhibitory capacity of KCZ on ROS and IL-8 production, and KCZ-induced Nrf2 activation was lost upon AhR knockdown demonstrating that the engagement of AhR by KCZ exhibits the cytoprotective effect mediated by the Nrf2 redox system, which potently downregulates either cytokine-induced (AhR-independent) or PAH-induced (AhR-dependent) oxidative stress. Interestingly, KCZ is a racemic mixture of two enantiomers, specifically (2R,4S)(+)-KCZ and (2S,4R)(−)-KCZ. An enantio-specific effect of KCZ on AhR activity was established by demonstrating that (+)-KCZ dose-dependently activated AhR in a human gene reporter cell line displaying up to

20-fold higher agonist activity as compared to (−)-KCZ. (+)-KCZ strongly induced CYP1A1 mRNA and protein in human HepG2 cells, while (−)-KCZ exerted less than 10 % of (+)-KCZ activity (Novotna et al. 2014).

Topical interventions using bio-compatible phytochemicals displaying dual AhR-Nrf2 agonistic activity for cytoprotection and skin barrier enhancement have now attracted increased attention (Furue et al. 2015) For example, an antioxidant opuntia (ficus indica) extract activates AhR-Nrf2 signaling and upregulates filaggrin and loricrin expression in human keratinocytes (Nakahara et al. 2015). Likewise, cynaropicrin, a sesquiterpene lactone phytochemical extracted from artichoke has recently been shown to activate the AhR-Nrf2-Nqo1 cytoprotective pathway, strengthening both skin barrier function, oxidative defenses, and facilitating suppression of inflammatory mediators (IL-6, TNFα) in UVB-exposed keratinocytes suggesting a potential utility in the prevention of UVB-induced photoaging (Takei et al. 2015). Remarkably, cynaropicrin-induced AhR-Nrf2-Nqo1 activation is AhR- and Nrf2-dependent, as demonstrated by the observation that keratinocytes transfected by siRNA against either AhR or Nrf2 are not responsive to this phytochemical. In accordance with these findings, cynaropicrin inhibits generation of ROS from keratinocytes irradiated with UVB in a Nrf2-dependent manner. Recently, topical application of a galactomyces-derived microbial fermentation filtrate has been shown to prevent T helper 2-mediated reduction of filaggrin, upregulating gene expression (*FLG, LOR*) in an AhR-dependent manner (Takei et al. 2015).

16.6.5 The Cutaneous AhR: A Key Regulator of Immune Function, Photoimmunosuppression, Inflammation, and Carcinogenesis

AhR activation in skin exposed to solar UV radiation has now been identified as a major mechanistic factor underlying systemic photoimmunosuppression, the UV-induced suppression of the immune system that occurs in an antigen-specific manner via induction of regulatory T cells (T_{regs}). Strikingly, induction of UV-induced T_{regs} is prevented by AhR antagonists demonstrating that UV-induced AhR activation is involved in UVR-mediated immunosuppression, and AhR-KO mice display resistance to UVR-induced immunosuppression (Navid et al. 2013). Recent evidence demonstrates that antigen-presenting cells are critically involved in AhR-induced immunosuppression, based on the finding that AhR activation switches antigen-presenting cells from a stimulatory into a regulatory phenotype controlling T_{reg} formation. Specifically, AhR activation triggers the release of IL-2 by DC inducing the expression of Foxp3 essential for maintaining T_{reg} as critical mediators of photo-immunosuppression (Turka and Walsh 2008; Kulhankova et al. 2012). Importantly, AhR has now been recognized as a ligand-specific modulator of TH17 and FoxP3+ T_{reg} differentiation, in which TCDD suppressed experimental autoimmune encephalomyelitis (EAE) in mice by promoting immunosuppressive T_{reg} differentiation (Quintana et al. 2008). Likewise, the tryptophan-derived endogenous AhR ligand ITE suppressed EAE in mice via induction of FoxP3+ T_{reg} differentiation in a retinoic acid-dependent manner, suggesting that AhR agonists may serve as potential therapeutic agents for autoimmune diseases (Quintana et al. 2010). It is now widely appreciated that therapeutic immunosuppression might be achieved through pharmacological AhR activation. For example, recent research has identified 4-n-nonylphenol (NP) as a synthetic drug-like AhR agonist that suppressed sensitization and induced T_{reg} reminiscent of the photoimmunosuppressive effects of UV exposure. Strikingly, injection of hapten-coupled dendritic cells treated with NP into mice did not result in sensitization but induced T_{regs} suggesting that AhR agonists may represent a viable therapeutic strategy to attenuate immunity, equipotent to UV exposure without causing adverse effects including sunburn and photomutagenicity (Navid et al. 2013). The identification of drug-like AhR agonists for therapeutic immunomodulation remains an ongoing area of research, and a new class of rapidly metabolized AhR ligands, benzimidazoisoquinolines [including 10-chloro-7H-benzimidazo[2,1-a]benzo[de] Iso-quinolin-7-one(10-Cl-BBQ)] that induce AhR-dependent T_{regs} and prevent murine graft-versus-host disease, has recently been identified (Punj et al. 2014).

Earlier research has demonstrated that the immunosuppressive effects of TCDD depend on AhR activity (Vorderstrasse et al. 2001), and subsequent studies reported that impaired Langerhans cell (LC) maturation in AhR-KO mice is due to a significant reduction in dendritic epidermal T-cells (DETC) that secrete GM-CSF necessary for LC maturation. Indeed, AhR deficient mice displayed a marked reduction of DETC levels and DETC lacked cell surface expression of c-Kit (Kadow et al. 2011). Based on cumulative experimental evidence that identifies AhR as a major orchestrator of immune function and inflammatory activity, AhR has become an attractive target for investigational therapeutic interventions targeting human skin pathologies associated with dysregulated inflammatory signaling.

16.6.5.1 Atopic Dermatitis

Atopic dermatitis (AD) is characterized by erythema, pruritus, intercellular epidermal edema, and keratinocyte apoptosis. In AD patients, important epidermal barrier proteins (filaggrin, involucrin, loricrin) are downregulated by IL-4, IL-5, and IL-13 through a STAT6-dependent process (Palmer et al. 2006; Kim et al. 2006; Jakasa et al. 2011). Furthermore, the terminal differentiation protein hornerin has also been associated with AD (Esparza-Gordillo et al. 2009; Henry et al. 2011). Tauchi et al. (2005) demonstrated transgenic mice with constitutive AhR activation developed inflammatory skin lesions and pruritus accompanied with up-regulated inflammation-associated gene expression resembling AD. Additionally, AD patients display higher protein levels of AhR and Arnt, and elevated AhR, Arnt and CYP1A1 mRNA levels have been detected in the epidermis of these patients (Kim et al. 2014). Interestingly, for many years, topical coal tar has been used treat various skin disease for its anti-inflammatory properties. Coal tar contains a diverse spectrum of hydrocarbons and aromatic compounds therefore its effects through AhR signaling has been investigated. In keratinocytes derived from AD patients and epidermal skin equivalents, coal tar improved epidermal differentiation and up-regulated epidermal barrier proteins including filaggrin, involucrin and hornerin expression with inhibition of IL/4/STAT-6 signaling resulting in downregulation of eosinophilic chemoattractant CCL26 expression (van den Boggard et al. 2013).

16.6.5.2 Psoriasis

Psoriasis, an immune-mediated chronic skin pathology associated with increased secretion of inflammatory cytokines (including IL-23, IL-17, IL-22) and infiltration of neutrophiles and T cells, undermines skin barrier structure and function, and formation of itchy, red, scaly plaques are a phenotypic hallmark of the disease. Evidence has now been generated indicating that environmental factors that activate AhR (e.g. solar UV-induced FICZ or coal tar-based topical treatment) attenuate keratinocyte responsiveness to inflammatory stimuli (IL-1β), thereby potentially limiting psoriatic pathology in human patients. Immunofluorescence staining performed on skin lesion biopsies from psoriatic patients displayed high AhR and Arnt levels throughout the epidermis, with nuclear colocalization of AhR and Arnt in the lower epidermis (Kim et al. 2014). AhR activation via FICZ treatment on psoriatic skin biopsies derived from patients revealed transcriptional suppression of pro-inflammatory psoriasis-associated genes (including interferon-induced genes such as *IFIT*, *RSAD2*, *IFIT3*, *CMPK2*, *MX2*), whereas pharmacological antagonism of AhR (using CH-223191, a drug-like synthetic AhR antagonist that prevents TCDD-caused cytochrome P450 induction, liver toxicity, and wasting syndrome in mice) upregulated expression of these genes, substantiating a new role of AhR in the modulation of the psoriasis-associated transcriptome (Di Meglio et al. 2014). Indeed, in an imiquimod-induced murine model of psoriasis (mimicking the human disease concerning acanthosis, parakeratosis, IL-23/IL-17/IL-22 pathway engagement, and neutrophil recruitment) psoriasiform exacerbation was observed in AhR-deficient mice resulting in scaling and parakeratosis of the stratum corneum, epidermal acanthosis, and inflammatory infiltration, compared to wild type mice. FICZ treatment prior to imiquimod attenuated inflammatory responses and also reduced epidermal thickness and parakeratosis. The hyper-inflammatory phenotype observed in AhR KO mice was replicated only in conditional KO mice lacking AhR expression in keratinocytes and fibroblasts but not in dendritic cells or macrophages, indicating that AhR deficiency in nonhematopoietic cells exacerbates skin inflammation (Di Meglio et al. 2014). Elevated levels of the AP-1 family member JunB were detected in human keratinocytes following imiquimod treatment, and AhR genetic status was a determinant of imiquimod responsiveness, suggesting a crucial role of AhR in suppressing skin inflammatory functions through the regulation of JunB expression.

16.6.5.3 Scleroderma

Scleroderma is a chronic fibrotic autoimmune disease that affects the connective tissue resulting in thickened and tightened skin associated with calcinosis, exaggerated vasoconstriction (Raynaud's phenomenon), esophageal dysfunction, sclerodactyly, and telangiectasias. Therapeutic studies are addressing factors involved in fibrotic progression such as the major cytokine transforming growth factor-β1 (TGFβ1), mediating myofibroblast differentiation and displaying altered expression in scleroderma (Denton and Abraham 2001). It has been reported that the AhR ligand ITE suppresses TGFβ1-driven myofibroblast differentiation by inhibiting the nuclear translocation of Smad2/3/4 but the specific involvement of AhR signaling remains to be elucidated (Lehman et al. 2011).

16.6.5.4 Seborrheic Dermatitis

Seborrheic dermatitis is a chronic inflammatory cutaneous disease characterized by erythematous patches, pruritus, and fine scaling found in sebum-rich areas. Interestingly, seborrheic dermatitis has been associated with tryptophan metabolites (including FICZ, ICZ, malassezin, and pityriacitrin) generated by commensal cutaneous yeasts (such as Malassezia globosa, Malassezia restricta, and Malassezia furfur), displaying activity as AhR agonists (Gaitanis et al. 2008; Del Rosso 2011; Gaitanis et al. 2012; Magiatis et al. 2013; Mexia et al. 2015). Skin scale extracts from patients with Malassezia-associated diseases displayed up to one thousand-fold higher AhR-activating capacity than control skin extracts, and LC-MS analysis of human skin extracts derived from seborrheic dermatitis patients revealed the presence of microbial AhR agonists including indirubin, FICZ, ICZ, malassezin, pityriacitrin, and the novel microbial indoloazepinone-metabolite pityriazepin (Mexia et al. 2015). As compared to TCDD, indirubin and FICZ caused AhR activation in HaCaT keratinocytes with high, yet transient potency, an observation consistent with metabolic susceptibility and rapid turnover of these microbial high affinity AhR agonists downstream of AhR-induced upregulation of CYP1A1. Interestingly, it has been suggested that a microbiome-related contribution to skin photocarcinogenesis in the context of basal cell carcinoma (BCC) may originate from the commensal generation of AhR-directed metabolites including FICZ, a tempting hypothesis envisioning the synergistic overlap between microbiome-derived AhR-directed metabolites and environmental toxicants (solar UV) in the causation of tissue damage to be substantiated by future experimentation (Gaitanis et al. 2012).

16.6.6 AhR in Melanogenesis, Vitiligo, and Malignant Melanomagenesis

Cutaneous hyperpigmentation is an established hallmark of human xenobiotic exposure. Early reports documented that accidental exposure to persistent organochlorine compounds including polychlorinated biphenyls (PCBs), polychlorinated di-benzofurans (PCDFs), and polychlorinated dibenzo-*p*-dioxin (PCDDs) through dietary consumption of contaminated cooking oil in the 1970s in Japan ('Yusho incident') and Taiwan ('Yu-Cheng incident') causes abnormal pigmentation (affecting skin, nail, and gingiva) together with the development of acne-like eruptions, developmental defects and endocrine dysfunction, immunotoxicity, and reproductive toxicity (Hashiguchi et al. 1987; Pluim et al. 1993; Weisglas-Kuperus et al. 2000; Ayotte et al. 2003; Tsukimori et al. 2011). Likewise, it is well established that the fetal PCB syndrome observed in prenatally exposed babies involves dark brown pigmentation of skin and mucous membranes (Yamashita and Hayashi 1985). Recently, the role of AhR in pigment formation by regulating the expression of genes coding for enzymes of the melanogenic pathway has been established at the molecular level. TCCD and FICZ-induced AhR signaling has been shown to stimulate melanogenesis in cultured human melanocytes causing upregulation of tyrosinase enzyme activity and total melanin content, and genomic sequence analysis revealed the presence of putative XRE-sequences in promoter regions, introns, and 3′ noncoding regions of human tyrosinase (*TYR*) and tyrosinase related genes [*TYRP1*, *TYRP2* (*DCT*)] (Luecke et al. 2010). Subsequent experiments demonstrated a role of AhR in UVB-induced skin tanning based on the observation that UVB-induced pigmentation was diminished in AhR KO mice (Jux et al. 2011).

Consistent with its emerging role in melanocyte function and melanogenesis, AhR signaling has recently been shown to be involved in the pathogenesis of vitiligo, a cutaneous condition characterized by progressive hypopigmentation and reduction of melanocyte numbers in lesional skin causing the loss of inherited skin pigmentation. It has been hypothesized that functional mutations of the AhR gene may have a negative impact on downstream genes including *TYR*, *TYRP2 (DCT)*, *KITLG* (*SCF*), and *KIT* impacting the risk of vitiligo in human patients. Indeed, the association of functional polymorphisms in the aryl hydrocarbon receptor gene with the risk of vitiligo has been reported in Han Chinese populations (Wang et al. 2012, 2015). Moreover, it has been demonstrated that AhR-mediated immune response signaling is compromised in vitiligo undergoing massive epidermal oxidative stress mediated by hydrogen peroxide and peroxynitrite with oxidative posttranslational modification and inactivation of indoleamine 2,3-dioxygenase and AhR (Schallreuter et al. 2012), and it was suggested that impaired epidermal AhR and IDO signaling could provide a molecular mechanism underlying the absence of T_{reg} cells in lesional, perilesional, and normal pigmented skin of patients with vitiligo (Klarquist et al. 2010). Importantly, it has been proposed that topical application of AhR agonists such as FICZ may be effective in inducing skin pigmentation in vitiligo patients (Jux et al. 2011), a rational awaiting clinical validation and also supported by the finding that hair follicle melanocytes can repopulate depigmented epidermis in transgenic mice constitutively expressing stem cell factor [SCF; kit ligand (*KITLG*) (Nishimura et al. 2002)].

In the context of AhR-engagement in cutaneous dyspigmentation, it is noteworthy that tinea (or 'pityriasis') versicolor, a common cutaneous mycosis located on sebaceous areas caused by overgrowth of various species of the commensal yeast Malassezia, is characterized by depigmented cutaneous lesions. Indeed, apoptotic elimination of melanocytes by the microbial metabolite and AhR agonist malassezin was recently proposed as the mechanistic basis of the marked depigmentation characteristic of tinea versicolor (Kramer et al. 2005; Prohic and Ozegovic 2007).

In malignant melanomagenesis, a complex role of AhR has now been recognized as supported by the fact that AhR can display either oncogenic or tumor suppressor functions, activities that depend on cellular context. AhR expression in human melanoma cells has been connected to AhR-dependent regulation of genes involved in melanoma progression (Villano et al. 2006). Normal melanocytes and melanoma cells express the AhR/Arnt, and activation of this pathway by TCDD in A2058 melanoma cells results in increased expression and activity of MMP-1, MMP-2 and MMP-9, as well as increased invasiveness. Interestingly, it has been demonstrated that human metastatic melanomas display reduced AhR expression levels as compared to benign nevi, and the observation that experimental AhR knockdown promotes primary tumorigenesis and metastasis in murine models of malignant melanoma suggests that AhR displays tumor suppressor activity in melanomagenesis. (Contador-Troca et al. 2015). Moreover, AhR activation antagonizes the tumorigenic effects of aldehyde dehydrogenase (Aldh1A1) expression, blocking melanoma tumorigenesis and metastasis providing clinically relevant evidence that the combined AhR^{low}-$Aldh1A1^{high}$ phenotype may predict poor prognosis in human melanoma patients (O'Donnell et al. 2012; Contador-Troca et al. 2013).

16.6.7 AhR and Cancer: Focus on Nonmelanoma Skin Photocarcinogenesis

The tumor promoting potential of AhR activation has been supported by experimental evidence indicating AhR-driven enhanced extracellular matrix degradation, anti-apoptotic and pro-inflammatory proteins (i.e. COX2, IL-1B, IL-8, IL-18) following ligand binding (Sutter et al. 1991; Tauch et al. 2005; Fritsche et al. 2007; Haarmann-Stemmann et al. 2009; Ono et al. 2013). Interestingly, in non-cutaneous malignancy, the oxidative tryptophan catabolite kynurenine has been identified as an endogenous tumour-promoting ligand of the human aryl hydrocarbon receptor, generated constitutively by human tumor cells involving indoleamine-pyrrole 2,3-dioxygenase (IDO) and tryptophan-2,3-dioxygenase (TDO). The TDO-AhR pathway, active in human brain tumors associated with malignant progression and poor survival, produces kynurenine blocking antitumor immune responses and promoting tumor-cell survival and motility through AhR engagement in an autocrine/paracrine fashion (Opitz et al. 2011). Targeting various immune cells involved in tumor evasion of immune surveillance, kynurenine-based AhR activation suppresses effector T cell function helping tumor immune evasion, and kynurenine-AhR interactions involving dendritic cells and regulatory B cells increase immune tolerance by initiating the formation of tumor promoting T_{regs} that facilitate metastasis.

It is well known that AhR may mediate genotoxicity through the generation of DNA adductors potentially serving as mutagenic initiators in tumorgenesis targeting diverse organ systems including skin (Chakravarti et al. 1998). Remarkably, AhR-deficient mice did not develop skin tumors following long term treatment by subcutaneously administered or topical BaP as seen only in AhR-wildtype mice indicating that AhR plays an essential role in BaP-induced cutaneous tumorigenicity (Shimizu et al. 2000). For physiological relevance, AhR activity by the PAH BaP at concentrations comparable to environmental or occupational exposure has been demonstrated to induce CYP1A1, operating upstream of oxidative stress and cytotoxic effects in human skin (Costa et al. 2010). Interestingly, a population-directed study investigating workers exposed to asphalt-derived PAHs indicated that the primary route of PAH exposure is cutaneous (McClean et al. 2004). This is corroborated by reports of enhanced AhR and CYP1A1 activity in skin biopsies from dioxin-exposed workers (Tang et al. 2008).

The photooxidative formation of the tryptophan-photoproduct and high-affinity AhR ligand FICZ is thought to underlie the known ability of solar UVB to activate AhR, a process originating from UVB absorption of free cytosolic tryptophan in epidermal keratinocytes (Fritsche et al. 2007). Subsequently, FICZ binding initiates the dissociation of the AhR multiprotein complex consisting of heat-shock protein 90 (Hsp90), tyrosine kinase c-src, and other co-chaperones followed by AhR nuclear translocation and expression of AhR target genes including CYP1A1 thought to be involved in redox dysregulation and and the metabolic activation of procarcinogens including BaP. Translocation of c-src to the cell membrane occurs with phosphorylation of the epidermal growth factor receptor (EGFR), activation of downstream MAPK signaling, and induction of XRE-independent target genes such as *COX2*, a mediator of inflammation and oxidative stress with an established role in skin photocarcinogenesis, a signaling pathway that has been referred to as 'non-genomic' AhR signaling.

More recent evidence indicates that in experimental NMSC, AhR plays the role of an UVB-sensitive transcription factor serving an anti-apoptotic/pro-survival function in human keratinocytes (Frauenstein et al. 2013). Consistent with this hypothesis pharmacological [3′-methoxy-4′-nitroflavone (MNF)] and genetic (shRNA-based) inhibition of AhR signaling sensitized cultured keratinocytes to UVB-induced apoptosis by decreasing the expression of E2F1 and its target gene checkpoint kinase 1 (CHK1). Importantly, the anti-apoptotic function of AhR was also observed in murine skin. Specifically, in contrast to AhR-proficient SKH-1 mice, an enhanced cleavage of caspase-3 in the skin of AhR-KO SKH-1 mice occurred after UVB exposure. Taken together, these data suggest that the AhR-E2F1-CHK1 axis may serve as a novel anti-apoptotic pathway in epidermal keratinocytes, representing a promising target for chemoprevention of non-melanoma skin cancer.

Consequently, AhR-antagonistic strategies have been under consideration for pharmacological UVB photoprotection, and prototype evidence has been presented indicating that the new aryl hydrocarbon receptor antagonist E/Z-2-benzylindene-5,6-dimethoxy-3,3-dimethylindan-1-one (BDDI) suppresses UVB-induced signal transduction (Tigges et al. 2014). Cutaneous administration of BDDI (0.5 % topical formulation) blocks XRE-binding of AhR/Arnt and represses UVB [1.5 MED (minimal erythema dose)]-induced gene expression (*CYP1A1*, *COX2*, *MMP1*) in a human in vivo study. Importantly, the UV-induced cutaneous erythema response was not significantly modulated by BDDI topical application indicating that UVB-induced AhR-dependent signaling can be blocked selectively in human skin without affecting the sunburn response.

16.7 Conclusions

Due to the fundamental role that AhR-controlled signaling plays in skin barrier formation, homeostasis, resilience to environmental stressors, and damage repair, AhR-directed pharmacological strategies that aim at modulation of AhR-orchestrated signaling for anti-inflammatory, immune-modulatory, cancer chemopreventive, and barrier enhancing intervention hold great therapeutic promise, delivering unique patient-directed benefit by targeting specific skin pathologies that have remained molecularly elusive and hard to treat so far (Haarmann-Stemmann et al. 2015). The ever expanding and accessible range of chemically diverse physiological and synthetic AhR-modulators that differ with regard to pharmacokinetic and pharmacodynamic profile, AhR-directed potency, metabolic stability, and off-target effects through engagement of other signaling pathways provides a versatile and accessible compound platform of prototype agents and therapeutic leads for experimental intervention through AhR engagement, potentially representing breakthrough therapeutics that can quickly be optimized, developed, and formulated into novel AhR-directed cutaneous therapeutic entities.

References

Adachi J, Mori Y, Matsui S, Takigami H, Fujino J, Kitagawa H, Miller CA III, Kato T, Saeki K, Matsuda T (2001) Indirubin and indigo are potent aryl hydrocarbon receptor ligands present in human urine. J Biol Chem 276:31475–31478

Afaq F, Zaid MA, Pelle E, Khan N, Syed DN, Matsui MS, Maes D, Mukhtar H (2009) Aryl hydrocarbon receptor is an ozone sensor in human skin. J Invest Dermatol 129:2396–2403

Ashida H (2000) Suppressive effects of flavonoids on dioxin toxicity. BioFactors 12(1–4):201–206

Aylward LL, Brunet RC, Carrier G, Hays SM, Cushing CA, Needham LL, Patterson DG, Gerthoux PM, Brambilla P, Mocarelli P (2005) Concentration-dependent TCDD elimination kinetics in humans: toxicokinetic modeling for moderately to highly exposed adults from Seveso, Italy, and Vienna, Austria, and impact on dose estimates for the NIOSH cohort. J Expo Anal Environ Epidemiol 15(1):51–65

Ayotte P, Muckle G, Jacobson JL, Jacobson SW, Dewailly E (2003) Inuit Cohort Study. Assessment of pre- and postnatal exposure to polychlorinated biphenyls: lessons from the Inuit Cohort Study. Environ Health Perspect 111(9):1253–1258

Banerjee G, Gupta N, Tiwari J, Raman G (2005) Ultraviolet-induced transformation of keratinocytes: possible involvement of long interspersed element-1 reverse transcriptase. Photodermatol Photoimmunol Photomed 21(1):32–39

Barouki R, Coumoul X, Fernandez-Salguero PM (2007) The aryl hydrocarbon receptor, more than a xenobiotic-interacting protein. FEBS Lett 581(19):3608–3615

Baudouin C, Charveron M, Tarroux R, Gall Y (2002) Environmental pollutants and skin cancer. Cell Biol Toxicol 18(5):341–348

Bergander L, Wincent E, Rannug A, Foroozesh M, Alworth W, Rannug U (2004) Metabolic fate of the Ah receptor ligand 6-formylindolo[3,2-b]carbazole. Chem Biol Interact 149(2–3): 151–164

Berghard A, Gradin K, Toftgård R (1992) The stability of dioxin-receptor ligands influences cytochrome P4501A1 expression in human keratinocytes. Carcinogenesis 13:651–655

Bisson WH, Koch DC, O'Donnell EF, Khalil SM, Kerkvliet NI, Tanguay RL, Abagyan R, Kolluri SK (2009) Modeling of the aryl hydrocarbon receptor (AhR) ligand binding domain and its utility in virtual ligand screening to predict new AhR ligands. J Med Chem 52:5635–5641

Bittinger MA, Nguyen LP, Bradfield CA (2003) Aspartate aminotransferase generates proagonists of the aryl hydrocarbon receptor. Mol Pharmacol 64(3):550–556

Bjeldanes LF, Kim JY, Grose KR, Bartholomew JC, Bradfield CA (1991) Aromatic hydrocarbon responsiveness-receptor agonists generated from indole-3-carbinol in vitro and in vivo: comparisons with 2,3,7,8-tetrachlorodibenzo-p-dioxin. Proc Natl Acad Sci USA 88(21): 9543–9547

Bruhs A, Haarmann-Stemmann T, Frauenstein K, Krutmann J, Schwarz T, Schwarz A (2015) Activation of the arylhydrocarbon receptor causes immunosuppression primarily by modulating dendritic cells. J Invest Dermatol 135(2):435–444

Carreira PE, Richardson SR, Faulkner GJ (2014) L1 retrotransposons, cancer stem cells and oncogenesis. FEBS J 281(1):63–73

Chakravarti D, Mailander P, Franzen J, Higginbotham S, Cavalieri EL, Rogan EG (1998) Detection of dibenzo[a,l]pyrene-induced H-ras codon 61 mutant genes in preneoplastic SENCAR mouse skin using a new PCR-RFLP method. Oncogene 16(24):3203–3210

Chang TK, Chen J, Yang G, Yeung EY (2010) Inhibition of procarcinogen-bioactivating human CYP1A1, CYP1A2 and CYP1B1 enzymes by melatonin. J Pineal Res 48:55–64

Ciolino HP, Daschner PJ, Wang TT, Yeh GC (1998) Effect of curcumin on the aryl hydrocarbon receptor and cytochrome P4501A1 in MCF-7 human breast carcinoma cells. Biochem Pharmacol 56:197–206

Ciolino HP, Daschner PJ, Yeh GC (1999) Dietary flavonols quercetin and kaempferol are ligands of the aryl hydrocarbon receptor that affect CYP1A1 transcription differentially. Biochem J 340:715–722

Contador-Troca M, Alvarez-Barrientos A, Barrasa E, Rico-Leo EM, Catalina-Fernández I, Menacho-Márquez M, Bustelo XR, García-Borrón JC, Gómez-Durán A, Sáenz-Santamaría J, Fernández-Salguero PM (2013) The dioxin receptor has tumor suppressor activity in melanoma growth and metastasis. Carcinogenesis 34(12):2683–2693

Contador-Troca M, Alvarez-Barrientos A, Merino JM, Morales-Hernández A, Rodríguez MI, Rey-Barroso J, Barrasa E, Cerezo-Guisado MI, Catalina-Fernández I, Sáenz-Santamaría J, Oliver FJ, Fernandez-Salguero PM (2015) Dioxin receptor regulates aldehyde dehydrogenase to block melanoma tumorigenesis and metastasis. Mol Cancer 14:148

Costa C, Catania S, De Pasquale R, Stancanelli R, Scribano GM, Melchini A (2010) Exposure of human skin to benzo[a]pyrene: role of CYP1A1 and aryl hydrocarbon receptor in oxidative stress generation. Toxicology 271(3):83–86

Davis AL, Qiao S, Lesson JL, Rojo de la Vega M, Park SL, Seanez CM, Gokhale V, Cabello CM, Wondrak GT (2015) The quinone methide aurin is a heat shock response inducer that causes proteotoxic stress and noxa-dependent apoptosis in malignant melanoma cells. J Biol Chem 290(3):1623–1638

Del Rosso JQ (2011) Adult seborrheic dermatitis: a status report on practical topical management. J Clin Aesthet Dermatol 5:32–38

Denison MS, Heath-Pagliuso S (1998) The Ah receptor: a regulator of the bio-chemical and toxicological actions of structurally diverse chemicals. Bull Environ Contam Toxicol 61:557–568

Denison MS, Nagy SR (2003) Activation of the aryl hydrocarbon receptor by structurally diverse exogenous and endogenous chemicals. Annu Rev Pharmacol Toxicol 43(1):309–334

Denison MS, Seidel SD, Rogers WJ, Ziccardi M, Winter GM, Heath-Pagliuso S (1998) Natural and synthetic ligands for the Ah receptor. In: Puga A, Wallace KB (eds) Molecular Biology Approaches to Toxicology, Taylor & Francis, Philadelphia, pp 393–410

Denton CP, Abraham DJ (2001) Transforming growth factor- and connective tissue growth factor: key cytokines in scleroderma pathogenesis. Curr Opin Rheumatol 13(6):505–511

Dere E, Lo R, Celius T, Matthews J, Zacharewski TR (2011) Integration of genome-wide computation DRE search, AhR ChIP-chip and gene expression analyses of TCDD-elicited responses in the mouse liver. BMC Genom 15(12):365

Devito MJ, Birnbaum LS (1994) Toxicology of dioxins and related chemicals. In: Schecter A (ed) Dioxins and Health, Plenum, New York, pp 139–162

Diani-Moore S, Ma Y, Labitzke E, Tao H, David WJ, Anderson J, Chen Q, Gross SS, Rifkind AB (2011) Discovery and biological characterization of 1-(1H- indol-3-yl)-9H-pyrido[3,4-b]indole as an aryl hydrocarbon receptor activator generated by photoactivation of tryptophan by sunlight. Chem Biol Interact 193(2):119–128

DiNatale BC, Murray IA, Schroeder JC, Flaveny CA, Lahoti TS, Laurenzana EM, Omiecinski CJ, Perdew GH (2010) Kynurenic acid is a potent endogenous aryl hydrocarbon receptor ligand that synergistically induces interleukin-6 in the presence of inflammatory signaling. Toxicol Sci 115:89–97

Di Meglio P, Duarte JH, Ahlfors H, Owens ND, Li Y, Villanova F, Tosi I, Hirota K, Nestle FO, Mrowietz U, Gilchrist MJ, Stockinger B (2014) Activation of the aryl hydrocarbon receptor dampens the severity of inflammatory skin conditions. Immunity 40(6):989–1001

Diry M, Tomkiewicz C, Koehle C, Coumoul X, Bock KW, Barouki R, Transy C (2006) Activation of the dioxin/aryl hydrocarbon receptor (AhR) modulates cell plasticity through a JNK-dependent mechanism. Oncogene 25:5570–5574

Esparza-Gordillo J, Weidinger S, Fölster-Holst R, Bauerfeind A, Ruschendorf F, Patone G, Rohde K, Marenholz I, Schulz F, Kerscher T, Hubner N, Wahn U, Franke A, Schreiber S, Vogler R, Heath S, Baurecht H, Novak N, Rodriguez E, Illig T, Lee-Kirsch MA, Ciechanowicz A, Kurek M, Piskackova T, Macek M, Lee YA, Ruether A (2009) A common variant on chromosome 11q13 is associated with atopic dermatitis. Nat Genet 41(5):596–601

Esser C, Rannug A (2015) The aryl hydrocarbon receptor in barrier organ physiology, immunology, and toxicology. Pharmacol Rev 67(2):259–279

Evans BR, Karchner SI, Allan LL, Pollenz RS, Tanguay RL, Jenny MJ, Sherr DH, Hahn ME (2008) Repression of aryl hydrocarbon receptor (AhR) signaling by AhR repressor: role of DNA binding and competition for AhR nuclear translocator. Mol Pharmacol 73:387–398

Flaveny CA, Murray IA, Perdew GH (2010) Differential gene regulation by the human and mouse aryl hydrocarbon receptor. Toxicol Sci 114(2):217–225

Forrester AR, Elias MS, Woodward EL, Graham M, Williams FM, Reynolds NJ (2014) Induction of a chloracne phenotype in an epidermal equivalent model by 2,3,7,8-tetrachlorodibenzo-p-dioxin (TCDD) is dependent on aryl hydrocarbon receptor activation and is not reproduced by aryl hydrocarbon receptor knock down. Dermatol Sci 73(1):10–22

Fraschini E, Bonati L, Pitea D (1996) Molecular polarizability as a tool for understanding the binding properties of polychlorinated dibenzo-p-dioxins: definition of a reliable computational procedure. J Phys Chem 100:10564–10569

Frauenstein K, Sydlik U, Tigges J, Majora M, Wiek C, Hanenberg H, Abel J, Esser C, Fritsche E, Krutmann J, Haarmann-Stemmann T (2013) Evidence for a novel anti-apoptotic pathway in human keratinocytes involving the aryl hydrocarbon receptor, E2F1, and checkpoint kinase 1. Cell Death Differ 20:1425–1434

Fritsche E, Schäfer C, Calles C, Bernsmann T, Bernshausen T, Wurm M, Hübenthal U, Cline JE, Hajimiragha H, Schroeder P, Klotz LO, Rannug A, Fürst P, Hanenberg H, Abel J, Krutmann J (2007) Lightening up the UV response by identification of the arylhydrocarbon receptor as a cytoplasmatic target for ultraviolet B radiation. Proc Natl Acad Sci USA 104:8851–8856

Furue M, Tsuji G, Mitoma C, Nakahara T, Chiba T, Morino-Koga S, Uchi H (2015) Gene regulation of filaggrin and other skin barrier proteins via aryl hydrocarbon receptor. J Dermatol Sci 80(2):83–88

Gaitanis G, Magiatis P, Stathopoulou K, Bassukas ID, Alexopoulos EC, Velegraki A, Skaltsounis AL (2008) AhR ligands, malassezin, and indolo[3,2-b]carbazole are selectively produced by Malassezia furfur strains isolated from seborrheic dermatitis. J Invest Dermatol 128(7):1620–1625

Gaitanis G, Magiatis P, Hantschke M, Bassuka ID, Velegrakid A (2012) The Malassezia genus in skin and systemic diseases. Clin Microbiol Rev 25(1):106–141

Gao Z, Perez-Perez GI, Chen Y, Blaser MJ (2010) Quantitation of major human cutaneous bacterial and fungal populations. J Clin Microbiol 48(10):3575–3581

Giorgi G, Marcantonio P, Del Re B (2011) LINE-1 retrotransposition in human neuroblastoma cells is affected by oxidative stress. Cell Tissue Res 346(3):383–391

Gradelet S, Astorg P, Le Bon A-M, Bergès R, Suschetet M (1997) Modulation of aflatoxin B1 carcinogenicity, genotoxicity and metabolism in rat liver by dietary carotenoids: evidence for a protective effect of CYP1A inducers. Cancer Lett 114:221–223

Gu YZ, Hogenesch JB, Bradfield CA (2000) The PAS superfamily: sensors of environmental and developmental signals. Annu Rev Pharmacol Toxicol 40:519–561

Guengerich P, Martin MV, McCormick WA, Nguyen LP, Glover E, Bradfield CA (2004) Aryl hydrocarbon receptor response to indigoids in vitro and in vivo. Arch Biochem Biophys 423:309–316

Gupta AK, Batra R, Bluhm R, Boekhout T, Dawson TL Jr (2004) Skin diseases associated with Malassezia species. J Am Acad Dermatol 51:785–798

Haarmann-Stemmann T, Bothe H, Abel J (2009) Growth factors, cytokines and their receptors as downstream targets of arylhydrocarbon receptor (AhR) signaling pathways. Biochem Pharmacol 77(4):508–520

Haarmann-Stemmann T, Abel J, Fritsche E, Krutmann J (2012) The AhR-Nrf2 pathway in keratinocytes: on the road to chemoprevention?. J Invest Dermatol 132(1):7–9

Haarmann-Stemmann T, Esser C, Krutmann J (2015) The janus-faced role of aryl hydrocarbon receptor signaling in the skin: consequences for prevention and treatment of skin disorders. J Invest Dermatol 135(11):2572–2576

Hashiguchi I, Akamine A, Miyatake S, Hara Y, Maeda K, Toriya Y, Aono M, Fukuyama H, Okumura H (1987) Histological study on the gingiva of the patient with yusho and of PCB-poisoned monkeys. Fukuoka Igaku Zasshi 78(5):259–265

Heath-Pagliuso S, Rogers WJ, Tullis K, Seidel SD, Cenijn PH, Brouwer A, Denison MS (1998) Activation of the Ah receptor by tryptophan and tryptophan metabolites. Biochemistry 37 (33):11508–11515

Helferich WG, Denison MS (1991) Ultraviolet photoproducts of tryptophan can act as dioxin agonists. Mol Pharmacol 40(5):674–678

Henry J, Hsu CY, Haftek M, Nachat R, de Koning HD, Gardinal-Galera I, Hitomi K, Balica S, Jean-Decoster C, Schmitt AM, Paul C, Serre G, Simon M (2011) Hornerin is a component of the epidermal cornified cell envelopes. FASEB J 25(5):1567–1576

Hu W, Sorrentino C, Denison MS, Kolaja K, Fielden MR (2007) Induction of Cyp1A1 is a nonspecific biomarker of aryl hydrocarbon receptor activation: results of large scale screening of pharmaceuticals and toxicants in vivo and in vitro. Mol Pharmacol 71(6):1475–1486

Hubbard TD, Murray IA, Bisson WH, Lahoti TS, Gowda K, Amin SG, Patterson AD, Perdew GH (2015) Adaptation of the human aryl hydrocarbon receptor to sense microbiota-derived indoles. Sci Rep 5:12689

Jagielski T, Rup E, Ziółkowska A, Roeske K, Macura AB, Bielecki J (2014) Distribution of Malassezia species on the skin of patients with atopic dermatitis, psoriasis, and healthy volunteers assessed by conventional and molecular identification methods. BMC Dermatol 14:3

Jakasa I, Koster ES, Calkoen F, McLean WH, Campbell LE, Bos JD, Verberk MM, Kezic S (2011) Skin barrier function in healthy subjects and patients with atopic dermatitis in relation to filaggrin loss-of-function mutations. J Invest Dermatol 131(2):540–542

Jin U, Lee S, Pfent C, Safe S (2014) The aryl hydrocarbon receptor ligand omeprazole inhibits breast cancer cell invasion and metastasis. BMC Cancer 14:498

Jux B, Kadow S, Esser C (2009) Langerhans cell maturation and contact hypersensitivity are impaired in aryl hydrocarbon receptor-null mice. J Immunol 182(11):6709–6717

Jux B, Kadow S, Luecke S, Rannug A, Krutmann J, Esser C (2011) The aryl hydrocarbon receptor mediates UVB radiation-induced skin tanning. J Invest Dermatol 131(1):203–210

Kadow S, Jux B, Zahner SP, Wingerath B, Chmill S, Clausen BE, Hengstler J, Esser C (2011) Aryl hydrocarbon receptor is critical for homeostasis of invariant gammadelta T cells in the murine epidermis. J Immunol 187:3104–3110

Kazlauskas A, Poellinger L, Pongratz I (1999) Evidence that the co-chaperone p23 regulates ligand responsiveness of the dioxin (Aryl hydrocarbon) receptor. J Biol Chem 274:13519–13524

Kazlauskas A, Poellinger L, Pongratz I (2001) The immunophilin-like protein XAP2 regulates ubiquitination and subcellular localization of the dioxin receptor. J Biol Chem 275 (52):41317–41324

Kim TJ, Upadhyay V, Kumar V, Lee KM, Fu YX (2014) Innate lymphoid cells facilitate NK cell development through a lymphotoxin-mediated stromal microenvironment. J Exp Med 211:1421–1431

Kim SH, Henry EC, Kim DK, Kim YH, Shin KJ, Han MS, Lee TG, Kang JK, Gasiewicz TA, Ryu SH, Suh PG (2006) Novel compound 2-methyl-2H-pyrazole-3-carboxylic acid (2-methyl-4-o-tolylazo-phenyl)-amide (CH-223191) prevents 2,3,7,8-TCDD-induced toxicity by antagonizing the aryl hydrocarbon receptor. Mol Pharmacol 69:1871–1878

Kim MJ, Pelloux V, Guyot E, Tordjman J, Bui LC, Chevallier A, Forest C, Benelli C, Clement K, Barouki R (2012) Inflammatory pathway genes belong to major targets of persistent organic pollutants in adipose cells. Environ Health Perspect 120:508–514

Klarquist J, Denman CJ, Hernandez C, Wainwright DA, Strickland FM, Overbeck A, Mehrotra S, Nishimura MI, Le Poole IC (2010) Reduced skin homing by functional Treg in vitiligo. Pigment Cell Melanoma Res 23(2):276–286

Kloypan C, Srisa-art M, Mutirangura A, Boonla C (2015) LINE-1 hypomethylation induced by reactive oxygen species is mediated via depletion of S-adenosylmethionine. Cell Biochem Funct 33(6):375–385

Knatko EV, Ibbotson SH, Zhang Y, Higgins M, Fahey JW, Talalay P, Dawe RS, Ferguson J, Huang JT, Clarke R, Zheng S, Saito A, Kalra S, Benedict AL, Honda T, Proby CM, Dinkova-Kostova AT (2015) Nrf2 Activation protects against solar-simulated ultraviolet radiation in mice and humans. Cancer Prev Res (Phila) 8(6):475–486

Kopf PG, Scott JA, Agbor LN, Boberg JR, Elased KM, Huwe JK, Walker MK (2010) Cytochrome P4501A1 is required for vascular dysfunction and hypertension induced by 2,3,7,8-tetrachloro-dibenzo-p-dioxin. Toxicol Sci 117:537–546

Kramer HJ, Podobinska M, Bartsch A, Battmann A, Thoma W, Bernd A, Kummer W, Irlinger B, Steglich W, Mayser P (2005) Malassezin, a novel agonist of the aryl hydrocarbon receptor from the yeast Malassezia furfur, induces apoptosis in primary human melanocytes. ChemBioChem 6:860–865

Kulhankova K, Rouse T, Nasr ME, Field EH (2012) Dendritic cells control CD4+CD25+ Treg cell suppressor function in vitro through juxtacrine delivery of IL-2. PLoS ONE 7(9):e43609

Kuo IH, Yoshida T, De Benedetto A, Beck LA (2013) The cutaneous innate immune response in patients with atopic dermatitis. J Allergy Clin Immunol 131(2):266–278

Kuratsune M, Yoshimura T, Matsuzaka J, Yamaguchi A (1971) Yusho, a poisoning caused by rice oil contaminated with polychlorinated biphenyls. HSMHA Health Rep 86(12):1083–1091

Kypriotou M, Huber M, Hohl D (2012) The human epidermal differentiation complex: cornified envelope precursors, S100 proteins and the 'fused genes' family. Exp Dermatol 21(9):643–649

Larangeira de Almeida H, Jr Mayser P (2006) Absence of sunburn in lesions of pityriasis versicolor alba. Mycoses 49(6):516

Lehmann GM, Xi X, Kulkarni AA, Olsen KC, Pollock SJ, Baglole CJ, Gupta S, Casey AE, Huxlin KR, Sime PJ, Feldon SE, Phipps RP (2011) The aryl hydrocarbon receptor ligand ITE inhibits TGFβ1-induced human myofibroblast differentiation. Am J Pathol 178(4):1556–1567

Lieder F, Reisen F, Goeppert T, Sollberger G, Beer HD, auf den Keller U, Schafer M, Detmar M, Schneider G, Werner S (2012) Identification of UV-protective activators of nuclear factor erythroid-derived 2-related factor 2 (Nrf2) by combining a chemical library screen with computer-based virtual screening. J Biol Chem 287:33001–33013

Loertscher JA, Sattler CA, Allen-Hoffmann BL (2001) 2,3,7,8- Tetrachlorodibenzo-p-dioxin alters the differentiation pattern of human keratinocytes in organotypic culture. Toxicol Appl Pharmacol 175(2):121–129

Loertscher JA, Lin TM, Peterson RE, Allen-Hoffmann BL (2002) *In utero* exposure to 2,3,7,8-tetrachlorodibenzo-p-dioxin causes accelerated terminal differentiation in fetal mouse skin. Toxicol Sci 68(2):465–472

Long M, Rojo de la Vega M, Wen Q, Bharara M, Jiang T, Zhang R, Zhou S, Wong PK, Wondrak GT, Zheng H, Zhang DD (2016) An essential role of Nrf2 in diabetic wound healing. Diabetes 65(3):780–793

Lowe MM, Mold JE, Kanwar B, Huang Y, Louie A, Pollastri MP, Wang C, Patel G, Franks DG, Schlezinger J, Sherr DH, Silverstone AE, Hahn ME, McCune JM (2014) Identification of cinnabarinic acid as a novel endogenous aryl hydrocarbon receptor ligand that drives IL-22 production. PLoS One 9, e87877

Luecke S, Wincent E, Backlund M, Rannug U, Rannug A (2010) Cytochrome P450 1A1 gene regulation by UVB involves crosstalk between the aryl hydrocarbon receptor and nuclear factor kB. Chem Biol Interact 184:466–473

Magiatis P, Pappas P, Gaitanis G, Mexia N, Melliou E, Galanou M, Vlachos C, Stathopoulou K, Skaltsounis AL, Marselos M, Velegraki A, Denison MS, Bassukas ID (2013) Malassezia yeasts produce a collection of exceptionally potent activators of the Ah (dioxin) receptor detected in diseased human skin. J Invest Dermatol 133(8):2023–2030

Mexia N, Gaitanis G, Velegraki A, Soshilov A, Denison MS, Magnates P (2015) Pityriazepin and other potent AhR ligands isolated from Malassezia furfur yeast. Arch Biochem Biophys 571:16–20

Moffett JR, Namboodiri MA (2003) Tryptophan and the immune response. Immunol Cell Biol 81 (4):247–265

Moura-Alves P, Faé K, Houthuys E, Dorhoi A, Kreuchwig A, Furkert J, Barison N, Diehl A, Munder A, Constant P, Skrahina T, Guhlich-Bornhof U, Klemm M, Koehler AB, Bandermann S, Goosmann C, Mollenkopf HJ, Hurwitz R, Brinkmann V, Fillatreau S, Daffe M, Tümmler B, Kolbe M, Oschkinat H, Krause G, Kaufmann SH (2014) AhR sensing of bacterial pigments regulates antibacterial defence. Nature (7515):387–392

McClean MD, Rinehart RD, Ngo L, Eisen EA, Kelsey KT, Herrick RF (2004) Inhalation and dermal exposure among asphalt paving workers. Ann Occup Hyg 48(8):663–671

McMahon M, Lamont DJ, Beattie KA, Hayes JD (2010) Keap1 perceives stress via three sensors for the endogenous signaling molecules nitric oxide, zinc, and alkenals. Proc Natl Acad Sci USA 107(44):18838–18843

Mezrich JD, Fechner JH, Zhang X, Johnson BP, Burlingham WJ, Bradfield CA (2010) An interaction between kynurenine and the aryl hydrocarbon receptor can generate regulatory T cells. J Immunol 185:3190–3198

Miao W, Hu L, Scrivens PJ, Batist G (2005) Transcriptional regulation of NF-E2 p45-related factor (Nrf2) expression by the aryl hydrocarbon receptor-xenobiotic response element signaling pathway: direct cross-talk between phase I and II drug-metabolizing enzymes. J Biol Chem 280(21):20340–20348

Mischke D, Korge BP, Marenholz I, Volz A, Ziegler A (1996) Genes encoding structural proteins of epidermal cornification and S100 calcium-binding proteins form a gene complex ("epidermal differentiation complex") on human chromosome 1q21. J Invest Dermatol 106 (5):989–992

Nakabayashi A, Sei Y, Guillot J (2000) Identification of Malassezia species isolated from patients with seborrhoeic dermatitis, atopic dermatitis, pityriasis versicolor and normal subjects. Med Mycol 38:337–341

Nakahara T, Mitoma C, Hashimoto-Hachiya A, Takahara M, Tsuji G, Uchi H, Yan X, Hachisuka J, Chiba T, Esaki H. Kido-Nakahara M, Furue M (2015) Antioxidant opuntia ficus-indica extract activates AhR-Nrf2 signaling and upregulates filaggrin and loricrin expression in human keratinocytes. J Med Food 18(10):1143–1149

Navid F, Bruhs A, Schuller W, Fritsche E, Krutmann J, Schwarz T, Schwarz A (2013) The Aryl hydrocarbon receptor is involved in UVR-induced immunosuppression. J Invest Dermatol 133 (12):2763–2770

Nguyen NT, Kimura A, Nakahama T, Chinen I, Masuda K, Nohara K, Fujii-Kuriyama Y, Kishimoto T (2010) Aryl hydrocarbon receptor negatively regulates dendritic cell immunogenicity via a kynurenine-dependent mechanism. Proc Natl Acad Sci USA 107:19961–19966

Nishimura EK, Jordan SA, Oshima H, Yoshida H, Osawa M, Moriyama M, Jackson IJ, Barrandon Y, Miyachi Y, Nishikawa S (2002) Dominant role of the niche in melanocyte stem-cell fate determination. Nature 416:854–860

Novotna A, Korhonova M, Bartonkova I, Soshilov AA, Denison MS, Bogdanova K, Kolar M, Bednar P, Dvorak Z (2014) Enantiospecific effects of ketoconazole on aryl hydrocarbon receptor. PLoS ONE 9(7):e101832

Nugent LF, Shi G, Vistica BP, Ogbeifun O, Hinshaw SJ, Gery I (2013) A novel endogenous nontoxic aryl hydrocarbon receptor ligand efficiently suppresses EAU and T-Cell–mediated immunity. Invest Ophthalmol Vis Sci 54(12):7463–7469

O'Donnell EF, Kopparapu PR, Koch DC, Jang HS, Phillips JL, Tanguay RL, Kerkvliet NI, Kolluri SK (2012) The aryl hydrocarbon receptor mediates leflunomide-induced growth inhibition of melanoma cells. PLoS ONE 7(7):e40926

Oberg M, Bergander L, Håkansson H, Rannug U, Rannug A (2005) Identification of the tryptophan photoproduct 6-formylindolo[3,2-b]carbazole, in cell culture medium, as a factor that controls the background aryl hydrocarbon receptor activity. Toxicol Sci 85(2):935–943

Ono Y, Torii K, Fritsche E, Shintani Y, Nishida E, Nakamura M, Shirakata Y, Haarmann-Stemmann T, Abel J, Krutmann J, Morita A (2013) Role of the aryl hydrocarbon receptor in tobacco smoke extract-induced matrix metalloproteinase-1 expression. Exp Dermatol 22(5):349–353

Opitz CA, Litzenburger UM, Sahm F, Ott M, Tritschler I, Trump S, Schumacher T, Jestaedt L, Schrenk D, Weller M, Jugold M, Guillemin GJ, Miller CL, Lutz C, Radlwimmer B, Lehmann I, von Deimling A, Wick W, Platten M (2011) An endogenous tumour-promoting ligand of the human aryl hydrocarbon receptor. Nature 478:197–203

Palmer CN, Irvine AD, Terron-Kwiatkowski A, Zhao Y, Liao H, Lee SP, Goudie DR, Sandilands A, Campbell LE, Smith FJ, O'Regan GM, Watson RM, Cecil JE, Bale SJ,Compton JG, DiGiovanna JJ, Fleckman P, Lewis-Jones S, Arseculeratne G, Sergeant A, Munro CS, El Houate B, McElreavey K, Halkjaer LB, Bisgaard H, Mukhopadhyay S, and McLean WH (2006) Common loss-of-function variants of the epidermal barrier protein filaggrin are a major predisposing factor for atopic dermatitis. *Nat Genet* 38(4): 441–446

Park JY, Shigenaga MK, Ames BN (1996) Induction of cytochrome P4501A1 by 2,3,7,8-tetrachlorodibenzo-p-dioxin or indolo(3,2-b)carbazole is associated with oxidative DNA damage. Proc Natl Acad Sci USA 93:2322–2327

Park SL, Justiniano R, Williams JD, Cabello CM, Qiao S, Wondrak GT (2015) The tryptophan-derived endogenous aryl hydrocarbon receptor ligand 6-formylindolo [3,2-b]carbazole is a nanomolar UVA photosensitizer in epidermal keratinocytes. J Invest Dermatol 135(6):1649–1658

Pluim HJ, de Vijlder JJ, Olie K, Kok JH, Vulsma T, van Tijn DA, van der Slikke JW, Koppe JG (1993) Effects of pre- and postnatal exposure to chlorinated dioxins and furans on human neonatal thyroid hormone concentrations. Environ Health Perspect 101(6):504–508

Poland A, Knutson JC (1982) 2,3,7,8-tetrachlorodibenzo-p-dioxin and related halogenated aromatic hydrocarbons: examination of the mechanism of toxicity. Annu Rev Pharmacol Toxicol 22:517–554

Poland A, Knutson JC, Poland A, Glover E, Kende AS (1976) Stereospecific, high affinity binding of 2,3,7,8-tetrachlorodibenzo-p-dioxin by hepatic cytosol. Evidence that the binding species is receptor for induction of aryl hydrocarbon hydroxylase. J Biol Chem 251:4936–4946

Pouillot A, Dayan N, Polla AS, Polla LL, Polla BS (2008) The stratum corneum: a double paradox. J Cosmet Dermal 7(2):143–148

Prochazkova J, Kozubik A, Machala M, Vondracek J (2011) Differential effects of indirubin and 2,3,7,8-tetrachlorodibenzo-p-dioxin on the aryl hydrocarbon receptor (AhR) signalling in liver progenitor cells. Toxicology 279:146–154

Prohic A, Ozegovic L (2007) Malassezia species isolated from lesional and non-lesional skin in patients with pityriasis versicolor. Mycoses 50:58–63

Punj S, Kopparapu P, Jang HS, Phillips JL, Pennington J, Rohlman D, O'Donnell E, Iversen PL, Kolluri SK, Kerkvliet NI (2014) Benzimidazoisoquinolines: a new class of rapidly metabolized aryl hydrocarbon receptor (AhR) ligands that induce AhR-dependent Tregs and prevent murine graft-versus-host disease. PLoS ONE 9(2):e88726

Quintana FJ, Basso AS, Iglesias AH, Korn T, Farez MF, Bettelli E, Caccamo M, Oukka M, Weiner HL (2008) Control of T(reg) and T(H)17 cell differentiation by the aryl hydrocarbon receptor. Nature 453:65–71

Quintana E, Shackleton M, Foster HR, Fullen DR, Sabel MS, Johnson TM, Morrison SJ (2010) Phenotypic heterogeneity among tumorigenic melanoma cells from patients that is reversible and not hierarchically organized. Cancer Cell 18(5):510–523

Rannug A, Rannug U, Rosenkranz HS, Winqvist L, Westerholm R, Agurell E, Grafström AK (1987) Certain photooxidized derivatives of tryptophan bind with very high affinity to the Ah receptor and are likely to be endogenous signal substances. J Biol Chem 262:15422–15427

Rannug U, Rannug A, Sjöberg U, Li H, Westerholm R, Bergman J (1995) Structure elucidation of two tryptophan-derived, high affinity Ah receptor ligands. Chem Biol 2(12):841–855

Ray SS, Swanson HI (2003) Alteration of keratinocyte differentiation and senescence by the tumor promoter dioxin. Toxicol Appl Pharmacol 192:131–145

Reggiani G (1978) Medical problems raised by the TCDD contamination in Seveso. Italy. Arch Toxicol 40(3):161–188

Rowlands JC, McEwan IJ, Gustafsson JA (1996) Trans-activation by the human aryl hydrocarbon receptor and aryl hydrocarbon receptor nuclear translocator proteins: direct interactions with basal transcription factors. Mol Pharmacol 50(3):538–548

Safe S (1990) Polychlorinated biphenyls (PCBs), dibenzo-p-dioxins (PCDDs), dibenzofurans (PCDFs), and related compounds: environmental and mechanistic considerations which support the development of toxic equivalency factors (TEFs). Crit Rev Toxicol 21:51–88

Saurat JH, Sorg O (2010) Chloracne, a misnomer and its implications. Dermatology 221(1):23–26

Saurat JH, Kaya G, Saxer-Sekulic N, Pardo B, Becker M, Fontao L, Mottu F, Carraux P, Pham XC, Barde C, Fontao F, Zennegg M, Schmid P, Schaad O, Descombes P, Sorg O (2012) The cutaneous lesions of dioxin exposure: lessons from the poisoning of Victor Yushchenko. Toxicol Sci 125(1):310–317

Saw CL, Huang MT, Liu Y, Khor TO, Conney AH, Kong AN (2011) Impact of Nrf2 on UVB-induced skin inflammation/photoprotection and photoprotective effect of sulforaphane. Mol Carcinog 50(6):479–486
Schäfer M and Werner S (2015) Nrf2-A regulator of keratinocyte redox signaling. Free Radic Biol Med 88(Pt B):243–252
Schäfer M, Dütsch S, auf dem Keller U, Navid F, Schwarz A, Johnson DA, Johnson JA, Werner S (2010) Nrf2 establishes a glutathione-mediated gradient of UVB cytoprotection in the epidermis. Genes Dev 24(10):1045–1058
Schäfer M, Willrodt AH, Kurinna S, Link AS, Farwanah H, Geusau A, Gruber F, Sorg O, Huebner AJ, Roop DR, Sandhoff K, Saurat JH, Tschachler E, Schneider MR, Langbein L, Bloch W, Beer HD, Werner S (2014) Activation of Nrf2 in keratinocytes causes chloracne (MADISH)-like skin disease in mice. EMBO Mol Med 6(4):442–457
Schäfer M, Farwanah H, Willrodt AH, Huebner AJ, Sandhoff K, Roop D, Hohl D, Bloch W, Werner S (2012) Nrf2 links epidermal barrier function with antioxidant defense. EMBO Mol Med 4:364–379
Schallreuter KU, Salem MA, Gibbons NC, Maitland DJ, Marsch E, Elwary SM, Healey AR (2012) Blunted epidermal L-tryptophan metabolism in vitiligo affects immune response and ROS scavenging by Fenton chemistry, part 2: epidermal H_2O_2/ONOO(−)-mediated stress in vitiligo hampers indoleamine 2,3-dioxygenase and aryl hydrocarbon receptor-mediated immune response signaling. FASEB J 26(6):2471–2485
Sheipouri D, Braidy N, Guillemin GJ (2012) Kynurenine Pathway in Skin Cells: Implications for UV-Induced Skin Damage. Int J Tryptophan Res 5:15–25
Sheipouri D, Grant R, Bustamante S, Lovejoy D, Guillemin GJ, Braidy N (2015) Characterisation of the kynurenine pathway in skin-derived fibroblasts and keratinocytes. J Cell Biochem 116 (6):903–922
Shimizu Y, Nakatsuru Y, Ichinose M, Takahashi Y, Kume H, Mimura J, Fujii-Kuriyama Y, Ishikawa T (2000) Benzowaxpyrene carcinogenicity is lost in mice lacking the aryl hydrocarbon receptor. Proc Natl Acad Sci USA 97:779–782
Smirnova A, Wincent E, Vikström Bergander L, Alsberg T, Bergman J, Rannug A, Rannug U (2016) Evidence for New Light-Independent Pathways for Generation of the Endogenous Aryl Hydrocarbon Receptor Agonist FICZ. Chem Res Toxicol 29(1):75–86
Song J, Clagett-Dame M, Peterson RE, Hahn ME, Westler WM, Sicinski RR (2002) A ligand for the aryl hydrocarbon receptor isolated from lung. Proc Natl Acad Sci USA 99:14694–14699
Sorg O, Zennegg M, Schmid P Fedosyuk R, Valikhnovskyi R, Gaide O, Kniazevych V, Saurat JH (2009) 2,3,7,8-Tetrachlorodibenzo-p- dioxin (TCDD) poisoning in Victor Yushchenko: identification and measurement of TCDD metabolites. Lancet 374:1179–1185
Soshilov AA, Denison MS (2014) Ligand promiscuity of aryl hydrocarbon receptor agonists and antagonists revealed by site-directed mutagenesis. Mol Cell Biol 34(9):1707–1719
Spink BC, Hussain MM, Katz BH, Eisele L, Spink DC (2003) Transient induction of cytochromes P4501A1 and 1B1 in MCF-7 human breast cancer cells by indirubin. Biochem Pharmacol 66 (12):2313–2321
Stribinskis V, Ramos KS (2006) Activation of human long interspersed nuclear element 1 retrotransposition by benzo(a)pyrene, an ubiquitous environmental carcinogen. Cancer Res 66:2616–2620
Sugita T, Takashima M, Shinoda T, Suto H, Unno T, Tsuboi R, Ogawa H, Nishikawa A (2002) New yeast species, Malassezia dermatis, isolated from patients with atopic dermatitis. J Clin Microbiol 40(4):1363–1367
Sutter TR, Guzman K, Dold KM, Greenlee WF (1991) Targets for dioxin: genes for plasminogen activator inhibitor-2 and interleukin-1i. Science 254:415–418
Sutter CH, Yin H, Li Y, Mammen JS, Bodreddigari S, Stevens G, Cole JA, Sutter TR (2009) EGF receptor signaling blocks aryl hydrocarbon receptor-mediated transcription and cell differentiation in human epidermal keratinocytes. Proc Natl Acad Sci USA 106(11):4266–4271

Sutter CH, Bodreddigari S, Campion C, Wible RS, Sutter TR (2011) 2,3,7,8-Tetrachlorodibenzo-p-dioxin increases the expression of genes in the human epidermal differentiation complex and accelerates epidermal barrier formation. Toxicol Sci 124(1):128–137

Syed DN, Mukhtar H (2015) FICZ: A Messenger of Light in Human Skin. J Invest Dermatol 135 (6):1478–1481

Takei K, Mitoma C, Hashimoto-Hachiya A, Takahara M, Tsuji G, Nakahara T, Furue M (2015) Galactomyces fermentation filtrate prevents T helper 2-mediated reduction of filaggrin in an aryl hydrocarbon receptor-dependent manner. Clin Exp Dermatol 40(7):786–793

Tang NJ, Liu J, Coenraads PJ, Dong L, Zhao LJ, Ma SW, Chen X, Zhang CM, Ma XM, Wei WG, Zhang P, Bai ZP (2008) Expression of AhR, CYP1A1, GSTA1, c-fos and TGF-alpha in skin lesions from dioxin-exposed humans with chloracne. Toxicol Lett 177(3):182–187

Tao S, Justiniano R, Zhang DD, Wondrak GT (2013) The Nrf2-inducers tanshinone I and dihydrotanshinone protect human skin cells and reconstructed human skin against solar simulated UV. Redox Biol 29(1):532–541

Tao S, Park SL, Rojo de la Vega M, Zhang DD, Wondrak GT (2015) Systemic administration of the apocarotenoid bixin protects skin against solar UV-induced damage through activation of Nrf2. Free Radic Biol Med 89:690–700

Tauchi M, Hida A, Negishi T, Katsuoka F, Noda S, Mimura J, Hosoya T, Yanaka A, Aburatani H, Fujii-Kuriyama Y, Motohashi H, Yamamoto M (2005) Constitutive expression of aryl hydrocarbon receptor in keratinocytes causes inflammatory skin lesions. Mol Cell Biol 25 (21):9360–9368

Thomas SR, Stocker R (1999) Redox reactions related to indoleamine 2,3-dioxygenase and tryptophan metabolism along the kynurenine pathway. Redox Rep 4(5):199–220

Tigges J, Haarmann-Stemmann T, Vogel CFA, Grindel A, Hübenthal U, Brenden H, Fritsche E (2014) The new aryl hydrocarbon receptor antagonist E/Z-2-benzylindene-5,6-dimethoxy-3,3-dimethylindan-1-one protects against UVB-induced signal transduction. J Invest Dermatol 134(2):556–559

Tsuchiya Y, Nakajima M, Itoh S, Iwanari M, Yokoi T (2003) Expression of aryl hydrocarbon receptor repressor in normal human tissues and inducibility by polycyclic aromatic hydrocarbons in human tumor-derived cell lines. Toxicol Sci 72:253–259

Tsuji G, Takahara M, Uchi H, Matsuda T, Chiba T, Takeuchi S, Yasukawa F, Moroi Y, Furue M (2012) Identification of ketoconazole as an AhR-Nrf2 activator in cultured human keratinocytes: the basis of its anti-inflammatory effect. J Invest Dermatol 132:59–68

Tsukimori K, Uchi H, Mitoma C, Yasukawa F, Fukushima K, Todaka T, Kajiwara J, Yoshimura T, Hirata T, Wake N, Furue M (2011) Comparison of the concentrations of polychlorinated biphenyls and dioxins in mothers affected by the Yusho incident and their children. Chemosphere 84(7):928–935

Turka LA, Walsh PT (2008) IL-2 signaling and CD4+ CD25+ Foxp3+ regulatory T cells. Front Biosci 13:1440–1446

van den Bogaard EH, Bergboer JGM, Vonk-Bergers M, van Vlijmen-Willems IMJJ, Hato SV, van der Valk PGM, Schroder JM, Joosten I, Zeeuwan JM, Schalkwijk J (2013) Coal tar induces AhR-dependent skin barrier repair in atopic dermatitis. J Clinical Invest 123(2):917–927

van den Bogaard EH, Podolsky MA, Smits JP, Cui X, John C, Gowda K, Desai D, Amin SG, Schalkwijk J, Perdew GH, Glick AB (2015) Genetic and pharmacological analysis identifies a physiological role for the AhR in epidermal differentiation. J Invest Dermatol 135(5):1320–1328

Villano CM, Murphy KA, Akintobi A, White LA (2006) 2,3,7,8- tetrachlorodibenzo-p-dioxin (TCDD) induces matrix metalloproteinase (MMP) expression and invasion in A2058 melanoma cells. Toxicol Appl Pharmacol 210(3):212–224

Vlachos C, Schulte BM, Magiatis P Adema GJ, Gaitanis G (2012) Malassezia-derived indoles activate the aryl hydrocarbon receptor and inhibit Toll-like receptor-induced maturation in monocyte-derived dendritic cells. Br J Dermatol 167:496–505

Vorderstrasse BA, Steppan LB, Silverstone AE, Kerkvliet NI (2001) Aryl hydrocarbon receptor-deficient mice generate normal immune responses to model antigens and are resistant to TCDD-induced immune suppression. Toxicol Appl Pharmacol 171:157–164

Wang XW, Li K, Guo S, Qiang HN, Liu L, Song P, Wei C, Yi XL, Jian Z, Li Q, Li CY, Gao TW (2012) The association of functional polymorphisms in the aryl hydrocarbon receptor (AhR) gene with the risk of vitiligo in Han Chinese populations. Br J Dermal 166(5):1081–1087

Wang XW, Li K, Liu L, Shi Q, Song P, Jian Z, Guo S, Wang G, Li C, Gao TW (2015) AhR promoter variant modulates its transcription and downstream effectors by allele-specific AhR-SP1 interaction functioning as a genetic marker for vitiligo. Sci Rep 5:13542

Wei YD, Bergander L, Rannug U, Rannug A (2000) Regulation of CYP1A1 transcription via the metabolism of the tryptophan-derived 6-formylindolo[3,2-b]carbazole. *Arch Biochem Biophys* 383(1):99–107

Weisglas-Kuperus N, Patandin S, Berbers GA, Sas TC, Mulder PG, Sauer PJ, Hooijkaas H (2000) Immunologic effects of background exposure to polychlorinated biphenyls and dioxins in Dutch preschool children. Environ Health Perspect 108(12):1203–1207

Wincent E, Amini N, Luecke S, Glatt H, Bergman J, Crescenzi C, Rannug A, Rannug U (2009) The suggested physiologic aryl hydrocarbon receptor activator and cytochrome P4501 substrate 6-formylindolo[3,2-b]carbazole is present in humans. J Biol Chem 284:2690–2696

Wincent E, Bengtsson J, Mohammadi Bardbori A, Alsberg T, Luecke S, A Rannug U, Rannug A (2012) Inhibition of cytochrome P4501-dependent clearance of the endogenous agonist FICZ as a mechanism for activation of the aryl hydrocarbon receptor. Proc Natl Acad Sci USA 109:4479–4484

Wondrak GT, (2014) Sunscreen-Based Skin Protection Against Solar Insult: Molecular Mechanisms and Opportunities. D. Alberts (Ed.), *Fundamentals of Cancer Prevention*, Springer Science & Business Media (2014), pp. 301–320

Wondrak GT, Jacobson MK, Jacobson EL (2006) Endogenous UVA photosensitizers: mediators of skin photodamage and novel targets for skin photoprotection. Photochem Photobiol Sci 5 (2):215–237

Wondrak GT, Cabello CM, Villeneuve NF, Zhang S, Ley S, Li Y, Sun Z, Zhang DD (2008) Cinnamoyl-based Nrf2-activators targeting human skin cell photo-oxidative stress. Free Radic Biol Med 45(4):385–395

Wu D, Potluri N, Kim Y, Rastinejad F (2013) Structure and dimerization properties of the aryl hydrocarbon receptor PAS-A domain. Mol Cell Biol 33(21):4346–4356

Yamashita F, Hayashi M (1985) Fetal PCB syndrome: clinical features, intrauterine growth retardation and possible alteration in calcium metabolism. Environ Health Perspect 59:41–45

Yeager RL, Reisman SA, Aleksunes LM, Klaassen CD (2009) Introducing the TCDD-inducible AhR-Nrf2 gene battery. Toxicol Sci 111(2):238–246

Zelante T, Iannitti RG, Cunha C, De Luca A, Giovannini G, Pieraccini G, Zecchi R, D'Angelo C, Massi-Benedetti C, Fallarino F, Carvalho A, Puccetti P, Romani L (2013) Tryptophan catabolites from microbiota engage aryl hydrocarbon receptor and balance mucosal reactivity via interleukin-22. Immunity 39(2):372–385

Zhang DD, Hannink M (2003) Distinct cysteine residues in Keap1 are required for Keap1-dependent ubiquitination of Nrf2 and for stabilization of Nrf2 by chemopreventive agents and oxidative stress. Mol Cell Biol 23:8137–8151

Chapter 17
Biological Cell Protection by Natural Compounds, a Second Line of Defense Against Solar Radiation

Ludger Kolbe

Abstract Human skin has to cope constantly with the harmful effects of solar radiation. With skin cancer rates worldwide on the rise, effective photoprotection is an urgent need. Sun care products are formulated with high efficacy in the entire UVB and UVA range to deliver broadband protection. However, UV-filters in topical sun care products cannot completely block UV radiation. Although products with SPF 50 reduce the UV dose 50-fold, this means that still 2 % of the radiation penetrate into the skin. Nevertheless, skin cells contain protective enzymatic and non-enzymatic antioxidant systems that scavenge harmful reactive oxygen species, detoxify reactive metabolites, and repair UV-induced damage to DNA, proteins and lipids. Activating these endogenous cellular protection mechanisms by natural compounds contributes to a comprehensive skin protection from solar radiation. Several studies, mainly with carotenoids or flavonoids, have been published during the last two decades, proving the validity of the concept. Licochalcone A from Glycyrrhiza inflata has been shown to inhibit NFκB and activate Nrf2 pathways and, thus, provides strong anti-oxidative and anti-inflammatory efficacy. In conclusion, topical products containing licochalcone A minimize UVA and high energy visible light-induced oxidative stress and reduce erythema after exposure to excessive solar radiation.

Keywords Photoprotection · Licorice · Polyphenols · Carotenoids · Licochalcone A · Vitamin C · Vitamin E · NFκB · Nrf2 · Antioxidant · Anti-inflammatory

17.1 Introduction

As the outermost barrier of the body, the human skin has to cope constantly with the harmful effects of solar radiation. However, several cytoprotective defense and repair mechanisms help skin cells to reduce the damages. The most important

L. Kolbe (✉)
Front End Innovation, BF 519, Beiersdorf AG, Unnastrasse 48, 20245 Hamburg, Germany
e-mail: Ludger.Kolbe@Beiersdorf.com

G.T. Wondrak (ed.), *Skin Stress Response Pathways*,
DOI 10.1007/978-3-319-43157-4_17

defense against UV radiation is the production of melanin. The pigment absorbs UV rays and, thus, protects skin cells from further damage. The production of melanin increases substantially after exposure to sun light, leading to a protective UV absorbing tan. Enhanced melanin production usually starts three to four days after UV exposure (delayed tanning) and remains elevated for several weeks. In addition, the epidermal layer thickens after repetitive exposure to UV radiation (epidermal hyperplasia) to develop a denser stratum corneum, which more readily absorbs and disperses solar radiation and thus protects the viable epidermal skin cells underneath. Epidermal hyperplasia starts within days after sun exposure and lasts for up to one month. Consequently, these slow adaptive mechanisms cannot prevent skin damage induced by acute UV exposure. However, skin cells also contain protective enzymatic and non-enzymatic antioxidant systems that scavenge harmful reactive oxygen species (ROS), detoxify reactive metabolites, and repair UV-induced damage to DNA, proteins and lipids. These adaptive mechanisms are up regulated within hours (Talalay et al. 2007).

Nevertheless, the endogenous protection of human skin against solar UV radiation is not at all sufficient to fully protect the skin from acute and chronic skin damages. Especially in lighter skin types with little epidermal melanin, excessive sun exposure results in sunburn after just a short period of time. On a sunny summer day, sun exposure for 15 min might be enough for very sensitive individuals to get a sunburn. Usually the sunburn develops within 5 h, peaks within the first 24 h, but can last for several days. Chronic sun exposure, even at suberythemal doses, results in premature skin aging with wrinkle formation, dryness, loss of elasticity, hyperkeratosis and hyperpigmentation (Kligman and Kligman 1986). UVB radiation at wavelength ranging from 290 to 320 nm is mainly responsible for sunburn, whereas UVA radiation at 320–400 nm is mainly responsible for long-term photodamage of the skin. While premature skin aging is primarily a cosmetic problem, the development of skin cancer after long-term exposure to UV radiation is a major health issue. With skin cancer rates worldwide on the rise (Lomas et al. 2012), effective photoprotection is an urgent need. Recent publications show that consistent use of sunscreen product indeed reduces the risk for skin cancer (Iannacone et al. 2014) but sunscreen use remains low among the general population. A broadband UV protection system is of outmost importance to block both, damaging UVA and UVB rays. In ophthalmology, the damaging effect of blue-violet light has been known for quite some time (Downes 2016) and sunglasses blocking these wavelengths are available. The effects of blue-violet light on skin are currently under discussion, while the effect of solar infrared radiation A (IRA) on skin is another topic of debate. In dermatology, we just begin to understand the impact of non-UV radiation on skin physiology (Liebel et al. 2012; Kolbe 2012; Grether-Beck et al. 2014; Barolet et al. 2016). Blue light filters are not available for topical use and, if so, would not be accepted by the consumers since products containing these filters would turn the skin yellow.

The avoidance of sun exposure during peak hours and wearing of protective clothing were the only protection measures for centuries. During the 1930s, topical products with UV filters that absorb or reflect UV radiation were developed. Today, these products are formulated with high efficacy in the entire UVB and UVA range to deliver broadband sun protection. The sun protection factor (SPF) refers to the factor by which the UV filters of the product reduce the UV radiation penetrating into the skin (ISO 24444 2010). Hence, a product with a SPF 50 reduces the dose 50-fold, but this also means that 2 % of the radiation still penetrate into the skin. Consumers tend to apply less than the amount of product necessary, therefore, the actual SPF is often less than the labelled SPF on the product and even more residual radiation might penetrate into the skin. Since UV-filters in topical sun care products cannot completely block UV radiation, there are many approaches published in the literature aiming at boosting endogenous cellular protection mechanisms for a comprehensive sun protection.

17.2 Photoprotection by Retinoids and Nonsteroidal Anti-inflammatory Drugs

17.2.1 Retinoids

Several studies documented the positive effect of oral retinoids on skin cancer development. A study with patients at moderate risk to develop skin cancer, due to actinic keratosis, showed a reduced risk to develop new squamous cell carcinoma after oral retinol (Moon et al. 1997). Other studies with renal transplant patients found that oral acitretin significantly reduced new non-melanoma skin cancers (Bavinck et al. 1995; George et al. 2002; McKenna and Murphy 1999). In summary, these studies showed that oral retinoids prevent squamous cell carcinomas and probably prevent basal cell carcinomas as well as actinic keratosis. However, due to the severe side effects of oral retinoids the use of these compounds is limited to high-risk patients only.

17.2.2 Nonsteroidal Anti-inflammatory Drugs (NSAIDS)

NSAIDS inhibit inflammation mainly by inhibiting the production of prostaglandins from cyclooxygenase activity. Prostaglandin E_2 (PGE_2) has been identified as an important mediator of UV-damage to human skin (Halliday 2005). Two studies from Australia found a lower incidence of actinic keratosis and squamous cell carcinomas with regular use of NSAIDS (Butler et al. 2005; Grau et al. 2006). Another study confirmed the protective effect of NSAIDS on basal cell carcinoma and squamous cell carcinoma development (Clouser et al. 2009). In conclusion, oral NSAIDS seem to be photoprotective by inhibiting UV-induced inflammation and thus reduce UV-induced skin cancer (Elmets et al. 2010). However, NSAIDS are drugs with certain side effects and for that reason should not be used for photoprotection in general but for high-risk patients only.

17.3 Photoprotection with Natural Compounds

Plants use solar light to generate metabolic energy via photosynthesis and, therefore, developed highly effective molecular systems to harvest photons. At the same time, they had to develop very effective mechanisms to protect the light harvesting photosynthetic system and all other cellular components from excessive solar radiation. Plant-derived natural compounds are part of our daily diet and, therefore, these compounds might be active in humans after ingestion. Over the past decades, many photoprotective molecules, such as carotenoids, other terpenoids, flavonoids, and other polyphenolic compounds have been identified in various plant species. Several published studies provided evidence that individuals with a diet containing high amounts of vegetables and fruits are somewhat protected from the development of actinic keratosis (Hughes et al. 2009). Patients with a history of squamous cell carcinoma consuming large amounts of vegetables seem to be protected from the development of new skin cancers (Hughes et al. 2006). Therefore, plant-derived dietary components appear to have the potential to contribute to the protection of human skin from photodamage.

17.3.1 Caffeine and Green Tea Catechins

Caffeine is present in leaves, fruits and seeds of various plant species. It is well known for its stimulatory effect on the sympathetic nervous system and consumed in large amounts in teas and coffee (Fisone et al. 2004). Data of large prospective observational studies showed that those with the highest intake of caffeine developed less basal cell carcinoma than those with the lowest consumption (Song et al. 2012).

Green tea contains high levels of antioxidants, especially catechins, which are very effective radical scavengers (Nanjo et al. 1999; Weisburg et al. 2004; Higdon and Frei 2003; Khan and Mukhtar 2007). These polyphenolic compounds were studied intensively for their photoprotective properties. Oral green tea has been shown to enhance repair of UV-induced DNA damage in vitro (Katiyar 2011). In a 12-week, double-blind, placebo-controlled study, 60 female volunteers consumed either a beverage with green tea polyphenols (1402 mg total catechins/d) or a control beverage. UV-induced erythema decreased significantly in the intervention group after 6 and 12 weeks, respectively (Heinrich et al. 2011). Another study showed protection against UV radiation-induced cutaneous inflammation in an open oral intervention study with sixteen healthy human subjects, given green tea catechins (540 mg) and vitamin C (50 mg) daily for 12 weeks. (Rhodes et al. 2013). However, in a larger study with higher dose of green tea catechins (1080 mg/d) the group could not confirm the initial results (Farrar et al. 2015). The efficacy of topical application of green tea phenols was evaluated in a small study involving six subjects. DNA-damage (cyclobutane pyrimidine dimers) and erythema development showed a dose-dependent reduction after relatively high amounts of green tea polyphenols (1–4 mg/2.5 cm^2). The UV-absorbing properties of green tea phenols likely contributed to the efficacy (Katiyar et al. 2000).

17.3.2 *ß-Carotene and Other Carotenoids*

Carotenoids are well known for their antioxidant activity, with the most prominent member of this chemical group being ß-carotene. A PubMed search with the search term "beta carotene antioxidant" at the beginning of 2016 revealed more than 9000 publications on this topic. Since ß-carotene is contained in many vegetable foodstuffs, it is consumed in relative large amounts with the normal diet. Therefore, ß-carotene can be detected in human skin and plasma (Stahl and Sies 2012). After sun exposure, ß-carotene levels in human skin decrease, leading to the conclusion that ß-carotene is protective and consumed by UV-induced ROS (Biesalski et al. 1996). Several human intervention studies showed the effectiveness of dietary carotenoids. Daily ingestion of 40 g tomato paste for 10 weeks elevated the plasma levels of lycopene, the tomato-specific carotenoid, and reduced erythema formation after irradiation with a solar light simulator. Significantly lower erythema intensity was found after 10 weeks but not after 4 weeks of treatment (Stahl and Sies 2002). A further study was conducted to examine whether tomato paste rich in lycopene protects against cutaneous photodamage (Rizwan et al. 2011). Lycopene was found to protect from acute and long-term photodamage. A recent study failed to reproduce significant results (Sokoloski et al. 2015) with only 20 volunteers; merely a tendency towards reduced erythema was seen. Already in 1972, the photoprotective efficacy of ß-carotene (180 mg/d) supplementation was demonstrated after 10 weeks (Mathews-Roth et al. 1972). Several studies showed protection against UV-induced erythema when ß-carotene was supplemented for at least 7 weeks and 12 mg or more per day (Lee et al. 2000; Stahl et al. 2000; Heinrich et al. 2003).

17.3.3 *Polypodium Leucotomos Extract*

Extracts from the tropical fern Polypodium leucotomos contain phenolic compounds like caffeic acid and ferulic acid. The extract has been shown to exert antioxidant and anti-inflammatory efficacy. In mice, P. leucotomos extract reduced the expression of COX-2, increased p53 expression and enhanced DNA repair. In a human study, the extracts showed antioxidant and anti-inflammatory activity and two oral doses of 7.5 mg/kg of the extract significantly reduced the sunburn reaction after irradiation with UVA + UVB as well as DNA damage (Middelkamp-Hup et al. 2004). The effects of Polypodium leucotomos extracts on human skin are currently studied intensively (Bhatia 2015; Gonzalez et al. 2011). While the oral efficacy was investigated in several studies (El-Haj and Goldstein

2015; Bhatia 2015), efficacy after topical treatment of human skin has not yet been shown convincingly.

17.3.4 Vitamin C and E

The fat-soluble Vitamin E and the water-soluble Vitamin C are a perfect combination for preventing UV-induced oxidative stress. Vitamin E molecules, i.e. tocopherols and tocotrienols, are excellent antioxidants preventing lipid oxidation (Thiele and Ekanayake-Mudiyanselage 2007). Vitamins C and E interact synergistically to protect each other and increase overall effectiveness (Halpner et al. 1998). Combinations of vitamin C and vitamin E are effective in photoprotection. Daily oral supplements of 3 g vitamin C and 2 g vitamin E increased the protection against photodamage in skin by approximately 1.5 times; either vitamin alone was ineffective (Fuchs and Kern 1998). Topical formulation of vitamins C and E deliver improved protection of skin against photodamage, achieving significantly greater protection than after oral application. A stable aqueous solution of 15 % vitamin C (L-ascorbic acid) and 1 % vitamin E (α-tocopherol) applied topically can provide fourfold photoprotection for skin (Lin et al. 2003). Topically applied vitamin C induced significant photoprotective effects at concentrations of at least 10 % in animals and humans, whereas a photoprotective effect has not been demonstrated by oral administration even at high doses in humans. Topical vitamin E reduced erythema, sunburn cells, chronic UV-B–induced skin damage and photocarcinogenesis in the majority of the published studies, whereas only high doses of oral vitamin E may affect the response to UV-B in humans. Combination of vitamins C and E, partly with other photoprotective compounds, did increase the photoprotective effects dramatically compared to monotherapies (Eberlein-König and Ring 2005).

17.3.5 Licochalcone A

Licorice is the extract from the dried roots and rhizomes of several plants of the genus Glycyrrhiza and is used as sweetener and as a traditional herbal medicine (Shibata 2000). It is added to candies, chewing gum, beverages (e.g., herbal teas), and herbal remedies for cough and stomach problems. Licorice candies are consumed worldwide and estimates suggest an annual consumption of about 1.5 kg/person (Spinks and Fenwick 1990). The Chinese pharmacopoeia accepts three species of licorice plants, Glycyrrhiza glabra, Glycyrrhiza uralensis, and Glycyrrhiza inflata, as sources for traditional medicines (State Pharmacopoeia Commission of the PRC 2010). The first written record of licorice use dates back to 2100 BC (Gibson 1978). Licorice is a rich source of antioxidant and anti-inflammatory substances. More than 20 triterpenoids and nearly 300 flavonoids

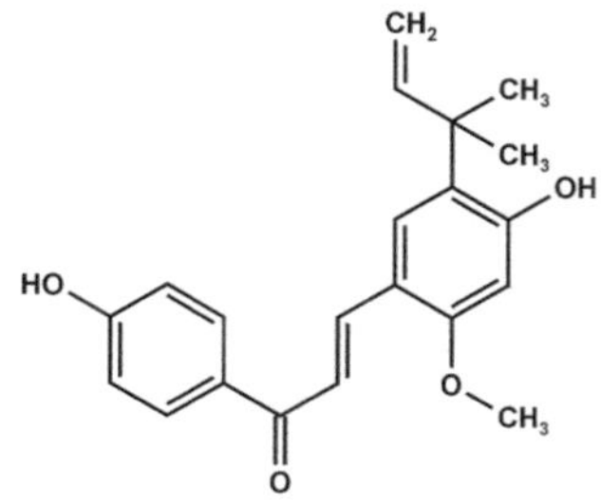

Fig. 17.1 Chemical structure of licochalcone A

have been identified so far (Wang et al. 2015). Glycyrrhiza inflata is one of the main botanical sources of licorice, and is chemically characterized by the presence of unusual chalcones, "retrochalcones", which are distinguished from ordinary chalcones by the absence of an oxygen functionality at the 2-position (Kondo et al. 2007). Licochalcones A was first isolated from Glycyrrhiza roots in 1975 and the structure of this compound (Fig. 17.1) was elucidated (Saitoh and Shibata 1975). From the above-mentioned three licorice plants, only G. inflata contains licochalcone A (Kondo et al. 2007).

17.3.5.1 In Vitro Efficacy of Licochalcone A

The retrochalcones from G. inflata are excellent antioxidants and superoxide scavenger (Haraguchi et al. 1998; Fu et al. 2013). In addition, licochalcone A has demonstrated anti-bacterial (Friis-Moller et al. 2002; Fukai et al. 2002), anti-fungal (Messier and Grenier 2011), anti-protozoan (Chen et al. 1993), and anti-tumor properties (Wang and Nixon 2001; Tsai et al. 2015). The anti-inflammatory activity of licochalcone A was first discovered when the compound was shown to inhibit mouse ear edema induced by arachidonic acid and phorbol 12-myristate 13-acetate (TPA) (Shibata et al. 1991). Concentrations of 500 μg/ear significantly reduced edema when the compound was applied no longer than 30 min after induction of the edema. The authors also found an inhibition of the tumor-promoting effect of TPA by licochalcone A. Various publications showed the comprehensive antioxidative and anti-inflammatory efficacy of licochalcone A. The compound is not only a classical radical scavenger, as shown by suppressing lipid peroxidation in several biological systems (Haraguchi et al. 1998), but also reduced the fMLP- and zymosan-induced oxidative burst and the migration of human mononuclear neutrophil granulocytes (Kolbe et al. 2006; Funatoshi-Tago et al. 2010). Licochalcone A was found to reduce the release of pro-inflammatory cytokines from various cell types. In human T cells, licochalcone A inhibited the proliferative activation by phytohemagglutinin and the production of TNF-α and IFN-γ (Barfod et al. 2002). In human dendritic cells, stimulated with LPS to produce the pro-inflammatory cytokines IL-6 and TNF-α, licochalcone A reduced both cytokines in a dose-dependent way down to control levels, or even below (Kolbe et al. 2006). In human fibroblasts, licochalcone

A inhibited PGE_2 and PGF2α production in response to interleukin 1β (IL-1β) stimulation (Furuhashi et al. 2005). However, licochalcone A had no effect on Cyclooxygenase (COX)-2 mRNA and protein expression in these cells and no effect on COX-1-dependent PGE_2 production. The authors concluded that licochalcone A induces an anti-inflammatory effect through the inhibition of COX-2-dependent PGE_2 and that this is quite different from the mechanism of corticosteroids. A recent study examined how licochalcone A inhibits UV-induced inflammatory responses in HaCaT cells (Song et al. 2015). Licochalcone A did not suppress COX-2 enzyme activity in vitro, but inhibited AP-1 activity and consequently reduced UV-induced COX-2 expression and PGE_2 release. In LPS stimulated mouse macrophages, licochalcone A dose-dependently inhibited the production of NO and PGE_2. Here, a reduction in iNOS and COX-2 expression was responsible for the inhibition (Kwon et al. 2008; Cui et al. 2008). In human EpiDerm™ skin models the inhibitory efficacy of licochalcone A on PGE_2 production was determined after UV-irradiation (Kolbe et al. 2006). PGE_2 release from human keratinocytes after UV-irradiation was reduced to control levels in the presence of 10 µg/mL licochalcone A-containing licorice extract (Fig. 17.2). Inhibiting prostaglandin production often results in increased leukotriene production, therefore, the release of Leukotriene B_4 (LTB_4) from human mononuclear neutrophil granulocytes was determined and licochalcone A was found to inhibit dose dependently the production of LTB_4.

In summary, Licochalcone A has a broad anti-oxidative and anti-inflammatory efficacy. It acts as a radical scavenger, inhibits the oxidative burst of neutrophils,

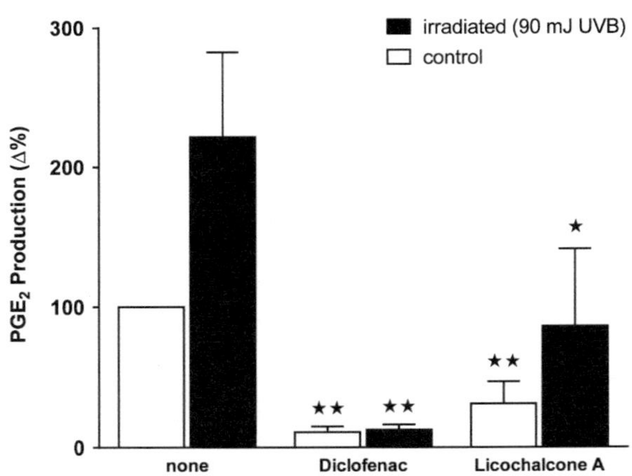

Fig. 17.2 Effects of licochalcone A on PGE_2 production of human keratinocytes. PGE_2 production of human keratinocytes in the EpiDerm™ skin model without UV irradiation (*open bars*) or after UV irradiation (90 mJ UVB/cm²) (*closed bars*) was measured. Keratinocyte cultures were set up in the presence of the G. inflata extract corresponding to 10 µg/ml licochalcone A, or 50 ng/ml diclofenac, or without the active compounds (none). Data represent means ± SD of three independent experiments. Statistics: two-sided t test (active compound versus none); $*P < 0.05$; $**P < 0.01$

reduces release of pro-inflammatory cytokines and decreases the production of pro-inflammatory prostanoids by various cell types.

17.3.5.2 Modulation of Anti-inflammatory and Anti-oxidative Pathways by Licochalcone A

The analysis of the mechanisms of the anti-inflammatory efficacy of licochalcone A focused on the inhibition of NFκB activation (Furusawa et al. 2009; Funakoshi-Tago et al. 2009). Licochalcone A was found to inhibit LPS-induced signaling through the inhibition of NFκB phosphorylation at serine 276 but licochalcone A had no effect on LPS-induced phosphorylation and degradation of IκBα indicating an inhibition downstream of IKK activation. It was shown that licochalcone A inhibited the interaction of NFκB p65 and the co-activator p300 leading to a reduction of NFκB transactivation. Interestingly, the inhibition of TNF-α-induced NFκB activation was found to be exerted by direct inhibition of IκB kinase complex activation (Funakoshi-Tago et al. 2009). Detailed analysis, using licochalcone A derivatives, revealed that the α,β-unsaturated ketone is very important for the effect of licochalcone A on the TNF-α and LPS signaling pathways. Reduced licochalcone A, lacking the double bond, had no effect on IKK activity. IKK was not inhibited by the addition of reduced licochalcone A (Funakoshi-Tago et al. 2010). The same group found that echinatin, a chalcone also from in G. inflata, was not able to inhibit TNFα-induced IKK activation, NFκB activation and chemokine expression (Funakoshi-Tago et al. 2009). In comparison to licochalcone A, echinatin lacks the 1,1-dimethyl-2-propenyl group. The authors concluded that not only the double bond but also the 1,1-dimethyl-2-propenyl group is required for IKK inhibition by licochalcone A (Funakoshi-Tago et al. 2010).

A key player in orchestrating the cytoprotective response in skin cells is the Nuclear Factor-E2-related factor 2 (Nrf2) (Schäfer and Werner 2015). Several studies demonstrated that Nrf2 activation efficiently protects cells from oxidative damage. Some studies suggested that PI3 K/Akt and MAPK pathways play a key role in regulating heme oxygenase 1 (HO-1) expression and Nrf2 dependent transcription (Zipper and Mulcahy 2000; Gong et al. 2004). In primary human fibroblasts, treatment with licochalcone A induced the nuclear translocation of Nrf2. This resulted in elevated HO-1 and glutamate-cysteine ligase (GCLM) expression leading to a higher ratio of reduced glutathione to oxidized glutathione and concomitant decrease of intracellular ROS concentration (Kühnl et al. 2015). Studies with RAW 264.7 cells revealed that inhibitors of PI3 K/Akt and ERK 1/2 abolished the nuclear translocation of Nrf2 by licochalcone A after chemically (tert-butyl hydroperoxide) induced oxidative stress. This suggest that licochalcone A induced HO-1 expression via the activation of PI3 K/Akt, ERK, and Keap1/Nrf2/ARE signaling (Lv et al. 2015), whereas JNK and p38 MAPK had no effect in these cells. Interestingly, in HaCaT cells, Licochalcone A effectively suppressed UV-induced phosphorylation of Akt and mTOR (Song et al. 2015). In this study, licochalcone A also did not influence the JNK or p38 MAPK signaling pathways. After carefully analyzing potential molecular targets, the authors found that licochalcone A effectively inhibits UV-induced PI3 K, MEK1, and B-Raf kinase activity, but not C-Raf. The effects of licochalcone A on the PI3/AKT, mTOR pathway were confirmed by another group (Tsai et al. 2015) in SiHa cells. They found induction of autophagy and apoptosis by licochalcone A, treatment with autophagy-specific inhibitors enhanced licochalcone A induced apoptosis. In transgenic mice, the effect of licochalcone A on JNK was analyzed in great detail (Yao et al. 2014). Licochalcone A inhibited JNK1-mediated, but not JNK2-mediated, c-Jun phosphorylation in vivo and in vitro. Licochalcone A competed with JIP1 for binding with JNK1. In some tumor cells, Licochalcone A seem to activate other MAPK pathways. In head and neck squamous cell carcinoma cells (FaDu cells) licochalcone A induced TNF-related apoptosis-inducing ligand (TRAIL) expression via ERK 1/2 and p38 MAPK pathways (Park et al. 2015). The stimulation of TRAIL expression induces apoptosis in cancer cells without toxicity to normal cells. In HeLa cells, licochalcone A enhanced TRAIL-induced apoptosis through increased expression of TRAIL-R2 (Szliszka et al. 2012). Two recent papers demonstrated that licochalcone A might not only activate detoxification enzymes through the Keap1/Nrf2 pathway but also by inhibiting the arylhydrocarbon receptor (AhR) pathway. Licochalcone A was shown to be a strong AhR receptor antagonist (Hajirahimkhan et al. 2015; Dunlap et al. 2015). Taken together, these mechanisms might explain the chemo-preventive efficacy of licochalcone A (Shibata 1994; Bode and Dong 2015).

In summary, Licochalcone acts via activation of the Nrf2 pathway and inhibition of NFκB and AhR pathways. The role of MAP-Kinases in Licochalcone signaling is not yet fully understood.

17.3.5.3 In Vivo Efficacy of Licochalcone A

Several studies, revealing the efficacy of licochalcone in inflammatory skin condition have been published (Weber et al. 2006; Wananukul et al. 2012; Angelova-Fischer et al. 2013; Angelova-Fischer et al. 2014). The photoprotective efficacy in vivo was determined in three different experimental settings. In the first study, using solar simulated radiation, the effect of licochalcone A on the sunburn reaction on the back of 12 human volunteers was determined. A licochalcone A-containing formulation (0.05 % of a licochalcone A-rich licorice extract) applied immediately and 5 h after irradiation with solar simulated radiation reduced the developing erythema significantly relative to the vehicle-treated test sites. At 5 h and 24 h after exposure, skin redness was visibly reduced (Kolbe et al. 2006). To investigate whether the effect of licochalcone A on ROS production in vitro translates into the inhibition of oxidative processes in vivo, a human intervention study was performed using ultraweak photon emission (UPE) as readout parameter. The UPE method detects photons generated mainly by oxidative processes in the skin (Khabiri et al. 2008; Hagens et al. 2008). The UVA-evoked UPE detects the photons from human skin after irradiation with a short pulse of UVA. Irradiation of

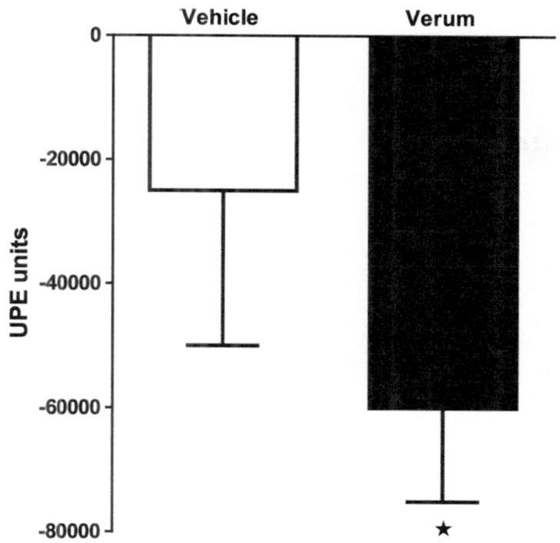

Fig. 17.3 Effect of topically applied licochalcone A on UVA-induced photon emission of the skin. In a study with 22 healthy volunteers, a test formulation containing licochalcone A-rich licorice extract and a corresponding vehicle without licorice extract were applied on the inner forearm for 2 weeks. The UVA-induced photon emission of untreated, verum and vehicle areas were quantified in vivo by utilizing a photomultiplier system. The total number of photons was counted and normalized to the corresponding measurements before the application of products. Data were analyzed using Wilcoxon's signed rank test for original data, $*P < 0.05$

endogenous chromophores, e.g. porphyrins and flavins, with UVA leads to the formation of reactive oxygen species (Dalle Carbonare and Pathak 1992). In the study, 22 volunteers applied a formulation containing licochalcone A and the corresponding vehicle twice daily to their inner forearms. Two weeks of treatment with the licochalcone A containing lotion significantly reduced the amount of skin-derived photons induced by a short stimulus of UVA radiation compared to untreated and vehicle-treated skin areas (Kühnl et al. 2015). The study confirmed that licochalcone A significantly reduced oxidative stress in vivo (Fig. 17.3). In the third study, the photoprotective efficacy in the visible range (400–700 nm, maximum at 440 nm) of a sunscreen formulation containing licochalcone A was investigated using resonance Raman spectroscopy (Vandersee et al. 2015) in a double blind, vehicle controlled pilot study performed on six healthy volunteers (Darvin et al. 2016). The sunscreens containing licochalcone A, or its vehicle, were topically applied on the volunteers' forearms and after 1 h the initial carotenoid values were measured. After irradiation with 100 J/cm^2 the measurements were repeated. In unprotected skin areas and areas treated with the vehicle, the carotenoid content dropped significantly by 15 %. The carotenoid content in areas treated with licochalcone A containing sunscreen remained unchanged, illustrating the anti-oxidative potency of licochalcone also against visible light induced oxidative stress (Fig. 17.4).

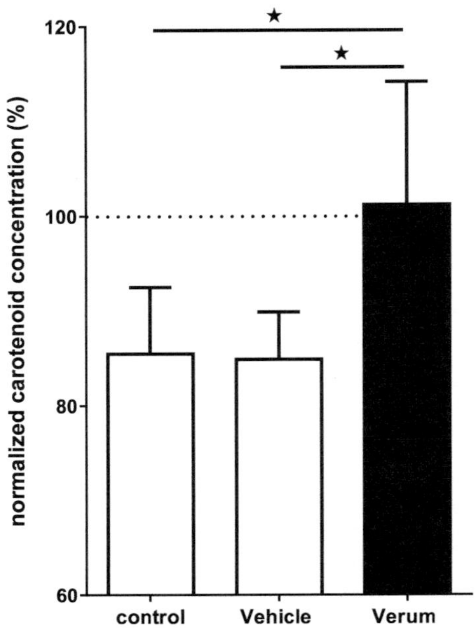

Fig. 17.4 Cutaneous carotenoids degradation after the irradiation with blue light. The protective efficacy of a sunscreen formulation containing Lica A was investigated in vivo in the visible range (400–700 nm, with a maximum at 440 nm) using resonance Raman spectroscopy in a double blind pilot study performed on six healthy volunteers. The sunscreens were topically applied to the forearms and 1 h later the absorption the initial carotenoid values were measured. After irradiation with 100 J/cm^2 the measurements were repeated. Pre-irradiation cutaneous carotenoid values were set to 100 %. Data were analyzed using Wilcoxon's signed rank test for original data, $*P < 0.05$ for verum versus control and verum versus vehicle

In summary, Licochalcone showed photoprotective efficacy in vivo against solar simulated radiation induced erythema and UVA- as well as VIS-induced oxidative stress.

17.4 Photoprotection with Natural Compounds—Systemic Versus Topical Application

Given the fact that protection by topical sunscreens even at SPF 50 still allows 2 % of UV-rays and all of the high energy visible light to penetrate into the skin, there is a need for complementary protection measures. Consequently, an additional line of defense against harmful sunrays within the skin by cellular protection mechanisms would enhance the overall resulting skin protection against solar radiation. Stimulating the endogenous cytoprotective mechanisms, e.g. by activating Nrf2, results in a higher resistance of skin cells to solar radiation induced oxidative stress.

However, biological photoprotection by small molecules, whether they are natural or synthetic, can only be complimentary to the classical sun protection by UV-filters.

Published studies on antioxidants mainly focus on the oral delivery of the actives because the investigators mostly were interested in systemic health benefits (Rani et al. 2016). With regard to endogenous photoprotection, oral treatment has certain disadvantages. Systemic treatment results in long pre-treatment periods before effective concentrations of the active are reached in the skin. In addition, high doses of active ingredients might be needed to achieve beneficial effects and this might lead to side effects in other organs. On the contrary, some of the most active antioxidants are very colorful, like lycopene or ß-carotene, and for this reason cannot be included in high concentrations in topical products. A diet rich in carotenoids and polyphenols may contribute to endogenous photoprotection in the long term. However, the long period of 7–10 weeks until protection becomes significant and the low level of protection make it impossible to rely on oral photoprotection alone. In conclusion, nutritional supplementation of photoprotective compounds can only be complementary to topical photoprotection.

Topical sun care products containing UV filters almost instantly protect against solar radiation. However, as mentioned above, even with a SPF 50 product 2 % of the sun light still penetrates into the skin. Therefore, adding active ingredients that stimulate the cellular protective mechanisms offer a second line of defense against UV radiation within the skin, coping with potential damage caused by residual penetrating solar radiation. Since topical sun protection products are applied directly on the target organ this allows effective concentrations of supplementary photoprotective ingredients much faster than via oral intake. Effective concentrations might be obtained within hours or days, not in weeks as shown for oral application. In addition, even with lower concentrations of the active ingredient in the product, compared to products for oral treatment, topical treatment can result in much higher effective doses in the skin. Most studies on endogenous photoprotection focused on increasing the minimal erythema dose as read-out for efficacy. However, effective endogenous photoprotection should not be seen as a method to provide additional sunburn protection. Prevention of sunburn, measured as the sun protection factor (SPF), should solely be achieved by UV-filters.

There are several ways to determine photoprotective efficacy of natural compounds in vivo, e.g. by measuring oxidized metabolites like isoprostane or 4-hydroxynonenal as markers of oxidative stress, assessing cyclobutane pyrimidine dimers, 6–4 photoproducts and 8-oxo-deoxyguanin as markers for DNA damage, or determining pro-inflammatory markers like TNFα, IL-6 and PGE_2, to name a few. These parameters are suitable as endpoints to determine photoprotective efficacy, but some more need to be defined.

17.5 Concluding Remarks

UV filters are the backbone of every effective sun care product; however, adding small natural compounds that activate endogenous cytoprotective mechanisms can significantly contribute to overall photoprotection. While formulating some of these natural compounds remains a challenge, some already made their way into topical suncare products. The era of biological photoprotection has just begun.

References

Angelova-Fischer I, Neufang G, Jung K, Fischer TW, Zillikens D (2014) A randomized, investigator-blinded efficacy assessment study of stand-alone emollient use in mild to moderately severe atopic dermatitis flares. J Eur Acad Dermatol Venereol 28(Suppl 3):9–15

Angelova-Fischer I, Rippke F, Fischer TW, Neufang G, Zillikens D (2013) A double-blind, randomized, vehicle-controlled efficacy assessment study of a skin care formulation for improvement of mild to moderately severe acne. J Eur Acad Dermatol Venereol 27(Suppl 2): 6–11

Barfod L, Kemp K, Hansen M, Kharazmi A (2002) Chalcones from Chinese liquorice inhibit proliferation of T cells and production of cytokines. Int Immunopharmacol 2:545–555

Barolet D, Christiaens F, Hamblin MR (2016) Infrared and skin: Friend or foe. J Photochem Photobiol B 155:78–85

Bavinck JN, Tieben LM, Van der Woude FJ, Tegzess AM, Hermans J, ter Schegget J, Vermeer BJ (1995) Prevention of skin cancer and reduction of keratotic skin lesions during acitretin therapy in renal transplant recipients: a double-blind, placebo-controlled study. J Clin Oncol 13:1933–1938

Bhatia N (2015) Polypodium leucotomos: a potential new photoprotective agent. Am J Clin Dermatol 16:73–79

Biesalski HK, Hemmes C, Hopfenmuller W, Schmid C, Gollnick HP (1996) Effects of controlled exposure of sunlight on plasma and skin levels of beta-carotene. Free Radical Res 24:215–224

Bode AM, Dong Z (2015) Chemopreventive effects of licorice and its components. Curr Pharmacol Rep 1:60–71

Butler GJ, Neale R, Green AC, Pandeya N, Whiteman DC (2005) Nonsteroidal anti-inflammatory drugs and the risk of actinic keratoses and squamous cell cancers of the skin. J Am Acad Dermatol 53:966–972

Chen M, Christensen SB, Blom J, Lemmich E, Nadelmann L, Fich K, Theander TG, Kharazmi A (1993) Licochalcone A, a novel antiparasitic agent with potent activity against human pathogenic protozoan species of Leishmania. Antimicrob Agents Chemother 37:2550–2556

Clouser MC, Roe DJ, Foote JA, Harris RB (2009) Effect of non-steroidal anti-inflammatory drugs on non-melanoma skin cancer incidence in the SKICAP-AK trial. Pharmacoepidemiol Drug Saf 18:276–283

Cui Y, Ao M, Li W, Hu J, Yu L (2008) Anti-inflammatory activity of licochalcone A isolated from glycyrrhiza inflata. Z Naturforsch C 63:361–365

Dalle Carbonare M, Pathak MA (1992) Skin photosensitizing agents and the role of reactive oxygen species in photoaging. J Photochem Photobiol, B 14:105–124

Darvin ME, Schanzer S, Lademann J, Tesch M, Buerger A, Rippke F, Meinke MC (2016) Protective efficacy of a licochalcone A containing sunscreen in the high energy visible spectral range in vivo. Exp Dermatol 25:E32

Downes SM (2016) Ultraviolet or blue-filtering intraocular lenses: what is the evidence? Eye 30:215–221

Dunlap TL, Wang S, Simmler C, Chen SN, Pauli GF, Dietz BM, Bolton JL (2015) Differential Effects of Glycyrrhiza Species on Genotoxic Estrogen Metabolism: Licochalcone A Downregulates P450 1B1, whereas Isoliquiritigenin Stimulates It. Chem Res Toxicol 28:1584–1594

Eberlein-König B, Ring J (2005) Relevance of vitamins C and E in cutaneous photoprotection. J Cosmet Dermatol 4:4–9

El-Haj N, Goldstein N (2015) Sun protection in a pill: the photoprotective properties of Polypodium leucotomos extract. Int J Dermatol 54:362–366

Elmets CA, Viner JL, Pentland AP, Cantrell W, Lin HY, Bailey H, Kang S, Linden KG, Heffernan M, Duvic M, Richmond E, Elewski BE, Umar A, Bell W, Gordon GB (2010) Chemoprevention of nonmelanoma skin cancer with celecoxib: a randomized, double-blind, placebo-controlled trial. J Natl Cancer Inst 102:1835–1844

Farrar MD, Nicolaou A, Clarke KA, Mason S, Massey KA, Dew TP, Watson RE, Williamson G, Rhodes LE (2015) A randomized controlled trial of green tea catechins in protection against ultraviolet radiation-induced cutaneous inflammation. Am J Clin Nutr 102:608–615

Fisone G, Borgkvist A, Usiello A (2004) Caffeine as a psychomotor stimulant: mechanism of action. Cell Mol Life Sci 61:857–872

Frei B, Higdon JV (2003) Antioxidant activity of tea polyphenols in vivo: evidence from animal studies. J Nutr 133:3275S–3284S

Friis-Møller A, Chen M, Fuursted K, Christensen SB, Kharazmi A (2002) In vitro antimycobacterial and antilegionella activity of licochalcone A from Chinese licorice roots. Planta Med 68:416–419

Fuchs J, Kern H (1998) Modulation of UV-light-induced skin inflammation by D-alpha-tocopherol and L-ascorbic acid: a clinical study using solar simulated radiation. Free Radical Biol Med 25:1006–1012

Fukai T, Marumo A, Kaitou K, Kanda T, Terada S, Nomura T (2002) Antimicrobial activity of licorice flavonoids against methicillin-resistant Staphylococcus aureus. Fitoterapia 73:536–539

Funakoshi-Tago M, Tanabe S, Tago K, Itoh H, Mashino T, Sonoda Y, Kasahara T (2009) Licochalcone A potently inhibits tumor necrosis factor alpha-induced nuclear factor-kappaB activation through the direct inhibition of IkappaB kinase complex activation. Mol Pharmacol 76:745–753

Funakoshi-Tago M, Nakamura K, Tsuruya R, Hatanaka M, Mashino T, Sonoda Y, Kasahara T (2010) The fixed structure of Licochalcone A by alpha, beta-unsaturated ketone is necessary for anti-inflammatory activity through the inhibition of NF-kappaB activation. Int Immunopharmacol 10:562–571

Furuhashi I, Iwata S, Shibata S, Sato T, Inoue H (2005) Inhibition by licochalcone A, a novel flavonoid isolated from liquorice root, of IL-1beta-induced PGE2 production in human skin fibroblasts. J Pharm Pharmacol 57:1661–1666

Furusawa J, Funakoshi-Tago M, Tago K, Mashino T, Inoue H, Sonoda Y, Kasahara T (2009) Licochalcone A significantly suppresses LPS signaling pathway through the inhibition of NF-kappaB p65 phosphorylation at serine 276. Cell Signal 21:778–785

Fu Y, Chen J, Li YJ, Zheng YF, Li P (2013) Antioxidant and anti-inflammatory activities of six flavonoids separated from licorice. Food Chem 141:1063–1071

George R, Weightman W, Russ GR, Bannister KM, Mathew TH (2002) Acitretin for chemoprevention of non-melanoma skin cancers in renal transplant recipients. Australas J Dermatol 43:269–273

Gibson MR (1978) Glycyrrhiza in old and new perspectives. Lloydia 41:348–354

Grau MV, Baron JA, Langholz B, Karagas M, Greenberg ER, Stukel TA, Mandel JS (2006) Effect of NSAIDs on the recurrence of nonmelanoma skin cancer. Int J Cancer 119, 682–686

Grether-Beck S, Marini A, Jaenicke T, Krutmann J (2014) Photoprotection of human skin beyond ultraviolet radiation. Photodermatol Photoimmunol Photomed 30:167–174

Gong P, Hu B, Cederbaum AI (2004) Diallyl sulfide induces heme oxygenase-1 through MAPK pathway. Arch Biochem Biophys 432:252–260

Gonzalez S, Gilaberte Y, Philips N, Juarranz A (2011) Fernblock, a nutriceutical with photoprotective properties and potential preventive agent for skin photoaging and photoinduced skin cancers. Int J Mol Sci 12:8466–8475

Hagens R, Khabiri F, Schreiner V, Wenck H, Wittern KP, Duchstein HJ, Mei W (2008) Non-invasive monitoring of oxidative skin stress by ultraweak photon emission measurement. II: biological validation on ultraviolet A-stressed skin. Skin Res Technol 14:112–120

Hajirahimkhan A, Simmler C, Dong H, Lantvit DD, Li G, Chen SN, Nikolić D, Pauli GF, van Breemen RB, Dietz BM, Bolton JL (2015) Induction of NAD(P)H: quinone oxidoreductase 1 (NQO1) by glycyrrhiza species used for women's health: differential effects of the Michael acceptors isoliquiritigenin and licochalcone A. Chem Res Toxicol 28:2130–2141

Halliday GM (2005) Inflammation, gene mutation and photoimmunosuppression in response to UVR-induced oxidative damage contributes to photocarcinogenesis. Mutat Res 571:107–120

Halpner AD, Handelman GJ, Harris JM, Belmont CA, Blumberg JB (1998) Protection by vitamin C of loss of vitamin E in cultured rat hepatocytes. Arch Biochem Biophys 359:305–309

Haraguchi H, Ishikawa H, Mizutani K, Tamura Y, Kinoshita T (1998) Antioxidative and superoxide scavenging activities of retrochalcones in glycyrrhiza inflata. Bioorg Med Chem 6:339–347

Heinrich U, Gärtner C, Wiebusch M, Eichler O, Sies H, Tronnier H, Stahl W (2003) Supplementation with beta-carotene or a similar amount of mixed carotenoids protects humans from UV-induced erythema. J Nutr 133:98–101

Heinrich U, Moore CE, De Spirt S, Tronnier H, Stahl W (2011) Green tea polyphenols provide photoprotection, increase microcirculation, and modulate skin properties of women. J Nutr 141:1202–1208

Hughes MC, van der Pols JC, Marks GC, Green AC (2006) Food intake and risk of squamous cell carcinoma of the skin in a community: the Nambour skin cancer cohort study. Int J Cancer 119:1953–1960

Hughes MC, Williams GM, Fourtanier A, Green AC (2009) Food intake, dietary patterns, and actinic keratoses of the skin: a longitudinal study. Am J Clin Nutr 89:1246–1255

Iannacone MR, Hughes MC, Green AC (2014) Effects of sunscreen on skin cancer and photoaging. Photodermatol Photoimmunol Photomed 30:55–61

International Standardisation Organisation (2010) Cosmetics—Sun protection test methods—in vivo determination of the sun protection factor (SPF). ISO 24444:2010

Khabiri F, Hagens R, Smuda C, Soltau A, Schreiner V, Wenck H, Wittern KP, Duchstein HJ, Mei W (2008) Non-invasive monitoring of oxidative skin stress by ultraweak photon emission (UPE)-measurement. I: mechanisms of UPE of biological materials. Skin Res Technol 14:103–111

Katiyar SK, Perez A, Mukhtar H (2000) Green tea polyphenol treatment to human skin prevents formation of ultraviolet light B-induced pyrimidine dimers in DNA. Clin Cancer Res 6:3864–3869

Katiyar SK (2011) Green tea prevents non-melanoma skin cancer by enhancing DNA repair. Arch Biochem Biophys 508:152–158

Khan N, Mukhtar H (2007) Tea polyphenols for health promotion. Life Sci 81:519–533

Kligman LH, Kligman AM (1986) The nature of photoaging: its prevention and repair. Photodermatology 3:215–227

Kolbe L (2012) How much sun protection is needed?: are we on the way to full-spectrum protection? J Invest Dermatol 132:1756–1757

Kolbe L, Immeyer J, Batzer J, Wensorra U, tom Dieck K, Mundt C, Wolber R, Stäb F, Schönrock U, Ceilley RI, Wenck H (2006) Anti-inflammatory efficacy of Licochalcone A: correlation of clinical potency and in vitro effects. Arch Dermatol Res 298:23–30

Kondo K, Shiba M, Nakamura R, Morota T, Shoyama Y (2007) Constituent properties of licorices derived from Glycyrrhiza uralensis, G. glabra, or G. inflata identified by genetic information. Biol Pharm Bull 30:1271–1277

Kühnl J, Roggenkamp D, Gehrke SA, Stäb F, Wenck H, Kolbe L, Neufang G (2015) Licochalcone A activates Nrf2 in vitro and contributes to licorice extract-induced lowered cutaneous oxidative stress in vivo. Exp Dermatol 24:42–47

Kwon HS, Park JH, Kim DH, Kim YH, Park JH, Shin HK, Kim JK (2008) Licochalcone A isolated from licorice suppresses lipopolysaccharide-stimulated inflammatory reactions in RAW264.7 cells and endotoxin shock in mice. J Mol Med (Berl) 86:1287–1295

Lee J, Jiang S, Levine N, Watson RR (2000) Carotenoid supplementation reduces erythema in human skin after simulated solar radiation exposure. Proc Soc Exp Biol Med 223:170–174

Liebel F, Kaur S, Ruvolo E, Kollias N, Southall MD (2012) Irradiation of skin with visible light induces reactive oxygen species and matrix-degrading enzymes. J Invest Dermatol 132: 1901–1907

Lin JY, Selim MA, Shea CR, Grichnik JM, Omar MM, Monteiro-Riviere NA, Pinnell SR (2003) UV photoprotection by combination topical antioxidants vitamin C and vitamin E. J Am Acad Dermatol 48:866–874

Lv H, Ren H, Wang L, Chen W, Ci X (2015) Lico A enhances Nrf2-mediated defense mechanisms against t-BHP-induced oxidative stress and cell death via Akt and ERK activation in RAW 264.7 Cells. Oxid Med Cell Longev, 709–845

Mathews-Roth MM, Pathak MA, Parrish J, Fitzpatrick TB, Kass EH, Toda K, Clemens W (1972) A clinical trial of the effects of oral beta-carotene on the responses of human skin to solar radiation. J Invest Dermatol 59:349–353

McKenna DB, Murphy GM (1999) Skin cancer chemoprophylaxis in renal transplant recipients: 5 years of experience using low-dose acitretin. Br J Dermatol 140:656–660

Messier C, Grenier D (2011) Effect of licorice compounds licochalcone A, glabridin and glycyrrhizic acid on growth and virulence properties of Candida albicans. Mycoses 54: e801–e806

Middelkamp-Hup MA, Pathak MA, Parrado C, Goukassian D, Rius-Díaz F, Mihm MC, Fitzpatrick TB, González S (2004) Oral polypodium leucotomos extract decreases ultraviolet-induced damage of human skin. J Am Acad Dermatol 51:910–918

Moon TE, Levine N, Cartmel B, Bangert JL, Rodney S, Dong Q, Peng YM, Alberts DS (1997) Effect of retinol in preventing squamous cell skin cancer in moderate-risk subjects: a randomized, double-blind, controlled trial. Southwest Skin Cancer Prevention Study Group. Cancer Epidemiol Biomarkers Prev 6:949–956

Nanjo F, Mori M, Goto K, Hara Y (1999) Radical scavenging activity of tea catechins and their related compounds. Biosci Biotechnol Biochem 63:1621–1623

Lomas A, Leonardi-Bee J, Bath-Hextall F (2012) A systematic review of worldwide incidence of nonmelanoma skin cancer. Br J Dermatol 166:1069–1080

Park MR, Kim SG, Cho IA, Oh D, Kang KR, Lee SY, Moon SM, Cho SS, Yoon G, Kim CS, Oh JS, You JS, Kim Do K, Seo YS, Im HJ, Kim JS (2015) Licochalcone-A induces intrinsic and extrinsic apoptosis via ERK1/2 and p38 phosphorylation-mediated TRAIL expression in head and neck squamous carcinoma FaDu cells. Food Chem Toxicol 77:34–43

Rani V, Deep G, Singh RK, Palle K, Yadav UC (2016) Oxidative stress and metabolic disorders: pathogenesis and therapeutic strategies. Life Sci 148:183–193

Rhodes LE, Darby G, Massey KA, Clarke KA, Dew TP, Farrar MD, Bennett S, Watson RE, Williamson G, Nicolaou A (2013) Oral green tea catechin metabolites are incorporated into human skin and protect against UV radiation-induced cutaneous inflammation in association with reduced production of pro-inflammatory eicosanoid 12-hydroxyeicosatetraenoic acid. Br J Nutr 110:891–900

Rizwan M, Rodriguez-Blanco I, Harbottle A, Birch-Machin MA, Watson RE, Rhodes LE (2011) Tomato paste rich in lycopene protects against cutaneous photodamage in humans in vivo: a randomized controlled trial. Br J Dermatol 164:154–162

Saitoh T, Shibata S (1975) New type chalcones from licorice root. Tetrahedron Lett 50:4461–4462

Schäfer M, Werner S (2015) Nrf2–A regulator of keratinocyte redox signaling. Free Radical Biol Med 88:243–252

Shibata S (1994) Anti-tumorigenic chalcones. Stem Cells 12:44–52

Shibata S (2000) A drug over the millennia: pharmacognosy, chemistry, and pharmacology of licorice. Yakugaku Zasshi 120:849–862

Shibata S, Inoue H, Iwata S, Ma RD, Yu LJ, Ueyama H, Takayasu J, Hasegawa T, Tokuda H, Nishino A, Nishino H, Iwashima A (1991) Inhibitory effects of licochalcone A isolated from Glycyrrhiza inflata root on inflammatory ear edema and tumour promotion in mice. Planta Med 57:221–224

Sokoloski L, Borges M, Bagatin E (2015) Lycopene not in pill, nor in natura has photoprotective systemic effect. Arch Dermatol Res 307:545–549

Song F, Qureshi AA, Han J (2012) Increased caffeine intake is associated with reduced risk of basal cell carcinoma of the skin. Cancer Res 72:3282–3289

Song NR, Kim JE, Park JS, Kim JR, Kang H, Lee E, Kang YG, Son JE, Seo SG, Heo YS, Lee KW (2015) Licochalcone A, a polyphenol present in licorice, suppresses UV-induced COX-2 expression by targeting PI3 K, MEK1, and B-Raf. Int J Mol Sci 16:4453–4470

Spinks EA, Fenwick GR (1990) The determination of glycyrrhizin in selected UK liquorice products. Food Addit Contam 7:769–778

Stahl W, Heinrich U, Jungmann H, Sies H, Tronnier H (2000) Carotenoids and carotenoids plus vitamin E protect against ultraviolet light-induced erythema in humans. Am J Clin Nutr 71:795–798

Stahl W, Sies H (2002) Carotenoids and protection against solar UV radiation. Skin Pharmacol Appl Skin Physiol 15:291–296

Stahl W, Sies H (2012) β-Carotene and other carotenoids in protection from sunlight. Am J Clin Nutr 96:1179S–1184S

State Pharmacopoeia Commission of the PRC (2010) Pharmacopoeia of the People's Republic of China. China Medico-Pharmaceutical Science and Technology Publishing, Bejing

Szliszka E, Jaworska D, Ksek M, Czuba ZP, Król W (2012) Targeting death receptor TRAIL-R2 by chalcones for TRAIL-induced apoptosis in cancer cells. Int J Mol Sci 13:15343–15359

Talalay P, Fahey JW, Healy ZR, Wehage SL, Benedict AL, Min C, Dinkova-Kostova AT (2007) Sulforaphane mobilizes cellular defenses that protect skin against damage by UV radiation. Proc Natl Acad Sci 104:17500–17505

Thiele JJ, Ekanayake-Mudiyanselage S (2007) Vitamin E in human skin: organ-specific physiology and considerations for its use in dermatology. Mol Aspects Med 28:646–667

Tsai JP, Lee CH, Ying TH, Lin CL, Lin CL, Hsueh JT, Hsieh YH (2015) Licochalcone A induces autophagy through PI3 K/Akt/mTOR inactivation and autophagy suppression enhances Licochalcone A-induced apoptosis of human cervical cancer cells. Oncotarget 6:28851–28866

Vandersee S, Beyer M, Lademann J, Darvin ME (2015) Blue-violet light irradiation dose dependently decreases carotenoids in human skin, which indicates the generation of free radicals. Oxid Med Cell Longev 2015:579675

Wananukul S, Chatproedprai S, Charutragulchai W (2012) Randomized, double-blind, split-side comparison study of moisturizer containing licochalcone vs. 1 % hydrocortisone in the treatment of infantile seborrhoeic dermatitis. J Eur Acad Dermatol Venereol 26:894–897

Wang ZY, Nixon DW (2001) Licorice and cancer. Nutr Cancer 39:1–11

Wang L, Yang R, Yuan B, Liu Y, Liu C (2015) The antiviral and antimicrobial activities of licorice, a widely-used Chinese herb. Acta Pharm Sin B 5:310–315

Weber TM, Ceilley RI, Buerger A, Kolbe L, Trookman NS, Rizer RL, Schoelermann A (2006) Skin tolerance, efficacy, and quality of life of patients with red facial skin using a skin care regimen containing Licochalcone A. J Cosmet Dermatol 5:227–232

Weisburg JH, Weissman DB, Sedaghat T, Babich H (2004) In vitro cytotoxicity of epigallocatechin gallate and tea extracts to cancerous and normal cells from the human oral cavity. Basic Clin Pharmacol Toxicol 95:191–200

Yao K, Chen H, Lee MH, Li H, Ma W, Peng C, Song NR, Lee KW, Bode AM, Dong Z, Dong Z (2014) Licochalcone A, a natural inhibitor of c-Jun N-terminal kinase 1. Cancer Prev Res 7:139–149

Zipper LM, Mulcahy RT (2000) Inhibition of ERK and p38 MAP kinases inhibits binding of Nrf2 and induction of GCS genes. Biochem Biophys Res Commun 278:484–492

Chapter 18
The Cutaneous Microbiota as a Determinant of Skin Barrier Function: Molecular Interactions and Therapeutic Opportunities

Julia J. van Rensburg, Lana Dbeibo and Stanley M. Spinola

Abstract As the largest organ of the human body, skin provides the first barrier against environmental insults, including invading pathogens. Many studies have defined commensal skin bacteria; more recent metagenomic studies have extended characterization of the microbiota to resident fungi and viruses. The skin is dominated by members of *Actinobacteria*, *Firmicutes*, *Proteobacteria*, *Bacteroidetes*, *Malassezia* spp., bacteriophages and human viruses. Defining the microbiota of both healthy and affected skin provides insight into the influence of the cutaneous microbiota on immune responses and disease states. Crosstalk between commensal microbiota and the innate immune system facilitates proper response and healing. Commensal bacteria appear to protect from pathogens directly by releasing antibacterial products and indirectly by stimulating innate immune responses. Skin pathologies such as atopic dermatitis, rosacea, psoriasis and acne are characterized by disruptions of certain immune pathways and imbalances of skin microbiota. Additionally, susceptibility to skin infection appears to be influenced by the microbial community present on the skin, while infection and the resultant immune

J.J. van Rensburg · S.M. Spinola
Department of Microbiology and Immunology,
Indiana University School of Medicine, Indianapolis, IN, USA

L. Dbeibo · S.M. Spinola
Department of Medicine,
Indiana University School of Medicine, Indianapolis, IN, USA

S.M. Spinola
Department of Pathology and Laboratory Medicine,
Indiana University School of Medicine, Indianapolis, IN, USA

S.M. Spinola
The Center for Immunobiology,
Indiana University School of Medicine, Indianapolis, IN, USA

S.M. Spinola (✉)
635 Barnhill Drive, Indianapolis, IN 46202, USA
e-mail: sspinola@iu.edu

G.T. Wondrak (ed.), *Skin Stress Response Pathways*,
DOI 10.1007/978-3-319-43157-4_18

response alters the skin microbiota. Understanding the role of the skin microbiota in skin disorders and infection may lead to novel therapies that aim to restore the balance of commensal skin microbes.

Keywords Skin · Microbiome · Atopic dermatitis · Rosacea · Psoriasis · Acne · Infection · Bacterial community

18.1 The Skin Habitat

The skin is the largest organ of the human body, covering 1.5–2 m^2. The skin and its associated microbiota serve as the primary physical barrier to the environment and protect the body from external insults, including pathogenic microorganisms. The skin is composed of the epidermis, which provides the main barrier function, and the dermis (Fig. 18.1). The top layer of the epidermis, the stratum corneum, is composed of enucleated, cornified squamous keratinocytes. This outer layer is constantly shedding and renewing; squamous cells migrate from the basal layer to the surface and terminally differentiate in approximately 4 weeks. The epidermis contains sweat pores and hair shafts, which create variable microenvironments. Hair follicles, sebaceous glands and sweat glands originate in the lower dermal layer and represent specialized ecological niches (Fig. 18.1).

Human skin is characterized by physiologically distinct environments, including sebaceous, moist and dry. Sebaceous glands produce sebum, an oily lipid-rich substance that has antimicrobial properties yet supports the growth of commensal microbiota (Elias 2007; Drake et al. 2008). Sebaceous glands are connected to hair follicles, forming the pilosebaceous unit. Certain anatomical regions contain high densities of sebaceous glands, including areas of the head, upper chest and back. Metabolism of sebum by resident microorganisms maintains an acidity of approximately pH 5, which inhibits the growth of some pathogenic bacteria (Elias 2007).

Moist skin sites contain abundant sweat glands, which are divided into eccrine and apocrine glands. Eccrine sweat glands cover the majority of the body and secrete water and salt. Their primary function is thermoregulation, but secretion of electrolytes helps acidify the skin, which can prevent microbial growth. Apocrine glands are found in the armpit, nipple and anogenital region. Apocrine glands secrete a milky, odorless substance that may contain pheromones. Microbial metabolism of apocrine secretions creates the malodor associated with sweat (Decreau et al. 2003). Moist areas of the body include creases and folds, such as at the elbows, knees, groin, and between toes.

Dry skin is less well defined than sebaceous or moist sites but contains lower densities of sebaceous and sweat glands and is more prone to desiccation (Grice and

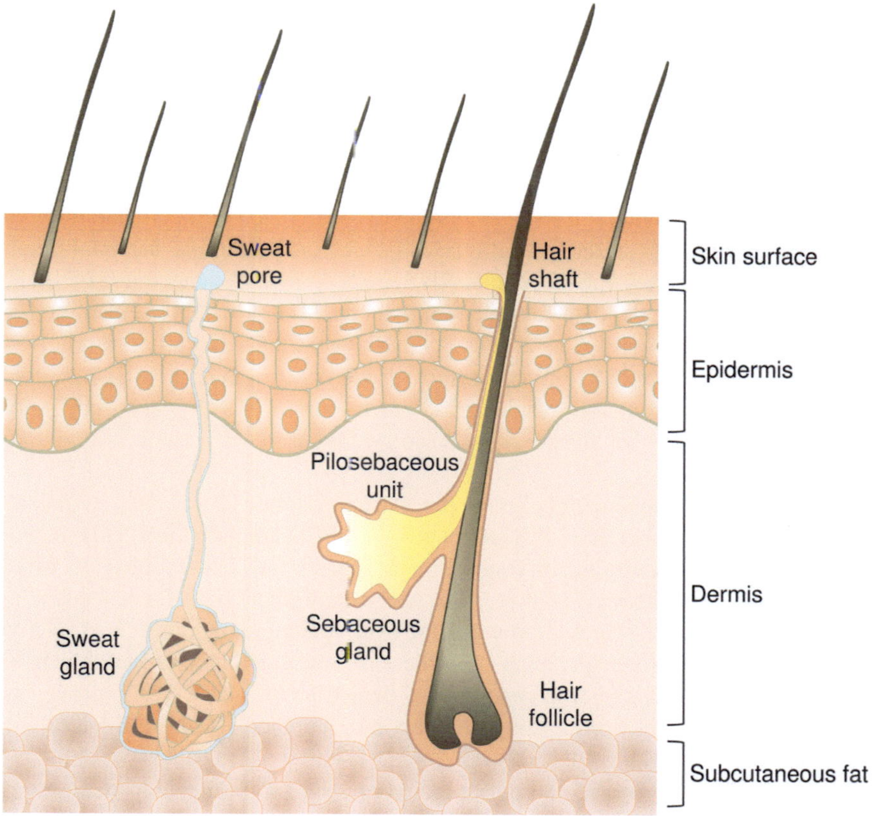

Fig. 18.1 Schematic representation of human skin. Multiple appendages form the skin topography, including hair follicles and shafts, and sweat and sebaceous glands. These structures and their products, sweat and sebum, create distinct ecological niches that select for specific bacteria, fungi and viruses

Segre 2011). Certain areas of dry skin, such as the arms and legs, tend to experience larger temperature fluctuations than more occluded areas. Commonly studied dry skin sites include the forearm, hypothenar palm and upper buttock.

The skin supports diverse microbiota, including bacteria, fungi and viruses. The microenvironment of each skin site selects for the growth of certain microorganisms, thus the anatomical site influences the skin microbiota. In turn, the interaction of the microbiota with host factors, such as metabolism of glandular secretions, affects the microenvironment and this reciprocal relationship creates unique skin habitats.

18.2 Methods to Identify Skin Microbiota

Culture-based analysis has been used for decades to characterize microorganisms residing on or in the skin. As this strategy only identifies culturable microbes, its use precludes a comprehensive survey of the cutaneous microbiota. Recent advances in high-throughput sequencing methods have enabled the identification of the metagenome, providing a more comprehensive approach to identification of the host microbiota. Most studies to date have focused on classifying bacterial inhabitants of the skin, using 16S ribosomal RNA (rRNA) gene sequencing (Fig. 18.2). Recent studies have extended classification to include fungi, which are identified by sequencing of the 18S rRNA gene (Fig. 18.2). Because the skin harbors a relatively low microbial density, PCR amplification of rRNA generates a robust sample. However, the amplification efficiency of each unique rRNA gene may vary, potentially resulting in over- or under-representation of certain community members.

Direct shot-gun sequencing, also known as metagenomic sequencing, of isolated DNA, removes the inherent biases associated with PCR amplification. This method is particularly useful for identifying resident viruses and bacteriophages, which contain no highly conserved marker gene. A current limitation of direct sequencing for characterization of skin microbiota is the overwhelming amount of host relative to microbial DNA. As sequencing costs decease and methods for enrichment of microbial nucleic acids and/or concomitant depletion of host DNA improve, the ability of metagenomics sequencing to detect rare members of the skin microbiota will improve.

A recent study compared the performance of shot-gun sequencing with amplification and sequencing of two commonly used targets of the 16S rRNA gene, hypervariable regions 1–3 and hypervariable region 4 (Meisel et al. 2016). All 3 methods were applied simultaneously to skin swab samples taken from healthy volunteers. Mock bacterial communities of known composition and concentration were used as a control for all three methods. Shotgun sequencing provides the most accurate representation of organisms at the species level, followed closely by amplification and sequencing of the V1–V3 region. Sequencing of V4 underperformed in terms of representation and speciation of organisms. For example, members of the genus *Propionobacterium* were underrepresented; this discrepancy could be explained by the fact that its V4 region was absent from some sequencing libraries. Due to the fact that the V4 region is highly conserved among *Staphylococcus* species, *Staphylococcus* speciation was also unreliable (Meisel et al. 2016). Thus, adequate primer selection and sequencing techniques are essential for obtaining accurate microbiome surveys.

Because the microbial load of the skin is relatively low, analysis of the skin microbiota is prone to confounding results introduced by contamination. Although contamination can be reduced by scrupulous handling of specimens throughout the entire process, DNA extraction kits and PCR reagents are usually contaminated with DNA from bacteria associated with water and soil (Salter et al. 2014).

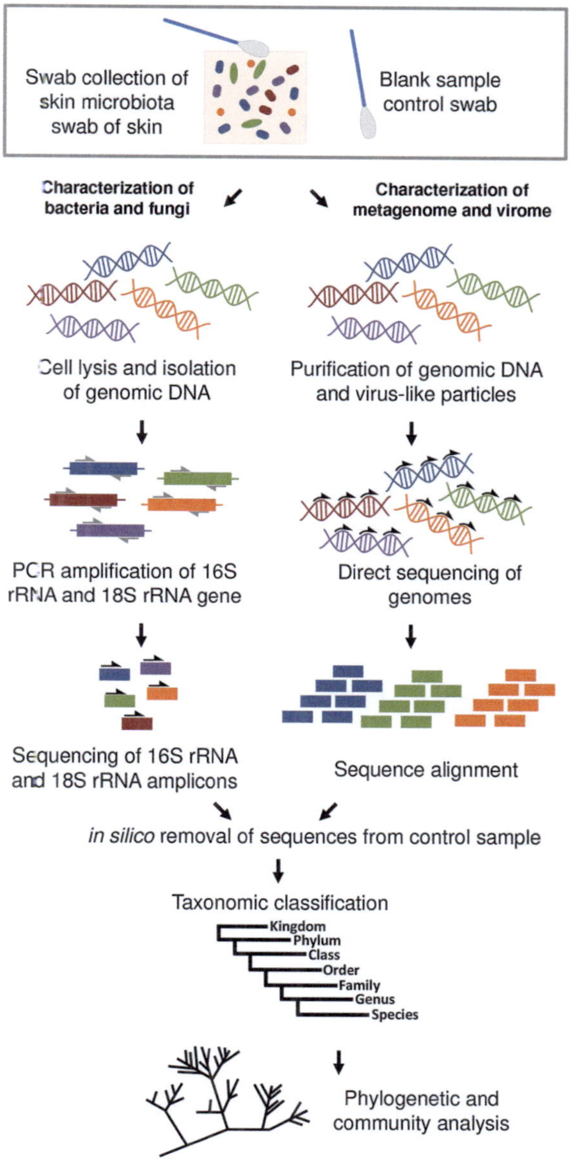

Fig. 18.2 Overview of process used to characterize skin microbiota and skin metagenome. DNA is isolated from bacteria, fungi and viruses. Amplification and sequencing of the 16S and 18S rRNA gene are used to identify bacteria and fungi, respectively. Direct sequencing of genomic DNA or virus-like particles is used to identify the metagenome or viruses, respectively. Sequences are classified based on alignment to existing genomes in the database. Blank controls are processed in parallel to facilitate in silico removal of contaminating taxa

Contaminating DNA becomes a major issue for samples that contain ~10^5 bacteria or less, such as skin (Salter et al. 2014). Ideally, potential contamination is controlled by including blank samples, which are processed and analyzed in parallel with the skin samples. Contaminating sequences are identified and removed in silico during data processing. Excluding negative sample controls may result in erroneous reporting of skin microbiota (Salter et al. 2014).

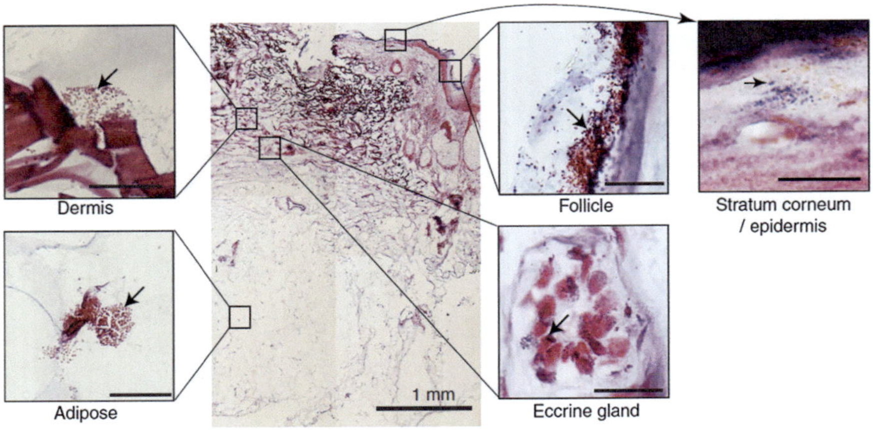

Fig. 18.3 Detection of skin bacteria. Gram-stained bacteria in frozen sections of facial skin from a healthy volunteer. Bacteria are observed in many structures, including hair follicles and eccrine sweat glands, and layers of the skin, including the epidermis, dermis and adipose. Image from Nakatsuji and colleagues (Nakatsuji et al. 2013) reproduced with permission from Nature Publishing Group

Although scraping and punch biopsy can be used to collect specimens, most studies rely on swabs to sample the skin. One study compared the microbiota identified in the antecubital fossa by swab, scrape and punch biopsy. The three methods sample the skin similarly; the identified microbiota overlaps by greater than 97 % (Grice et al. 2008). However, the bacterial load differs by collection method. The load collected by swab, scrape and biopsy is 10,000, 50,000 and 1,000,000 bacteria/cm^2, respectively (Grice et al. 2008). Because samples collected by swab and scrape contain $\sim 10^4$ microbial cells, they are more susceptible to contamination issues than biopsy samples. Bacteria also exist in the subepidermal compartments, including dermal and adipose tissue, regions previously thought to be devoid of microbes (Nakatsuji et al. 2013) (Fig. 18.3). Quantification of bacteria from skin cross sections shows that hair follicles contain the highest bacterial load, followed by the epidermis, and finally the dermis and adipose tissue, which contain equal loads (Nakatsuji et al. 2013). Although swabbing misses the less colonized subepidermal microbes, it adequately surveys the dominant skin microbiota.

18.3 Characterization of the Skin Microbiota

Four bacterial phyla dominate the human microbiota. *Actinobacteria*, *Firmicutes*, *Proteobacteria* and *Bacteroidetes* are found throughout the body, but the relative abundance of each phylum varies based on niche (Costello et al. 2009). Despite low phyletic diversity, the dominant species inhabiting each anatomical site vary widely. The physiological characteristics that differentiate the three cutaneous microenvironments select for microbiota that vary in terms of composition, load and diversity.

The microaerophilic, sebum-rich environment of sebaceous skin selects for facultatively anaerobic, lipid-metabolizing microorganisms. Sebaceous sites, including the glabella, forehead, alar crease, external auditory canal, manubrium, retroauricular crease and upper back are dominated by *Propionibacterium* and *Staphylococcus* (Grice et al. 2009; Staudinger et al. 2011; Oh et al. 2014). Modest proportions of *Corynebacteria* and *β-Proteobacteria* also inhabit these sebaceous sites (Grice et al. 2009; Oh et al. 2014). Overall, sebaceous sites have lower richness (number of taxa), evenness (uniform distribution of taxa) and diversity (factors both richness and evenness) but higher biomass than moist and dry skin sites (Grice et al. 2009; Oh et al. 2014).

Dry skin tends to support bacterial communities with relatively high richness, evenness and diversity, but lower biomass than moist or sebaceous sites (Grice et al. 2009; Oh et al. 2014). One study found a high relative abundance of *β-Proteobacteria* and *Flavobacteriales* on the dry skin of the volar forearm, hypothenar palm, and buttock (Grice et al. 2009). Other surveys found that the forearms and palms harbor a high relative abundance of *Actinobacteria*, (predominately *Propionibacterium* and *Corynebacterium*), followed by *Firmicutes* (primarily *Staphylococcus* and *Streptococcus*) and *β-Proteobacteria* (Gao et al. 2007; Fierer et al. 2008; Staudinger et al. 2011).

The community composition of moist skin sites varies widely. In general, the moist and/or occluded sites select for *Staphylococcus* and *Corynebacterium*, which tend to thrive in high humidity (Grice 2014). However, the microbial composition is highly variable across moist sites The inguinal crease and gluteal crease, umbilicus, and toe web space are dominated by *Corynebacterium*, followed by *Flavobacteriales* and *Staphylococcus* (Grice et al. 2009). The axilla harbors *Corynebacterium*, *Staphylococcus* and *β-Proteobacteria* and the antecubital fossa harbors *Proteobacteria*, *Flavobacteriales* and *Staphylococcus* (Grice et al. 2008, 2009). The popliteal fossa and plantar heel are dominated by *Staphylococcus*, along with low levels of *β-Proteobacteria* and *Flavobacteriales* (Grice et al. 2009). The richness, evenness and diversity of moist skin sites vary widely, but are higher on average than sebaceous skin (Grice et al. 2009).

Recent studies characterizing the cutaneous metagenomes found that bacteria dominate the microbial communities of most skin sites, but fungi are present as well. In general, fungi constitute a relatively low fraction of the microbiota across all sites; however, relatively higher proportions of fungi inhabit the glabella, external auditory canal, and retroauricular crease (Oh et al. 2014) (Fig. 18.4). Although bacteria outnumber fungi, the metabolic capacity of each fungal cell exceeds that of each bacterial cell; the relative metabolic impact of fungal taxa versus bacterial taxa in the skin is unknown. Fungal diversity is dependent on regional location, with foot sites harboring the greatest number of fungal taxa, followed by the arm and then the external auditory canal, inguinal crease, manubrium, retroauricular crease, back, glabella, nares, and occiput (Findley et al. 2013).

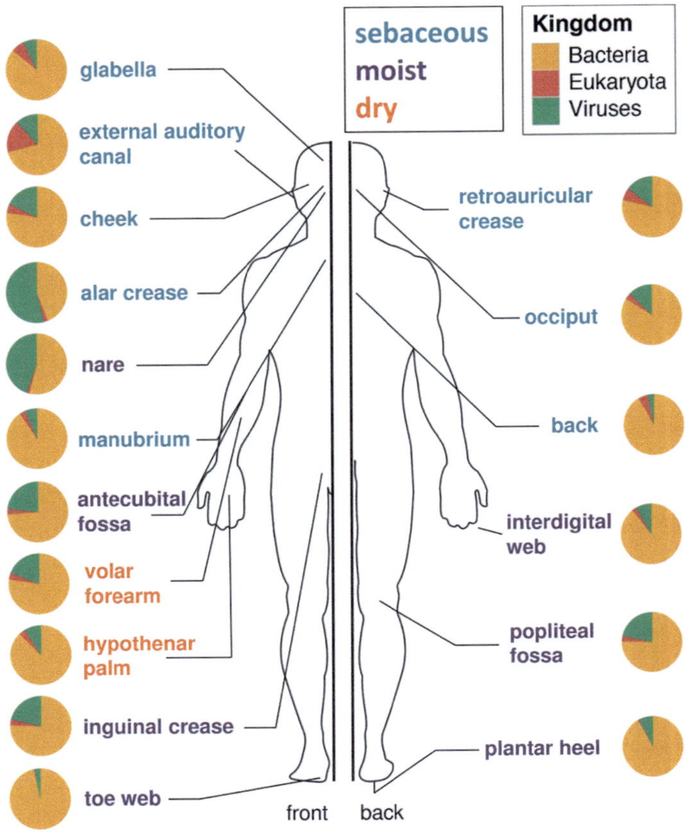

Fig. 18.4 Representation of the skin metagenome. Pie charts show the relative abundance of bacteria, eukaryota (*fungi*) and viruses from sebaceous (*aqua*), moist (*purple*), and dry (*orange*) sites. Bacteria dominate the skin, and fungi and viruses are detected to a lesser extent at all sites. Image adapted from Oh and colleagues (Oh et al. 2014) with permission from Nature Publishing Group

Malassezia is the predominant fungal genus found on the human body, except for the feet which harbor *Malassezia*, *Aspergillus*, *Cryptococcus*, *Rhodotorula*, and *Epicoccum* (Findley et al. 2013; Oh et al. 2014; Hannigan et al. 2015). Sebaceous sites such as the external auditory canal, retroauricular crease and glabella are dominated by *M. restricta*, whereas *M. globosa* is highly abundant on the back, occiput and inguinal crease (Findley et al. 2013). The nares, antecubital fossa, volar forearm and hypothenar palm harbor a mixed *Malassezia* spp. population (Findley et al. 2013).

Recent studies have focused on identifying viral sequences as part of the metagenome; however, several factors preclude comprehensive characterization of the virome. Current methods only sample DNA viruses, missing RNA viruses and potentially missing ssDNA or enveloped viruses. Additionally, the lack of viral genomes in the database complicates the identification of viral sequences; these uncharacterized or unmatched sequences are known as viral dark matter (Pedulla et al. 2003). Furthermore, small viral genomes tend to underrepresent viruses in metagenomics sequencing data (Hannigan et al. 2015). These issues can be partially circumvented by purification of virus-like particles, which improves specificity, and by using reference-independent assembly of viral contigs, which improves identification of viral genomes (Hannigan et al. 2015). However, the isolation method may also introduce biases. Despite these inherent challenges, bacteriophages and viruses are found at all skin sites surveyed thus far (Fig. 18.4). The most abundant viruses detected include bacteriophages, primarily those that infect *Propionibacterium*, *Staphylococcus*, and also *Pseudomonas* and *Bacillus* to a lesser extent (Oh et al. 2014; Hannigan et al. 2015). Additionally, human pathogens such as the human papillomavirus, Merkel cell polyomavirus, and molluscum contagiosum and animal pathogens such as *Circovirus* can be present (Foulongne et al. 2012; Oh et al. 2014; Hannigan et al. 2015). Sebaceous skin sites harbor less diverse viromes than moist or intermittently moist sites, and intermittently occluded sites had the most diverse viromes (Hannigan et al. 2015).

18.4 Factors Influencing Microbial Composition

Skin site and microenvironment appear to be the biggest drivers of microbial diversity (Costello et al. 2009) with sebaceous sites and dry sites imparting the strongest and weakest selection, respectively. The permissiveness of two skin microenvironments is addressed by transplantation experiments, in which tongue bacteria are inoculated onto the forehead or forearm. Twenty-four hours after transplantation, samples from foreheads resemble the forehead microbiota, but samples from forearms resemble tongue bacteria (Costello et al. 2009). These results suggest that the sebaceous environment supports a smaller subset of bacteria than dry skin; in other words, dry skin is more permissive than sebaceous skin.

In addition to microenvironment, individual variation contributes to differences in community composition (Costello et al. 2009; Oh et al. 2014). Intrapersonal variation is lower than interpersonal variation; the microbiota of multiple sites and environments within a volunteer are more likely to resemble each other than the microbiota of other volunteers (Gao et al. 2007; Grice et al. 2009). For example, only 17 % of taxa are shared between the palms of 51 volunteers, but samples obtained from both palms within a person are more similar than what is expected by chance (Fierer et al. 2008). Additionally, the community composition varies less in individuals sampled over time than between individuals sampled on the same day (Costello et al. 2009). A recent study found that host effects shape individual metagenomic signatures and that several low-abundance taxa can differentiate between individual hosts (Oh et al. 2014).

In general, skin bacterial membership and community composition remain fairly stable over time. Bacterial temporal stability depends on site. The nares, alar crease, inguinal crease and external auditory canal display the least variability while the buttock, volar forearm and popliteal fossa display the most variability over 4–6 months (Grice et al. 2009). The presence and community membership of *Malassezia* spp. remains fairly stable over a 4 week period (Findley et al. 2013; Hannigan et al. 2015). In comparison to the bacterial community, the human virome appears to be less stable over time (Hannigan et al. 2015). However, the temporal variability of the bacterial and viral skin communities remains significantly lower than interpersonal variation.

Age also affects skin microbiota. Although the womb is sterile, colonization of the infant begins during birth. The mode of delivery determines the bacterial community; infants born vaginally harbor microbiota that resemble their mother's vaginal microbiota, including *Lactobacillus*, *Prevotella* and *Sneathia*, whereas children born via Caesarean section harbor microbiota that resemble skin microbiota, including *Propionibacterium*, *Staphylococcus*, and *Corynebacterium* (Dominguez-Bello et al. 2010). The forearm, forehead and buttock skin of babies aged 1–12 months is dominated by *Staphylococcus* and *Streptococcus*, but the proportion of these genera decreases over the first year (Capone et al. 2011). Maturation-related differences occur in the microbiota of the antecubital and popliteal fossae, nares and volar forearms of children and adults. Children harbor higher proportions of *Bacteroidetes*, *Proteobacteria*, *Firmicutes*, particularly *Staphylococcus* and *Streptococcus* than adults. Puberty triggers increased sebum production that selects for lipophilic bacteria including *Propionibacterium* and *Corynebacterium* (Oh et al. 2012).

Other host factors, such as ethnicity, geography, and lifestyle contribute to the skin microbiota. For example, volar forearm bacteria differ among volunteers from Colorado, New York, and the Venezuelan Amazon. *Actinobacteria*, particularly *Propionibacterium*, dominate the microbiota from US volunteers, but the microbiota of Venezuelan Amerindians is either dominated by *Firmicutes*, particularly *Staphylococcus*, or is characterized by a diverse array of *Proteobacteria*, including *Pseudomonas*, *Xanthomonadaceae* and *Methylophilus* (Blaser et al. 2013). Similarly, another isolated group of Venezuelan Amerindians harbor more diverse volar forearm microbiota than US volunteers (Clemente et al. 2015). These Amerindians have higher proportions of bacteria classified as environmental taxa, including *Knoellia* and *Solibacteraceae*. These taxa may reflect the increased environmental exposure of Amerindians compared to US citizens (Clemente et al. 2015); however the lack of no-template controls for the skin microbiome in this study presents the possibility that environmental contamination confounded these results.

Gender also influences skin microbial communities. The diversity of the hand bacterial community is significantly higher in women than men (Fierer et al. 2008). However, the bacterial diversity of the upper buttock is higher in men than women (Zeeuwen et al. 2012). Women who use makeup daily have higher bacterial diversity on the forehead than men or women who do not use makeup (Staudinger et al. 2011).

Hygiene influences skin microbiota as well. In a survey of bacterial communities on the palm, *Staphylococcaceae*, *Streptococcaceae* and *Lactobacillaceae* are more abundant on recently washed hands, while *Propionibacterium*, *Neisseriales*, *Burkholderiales* and *Pasteurellaceae* increase over time after hand washing (Fierer et al. 2008).

18.5 Crosstalk of Microbiota and Immune System

Recent studies have shown that our commensal microbiota is closely linked to the proper functioning of the immune system. Germ free mice are susceptible to cutaneous infection with the protozoan *Leishmania major*, but colonization of the skin with *S. epidermidis* affords protective immunity against *Leishmania* (Naik et al. 2012). Colonization with *S. epidermidis* rescues IL-17A production in the skin, through an IL-1-dependent signaling pathway (Naik et al. 2012). Thus, *S. epidermidis* tunes resident T cells to respond to invading pathogens. However, *S. epidermidis* also decreases skin inflammation in mice. Following skin injury, the lipoteichoic acid of *S. epidermidis* suppresses TLR3-mediated release of the inflammatory cytokines IL-6 and TNF-α from keratinocytes, which is essential for the normal skin inflammatory response to injury (Lai et al. 2009). This suppression is mediated by TLR2, which induces TNF receptor-associated factor-1 (TRAF1), a negative regulatory factor (Lai et al. 2009). These findings indicate that *S. epidermidis* can modulate inflammation in the skin, and can induce a proinflammatory or anti-inflammatory response depending on the stimulus and type of injury to the skin (Fig. 18.5).

Analysis of the skin microbiota from patients with immunodeficiencies provides an opportunity to understand how altered immune function shapes the resident microbial community. Primary immunodeficiencies (PID) are caused by mutations in key immune regulators, which result in impaired in T- and B-cell function, differentiation, maturation, as well as other immune system defects. Thus, PID patients commonly experience skin infections. One study found that patients with hyper-IgE syndrome (HIES) and chronic mucocutaneous candidiasis have higher proportions of Gram-negative bacteria such as *Acinetobacter* and decreased abundance of *Corynebacterium* compared to healthy controls (Smeekens et al. 2014). Similarly, another group of HIES patients have higher levels of the Gram-negative opportunistic pathogen *Serratia marcescens* (Oh et al. 2013). These HIES patients, along with those suffering from other immunodeficiencies including Wiskott-Aldrich syndrome and DOCK8 deficiency had higher levels of *Firmicutes*, *Corynebacterium* and *Staphylococcus*, decreased abundance of *Bacteroidetes* and *Propionibacterium* and increased fungal richness (Oh et al. 2013). Interestingly, the site-to-site variation was lower in PID patients and the microbial communities were less stable over time compared to healthy skin (Oh et al. 2013). These results suggest that dysbiosis (imbalance in proportions of microbiota) in PID patients contributes to recurrent skin pathologies.

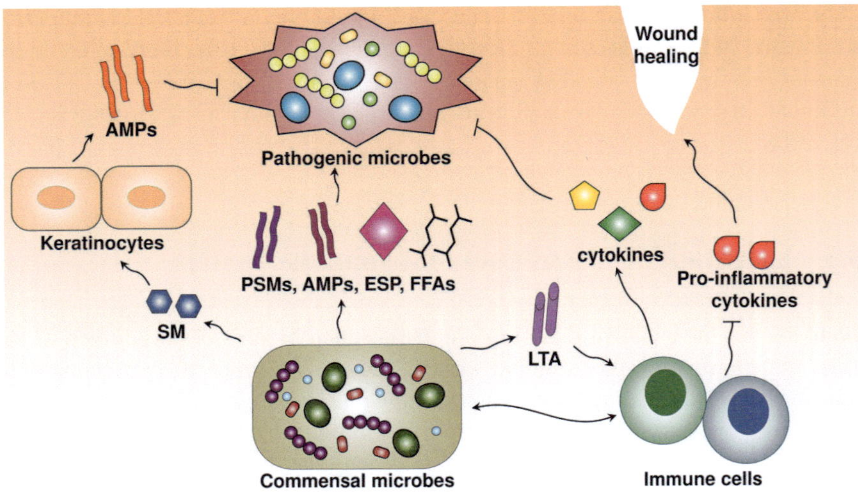

Fig. 18.5 Commensal microbes and the innate immune system coordinate processes in the skin. Cutaneous microbiota produce phenol soluble modulins (*PSMs*), antimicrobial peptides (*AMPs*), free fatty acids (*FFAs*), and a serine protease (*ESP*) that directly inhibit pathogenic bacteria. Crosstalk between commensal microbes and immune cells tunes the immune system and triggers production of pro- and anti-inflammatory cytokines that control pathogens. A small molecule (*SM*) produced by commensal bacteria stimulates keratinocytes to produce AMPs. Following skin injury microbiota-derived lipotechoic acid (*LTA*) suppresses the production of pro-inflammatory cytokines

Murine models have been used to delineate the effect of the immune system on the skin microbiota. Mice deficient in Langerhans cells, Rag1, or MyD88/TRIF have similar skin microbiota to wild-type mice (Scholz et al. 2014). Thus, these pathways do not affect the skin microbiota of mice housed under pathogen-free conditions. However, inhibition of C5A in mice modulates the diversity and composition of the skin bacteria, suggesting that complement pathways help shape the skin microbial diversity (Chehoud et al. 2013). In diabetic mice, chronic wounds are associated with altered skin microbiota composition and differential expression of genes involved in immune response and wound repair (Grice et al. 2010). Furthermore, increased expression of cutaneous host defense genes correlates with increased relative abundance of *S. aureus*. Thus, a persistent inflammatory response is directly linked to colonizing bacteria. Although it is clear that a relationship exists between the immune system and resident microbiota, additional studies are needed to understand how the immune system shapes cutaneous microbial communities.

Antimicrobial peptides (AMPs) are an important first-line of defense against invading pathogens. Recent evidence suggests that commensal bacteria make AMPs and influence the production of host AMPs. For example, phenol-soluble modulins isolated from *S. epidermidis* exhibit selective bactericidal activity against skin pathogens, including *S. aureus*, group A streptococcus, and *E. coli* (Cogen et al. 2010; Gallo and Nakatsuji 2011). Such phenol-soluble modulins may enhance the activity of human cutaneous AMPs. A yet-to-be-identified <10 kDa small molecule from *S. epidermidis* conditioned culture medium increases the expression of human beta-defensin (hBD) 2 and hBD3 in cultured keratinocytes via a TLR2-dependent mechanism (Lai et al. 2010). hBD2 and hBD3 are produced by human keratinocytes and have activity against many bacteria, fungi and viruses (Cogen et al. 2012) (Fig. 18.5).

The cutaneous microbiota plays a crucial role in immune function, by stimulating pathways that provide protection from invading pathogens or aid in proper wound healing. Disturbances in the cutaneous microbiota may contribute to both infectious and non-infectious skin pathologies. The following section discusses recent studies that identify differences in the skin microbiota of patients exhibiting skin disorders or infections.

18.6 The Role of Skin Microbiota in Skin Pathologies

18.6.1 Atopic Dermatitis

Atopic dermatitis (AD) is a chronic, recurrent inflammatory condition affecting approximately 15 % of children and 2 % of adults in the US (Grice and Segre 2011). The highly pruritic AD lesions are commonly found on moist skin, especially the antecubital and popliteal regions (Grice 2014). Dilute bleach baths, antibiotics and steroids help control the severity of lesions, suggesting that bacterial overgrowth and an uncontrolled immune response contribute to AD (Huang et al. 2009; Grice 2014).

S. aureus is associated with AD and is recovered from lesional and nonlesional skin of patients with AD flares (Leyden et al. 1975; Gallo and Nakatsuji 2011). A recent longitudinal study found that *Staphylococcus* spp. increases from 35 to 90 % of the microbiota during AD flares in children (Kong et al. 2012). Interestingly, proportions of both pathogenic *S. aureus* and commensal *S. epidermidis* increases during flares. Some strains of *S. epidermidis* produce Esp protein that inhibits *S. aureus* colonization in the nares (Iwase et al. 2010); whether the outgrowth of *S. epidermidis* in AD flares antagonizes *S. aureus* is unclear. The disease flare state also coincides with a decrease in microbial diversity and a decrease in the relative abundance of *Streptococcus*, *Corynebacterium* and *Propionibacterium* (Kong et al. 2012). Delineating whether the outgrowth of *S. aureus* and decreased microbial diversity directly contribute to disease severity or are the result of cutaneous inflammation will require detailed longitudinal analyses. Intermittent topical decolonization regimens directed against *S. aureus* result in improvement of AD without complete elimination of *S. aureus* (Huang et al. 2009). Effective treatment of AD may need to focus both on reducing *S. aureus* colonization and maintaining or restoring balance among the resident microbiota (Grice 2014).

In addition to the cutaneous microbiota, low diversity of gut bacteria in infants one month of age is associated with development of AD later in life (Abrahamsson et al. 2012; Grice 2014). Some studies show that giving probiotics to pregnant mothers reduces the incidence of AD in their infants (Foolad et al. 2013). One study showed that treatment of children with AD with probiotics reduces the severity of the disease (Foolad et al. 2013). Furthermore, prebiotic supplementation in infants has also been associated with a reduction in AD incidence in the first year of life (Foolad et al. 2013). The connection between gut microbial diversity and AD remains unknown, but gut microbiota may help tune the cutaneous immune system (Grice 2014).

18.6.2 Rosacea

Rosacea is a chronic cutaneous illness characterized by facial erythema, telangiectasias, and inflammatory papules and pustules (Crawford et al. 2004). It affects approximately 3 % of individuals in the US over the age of 30 (Berg and Liden 1989; Yamasaki et al. 2007). Although its pathophysiology is unknown, potential factors influencing the disease are aberrant inflammatory responses and vascular and sebaceous gland abnormalities. The epidermis of patients with rosacea is abundant in an enzymatically-altered form of the AMP cathelicidin and its activating serine protease kallikrein 5 (KLK5) (Yamasaki et al. 2007). This abnormal form of cathelicidin causes increased local inflammation and vascular dilation in the skin of mice injected with this molecule (Yamasaki et al. 2007). Expression of TLR-2, which enhances production of KLK5 from keratinocytes, is also increased in patients with rosacea (Yamasaki et al. 2011). Additionally, skin samples from rosacea patients have higher levels of genes encoding pro-inflammatory cytokines and inflammasome-related genes than controls (Casas et al. 2012). This overactive immune response may affect the resident commensals in patients affected by this disease (Holmes 2013).

Although a microbial component of rosacea is suspected, identification of contributing or causative microbiota remains inconclusive and controversial (Holmes 2013; Picardo and Ottaviani 2014). Studies have linked the presence or density of the following microorganisms in the skin to rosacea: the skin mite *Demodex folliculorum* (Holmes 2013), the mite symbiont *Bacillus oleronius* (Lacey et al. 2007) and *S. epidermidis* (Dahl et al. 2004). *Chlamydia pneumoniae* antigen is detectable in up to 40 % of biopsies of lesions, but the significance of this finding is unclear (Fernandez-Obregon and Patton 2007). Some studies have suggested a relationship between rosacea and *Helicobacter pylori* infection due to the high prevalence of *H. pylori* seropositivity in these patients (Tuzun et al. 2010). However, this issue remains controversial, as other studies have failed to show a similar association (Tuzun et al. 2010). To the best of our knowledge, characterization of the microbiota of rosacea patients has not been described. Perhaps metagenomics analysis would reveal insights into the causative agents of this common disease.

18.6.3 Psoriasis

Psoriasis is a chronic inflammatory condition observed primarily on dry areas of the skin, including the trunk, knees and elbows. It affects approximately 2 % of the world's population (Christophers 2001) and is characterized by hyperproliferation of keratinocytes and inflammation (Gao et al. 2008). Psoriasis vulgaris, which is thought to result from an immune intolerance to microbiota, is more common than guttate psoriasis, which is associated with streptococcal colonization and superantigen production (Leung et al. 1995; Fry et al. 2013).

Characterization of the microbiota in psoriasis patients reveals a higher abundance of *Firmicutes* and lower abundance of *Actinobacteria* and *Proteobacteria* (Gao et al. 2008) in lesional skin compared to healthy skin. The relative abundance of *P. acnes* is lower in psoriatic lesions (Gao et al. 2008; Fahlen et al. 2012), whereas *Streptococcus* is higher (Gao et al. 2008). A separate study that compared 51 psoriatic lesions with the unaffected skin of psoriasis patients and healthy skin of control volunteers found that the combined relative abundance of *Corynebacterium*, *Streptococcus*, *Staphylococcus* and *Propionibacterium* is higher in lesional than unaffected or healthy skin (Alekseyenko et al. 2013). This study also found that lesional skin trends towards decreased microbial diversity (Alekseyenko et al. 2013), whereas the former study found that diversity is higher in psoriatic lesions (Gao et al. 2008). Thus, differences between psoriatic lesions and healthy skin have been observed and additional studies are needed to determine the relevance of these differences to the disease state.

18.6.4 Acne Vulgaris

Acne is a widespread skin condition that affects up to 80 % of adolescents and often continues into adulthood. It is characterized by inflamed sebaceous follicles that present as papules, pustules or cysts (Ayer and Burrows 2006). Acne commonly responds to topical and oral antibiotics (Leyden and Del Rosso 2011), pointing to a bacterial component of the disease.

An association between the levels of *P. acnes* and acne vulgaris in adolescents was established long ago (Leyden et al. 1975; Grice 2014). However, because *P. acnes* is a member of the commensal microbiota and is abundant on healthy skin, understanding its specific role in acne has proven challenging. A small study showed that the sebaceous/hair follicles of 3 healthy volunteers contain only *P. acnes*, whereas those of 5 acne patients contain *P. acnes* and *S. epidermidis*

(Bek-Thomsen et al. 2008). A larger study including 49 healthy volunteers and 52 acne patients found both *P. acnes* and *S. epidermidis* in the pilosebaceous units of both groups (Fitz-Gibbon et al. 2013). Both studies found that *P. acnes* dominates the pilosebaceous unit microbiota (Bek-Thomsen et al. 2008; Fitz-Gibbon et al. 2013), but the latter study found no difference in proportions of taxa between healthy skin and skin of acne patients (Fitz-Gibbon et al. 2013). Quantitative culture analysis of the acne lesion surface from 100 patients revealed no difference in *Propionibacterium* or *Staphylococcus* compared to healthy controls, but culture-independent methods showed a higher proportion of *M. globosa* in acne patients (Numata et al. 2014).

Although the relative abundance of *P. acnes* does not differ between healthy and acne-prone skin, strain-level variations may contribute to the development of acne. Of 71 sequenced *P. acnes* genomes, four of the 10 most abundant ribotypes (RT), RT4, 5, 8 and 10, are significantly enriched in acne-prone skin, whereas RT6 is more commonly associated with the pilosebaceous units of healthy volunteers (Fitz-Gibbon et al. 2013). RT4 and 5 encode for a plasmid that carries genes associated with virulence in other bacterial species (Fitz-Gibbon et al. 2013). Whether these acne-associated RTs have enhanced virulence is not clear. It is important to note that this study focused on non-lesional skin in both patients and controls; characterizing the microbiota and genomes from acne lesions may provide additional insight into strain-level differences that contribute to disease.

18.7 Role of Skin Microbiota in Infectious Disease

The skin microbiota is thought to protect against infection by competing for resources, priming the immune system, and secreting molecules that inhibit the growth of pathogens. However, relatively few studies have analyzed whether microbial communities influence susceptibility or resistance to infection. This section highlights two studies that assessed the skin microbiota in relation to cutaneous infection.

S. aureus is a major cause of skin abscesses, especially in people who have recently used antibiotics (Moran et al. 2006; Horton et al. 2015). To test if perturbed microbiota contributes to infection susceptibility, the microbiota of peri-abscess and contralateral skin of 25 patients with *S. aureus* abscesses was compared to microbiota of analogous sites of 25 healthy volunteers. The peri-abscess and contralateral bacterial communities of the infected patients are similar to each other and significantly different than the microbiota of healthy controls, which are more distinct from one another than are the samples from patients. No major differences in taxa at the phylum level exist, but samples from healthy volunteers are enriched for *Brevibacillus* and *Lactococcus*, both members of the phylum *Firmicutes* (Horton et al. 2015). Interestingly, the patients who tested positive for *S. aureus* by culture also harbor high proportions of *S. aureus* in the peri-abscess and contralateral sites, suggesting that these patients were highly colonized with *S. aureus*.

Since preinfection samples were not available for the infected group, whether their similar microbiota enhances susceptibility to *S. aureus* infection or is the result of the infection is unclear.

Haemophilus ducreyi causes the sexually transmitted genital ulcer disease chancroid in adults and nonsexually transmitted cutaneous ulcers in children in the tropics (Marks et al. 2014; Mitjà et al. 2014; Ghinai et al. 2015). In experimental infection of human volunteers in the skin overlying the deltoid, papules occur at virtually all inoculated sites; these papules spontaneously resolve or progress to pustules in ~30 and 70 %, respectively, of the volunteers (Janowicz et al. 2009). To assess the potential role of microbiota in infection outcome, skin swab samples collected before and after infection were compared between 4 sets of dose-matched resolvers and pustule formers. At preinfection, resolvers have significantly different bacterial biota than pustule formers (van Rensburg et al. 2015) (Fig. 18.6). Although the taxa varied, resolvers harbor significantly higher proportions of *P. acnes* at preinfection than pustule formers. *P. acnes* may outcompete or inhibit *H. ducreyi*, or this observation may reflect an immune bias that favors clearance of *H. ducreyi*. Whereas the preinfection microbiota of resolvers more closely resembles each other than that of pustule formers, the latter group has a more similar microbiota at the clinical endpoint (Fig. 18.6), suggesting that infection with, or the immune response to *H. ducreyi* drives the microbiota to a common composition. Certain bacteria are overrepresented in pustule formers throughout the experiment, including members of the phyla *Proteobacteria* and *Bacteroidetes*, as well as *Micrococcus*, *Corynebacterium*, and *Staphylococcus*. These taxa may impart a growth advantage to *H. ducreyi*, reflect an immune status that is permissible to *H. ducreyi* infection, or thrive in the moist pustular environment that results from a failed immune response. As this study did contain preinfection samples from both groups, it seems to indicate that the common microbiota of resolvers prior to

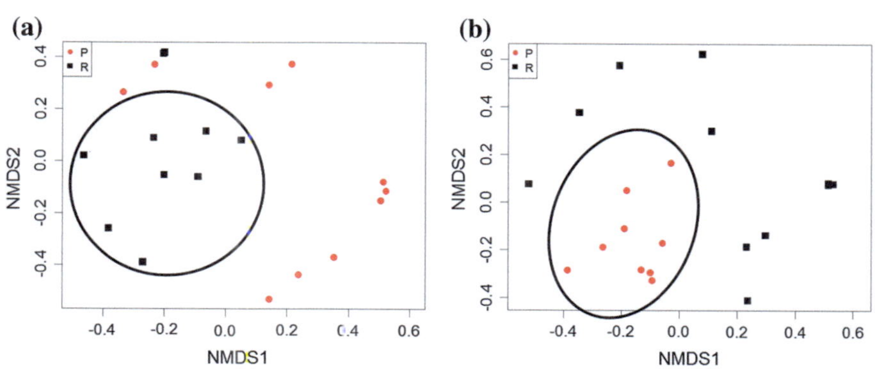

Fig. 18.6 Non-metric multidimensional scaling using normalized weighted UniFrac distances of OTUs detected in preinfection samples from resolvers (n = 10) and pustule formers (n = 10) (**a**) and in endpoint samples from resolved sites (n = 11) and pustule sites (n = 9) (**b**). For both comparisons, $P = 0.001$, PERMANOVA. At preinfection, resolver sites and sites within volunteers cluster. At endpoint, pustule sites and sites within volunteers cluster. *P*, pustule former; *R*, resolver

infection is associated with protection while the microbiota of pustule formers is driven to a common composition by the infection and the host immune response. Perhaps this is why persons with *S. aureus* abscesses also share a common microbiome.

18.8 Using the Microbiota to Prevent or Treat Skin Diseases

Understanding how certain skin microbial communities inhibit the colonization of or change in response to invading pathogens may influence our ability to prevent or treat skin infections. Studies of the microbiota of healthy and diseased skin show that dysbiosis can affect susceptibility to infection or exacerbate existing inflammatory dermatoses. Restoring a balanced microbial community may help prevent infectious and non-infectious skin conditions.

S. epidermidis ferments glycerol to produce several short chain fatty acids, including succinic acid, which inhibits the growth of *P. acnes* in acneiform lesions in mice (Wang et al. 2014). Injection of 5 mM or topical application of 100 mM succinic acid significantly reduces the counts of *P. acnes* and suppresses the inflammation associated with *P. acnes* overgrowth (Wang et al. 2014). As mentioned previously, the *S. epidermidis* serine protease Esp inhibits *S. aureus* colonization of the nares and disrupts existing *S. aureus* biofilms (Iwase et al. 2010). Inoculation with *S. epidermidis* or application of purified Esp eliminates nasal *S. aureus* carriage in humans who are chronic carriers (Iwase et al. 2010). A separate study showed that nasal inoculation with *Corynebacterium* sp. strain Co304 eliminates *S. aureus* from persistent carriers, perhaps by outcompeting *S. aureus* for adherence to nasal epithelium (Uehara et al. 2000). Persistent nasal carriage of *S. aureus* is a risk factor for skin infections (Toshkova et al. 2001); thus, using commensal bacteria or their metabolic byproducts to prevent colonization with *S. aureus* may have important public health implications.

Although topical application of probiotics to the skin has not been widely explored, many studies have evaluated the utility of oral probiotics to improve skin conditions. A systematic review of 16 randomized controlled trials concluded that oral administration of *Lactobacillus* to pregnant women is effective in preventing AD in their infants; but this result should be interpreted with caution due to the high degree of heterogeneity in the included studies (Fuchs-Tarlovsky et al. 2015). Additional studies are needed to ascertain the role of probiotics in treating skin pathologies such as eczema, acne, and cutaneous candidiasis. Oral probiotics promote gut homeostasis by regulating immune responses and inhibiting pathogen growth (Fuchs-Tarlovsky et al. 2015); however, the effect of oral probiotics and gut homeostasis on the skin microbiota and immune regulation remains unclear. Understanding this connection may provide insight into effective prevention strategies and treatment options for skin pathologies.

18.9 Summary and Concluding Remarks

The skin is home to a diverse array of bacteria, fungi, and viruses. Many factors influence the microbial composition of the skin, including the microenvironment, host genetics, age, ethnicity, lifestyle, gender, and daily habits. Recent studies have begun to elucidate the intimate relationship between resident skin microbiota and the immune system, which has furthered our understanding of the role of skin microbiota in skin pathologies. Prevalent taxa differ between patients with infectious and non-infectious skin conditions; however, whether the microbial community directly affects and/or reflects the host immune status remains to be determined. As many skin diseases and disorders potentially arise from dysbiosis, restoring balance by introducing beneficial microbes or applying their active metabolites may prove to be a worthwhile prevention or treatment strategy. Fully realizing this strategy requires a more detailed understanding of the variability of the skin microbiota, the link between specific taxa and disease, and the effect of certain taxa on the immune system and the microbiome as a whole.

Acknowledgments We thank David Nelson for critical reading of this chapter.

References

Abrahamsson TR, Jakobsson HE, Andersson AF, Bjorksten B, Engstrand L, Jenmalm MC (2012) Low diversity of the gut microbiota in infants with atopic eczema. J Allergy Clin Immunol 129:434–440, 440 e431–e432

Alekseyenko AV, Perez-Perez GI, De Souza A, Strober B, Gao Z, Bihan M, Li K, Methe BA, Blaser MJ (2013) Community differentiation of the cutaneous microbiota in psoriasis. Microbiome 1:31

Ayer J, Burrows N (2006) Acne: more than skin deep. Postgrad Med J 82:500–506

Bek-Thomsen M, Lomholt HB, Kilian M (2008) Acne is not associated with yet-uncultured bacteria. J Clin Microbiol 46:3355–3360

Berg M, Liden S (1989) An epidemiological study of rosacea. Acta Derm Venereol 69:419–423

Blaser MJ, Dominguez-Bello MG, Contreras M, Magris M, Hidalgo G, Estrada I, Gao Z, Clemente JC, Costello EK, Knight R (2013) Distinct cutaneous bacterial assemblages in a sampling of South American Amerindians and US residents. ISME J 7:85–95

Capone KA, Dowd SE, Stamatas GN, Nikolovski J (2011) Diversity of the human skin microbiome early in life. J Invest Dermatol 131:2026–2032

Casas C, Paul C, Lahfa M, Livideanu B, Lejeune O, Alvarez-Georges S, Saint-Martory C, Degouy A, Mengeaud V, Ginisty H, Durbise E, Schmitt AM, Redoules D (2012) Quantification of Demodex folliculorum by PCR in rosacea and its relationship to skin innate immune activation. Exp Dermatol 21:906–910

Chehoud C, Rafail S, Tyldsley AS, Seykora JT, Lambris JD, Grice EA (2013) Complement modulates the cutaneous microbiome and inflammatory milieu. Proc Natl Acad Sci USA 110:15061–15066

Christophers E (2001) Psoriasis—epidemiology and clinical spectrum. Clin Exp Dermatol 26: 314–320

Clemente JC, Pehrsson EC, Blaser MJ, Sandhu K, Gao Z, Wang B, Magris M, Hidalgo G, Contreras M, Noya-Alarcon O, Lander O, McDonald J, Cox M, Walter J, Oh PL, Ruiz JF, Rodriguez S, Shen N, Song SJ, Metcalf J, Knight R, Dantas G, Dominguez-Bello MG (2015) The microbiome of uncontacted Amerindians. Sci Adv 1:e1500183

Cogen AL, Yamasaki K, Sanchez KM, Dorschner RA, Lai Y, MacLeod DT, Torpey JW, Otto M, Nizet V, Kim JE, Gallo RL (2010) Selective antimicrobial action is provided by phenol-soluble modulins derived from *Staphylococcus epidermidis*, a normal resident of the skin. J Invest Dermatol 130:192–200

Cogen AL, Walker SL, Roberts CH, Hagge DA, Neupane KD, Khadge S, Lockwood DN (2012) Human beta-defensin 3 is up-regulated in cutaneous leprosy type 1 reactions. PLoS Negl Trop Dis 6:e1869

Costello EK, Lauber CL, Hamady M, Fierer N, Gordon JI, Knight R (2009) Bacterial community variation in human body habitats across space and time. Science 326:1694–1697

Crawford GH, Pelle MT, James WD (2004) Rosacea: I. Etiology, pathogenesis, and subtype classification. J Am Acad Dermatol 51:327–341; quiz 342–344

Dahl MV, Ross AJ, Schlievert PM (2004) Temperature regulates bacterial protein production: possible role in rosacea. J Am Acad Dermatol 50:266–272

Decreau RA, Marson CM, Smith KE, Behan JM (2003) Production of malodorous steroids from androsta-5,16-dienes and androsta-4,16-dienes by Corynebacteria and other human axillary bacteria. J Steroid Biochem Mol Biol 87:327–336

Dominguez-Bello MG, Costello EK, Contreras M, Magris M, Hidalgo G, Fierer N, Knight R (2010) Delivery mode shapes the acquisition and structure of the initial microbiota across multiple body habitats in newborns. Proc Natl Acad Sci USA 107:11971–11975

Drake DR, Brogden KA, Dawson DV, Wertz PW (2008) Thematic review series: skin lipids. Antimicrobial lipids at the skin surface. J Lipid Res 49:4–11

Elias PM (2007) The skin barrier as an innate immune element. Semin Immunopathol 29:3–14

Fahlen A, Engstrand L, Baker BS, Powles A, Fry L (2012) Comparison of bacterial microbiota in skin biopsies from normal and psoriatic skin. Arch Dermatol Res 304:15–22

Fernandez-Obregon A, Patton DL (2007) The role of Chlamydia pneumoniae in the etiology of acne rosacea: response to the use of oral azithromycin. Cutis 79:163–167

Fierer N, Hamady M, Lauber CL, Knight R (2008) The influence of sex, handedness, and washing on the diversity of hand surface bacteria. Proc Natl Acad Sci USA 105:17994–17999

Findley K, Oh J, Yang J, Conlan S, Deming C, Meyer JA, Schoenfeld D, Nomicos E, Park M, Program NIHISCCS, Kong HH, Segre JA (2013) Topographic diversity of fungal and bacterial communities in human skin. Nature 498:367–370

Fitz-Gibbon S, Tomida S, Chiu BH, Nguyen L, Du C, Liu M, Elashoff D, Erfe MC, Loncaric A, Kim J, Modlin RL, Miller JF, Sodergren E, Craft N, Weinstock GM, Li H (2013) Propionibacterium acnes strain populations in the human skin microbiome associated with acne. J Invest Dermatol 133:2152–2160

Foolad N, Brezinski EA, Chase EP, Armstrong AW (2013) Effect of nutrient supplementation on atopic dermatitis in children: a systematic review of probiotics, prebiotics, formula, and fatty acids. JAMA Dermatol 149:350–355

Foulongne V, Sauvage V, Hebert C, Dereure O, Cheval J, Gouilh MA, Pariente K, Segondy M, Burguiere A, Manuguerra JC, Caro V, Eloit M (2012) Human skin microbiota: high diversity of DNA viruses identified on the human skin by high throughput sequencing. PLoS ONE 7: e38499

Fry L, Baker BS, Powles AV, Fahlen A, Engstrand L (2013) Is chronic plaque psoriasis triggered by microbiota in the skin? Br J Dermatol 169:47–52

Fuchs-Tarlovsky V, Marquez-Barba MF, Sriram K (2015) Probiotics in dermatologic practice. Nutrition 32:289–295

Gallo RL, Nakatsuji T (2011) Microbial symbiosis with the innate immune defense system of the skin. J Invest Dermatol 131:1974–1980

Gao Z, Tseng CH, Pei Z, Blaser MJ (2007) Molecular analysis of human forearm superficial skin bacterial biota. Proc Natl Acad Sci USA 104:2927–2932

Gao Z, Tseng CH, Strober BE, Pei Z, Blaser MJ (2008) Substantial alterations of the cutaneous bacterial biota in psoriatic lesions. PLoS ONE 3:e2719

Ghinai R, El-Duah P, Chi KH, Pillay A, Solomon AW, Bailey RL, Agana N, Mabey DC, Chen CY, Adu-Sarkodie Y, Marks M (2015) A cross-sectional study of 'yaws' in districts of ghana which have previously undertaken azithromycin mass drug administration for trachoma control. PLoS Negl Trop Dis 9:e0003496

Grice EA (2014) The skin microbiome: potential for novel diagnostic and therapeutic approaches to cutaneous disease. Semin Cutan Med Surg 33:98–103

Grice EA, Segre JA (2011) The skin microbiome. Nat Rev Microbiol 9:244–253

Grice EA, Kong HH, Renaud G, Young AC, Bouffard GG, Blakesley RW, Wolfsberg TG, Turner ML, Segre JA (2008) A diversity profile of the human skin microbiota. Genome Res 18:1043–1050

Grice EA, Kong HH, Conlan S, Deming CB, Davis J, Young AC, Program NCS, Bouffard GG, Blakesley RW, Murray PR, Green ED, Turner ML, Segre JA (2009) Topographical and temporal diversity of the human skin microbiome. Science 324:1190–1192

Grice EA, Snitkin ES, Yockey LJ, Bermudez DM, Program NCS, Liechty KW, Segre JA (2010) Longitudinal shift in diabetic wound microbiota correlates with prolonged skin defense response. Proc Natl Acad Sci USA 107:14799–14804

Hannigan GD, Meisel JS, Tyldsley AS, Zheng Q, Hodkinson BP, SanMiguel AJ, Minot S, Bushman FD, Grice EA (2015) The human skin double-stranded DNA virome: topographical and temporal diversity, genetic enrichment, and dynamic associations with the host microbiome. MBio 6:e01578-15

Holmes AD (2013) Potential role of microorganisms in the pathogenesis of rosacea. J Am Acad Dermatol 69:1025–1032

Horton JM, Gao Z, Sullivan DM, Shopsin B, Perez-Perez GI, Blaser MJ (2015) The cutaneous microbiome in outpatients presenting with acute skin abscesses. J Infect Dis 211:1895–1904

Huang JT, Abrams M, Tlougan B, Rademaker A, Paller AS (2009) Treatment of *Staphylococcus aureus* colonization in atopic dermatitis decreases disease severity. Pediatrics 123:e808–e814

Iwase T, Uehara Y, Shinji H, Tajima A, Seo H, Takada K, Agata T, Mizunoe Y (2010) *Staphylococcus epidermidis* Esp inhibits *Staphylococcus aureus* biofilm formation and nasal colonization. Nature 465:346–349

Janowicz DM, Ofner S, Katz BP, Spinola SM (2009) Experimental infection of human volunteers with *Haemophilus ducreyi*: fifteen years of clinical data and experience. J Infect Dis 199: 1671–1679

Kong HH, Oh J, Deming C, Conlan S, Grice EA, Beatson MA, Nomicos E, Polley EC, Komarow HD, Program NCS, Murray PR, Turner ML, Segre JA (2012) Temporal shifts in the skin microbiome associated with disease flares and treatment in children with atopic dermatitis. Genome Res 22:850–859

Lacey N, Delaney S, Kavanagh K, Powell FC (2007) Mite-related bacterial antigens stimulate inflammatory cells in rosacea. Br J Dermatol 157:474–481

Lai Y, Di Nardo A, Nakatsuji T, Leichtle A, Yang Y, Cogen AL, Wu ZR, Hooper LV, Schmidt RR, von Aulock S, Radek KA, Huang CM, Ryan AF, Gallo RL (2009) Commensal bacteria regulate Toll-like receptor 3-dependent inflammation after skin injury. Nat Med 15:1377–1382

Lai Y, Cogen AL, Radek KA, Park HJ, Macleod DT, Leichtle A, Ryan AF, Di Nardo A, Gallo RL (2010) Activation of TLR2 by a small molecule produced by *Staphylococcus epidermidis* increases antimicrobial defense against bacterial skin infections. J Invest Dermatol 130: 2211–2221

Leung DY, Travers JB, Giorno R, Norris DA, Skinner R, Aelion J, Kazemi LV, Kim MH, Trumble AE, Kotb M et al (1995) Evidence for a streptococcal superantigen-driven process in acute guttate psoriasis. J Clin Invest 96:2106–2112

Leyden JJ, Del Rosso JQ (2011) Oral antibiotic therapy for acne vulgaris: pharmacokinetic and pharmacodynamic perspectives. J Clin Aesthetic Dermatol 4:40–47

Leyden JJ, McGinley KJ, Mills OH, Kligman AM (1975) Propionibacterium levels in patients with and without acne vulgaris. J Invest Dermatol 65:382–384

Marks M, Chi KH, Vahi V, Pillay A, Sokana O, Pavluck A, Mabey DC, Chen CY, Solomon AW (2014) *Haemophilus ducreyi* associated with skin ulcers among children, Solomon Islands. Emerg Infect Dis 20:1705–1707

Meisel JS, Hannigan GD, Tyldsley AS, SanMiguel AJ, Hodkinson BP, Zheng Q, Grice EA (2016) Skin microbiome surveys are strongly influenced by experimental design. J Invest Dermatol 136:947–956

Mitjà O, Lukehart SA, Pokowas G, Moses P, Kapa A, Godornes C, Robson J, Cherian S, Houinei W, Kazadi W, Siba P, de Lazzari E, Bassat Q (2014) *Haemophilus ducreyi* as a cause of skin ulcers in children from a yaws-endemic area of Papua New Guinea: a prospective cohort study. Lancet Glob Health 2:e235–e241

Moran GJ, Krishnadasan A, Gorwitz RJ, Fosheim GE, McDougal LK, Carey RB, Talan DA, Group EMINS (2006) Methicillin-resistant *S. aureus* infections among patients in the emergency department. N Engl J Med 355:666–674

Naik S, Bouladoux N, Wilhelm C, Molloy MJ, Salcedo R, Kastenmuller W, Deming C, Quinones M, Koo L, Conlan S, Spencer S, Hall JA, Dzutsev A, Kong H, Campbell DJ, Trinchieri G, Segre JA, Belkaid Y (2012) Compartmentalized control of skin immunity by resident commensals. Science 337:1115–1119

Nakatsuji T, Chiang HI, Jiang SB, Nagarajan H, Zengler K, Gallo RL (2013) The microbiome extends to subepidermal compartments of normal skin. Nat Commun 4:1431

Numata S, Akamatsu H, Akaza N, Yagami A, Nakata S, Matsunaga K (2014) Analysis of facial skin-resident microbiota in Japanese acne patients. Dermatology 228:86–92

Oh J, Conlan S, Polley EC, Segre JA, Kong HH (2012) Shifts in human skin and nares microbiota of healthy children and adults. Genome Med 4:77

Oh J, Freeman AF, Program NCS, Park M, Sokolic R, Candotti F, Holland SM, Segre JA, Kong HH (2013) The altered landscape of the human skin microbiome in patients with primary immunodeficiencies. Genome Res 23:2103–2114

Oh J, Byrd AL, Deming C, Conlan S, Program NCS, Kong HH, Segre JA (2014) Biogeography and individuality shape function in the human skin metagenome. Nature 514:59–64

Pedulla ML, Ford ME, Houtz JM, Karthikeyan T, Wadsworth C, Lewis JA, Jacobs-Sera D, Falbo J, Gross J, Pannunzio NR, Brucker W, Kumar V, Kandasamy J, Keenan L, Bardarov S, Kriakov J, Lawrence JG, Jacobs WR Jr, Hendrix RW, Hatfull GF (2003) Origins of highly mosaic mycobacteriophage genomes. Cell 113:171–182

Picardo M, Ottaviani M (2014) Skin microbiome and skin disease: the example of rosacea. J Clin Gastroenterol 48(Suppl 1):S85–S86

Salter SJ, Cox MJ, Turek EM, Calus ST, Cookson WO, Moffatt MF, Turner P, Parkhill J, Loman NJ, Walker AW (2014) Reagent and laboratory contamination can critically impact sequence-based microbiome analyses. BMC Biol 12:87

Scholz F, Badgley BD, Sadowsky MJ, Kaplan DH (2014) Immune mediated shaping of microflora community composition depends on barrier site. PLoS ONE 9:e84019

Smeekens SP, Huttenhower C, Riza A, van de Veerdonk FL, Zeeuwen PL, Schalkwijk J, van der Meer JW, Xavier RJ, Netea MG, Gevers D (2014) Skin microbiome imbalance in patients with STAT1/STAT3 defects impairs innate host defense responses. J Innate Immun 6:253–262

Staudinger T, Pipal A, Redl B (2011) Molecular analysis of the prevalent microbiota of human male and female forehead skin compared to forearm skin and the influence of make-up. J Appl Microbiol 110:1381–1389

Toshkova K, Annemuller C, Akineden O, Lammler C (2001) The significance of nasal carriage of Staphylococcus aureus as risk factor for human skin infections. FEMS Microbiol Lett 202: 17–24

Tuzun Y, Keskin S, Kote E (2010) The role of Helicobacter pylori infection in skin diseases: facts and controversies. Clin Dermatol 28:478–482

Uehara Y, Nakama H, Agematsu K, Uchida M, Kawakami Y, Abdul Fattah AS, Maruchi N (2000) Bacterial interference among nasal inhabitants: eradication of *Staphylococcus aureus* from nasal cavities by artificial implantation of *Corynebacterium* sp. J Hosp Infect 44:127–133

van Rensburg JJ, Lin H, Gao X, Toh E, Fortney KR, Ellinger S, Zwickl B, Janowicz DM, Katz BP, Nelson DE, Dong Q, Spinola SM (2015) The human skin microbiome associates with the outcome of and is influenced by bacterial infection. MBio 6:e01315-15

Wang Y, Kuo S, Shu M, Yu J, Huang S, Dai A, Two A, Gallo RL, Huang CM (2014) *Staphylococcus epidermidis* in the human skin microbiome mediates fermentation to inhibit the growth of Propionibacterium acnes: implications of probiotics in acne vulgaris. Appl Microbiol Biotechnol 98:411–424

Yamasaki K, Di Nardo A, Bardan A, Murakami M, Ohtake T, Coda A, Dorschner RA, Bonnart C, Descargues P, Hovnanian A, Morhenn VB, Gallo RL (2007) Increased serine protease activity and cathelicidin promotes skin inflammation in rosacea. Nat Med 13:975–980

Yamasaki K, Kanada K, Macleod DT, Borkowski AW, Morizane S, Nakatsuji T, Cogen AL, Gallo RL (2011) TLR2 expression is increased in rosacea and stimulates enhanced serine protease production by keratinocytes. J Invest Dermatol 131:688–697

Zeeuwen PL, Boekhorst J, van den Bogaard EH, de Koning HD, van de Kerkhof PM, Saulnier DM, van Swam II, van Hijum SA, Kleerebezem M, Schalkwijk J, Timmerman HM (2012) Microbiome dynamics of human epidermis following skin barrier disruption. Genome Biol 13:R101

Chapter 19
Sensing Environmental Factors: The Emerging Role of Receptors in Epidermal Homeostasis and Whole-Body Health

Mitsuhiro Denda

Abstract Epidermal keratinocytes have been recognized to form the water-impermeable structure and this barrier function is critical, especially for terrestrial animals. However, recent findings have dramatically changed the picture of epidermal keratinocytes, placing them at the forefront of the sensory system. Keratinocytes contains environmental sensors and a sensory information-processing system, and it generates a variety of hormones and neurotransmitters that influence whole-body states and emotions. Specifically, epidermal keratinocytes contain sensors of mechanical stress, temperature and chemical stimuli. Moreover, all the components of the hypothalamo-pituitary-adrenal (HPA) axis appear to be present in epidermal keratinocytes. These results suggest that the epidermis plays an important role in adapting whole-body physiology, and probably also emotional response, to changing environments.

Keywords Keratinocyte · Stratum corneum · Neurotransmitter

19.1 Introduction

In humans, the epidermis is the outermost part of the skin, and consists predominantly of keratinocytes, which differentiate as they move from the basal layer to the surface, from which dead keratinocytes (corneocytes) are finally lost by desquamation. The outermost layer of the epidermis (stratum corneum), which consists of corneocytes and intercellular lipids, serves as a water-impermeable barrier, protecting the organism against environmental dryness, as well as chemicals, ultraviolet light, mechanical stress and infectious agents. Other terrestrial vertebrates have a variety of skin coverings, such as scales in the case of reptiles, feathers on birds,

M. Denda (✉)
Japan Science and Technology Agency, CREST, Kawaguchi, Japan
e-mail: mitsuhiro.denda@to.shiseido.co.jp

M. Denda
Shiseido Research Center, Yokohama, Japan

G.T. Wondrak (ed.), *Skin Stress Response Pathways*,
DOI 10.1007/978-3-319-43157-4_19

and hair on most mammals, that may have a skin-protective function. On the other hand, humans have famously been called 'naked apes'. So, might there be an evolutionary advantage to this situation?

It is noteworthy that aquatic cnidarians (such as jellyfish) have sensory systems and dispersed nerve systems on the surface of their body. Thus, it is plausible that sensory systems on the skin surface provide a survival advantage, at least in the aqueous environment. Similarly, the presence of sophisticated sensory systems located close to the skin surface in humans, protected only by the stratum corneum consisting of 15–20 layers of corneocytes, might also be advantageous for sensitively detecting and rapidly responding to changes in the terrestrial environment. Indeed, we have demonstrated that multiple sensory systems are functionally expressed in human epidermal keratinocytes. Some are associated with homeostasis of the epidermal water-impermeable barrier, but others respond to a broad range of environmental factors. We also found a series of neurotransmitter receptors, which are known to play key roles in information processing in nerve systems, including the brain. Moreover, we demonstrated that various hormones and neuropeptides that can potentially influence whole-body physiology and emotion, are generated and released from epidermal keratinocytes. This situation is actually quite reasonable, because both neural systems and epidermis are originally derived from ectoderm at an early stage of development.

These discoveries led us to hypothesize that multiple receptors expressed in epidermal keratinocytes play an important role not only in epidermal homeostasis, but also in whole-body physiological responses, including emotion. In this chapter, I would like to introduce these receptors, and discuss the potential roles of the epidermis as an active interface between our body and the environment.

19.2 Effects of Environmental Factors on Epidermal Keratinocytes and Candidate Receptors Mediating These Effects

19.2.1 The Transient Receptor Potential (TRP) Receptor Family as a Sensory System for Temperature and Chemical Factors

A series of receptors named the transient receptor potential (TRP) family, the members of which are activated at defined temperatures, have been cloned in the past two decades. These receptors were first discovered in the nervous system (Dhaka et al. 2006). However, several thermo-sensitive TRP receptors were subsequently found to be expressed in epidermal keratinocytes (Denda and Tsutsumi 2011). We first discovered the expression and function of TRPV1 (VR1) in epidermal keratinocytes (Denda et al. 2001; Inoue et al. 2002). TPRV1 is activated by heat (>43 °C), acidic basic pH and capsaicin (Caterina et al. 1997; Dhaka et al. 2009). TRPV3 and TRPV4,

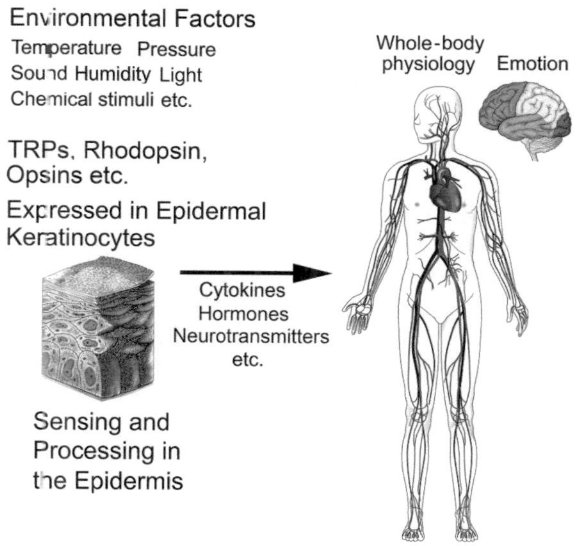

Fig. 19.1 Schematic illustration of the putative roles of epidermal keratinocytes. Epidermal keratinocytes sense a variety of environmental factors via a series of receptors, and environmental information from these receptors is processed in the epidermis, leading to release of effector molecules that may influence whole-body and brain homeostasis

which are both activated by heat (at around 30–40 °C), were also found in keratinocytes (Peier et al. 2002a; Chung et al. 2003) (Fig. 19.1).

Two cold-sensitive proteins, TRPA1 and TRPM8, which are activated by low temperature, have been cloned from peripheral nerve cells (Story et al. 2003; Peier et al. 2002b). TRPA1 is activated at temperatures lower than 17 °C and TRPM8 is activated at temperatures lower than 22 °C. Both of them are also functionally expressed in human epidermal keratinocytes (Tsutsumi et al. 2010; Denda et al. 2010a, b) We also reported expression of TRPV2, which is activated at temperatures above 52 °C (Tsutsumi et al. 2011).

Interestingly, some of the TRPs are associated with epidermal barrier homeostasis. To evaluate the influence of these receptors on barrier homeostasis, we kept hairless mouse skin and human skin at various temperatures immediately after tape stripping. At temperatures from 36 to 40 °C, barrier recovery was accelerated in both cases compared with that at 34 °C. At 34 or 42 °C, barrier recovery was delayed. Topical application of 4αPDD, a specific TRPV4 agonist, accelerated barrier recovery, while ruthenium red, a TRPV4 blocker, delayed barrier recovery. Capsaicin, a TRPV1 activator, delayed barrier recovery, while capsazepin, a TRPV1 antagonist, blocked this delay (Denda et al. 2007a, b).

We also examined the effects of topical application of TRPA1 agonists and brief cold exposure on the barrier recovery rate after barrier disruption (Denda et al. 2010a). Topical application of a TRPA1 agonist, allyl isothiocyanate or cinnamaldehyde, accelerated barrier recovery after tape stripping. The effects of both agonists were blocked by HC030031, an antagonist of TRPA1. Brief exposure (1 min) to cold (10–15 °C) also accelerated barrier recovery and this acceleration was also blocked by HC030031.

We next examined the effect of topical application of TRPM8 modulators on epidermal permeability barrier homeostasis (Denda et al. 2010b). Topical application of TRPM8 agonists, menthol and WS 12, accelerated barrier recovery after tape stripping. The effect of WS12 was blocked by Ruthenium Red, a non-selective TRP antagonist, and by BTCT, a TRPM8-specific antagonist. Topical application of WS12 also reduced epidermal proliferation associated with barrier disruption under low humidity, and this effect was blocked by BTCT. Overall, our results indicate that these TRPs expressed in epidermal keratinocytes play a role in epidermal permeability barrier homeostasis.

It has been reported that activation of TRP on keratinocytes induced generation and release of prostaglandin (Huang et al. 2008). Moreover, a recent study suggested that TRPV1 expressed in keratinocytes plays an important role in acute nociception-related pain (Pang et al. 2015). Thus, TRPs expressed on keratinocytes might be associated with a variety of patho-physiological conditions of whole skin.

19.2.2 Keratinocytes as a Sensory System Responsive to Mechanical Stimuli and Their Influence on Peripheral Circulation

It had long been believed that nerve endings in the dermis are involved in tactile sensation. However, although pressure points are located with a separation of millimeter order of magnitude, our fingertips can recognize micron- or even nanometer-scale patterns (Nakatani et al. 2011). Thus, we hypothesized that individual keratinocytes play a role in tactile sensation.

We first evaluated the changes of intracellular calcium concentration ($[Ca^{2+}]_i$) of cultured keratinocytes in response to external hydraulic pressure (Goto et al. 2010). First, we compared the responses of undifferentiated and differentiated keratinocytes with those of fibroblasts, vascular endothelial cells and lymphatic endothelial cells. Calcium propagation extended over a larger area and continued for a longer period of time in differentiated keratinocytes, as compared to the other cells. The response of the keratinocytes was dramatically reduced when the cells were incubated in medium without calcium. These results suggested that a mechano-sensitive calcium channel expressed in keratinocytes might play an important role in tactile sensation.

We next studied the intracellular calcium responses of individual cultured human keratinocytes, fibroblasts, endothelial cells, and neurons from dorsal root ganglion to air pressure. The $[Ca^{2+}]_i$ of differentiated keratinocytes was changed significantly when the pressure was increased, remained at the same level for a while, and then decreased, whereas undifferentiated keratinocytes and other cells derived from skin or dorsal root ganglion showed no response. The threshold of air pressure increase from the original level for inducing $[Ca^{2+}]_i$ response was 5–20 hPa (Ikeyama et al. 2013).

The keratinocyte receptors that respond to mechanical stimuli have not yet been identified. It has been suggested that TRPV4 and/or TRPA1 might be activated by mechanical stimuli (Dhaka et al. 2006), but we could not confirm any relationship between mechanical stimuli and these TRPs expressed in keratinocytes.

On the other hand, we studied the effects of mechanical stimulation on nitric oxide (NO) synthesis and release from epidermal keratinocytes and its influence on the cutaneous circulation (Ikeyama et al. 2007, 2010). Mechanical stimulation resulted in NO release from a skin organ culture. NO release also occurred from a reconstructed skin model containing only keratinocytes and fibroblasts, and was suppressed after detachment of the epidermal layer. Moreover, stimulation-induced NO release was significantly lower in skin organ culture of neuronal NO synthase knockout (nNOS-KO) mice, compared with wild-type (WT) mice. Mechanical stimulation of skin organ cultures of WT, nNOS-KO, endothelial NOS-KO (eNOS-KO) and WT mice caused enlargement of cutaneous lymphatic vessels. The degree of enlargement was significantly decreased after detachment of the epidermal layer, and was significantly lower for nNOS-KO than for WT mice. Skin blood flow in nNOS-KO mice after stimulation was significantly lower than in WT mice. eNOS-KO mice also showed lower responses than WT mice, and the difference was similar to that in the case of nNOS-KO mice. These results suggested that NO generated by nNOS expressed in the epidermis influences the cutaneous circulatory response to mechanical stimulation.

19.2.3 Responses to Humidity Changes

Seasonal changes affect the condition of normal skin and may trigger various cutaneous disorders (Wilkinson and Rycroft 1992; Sauer and Hall 1996). We demonstrated that low humidity stimulates epidermal DNA synthesis and amplifies the hyperproliferative response to barrier disruption (Denda et al. 1998a). The morphology of the stratum corneum is also influenced by dry environments (Denda et al. 1998b; Sato et al. 2000). When animals were kept in a dry condition for more than 1 week, barrier function was enhanced (Denda et al.1998b). On the other hand, a drastic decrease of environmental humidity induced barrier abnormality (Sato et al. 2002), and a decrease in the water retention capacity of the stratum corneum (Katagiri et al. 2003). Ashida et al. found an increase of IL-1α in the epidermis (Ashida et al. 2001a) and an increase of histamine and mast cells in the dermis (Ashida et al. 2001b) in a dry environment. Allergic response was also enhanced (Hosoi et al. 2000).

We investigated the signaling system of epidermal keratinocytes in response to low humidity, and found that calcium propagation was induced by exposure of cultured human keratinocytes to air (Denda and Denda 2007). A transient increase of intracellular calcium concentration, $[Ca^{2+}]_i$, was induced, followed by a wave-like increase in adjacent unexposed keratinocytes, which showed oscillations of $[Ca^{2+}]_i$ with a frequency that varied from cell to cell. The increase of $[Ca^{2+}]_i$ did not appear when calcium was removed from the medium or in the presence of suramin, a purinergic receptor antagonist. The ATP concentration also increased immediately after keratinocytes were exposed to air. Thus, we speculated that ATP is secreted from keratinocytes upon exposure to air, and induces an increase of intracellular calcium concentration. The receptor involved has not been identified, though it has been suggested that TRPV4 is a sensor of osmotic pressure (Liedtke 2007).

19.2.4 Responses to Visible Radiation

The effects of ultraviolet or infrared radiation on skin are well known, but relatively little is known about the effect of visible light. We showed that visible light influenced the epidermal barrier recovery rate after disruption (Denda and Fuziwara 2008). Irradiation with red light significantly accelerated the barrier recovery, while irradiation with blue light delayed it, compared with the control. White or green light did not affect the barrier recovery rate. An electron-microscopic study suggested that red light accelerated lamellar body secretion, while blue light blocked it. These results indicate that visible radiation influences skin barrier homeostasis, i.e., epidermal keratinocytes appear to have a sensory system for visible radiation.

Rhodopsin is a well-known photosensitive protein present in rod cells of the retina, and detects light/dark contrast. Cone opsins are photosensitive receptors in cone cells of the retina, and detect color. We found that these proteins are expressed in human epidermis (Tsutsumi et al. 2009a). Since transducin and phosphodiesterase 6 play key roles in signal transmission in the retina, we hypothesized that these proteins might also be present in epidermal keratinocytes and be associated with barrier homeostasis. First, we confirmed the expression of both transducin and phosphodiesterase 6 in epidermal keratinocytes (Goto et al. 2011). Topical application of zaprinast, a specific inhibitor of phosphodiesterases 5 and 6, blocked the acceleration of barrier recovery by red light, while T0156, a specific inhibitor of phosphodiesterase 5, had no effect. These results indicate that phosphodiesterase 6 is involved in the recovery-accelerating effect of red light on the disrupted epidermal permeability barrier, and suggest that epidermal keratinocytes have a similar energy conversion system to the retina.

In our studies described above, we focused on the effect of visible light on epidermal barrier homeostasis. However, several other reports have described non-visual photoreceptors. Reptiles have photoreceptors in the brain, and they form the parietal eye (Solessio and Engbretson 1993). Several photoreceptors were found in pineal body of chicken and rat (Okano et al. 1994; Zhao et al. 1997). However, in humans, the pineal body is located in a deeper area of the brain. On the other hand, exposure to bright light was shown to influence the circadian rhythm of blind patients (Czeisler et al. 1995). This result supports the idea that a photo-sensitive system exists on the surface of the human body. Thus, visible light might influence endocrinological condition via photoreceptor proteins and the energy transduction system in epidermal keratinocytes.

19.2.5 *Responses to Sound*

The frequency range of audible acoustic sound for adult humans is approximately 20–16000 Hz (Heffner 2004). However, Oohashi and his coworkers demonstrated that ultrasound at a frequency above 20000 Hz (20 kHz) influences human brain electrical activity and systemic hormonal levels (Oohashi et al. 2000, 2006; Kawai et al. 2001; Yagi et al. 2003). Interestingly, these effects did not occur via the ears (Oohashi et al. 2006). On the other hand, a recent study demonstrated that a slight, inaudible puff of air on the skin influenced auditory perception (Gick and Derrick 2009). These findings suggested that a so-far-unidentified system that is responsive to ultrasound exists at the human body surface. Based on the above findings, we speculated that audible or inaudible sound frequencies might influence epidermal barrier homeostasis.

To test this idea, we first evaluated the effects of 5, 10, 20 and 30 kHz sound on intact skin of hairless mice (Denda and Nakatani 2010). We disrupted the permeability barrier by tape stripping and immediately exposed the skin to sound for one hour. The speaker cone lightly touched one side of the flank, and we attached a silent speaker cone to the other flank as a control. Application of sound at a frequency of 10, 20 or 30 kHz accelerated barrier recovery, while 5 kHz sound had no effect.

The sound-sensitive receptors of keratinocytes have not been identified. Presumably mechano-sensitive receptor(s) play a role in the ability of skin to sense sound.

19.3 Information Processing in the Epidermis

There is evidence that information processing takes place in the skin (Pruszynski and Johansson 2014). Specifically, when different-shaped molds were pressed on the fingertip, different electrophysiological patterns were observed in the peripheral nerves in the forearm. That is, when we touch a shape, geometrical information might be recognized in the skin.

As already mentioned, epidermal keratinocytes appear to play an important role in tactile sensation. Information derived from the environment is transferred by afferent nerve fibers to the central nervous system, and processed in the brain with the aid of multiple neurotransmitters and specific receptors. We have shown that many of the neurotransmitter receptors originally found in the central nervous system are also expressed in epidermal keratinocytes (Denda et al. 2007a, b). We also showed that neurotransmitters, such as glutamate, dopamine and nitric oxide are released from keratinocytes (Fuziwara et al. 2003, 2005; Ikeyama et al. 2007), and these molecules are candidate messengers from keratinocytes to the nervous system.

In the brain, a spatiotemporally variable electro-physiological pattern is observed on the cortex, and this might represent information processing (Iijima et al. 1996). Interestingly, we also observed distinct spatiotemporal patterns of calcium concentration in monolayer-cultured human keratinocytes after physical or chemical stimulation (Tsutsumi et al. 2009b, 2013; Denda and Tsutsumi 2014). Thus, epidermal keratinocytes might be involved in information processing related to tactile sensation in the skin.

19.4 Signals from Epidermal Keratinocytes to the Whole Body and Brain

The role of the brain is not only information processing, but also control of whole-body homeostasis via signaling mediated by release of molecules such as neuropeptides and hormones. A variety of studies suggest that epidermal keratinocytes might also have a similar role; i.e., signals from epidermal keratinocytes might act on not only whole-body physiology, but also on emotion.

Immediately after barrier disruption, epidermal keratinocytes secrete multiple cytokines, including IL-1α,β, IL-6, TNFα, and INFγ (Wood et al. 1992). For example, skin surface dryness induces IL-1α generation (Ashida et al. 2001a). UVB-exposed keratinocytes secrete ATP, which induces IL-6 release (Inoue et al. 2007). Thus, barrier abnormality, insult or UVB irradiation may lead to release of multiple cytokines from epidermal keratinocytes. This is significant, because elevated serum cytokine levels are associated with impaired mental state, such as depression, in cancer patients (Miller et al. 2009; Capuron and Miller 2011). Also, in patients with severe dermatitis, a large area of skin may be involved, and secretion of cytokines might be sufficient to influence mental state. This idea is consistent with a report that etanercept, a TNFα inhibitor, improved symptoms of depression and fatigue in psoriasis patients (Tyring et al. 2006).

Dermatologists have found a correlation between the severity of atopic dermatitis and the level of patients' depression or anxiety (Hashiro and Okumura 1997; Arima et al. 2005). Sleep disturbance due to itching and concern over appearance might be associated with depression and anxiety. On the other hand, it has also been reported that cortisol plays an important role in depression and post-traumatic stress disorder (PTSD) and might directly affect the hippocampus (Sapolsky 1996; Sorrells et al. 2009).

These studies led us to hypothesize that environmental dryness might induce increased cortisol secretion in the epidermis. Therefore, we incubated a skin-equivalent model under dry (relative humidity less than 10 %) and humid (relative humidity approximately 100 %) conditions for 48 h and evaluated cortisol secretion and mRNA levels of cortisol-related enzymes (steroid 11β-hydroxylase, CYP11B1) and IL-1β. Under the dry condition, cortisol secretion and expression of both CYP11B1 and IL-1β mRNAs were much higher than those under the humid condition. Occlusion of the model with a water-impermeable plastic membrane partially blocked the increases of cortisol secretion and CYP11B1 and IL-1β mRNA expression in the dry condition (Takei et al. 2013). These results suggest that environmental dryness might induce increased cortisol secretion in epidermis of diseased skin characterized by epidermal barrier dysfunction (Denda et al. 2013).

We also found that keratinocytes generate and secrete oxytocin in response to stimulation with a stable ATP analog (Denda et al. 2012). Oxytocin is involved in behavior, memory and social bonding (Ferguson et al 2000; Kirsch et al. 2005). Further, systemic oxytocin infusion reduced repetitive behavior in patients with autism and Asperger's syndrome (Hollander et al 2003). Therefore, oxytocin produced in epidermal keratinocytes could potentially influence mental state.

19.5 Conclusion

Many studies, including ours, over the past decade or so have revealed that epidermal keratinocytes functionally express multiple receptors that respond to a variety of environmental factors. There is also increasing evidence that environmental information is processed in the epidermis and that the keratinocytes generate signals that may influence whole-body homeostasis and emotion in response to the changing environment. Thus, in addition to its protective role, the epidermis also appears to serve as a sophisticated, brain-like interface between our body and the environment. From this standpoint, systematic studies of the epidermis might lead to novel strategies for whole-body healthcare and even mental problems.

References

Arima M, Shimizu Y, Sowa J, Narita T, Nishi I, Iwata N, Ozaki N, Hashimoto S, Matsunaga K (2005) Psychosomatic analysis of atopic dermatitis using a psychological test. J Dermatol 32:160–168

Ashida Y, Ogo M, Denda M (2001a) Epidermal IL-1 alpha generation is amplified at low humidities: Implications for the pathogenesis of inflammatory dermatoses. Br J Dermatol 144:238–243

Ashida Y, Denda M, Hirao T (2001b) Histamine H1 and H2 receptor antagonists accelerate skin barrier repair and prevent epidermal hyperplasia induced by barrier disruption in a dry environment. J Invest Dermatol 116:261–265

Capuron L, Miller AH (2011) Immune system to brain signaling: neuropsychopharmacological implications. Pharmacol Ther 130:226–238

Caterina MJ, Schumacher MA, Tominaga M, Rosen TA, Levine JD, Julius D (1997) The capsaicin receptor: a heat-activated ion channel in the pain pathway. Nature 389:816–824

Chung MK, Lee H, Caterina MJ (2003) Warm temperatures activate TRPV4 in mouse 308 keratinocytes. J Biol Chem 278:32037–32046
Czeisler CA, Shanahan TL, Klerman EB, Martens H, Brotman DJ, Jonathan SE, Klein T, Rizzo JF (1995) Suppression of melatonin secretion in some blind patients by exposure to bright light. N Eng J Med 332:6–11
Denda M, Denda S (2007) Air-exposed keratinocytes exhibited intracellular oscillation. Skin Res Technol 13:195–201
Denda M, Fuziwara S (2008) Visible radiation affects epidermal permeability barrier recovery: selective effects of red and blue light. J Invest Dermatol 128:1335–1336
Denda M, Nakatani M (2010) Acceleration of permeability barrier recovery by exposure of skin to 10-30 kilohertz sound. Br J Dermatol 162:503–507
Denda M, Tsutsumi M (2011) Roles of transient receptor potential proteins (TRPs) in epidermal keratinocytes transient receptor potential channels. Advan Exp Med Biol 704:847–860
Denda M, Tsutsumi M (2014) Possible role of epidermal keratinocytes in the construction of acupuncture meridians. J Acupunct Meridian Stud 7:92–94
Denda M, Sato J, Masuda Y, Tsuchiya T, Koyama J, Kuramoto M, Elias PM, Feingold KR (1998a) Exposure to a dry environment enhances epidermal permeability barrier function. J Invest Dermatol 111:858–863
Denda M, Sato J, Tsuchiya T, Elias PM, Feingold KR (1998b) Low humidity stimulates epidermal DNA synthesis and amplifies the hyperproliferative response to barrier disruption: implication for seasonal exacerbations of inflammatory dermatoses. J Invest Dermatol 111:873–878
Denda M, Fuziwara S, Inoue K, Denda S, Akamatsu H, Tomitaka A, Matsunaga K (2001) Immunoreactivity of VR1 on epidermal keratinocyte of human skin. Biochem Biophys Res Commun 285:1250–1252
Denda M, Nakatani M, Ikeyama K, Tsutsumi M, Denda S (2007a) Epidermal keratinocytes as the forefront of the sensory system. Exp Dermatol 16:157–161
Denda M, Sokabe T, Tominaga T, Tominaga M (2007b) Effects of skin surface temperature on epidermal permeability barrier homeostasis. J Invest Dermatol 127:654–659
Denda M, Tsutsumi M, Goto M, Ikeyama K, Denda S (2010a) Topical application of TRPA1 agonists and brief cold exposure accelerate skin permeability barrier recovery. J Invest Dermatol 130:1942–1945
Denda M, Tsutsumi M, Denda S (2010b) Topical application of TRPM8 agonists accelerates skin permeability barrier recovery and reduces epidermal proliferation induced by barrier insult: the role of cold-sensitive TRP receptors in epidermal permeability barrier homeostasis. Exp Dermatol 19:791–795
Denda S, Takei K, Kumamoto J, Goto M, Tsutsumi M, Denda M (2012) Oxytocin is expressed in epidermal keratinocytes and released upon stimulation with adenosine 5'-[gamma-thio] triphosphate in vitro. Exp Dermatol 21:535–537
Denda M, Takei K, Denda S (2013) How does epidermal pathology interact with mental state? Med Hypothesis 80:194–196
Dhaka A, Viswanath V, Patapoutian A (2006) TRP ion channels and temperature sensation. Ann Rev Neurosci 29:135–161
Dhaka A, Uzzell V, Dubin AE, Mathur J, Petrus M, Bandell M, Patapoutian A (2009) TRPV1 is activated by both acidic and basic pH. J Neurosci 29:153–158
Ferguson JN, Young LJ, Hearn EF (2000) Social amnesia in mice lacking the oxytocin gene. Nat Genet 25:284–288
Fuziwara S, Inoue K, Denda M (2003) NMDA-type glutamate receptor is associated with cutaneous barrier homeostasis. J Invest Dermatol 120:1023–1029
Fuziwara S, Suzuki A, Inoue K, Denda M (2005) Dopamine D2-like receptor agonists accelerate barrier repair and inhibit the epidermal hyperplasia induced by barrier disruption. J Invest Dermatol 125:783–789
Gick B, Derrick D (2009) Aero-tactile integration in speech perception. Nature 462:502–504

Goto M, Ikeyama K, Tsutsumi M, Denda S, Denda M (2010) Calcium ion propagation in cultured keratinocytes and other cells in skin in response to hydraulic pressure stimulation. J Cell Physiol 224:229–233

Goto M, Ikeyama K, Tsutsumi M, Denda S, Denda M (2011) Phosphodiesterase inhibitors block the acceleration of skin permeability barrier repair by red light. Exp Dermatol 20:568–571

Hashiro M, Okumura M (1997) Anxiety, depression and psychosomatic symptoms in patients with atopic dermatitis: comparison with normal controls and among groups of different degrees of severity. J Dermatol Sci 14:63–67

Heffner RS (2004) Primate hearing from a mammalian perspective. Anat Rec A Discov Mol Cell Evol Biol 281:1111–1122

Hollander E, Notny S, Hanratty M (2003) Oxytocin infusion reduces repetitive behaviors in adults with autistic and Asperger's disorders. Neuropsychopharmacology 28:193–198

Hosoi J, Hariya T, Denda M, Tsuchiya T (2000) Regulation of the cutaneous allergic reaction by humidity. Contact Dermatitis 42:81–84

Huang SM, Lee H, Chung MK et al (2008) Overexpressed transient receptor potential vanilloid 3 ion channels in skin keratinocytes modulate pain sensitivity via prostaglandin E2. J Neurosci 28:13727–13737

Iijima T, Witter MP, Ichikawa M, Tominaga T, Kajiwara R, Matsumoto G (1996) Entorhinal-hippocampal interactions revealed by real-time imaging. Science 72:1176–1179

Ikeyama K, Fuziwara S, Denda M (2007) Topical application of neuronal nitric oxide synthase inhibitor accelerates cutaneous barrier recovery and prevents epidermal hyperplasia induced by barrier disruption. J Invest Dermatol 127:1713–1719

Ikeyama K, Denda S, Tsutsumi M, Denda M (2010) Neuronal nitric oxide synthase in epidermis is involved in cutaneous circulatory response to mechanical stimulation. J Invest Dermatol 130:1158–1166

Ikeyama K, Nakatani M, Kumamoto J, Denda M (2013) Distinct intracellular calcium responses of individual cultured human keratinocytes to air pressure changes. Skin Res Tech 19:346–351

Inoue K, Koizumi S, Fuziwara S, Denda S, Inoue K, Denda M (2002) Functional vanilloid receptors in cultured normal human keratinocytes. Biochem Biophys Res Commun 291:124–129

Inoue K, Hosoi J, Denda M (2007) Extracellular ATP has stimulatory effects on the expression and release of IL-6 via purinergic receptors in normal human keratinocytes. J Invest Dermatol 127:362–371

Katagiri C, Sato J, Nomura J, Denda M (2003) Changes in environmental humidity affect the water-holding property of the stratum corneum and its free amino acid content, and the expression of filaggrin in the epidermis of hairless mice. J Dermatol Sci 31:29–35

Kawai N, Honda M, Nakamura S et al (2001) Catecholamines and opioid peptides increase in plasma in humans during possession trances. NeuroReport 12:3419–3423

Kirsch P, Esslinger C, Chen Q (2005) Oxytocin modulates neural circuitry for social cognition and fear in humans. J Neurosci 25:11489–11493

Liedtke W (2007) Role of TRPV ion channels in sensory transduction of osmotic stimuli in mammals. Exp Physiol 92:507–512

Miller AH, Maletic V, Raison CL (2009) Inflammation and its discontents: the role of cytokines in the pathophysiology of major depression. Biol Psychiatry 65:732–741

Nakatani M, Kawasoe T, Denda M (2011) Sex difference in human fingertip recognition of micron-level randomness as unpleasant. Int J Cosmet Sci 33:346–350

Okano T, Yoshizawa T, Fukada Y (1994) Pinopsin is a chicken pineal photoreceptive molecule. Nature 372:94–97

Oohashi T, Nishina E, Honda M et al (2000) Inaudible high-frequency sounds affect brain activity: hypersonic effect. J Neurophysiol 83:3548–3558

Oohashi T, Kawai N, Nishina E et al (2006) The role of biological system other than auditorair-conduction in the emergence of the hypersonic effect. Brain Res 1073–1074:339–347

Pang Z, Sakamoto T, Tiwari V, Kim YS, Yang F, Dong X, Güler AD, Guan Y, Caterina MJ (2015) Selective keratinocyte stimulation is sufficient to evoke nociception in mice. Pain 156:656–665
Peier AM, Moqrich A, Hergarden AC et al (2002a) A trp channel that senses cold stimuli and menthol. Cell 108:705–715
Peier AM, Reeve AJ, Andersson DA, Moqrich A, Earley TJ, Hergarden AC, Story GM, Colley S, Hogenesch JB, McIntyre P, Bevan S, Patapoutian A (2002b) A heat-sensitive TRP channel expressed in keratinocytes. Science 296:2046–2049
Pruszynski JA, Johansson RS (2014) Edge-orientation processing in first-order tactile neurons. Nat Neurosci 17:1404–1409
Sapolsky RM (1996) Why stress is bad for your brain. Science 273:749–750
Sato J, Yanai M, Hirao T, Denda M (2000) Water content and thickness of stratum corneum contribute to skin surface morphology. Arch Dermatol Res 292:412–417
Sato J, Denda M, Chang S, Elias PM, Feingold KR (2002) Abrupt decreases in environmental humidity induce abnormalities in permeability barrier homeostasis. J Invest Dermatol 119:900–904
Sauer GC, Hall JC (1996) Seasonal skin diseases. In: Sauer GC, Hall JC (eds) Manual of skin diseases. Lippincott-Raven, Philadelphia, pp 23–28
Solessio E, Engbretson GA (1993) Antagonistic chromatic mechanisms in photoreceptors of the parietal eye of lizards. Nature 364:442–445
Sorrells SF, Caso JR, Munhoz CD, Sapolsky RM (2009) The stressed CNS: when glucocorticoids aggravate inflammation. Neuron 64:33–39
Story GM, Peier AM, Reeve AJ et al (2003) ANKTM1, a TRP-like channel expressed in nociceptive neurons, is activated by cold temperatures. Cell 112:819–829
Takei K, Denda S, Kumamoto J, Denda M (2013) Low environmental humidity induces synthesis and release of cortisol in an epidermal organotypic culture system. Exp Dermatol 22:662–664
Tsutsumi M, Ikeyama K, Denda S, Nakanishi J, Fuziwara S, Aoki H, Denda M (2009a) Expressions of rod and cone photoreceptor-like proteins in human epidermis. Exp Dermatol 18:567–570
Tsutsumi M, Inoue K, Denda S, Ikeyama K, Goto M, Denda M (2009b) Mechanical-stimulation-evoked calcium waves in proliferating and differentiated human keratinocytes. Cell Tissue Res 338:99–106
Tsutsumi M, Denda S, Ikeyama K, Goto M, Denda M (2010) Exposure to low temperature induces elevation of intracellular calcium in cultured human keratinocytes. J Invest Dermatol 130:1945–1948
Tsutsumi M, Kumamoto J, Denda M (2011) Intracellular calcium response to high temperature is similar in undifferentiated and differentiated cultured human keratinocytes. Exp Dermatol 20:839–840
Tsutsumi M, Goto M, Denda M (2013) Dynamics of intracellular calcium in cultured human keratinocytes after localized cell damage. Exp Dermatol 22:367–369
Tyring S, Gottlieb A, Papp K, Gordon K, Leonardi C, Wang A, Lalla D, Woolley M, Jahreis A, Zitnik R, Cella D, Krishnan R (2006) Etanercept and clinical outcomes, fatigue, and depression in psoriasis: double-blind placebo-controlled randomised phase III trial. Lancet 367:29–35
Wilkinson JD, Rycroft RJ (1992) Contact dermatitis. In: Burton JL, Ebling FJG (eds) Textbook of dermatology, 5th edn. Blackwell Scientific Publications, Oxford, pp 614–615
Wood LC, Jackson SM, Elias PM, Grunfeld C, Feingold KR (1992) Cutaneous barrier perturbation stimulates cytokine production in the epidermis of mice. J Clin Invest 90:482–487
Yagi R, Nishina E, Honda M et al (2003) Modulatory effect of inaudible high-frequency sounds on human acoustic perception. Neurosci Lett 351:191–195
Zhao X, Haeseleer F, Fariss RN, Huang J, Baehr W, Milam AH, Palczewski K (1997) Molecular cloning and localization of rhodopsin kinase in the mammalian pineal. Vis Neurosci 114: 225–232

Chapter 20
The Cutaneous Circadian Clock as a Determinant of Environmental Vulnerability: Molecular Pathways and Chrono-pharmacological Opportunities

Kyongshin Cho, Rajendra P. Gajula, Kenneth I. Porter and Shobhan Gaddameedhi

Abstract Circadian clocks have received consistent attention for decades due to their great potential for elucidating the mechanisms underlying psychiatric and neurodegenerative diseases. More recently, attention has been focused on molecular mechanisms contributing to other health outcomes, especially malignancies. The circadian system is essential for normal cellular homeostasis and maintenance of biological rhythms at cellular and systemic levels. Since circadian regulation has implications in a wide range of physiological functions, disrupted clocks can lead to metabolic diseases, including cancer. In addition, emerging evidence indicates that circadian regulation is critically involved in the pathogenesis of several cutaneous diseases. Solar radiation is the main cause of skin cancer as well as other skin conditions and, coincidentally, it is an important environmental time cue for human circadian rhythms. Moreover, circadian regulation of melatonin production can protect or repair solar UV-induced DNA damage, which has therapeutic prospects for skin cancer owing to endocrine and physiological functions of melatonin. Circadian mechanisms also have multidisciplinary interventions with epigenetic mechanisms in the rhythmic expression of clock genes. Considering the vulnerability of skin cells to environmental changes, skin can be a principal target of current therapeutic approaches based on circadian mechanisms. Therefore, chronotherapeutic intervention studies may yield more clinically meaningful results for curing or preventing cutaneous diseases including skin cancer. In this review, we discuss recent progress in our understanding of skin circadian mechanisms as they are challenged by environmental factors and future directions in designing strategies for chronotherapeutic applications.

K. Cho · R.P. Gajula · K.I. Porter · S. Gaddameedhi (✉)
Experimental and Systems Pharmacology, College of Pharmacy, Spokane, USA
e-mail: shobhan.gaddameedhi@wsu.edu

S. Gaddameedhi
Sleep and Performance Research Center, Washington State University, Spokane, WA 99210, USA

G.T. Wondrak (ed.), *Skin Stress Response Pathways*,
DOI 10.1007/978-3-319-43157-4_20

Keywords Skin · Circadian clock · Circadian rhythm · Clock genes · Ultraviolet radiation · Skin cancer · Circadian disruption · Melatonin · Chronotherapy · Epigenetics

20.1 Circadian Clock

All living organisms interact with the environment that provides fundamental sources for sustaining life on the earth. Light from the sun is one of the energy sources of the planet's ecosystems and shows a 24-h day/night periodicity due to the earth's rotation. In response to this predictable daily cycle, humans and other organisms including plants have evolved the circadian (from the Latin phrase circa diem, meaning about a day) system by which they can coordinate homeostatic processes including photosynthesis and respiration to maintain their growth and metabolism under the influence of solar radiation (Hastings et al. 2007; Mohawk et al. 2012). The circadian rhythm is a self-sustained system that plays important roles in a wide variety of behavioral and physiological adaptations (Mohawk et al. 2012). The circadian clock is an endogenous oscillator that enables organisms to respond appropriately to the daily and seasonally changing environment (Schultz and Kay 2003; Hastings et al. 2007). The circadian rhythmicity arises at molecular to cellular to systemic levels, and ubiquitous circadian mechanisms driven by autonomous biological clocks are closely related to many aspects of cell cycle regulation, DNA damage repair responses and metabolic functions (Sancar et al. 2004, 2015; Takahashi et al. 2008). Basically, the 24-h circadian rhythm is generated through the interplay between external stimuli (environmental zeitgebers) and intrinsic circadian oscillations, and it serves a defensive role to protect organisms against diverse diseases (Sancar et al. 2004; Mohawk et al. 2012). Indeed, circadian rhythmicity has a profound influence on human health; therefore, chronic circadian disturbance exhibits prolonged adverse consequences such as sleep and psychiatric disorders, heart disease, and cancer (Boivin 2000; Mohawk et al. 2012). It is now generally believed that more than 43 % of the genes in a given tissue are circadian-controlled and transcriptionally rhythmic (Zhang et al. 2014), suggesting that circadian disruption may be at least partially responsible for such adverse health consequences (Storch et al. 2002; Scheer et al. 2009; FitzGerald 2014).

20.2 Mammalian Circadian System

In mammals, the circadian system is composed of a hierarchy of functionally interconnected oscillators (central and peripheral clocks) distributed throughout the brain and peripheral tissues (Reppert and Weaver 2002; Mohawk et al. 2012). The central clock is located within the hypothalamic suprachiasmatic nuclei (SCN) as the master circadian pacemaker, orchestrating endogenous circadian rhythms in peripheral tissues (King and Takahashi 2000; Mohawk et al. 2012). The central neural and peripheral tissue clocks are interlocked by transcriptional-translational feedback loops (TTFL) that precisely synchronize their intrinsic circadian oscillators to the daily light/dark cycle through neural and hormonal cues (Reppert and Weaver 2002; Mohawk et al. 2012). Nevertheless, mechanisms that involve the circadian oscillators in both SCN and peripheral tissues are similar, yet the mechanism of such hierarchy in human pathogenesis still remains largely unknown. Light exposure is the most efficient environmental synchronizer of the circadian system, thus, though the circadian rhythmicity is also attributable to other factors such as temperature, locomotor behaviors, metabolites, hormones, and chronotherapeutic interventions, mammalian circadian rhythms are mainly affected by the 24-h ambient light/dark cycle (Smolensky and Peppas 2007; Takahashi et al. 2008; Mohawk et al. 2012).

20.3 Circadian Molecular Pathways

The molecular mechanisms of circadian rhythms have been studied mostly in rodent models, where the cell-based circadian machinery governs rhythmic oscillations by autoregulatory TTFL (King and Takahashi 2000; Shearman et al. 2000). The mammalian circadian clock comprises a series of interlinking positive and negative feedback loops of transcriptional regulation of clock genes which act as activators or repressors, such as circadian locomotor output cycles kaput (*Clock*), brain muscle ARNT-like 1 (*Bmal1*), period circadian protein homolog 1-3 (*Per1-3*), cryptochrome 1-2 (*Cry1-2*), retinoic acid-related orphan receptor (*Ror*), and Rev-erbα (*Nr1d1*) (Huang et al. 2011; Albrecht 2012). The principal CLOCK/BMAL1 activating complex binds to *cis*-acting E-box elements to activate clock-controlled genes, including *Cry* and *Per* genes whose protein products form the CRY/PER repressor complex (Albrecht 2012; Mohawk et al. 2012). Next, the CRY/PER repressor complex actively suppresses the CLOCK/BMAL1 activating complex, resulting in indirectly inhibiting its own synthesis (Albrecht 2012; Mohawk et al. 2012). Additionally, the feedback loop is fine-tuned by a secondary feedback loop composed of the nuclear receptors, ROR and REV-ERBα (Akashi and Takumi 2005; Albrecht 2012). Moreover, the mammalian circadian clock is regulated not only by interconnected post-transcriptional feedback loops but also by post-translational mechanisms involving casein kinase 1 delta and epsilon (CK1δ/ε) and glycogen synthase kinase 3 (GSK3) (Harmer et al. 2001; Lee et al. 2001; Lowrey and Takahashi 2011).

Substantial evidence has accumulated supporting the overall role of circadian rhythms in influencing metabolic and physiological disorders. The recent insights on genetic mouse studies have revealed that the circadian TTFL is a key component of the molecular clock (Albrecht 2012; Mohawk et al. 2012). In mice, homozygous dominant-negative mutation ($Clock^{\Delta19/\Delta19}$) shows disrupted circadian rhythms, leading to increasing susceptibility to metabolic syndrome (Ko and Takahashi 2006; Maury et al. 2010). The mutated CLOCK protein causes forming functionally impaired CLOCK/BMAL1 heterodimers which bind to E-box elements in *Cry* and *Per* genes (Ko and Takahashi 2006; Maury et al. 2010). Mice homozygous for *Bmal1* deletion (Bmal1$^{-/-}$) also exhibit severely disrupted circadian rhythms with characteristic phenotypes, such as aberrant levels of reactive oxygen species which are essential for homeostasis, infertility, arthropathy, and aging (Bunger et al. 2005; Dubrovsky et al. 2010). This suggests that CLOCK and BMAL1 proteins play a crucial role in circadian rhythmicity. However, the circadian rhythm remains functional when any single negative regulator (*Cry1*, *Cry2*, or *Per1*, *Per2* alone) is mutated, but simultaneous defects in both genes result in behavioral and molecular arrhythmicity (Vitaterna et al. 1999; Zheng et al. 2001; Asher and Schibler 2011). These data indicate that compensation or substitution for the function of each mutated clock gene may be absent, partial, or complete for maintaining circadian periodicity, and it may be determined by the presence of alternative pathways (Asher and Schibler 2011; Johnson and Egli 2014).

20.4 Tissue-Specific Expression Patterns of Circadian Genes

The molecular basis for mammalian circadian clocks involves the central, or master, circadian pacemaker located in the SCN of the brain, which is responsible for coordinating peripheral clocks present in other tissues (Huang et al. 2011; Albrecht 2012). This organization of the circadian system helps orchestrating biological oscillators at the organismal level as well as local levels (Albrecht 2012). However, recent studies showed that peripheral tissues have their own autonomous and self-sustained oscillators to generate SCN-independent rhythms (Albrecht 2012). For example, constitutive *Clock* mRNA expression is observed in the SCN, but it is also detected at various levels in the peripheral tissues (Dibner et al. 2010; Mohawk et al. 2012). In addition, the *Ror* family which comprises three members, *Rorα*, *Rorβ*, and *Rorγ* shows variations in gene expression patterns and circadian peak times across different tissues (Jetten and Ueda 2001; Guillaumond et al. 2005). *Rorα* is most specific to the SCN but less specific to peripheral tissues, whereas *Rorβγ* are most specific to peripheral tissues but less specific to the SCN (Jetten and Ueda 2001; Guillaumond et al. 2005). Moreover, RORα-deficient staggerer mice (RORα$^{sg/sg}$) display normal clock gene expression in peripheral tissues, suggesting that RORs affect the expression of molecular clock components in a tissue-dependent manner (Akashi and Takumi 2005; Kang et al. 2007). The way that the expression of clock genes and clock-controlled genes contributes to the amplitude of circadian oscillation can also vary greatly among tissues (Partch et al. 2014). For example, CLOCK-deficient mice (clock$^{-/-}$) show gene-specific and tissue-specific regulation of circadian transcription (Ko and Takahashi 2006).

Whereas CLOCK deficiency displays the critically reduced amplitude of the *Rev-erbα* transcript oscillation in the liver, the deficiency results in the partially affected amplitude of the *Rev-erbα* mRNA oscillation in the SCN (Triqueneaux et al. 2004; Ko and Takahashi 2006). However, CLOCK deficiency less affects *Per1* transcription less, having an almost similar level compared with the wild-type, whereas the deficiency shows a lower *Per1* level in the SCN (Chen et al. 2005; Gery et al. 2006; Ko and Takahashi 2006). Furthermore, *Per2* transcription also displays cell- and tissue-dependent manners by *Clock* gene mutation (Chen et al. 2005; Gery et al. 2006; Ko and Takahashi 2006). Together, these findings imply that the mammalian circadian hierarchy system is much more complicated than our current understanding, and investigating circadian gene expression patterns in gene- and tissue-specific manners is particularly important to understanding the circadian oscillation network at the systems level.

20.5 Circadian Physiological Effects

Circadian clocks are linked intimately with all aspects of physiological and behavioral homeostasis, including sleep-wake cycle, hormone release, body temperature, and cardiovascular function, which is almost certainly relevant for the pathogenesis of diseases, such as cancer, cardiovascular disease, and immune system decline (Laposky et al. 2008; Morris et al. 2012). Given the marked difference in circadian gene expression and phase distribution between tissues, studies comparing two or more tissues suggest that circadian gene expression patterns are regulated in a tissue-specific manner showing little overlap of the transcribed regions (Reppert and Weaver 2002; Lamia et al. 2008). Interestingly, a number of genes associated with circadian expression are preferentially silenced or expressed depending on the type of tissue (Lamia et al. 2008). Since circadian rhythms in peripheral tissues are important for maintaining normal cellular homeostasis, circadian fluctuations in the degree of both core clock genes and clock-controlled genes are believed to play an important role in the transcriptional and post-transcriptional control of metabolism in response to a wide variety of stress conditions (Albrecht 2012; Mohawk et al. 2012).

Circadian rhythm sleep disorder (CRSD) in humans is a clear example of how circadian regulation impacts physiology and metabolism, particularly in the context of specific sleep disorders including delayed and advanced sleep phase syndromes and free-running disorder (Dagan 2002; Sack et al. 2007). A number of animal studies have shown that CRSD is linked to mutations in circadian genes, resulting in altered sleep homeostatic features such as irregular sleep time and sleep fragmentation, lack of adequate sleep compensation, and sleep deprivation (Dagan 2002; Sack et al. 2007). These findings indicate that circadian gene expression is a key regulator conferring the susceptibility to sleep disorders and sleep homeostasis.

Circadian regulation of clock gene expression also underlies a variety of metabolic pathways, which reveals that circadian rhythms regulate metabolic regulation affecting the susceptibility to metabolic disorders (Mohawk et al. 2012). For example, *Clock* gene mutation in mice mediates changes in food intake and causes obesity and metabolic syndrome including hepatic steatosis, hyperlipidemia, hyperglycemia, and hypoinsulinemia (Zvonic et al. 2007; Takahashi et al. 2008). Moreover, BMAL1 deficiency in mice induces obesity and metabolic syndrome including hypoinsulinaemia and diabetes (Zvonic et al. 2007; Marcheva et al. 2010). Both genes, Clock and Bmal1, are also involved in lipid metabolism through activation of adipocyte-related genes, such as peroxisome proliferators-activated receptor (PPAR) (Inoue et al. 2005).

20.6 Skin Circadian Clock

The cutaneous circadian clock seems to create its own oscillation in skin cells (Tanioka et al. 2009), which is important for maintaining skin homeostasis from UV- and visible light-induced direct DNA damage response signaling and oxidative stress (Slominski et al. 2005; Gaddameedhi et al. 2011, 2015; Geyfman et al. 2012). While it has been reported that UVB radiation may involve multiple pathways down-regulating the expression of circadian genes, the core clock genes such as *Clock*, *Bmal1*, *Per1*, *Cry1* have been described at the molecular and genetic level in various human skin melanocytes, fibroblasts, and keratinocytes (Bjarnason et al. 2001; Hardeland et al. 2003). A circadian transcription factor Kruppel-like factor 9 (KLF9) in human epidermis is found to oscillate in a cortisol dependent manner and effects keratinocyte proliferation/differentiation through its downstream targets (Spörl et al. 2012). Collectively, these studies suggest that the cutaneous peripheral clock may participate in defense mechanisms against environment stresses (Fig. 20.1).

20.7 DNA Damage Repair and Skin Circadian Control

UV radiation that reaches earth's surface from sunlight is comprised of ~95 % UVA (320–400 nm) and ~5 % UVB (280–320 nm) and induces DNA damage by generating two major photoproducts: cyclobutane pyrimidine dimers (CPDs) and (6-4) photoproducts [(6-4) PPs] that are mutagenic and carcinogenic (Bowden 2004). Melanin, a pigment synthesized in melanocytes is well established for its protective role against UV radiation (Sinha and Häder 2002). However, there are independent reports that show melanin contributing to additional DNA damage and promoting development of melanoma in response to UV (Noonan et al. 2012). Melanoma induction by UVA is dependent and UVB is independent of the melanin pigment (Noonan et al. 2012). In another study, UVA was found to induce UV signature mutations, C $\longrightarrow$ T CPDs even hours after exposure to radiation called "Dark CPDs." Here, melanin acts as a molecular vector by exciting to triplet state

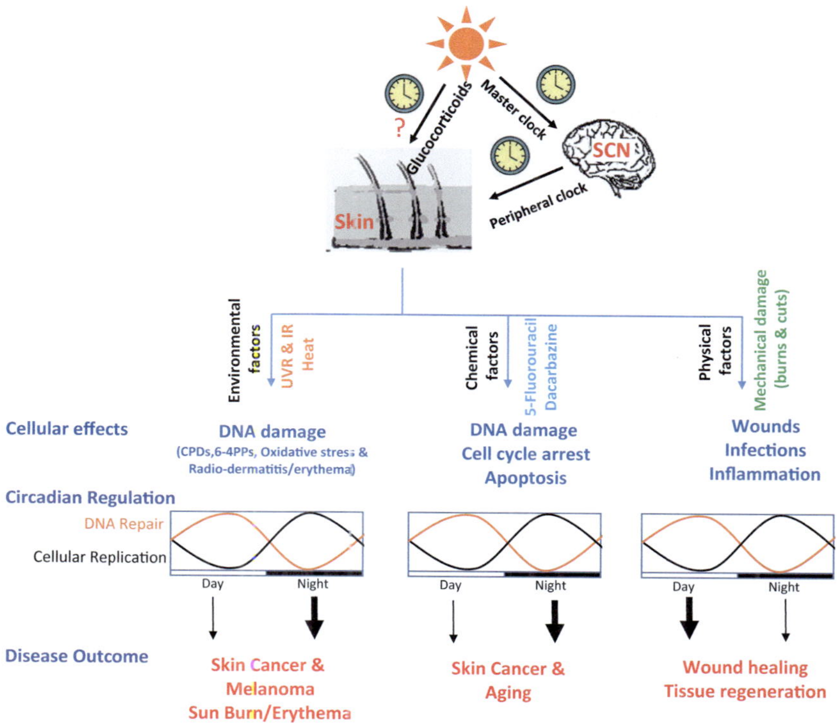

Fig. 20.1 Circadian modulation of skin stresses. Skin circadian rhythm has a peripheral clock and is regulated by the master clock controlled by the suprachiasmatic nuclei in the lower hypothalamus region of the brain. Also, skin cells are capable of synthesizing glucocorticoids (Slominski et al. 2013) and a study in zebrafish suggests that there might be a concert between the master clock and the independent clock regulated by glucocorticoids (Dickmeis et al. 2007). Skin is the primary barrier against external insults like environmental, chemical and physical or mechanical factors. These external factors will greatly affect the health or physiology, proliferation (growth) and aging of the skin. UV radiation is known to induce DNA damage by generating CPDs and 6-4PPs by UVB and oxidative stress (8-oxoG) by UVA. There are repair mechanisms such as nucleotide excision repair (repairs photoproducts) and base excision repair (repairs oxidative damage), which oscillate in a circadian manner. Chemotherapeutic drugs such as Dacarbazine, 5-FU are used to treat skin cancers and melanoma in conjunction with radiation therapy. Hence, exposure to such radiation or chemo drugs at low DNA repair activity would predispose skin cells to development of skin cancers or aging. For physical insults such as wounds, infections and inflammation the best time for recovery is during the night hours where the cells divide at their zenith

and transferring energy to DNA in a radiation-independent manner and this suggests that melanin contributes to additional DNA damage (Premi et al. 2015). Moreover, a recent report suggests that silencing the BMAL1 or PER1 expression in human hair follicles increases melanin synthesis as well as tyrosinase enzyme expression and activity suggesting that pigmentation is circadian-clock controlled (Hardman et al. 2015). However, understanding the molecular mechanisms of how the skin clock regulates melanin lineage pathway gene expression would be interesting.

In humans, CPDs and (6-4) PPs are solely repaired by nucleotide excision repair (NER), which is circadian regulated (Kang et al. 2009; Gaddameedhi et al. 2011). Defective NER is highly correlated with increased melanoma (Wang et al. 2009). Observations in mouse-cortex and skin cancer models show that NER activity is high in the afternoon/evening hours and is lowest in the morning hours. The *Xeroderma Pigmentosum A* (XPA) gene, a rate limiting factor in the NER pathway, exhibits daily rhythmicity in mouse skin with a minimum in the morning and a maximum in the afternoon/evening and hence influences DNA repair activity (Kang et al. 2009; Gaddameedhi et al. 2011). This suggests that humans probably have more repair activity in the morning hours compared to the afternoon/evening hours, as mice are nocturnal and humans are diurnal, however, there is no experimental evidence in humans.

Melanin is also involved in inducing oxidative DNA damage by generating 8-Oxo-7, 8-dihydro-2′-deoxyguanosine (8-oxodG) in response to UVA radiation. The eumelanin containing black mice and cultured melanocytes have showed rapid accumulation of nuclear 8-oxodG (Yarosh et al. 2005). However, eumelanin lacking albino mice or melanocytes did not show any DNA damage. The enzyme 8-oxo-guanine glycosylase (OGG1), a key gene in DNA base excision repair (BER) is involved in repairing these common DNA adducts generated by UV radiation, and defects in this gene lead to an increased risk of skin cancer (Yarosh et al. 2005). In a recent study OGG1 was shown to follow a circadian pattern in clearing 8-oxoG adducts at the mRNA level. In a recent study on human volunteers, it was elegantly shown that OGG1, a rate limiting gene in base excision repair (BER) pathway, oscillates in a circadian pattern, suggesting that human circadian clock might regulate the BER that removes oxidative DNA damage (Manzella et al. 2015).

20.8 Circadian Clock and Skin Cancer

Living organisms on the earth, including humans, are exposed to solar radiation, which has a 24-h cycle and a seasonal variation. These organisms respond to environmental changes, which have an enormous impact on their biological functions. The solar radiation is essential for the survival of all organisms, but some ultraviolet (UV) wavebands have been identified as risk factors for human health (Jhappan et al. 2003). Two ranges of UV wavebands (UVB and UVA) have been reported to penetrate to considerable depths in the skin, and DNA damage is attributed directly to UVB and indirectly to UVA photosensitization, both contributing to skin cancer development (Bowden 2004; Nichols and Katiyar 2010). Hence, while acute UV radiation participates in vitamin D3 photosynthesis and subsequent systemic immune function, chronic exposure has unwanted adverse effects such as skin cancer (Sinha and Häder 2002; Narayanan et al. 2010). Solar UV radiation has long been considered a significant risk factor for skin cancer and, as a major environmental cue, it can lead to cutaneous melanoma at a wide range of human body sites through DNA damage (de Gruijl et al. 2001; Nichols and Katiyar 2010).

Skin cancer is the most common form of malignancy in many human populations worldwide, and the incidence of melanoma and non-melanoma skin cancers has recently been increasing rapidly (Siegel et al. 2015). Although genetic, physiological, and environmental influences contribute to the etiology of skin cancer, environmental factors are gaining much interest to decrease the risk of this disease (Narayanan et al. 2010). Further efforts at identifying environmental risk factors for skin health allow a systematic approach for incorporating qualitative methods in the treatment and prevention of skin cancer, because the cancer risk can be easily modified by ensuring adequate conditions such as decreasing levels of exposure to UV radiation from sunlight (Smedby et al. 2005; Hardman et al. 2015).

Such considerations suggest that under certain circumstances, chronotherapeutic regimens based on circadian rhythms could be a novel approach in the treatment of skin cancer (Mormont and Levi 2003). The evidence presented in recent years shows that of endogenous repair mechanisms, the skin circadian clock principally controls the pathogenesis of UV-induced skin cancer, sunburn, and erythema (Sancar et al. 2015; Gaddameedhi et al. 2011, 2015; Desotelle et al. 2012; Geyfman et al. 2012). Several studies also showed that low levels of melatonin inversely associate with the risk for developing skin cancer, and more recent studies have shown that through sirtuin-1(Sirt1) inhibition, melatonin induces apoptotic cell death in melanoma cells (Jung-Hynes et al. 2010; Lévi et al. 2010).

20.9 Circadian Melatonin Regulation

Melatonin (5-methoxy-N-acetyltryptamine) plays a critical role in homeostatic regulation of circadian rhythmicity, which is closely associated with the light/dark and sleep/wake cycles (Jung-Hynes et al. 2010). While melatonin can be synthesized from pineal and extra-pineal sources, the nocturnal melatonin, which is almost exclusively released in the pineal gland and regulated by the SCN, is largely light responsive, so that its concentration remains relatively low during the daytime, rises in the evening, and peaks near the middle of the night (Reiter 1991; Simonneaux and Ribelayga 2003). The pineal melatonin secretion with the neuronal connectivity of the SCN, dorsomedial hypothalamic nucleus (DMH), and locus coeruleus (LC) importantly influences the central and peripheral circadian timing system (Aston-Jones et al. 2001; Colwell 2011). Since the nocturnal melatonin increase inhibits the wake-promoting activity of the SCN-DMH-LC circuit, exogenous melatonin is generally used as a sleep aid with appropriate dosage and timing (Aston-Jones et al. 2001; Colwell 2011). This inhibitory and phase shifting effect on the neuronal firing rate is mediated by membrane bound G protein-coupled melatonin receptors in the SCN to compensate sleep debt which is accumulated during wake (Aston-Jones et al. 2001; Colwell 2011).

Light during the night suppresses melatonin production, which is widely thought to be the cause of many different physiological and medical problems in night shift workers (Burgess et al. 2002). Exposure to bright light at night, which was a very uncommon event before the introduction of electric lighting, is a major concern of modern nocturnal physiology, because it disrupts the human endogenous circadian rhythmicity (Burgess et al. 2002). Recent studies showed that melatonin and circadian disruption by exposure to light at night stimulates tumor growth and metabolism, and cancer risk decreases by using optical filter shields or goggles to reduce low-wavelength light reaching the retina (Rahman et al. 2008). Melatonin has also been reported to have a protective effect against oxidative DNA damage by influencing the DNA repair pathway (Fischer et al. 2008). Such a mechanism could partially explain how melatonin inhibits tumorigenesis and why its levels inversely correlate with the risk of developing cancer (Fischer et al. 2008). Indeed, blind women without light perception show lower breast cancer incidence than blind women who have ability to process some degree of light perception (Davis et al. 2001; Kliukiene et al. 2001).

It has also been recognized in the mammalian system that melatonin markedly influences coordinating photoperiodic changes in immune defense responses, seasonal body weight and reproductive responses, diabetes and other chronic health conditions (Burgess et al. 2002; Rahman et al. 2008). Certainly, high concentrations of melatonin and large numbers of cell surface melatonin receptors are found in the bile, cerebrospinal fluid, saliva, bone marrow, lymphocytes, skin, and other organs (Reiter et al. 2000; Rahman et al. 2008). Considering that melatonin concentrations vary greatly among different organs and show a wide range of antioxidant potential and physiological efficacy, melatonin seems to have a tissue-specific manner for responding to regional stressors and overcoming circadian arrhythmicity, suggesting the existence of a localized melatoninergic system (Reiter 1991). In the skin, it was recently demonstrated that melatonin is involved in a melatoninergic antioxidative system to prevent and repair UV-induced skin damage by facilitating the gene expression of key antioxidant enzymes (Fischer et al. 2008).

Melatonin synthesis in the skin involves the amino acid tryptophan (Trp) and its derivative serotonin (5-hydroxytryptamine), which is finally converted to melatonin by hydroxyindole-O-methyltransferase (Simonneaux and Ribelayga 2003; Fischer et al. 2008). Interestingly, both the key precursors have antioxidant properties (Simonneaux and Ribelayga 2003; Fischer et al. 2008). Melatonin receptors, including both subtype 1 (MT1) and subtype 2 (MT2), are expressed in a cell type- and subcellular compartment-dependent manner, while MT1 exists predominantly as a melatonin receptor in both human skin and cultured melanoma cells (Simonneaux and Ribelayga 2003; Fischer et al. 2008).

20.10 Circadian Clock and Chronotherapy

Chronotherapy is commonly defined as the application of biological rhythms to medical treatment to improve the therapeutic efficacy of a given treatment (Mormont and Levi 2003). These new approaches offer very attractive therapeutic strategies for treatment of cancer and other diseases (Mormont and Levi 2003). Moreover, skin cancer is well suited for chronotherapy because the discrepancy in the risk of developing melanoma by the timing of UV exposure is well documented in epidermal carcinogenesis (Rigel 2008). Chronotherapeutic interventions are prominent and essential in developing risk-reducing strategies for treatment and prevention of several diseases (Mormont and Levi 2003; Smolensky and Peppas 2007). Recent research advancements show that the chronotherapeutic approaches as well as experimental and computational approaches are most promising systematic approaches in drug discovery, by exploring both favorable and unfavorable environments for drug metabolism (Mormont and Levi 2003; Smolensky and Peppas 2007). The levels of certain types of target receptors (proteins) for drugs have circadian fluctuations, resulting in time-dependent adverse events; chronotherapeutic interventions have recently gained much attention for their potential roles in assessing optimal timing of drug application and reducing adverse drug reactions (Ohdo 2010).

In fact, recent findings show that the majority (56/100) of best-selling drugs in the United States are direct targets of circadian clock regulated genes (Zhang et al. 2014; FitzGerald 2014). However, considering that many attempts have been made to define conditions for optimal therapeutic range of drugs, the possibility of circadian variation in adverse drug reactions has not yet been widely characterized (Ohdo 2010). On the other hand, we are obtaining more evidence that circadian disruption could be a major target for chronotherapy, since the hierarchical circadian system can amplify its rhythmic disruption through TTFL of clock genes (Ohdo 2010; Albrecht 2012; Mohawk et al. 2012). Therefore, some pathological symptoms can be alleviated by manipulating timing cues such as bright light treatment, exogenous melatonin, and sedative/hypnotic drugs (Srinivasan et al. 2009).

Radiation therapy is gaining importance in chronotherapy of skin cancers including melanoma (Desotelle et al. 2012). Chemo-sensitization of tumors using radiation and radio-sensitization of tumors with chemotherapy are the two ways that ionizing radiation (IR) can be used for therapeutic means. The strategic time to administer IR or any chemotherapeutic drug is during periods of low DNA replication combined with high DNA repair capacity of the normal cells which would be ideal to reduce the toxicity associated with radiation therapy. Recently published studies on genetic mouse models suggest that the cutaneous circadian clock regulates the DNA repair and replication where the repair capacity is high during evening hours compared to morning hours. The circadian rhythmicity of DNA replication is antiphase to that of DNA repair (Gaddameedhi et al. 2011; Geyfman et al. 2012). Interestingly another recent finding has shown that mice irradiated in

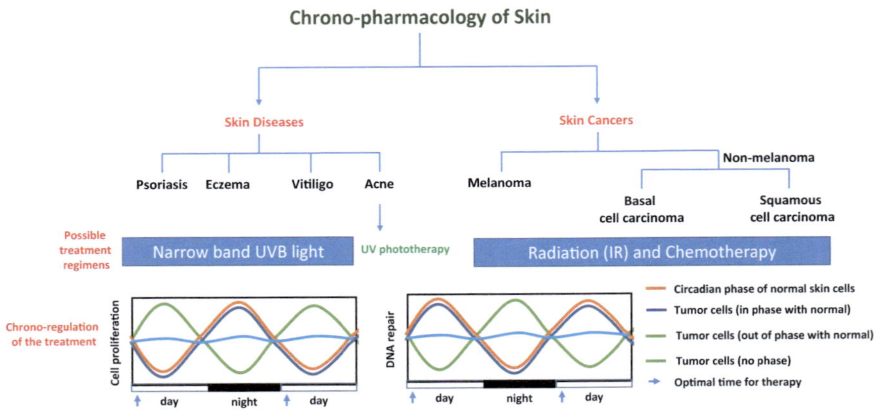

Fig. 20.2 Chronoradiotherapy of skin. The chronoradiotherapy or the time of administration of therapeutic modalities might be highly influential on the effectiveness of treating skin diseases such as Psoriasis, Eczema, Vitiligo and Acne. Apart from topical creams, narrow band UVB light or UV phototherapy is used for treatment. Skin cancers include melanoma and non-melanoma skin cancers- basal cell carcinoma and squamous cell carcinoma. As a treatment of skin cancers, most frequently, ionizing radiation is used and time of administration is exceedingly vital for the best outcome. Administering the treatment modalities with respect to low basal DNA repair activity of tumor cells is vital. For in phase tumor cells administering during morning hours should give good results. For out of phase tumor cells treatment should be given during late evening hours, when they are highly dividing and DNA repair activity is low. This is advantageous and highly effective treatment as normal skin cells are least effected by the treatment. As treating normal skin cells with radiation when their repair activity is low will dispose them to development of cancer. Out of phase tumor cells are mostly treated in the morning would probably be more succinct

the morning with a single dose of ionizing radiation (up to 5 Gy) had more hair loss than the evening group (Plikus et al. 2013).

The skin cell proliferation and radiation sensitivity using concurrent 5-Flourouracil (5-FU) and radiation show circadian fluctuations when the tumor cell proliferation is opposite to that of normal skin cells (Lévi et al. 1997). The main side effects of radiation therapy of skin cancers include radio-dermatitis. In a recent clinical study, administering radiation with concomitant BRAF inhibitors showed significant increase in acute radio-dermatitis in 36 % of a total 161 melanoma patients enrolled (Hecht et al. 2015). Understanding the role of the circadian clock in radio-dermatitis might be helpful in minimizing radiation associated melanoma therapy (Fig. 20.2).

20.11 Circadian Immune Regulation

There are other aspects of the circadian system that are relevant not only to preventing but also to curing various diseases, which are very closely linked to the immune system (Scheiermann et al. 2013; Plikus et al. 2013). The immune system is remarkable in its ability to trigger a sophisticated network of defense mechanisms against external challenges (Logan and Sarkar 2012). It has long been assumed that diurnal and nocturnal fluctuations of immune components can also affect immunity (Petrovsky and Harrison 1997; Plikus et al. 2013). Recent studies show that immune cells are a major source of autonomous circadian phenotypes (Logan and Sarkar 2012; Scheiermann et al. 2013). For example, the response of immune cells to environmental stimulation shows circadian cyclic elevation in circadian gene expression, though the variations display a wide range of transcriptional activities depending on cell types (Logan and Sarkar 2012; Scheiermann et al. 2013). As a key regulator of the circadian system, melatonin has been known to interact with the circadian daily and seasonal rhythms in immune responses, showing that chronotherapeutic interventions may be prominent and essential in developing preventive strategies for immune-related diseases (Fu and Lee 2003).

20.12 Circadian Clock and Epigenetics

Epigenetics is generally considered a hallmark of a series of oncogenic transformation processes since its mechanisms, such as DNA methylation and histone modification, create heritable changes in gene expression without changes in DNA sequence (Jaenisch and Bird 2003; Sharma et al. 2010). Epigenetic mechanisms have been well documented in transgenerational effects of intrauterine environmental factors in cancer, and those mechanisms are especially important for supporting defensive roles in pathogenesis against diverse diseases (Jaenisch and Bird 2003; Cho et al. 2012). Circadian and epigenetic mechanisms are prone to be vulnerable to external stimuli, and both can be modified relatively easily by changing environmental conditions (Masri and Sassone-Corsi 2013). Recent efforts have focused on epigenetic approaches in the transcriptional control of circadian clock genes, and genome-wide comparisons reveal that there is a reciprocal connectivity between circadian and epigenetic mechanisms and high chance of synergistic interactions (Masri and Sassone-Corsi 2013). The mammalian circadian rhythm is generated through TTFLs by the central CLOCK/BMAL1 activating complex which can act as a transcriptional activator of *Cry* and *Per* genes, causing the CRY/PER repressor complex to repress their own transcription by binding to the activating complex (Shearman et al. 2000; Sahar and Sassone-Corsi 2009). The steps of TTFL require a variety of phosphorylation, acetylation/deacetylation and methylation/demethylation of genes histones and in some cases proteins, which regulates chromatin structure and post-translational modifications of clock genes (Shearman et al. 2000; Sancar 2008; Sahar and Sassone-Corsi 2009). This indicates that exploring the emerging complexity in TTFL is a key step in understanding the molecular mechanisms of mammalian circadian rhythms. Given these, growing multidisciplinary research on circadian rhythmicity and epigenetic regulation across human cancers will be helpful to delineate the underlying mechanisms to develop new cancer chronotherapeutics.

20.13 Conclusions

This review encompasses molecular mechanisms and therapeutic applications emerging from studies of the cutaneous circadian system. Despite recent progress in understanding the mechanisms of mammalian circadian clocks which consist of hierarchically organized systems, the systemic and peripheral mechanisms which produce rhythmic abundance have remained largely unknown. There is also increasing evidence that in some cases the circadian system is a crucial driving force behind the diverse aspects of mammalian behavioral and physiological responses, which indicates that the endogenous circadian clock oscillates many pathways associated in chronobiological properties involved in pharmacodynamics of drug absorption, distribution, metabolism, and excretion (Rigel 2008; Albrecht 2012; Mohawk et al. 2012). Such collective properties should be investigated further to better understand the many facets of time-dependent rhythms in the pathogenesis and treatment strategies of a variety of diseases (Rigel 2008; Albrecht 2012; Mohawk et al. 2012). Moreover, skin stress represents one of the most feasible models of circadian regulation since skin is continuously exposed to solar radiation so that it is extremely vulnerable to external stimuli (i.e., environmental zeitgebers) compared with other body sites (Bjarnason et al. 2001; Rigel 2008). Therefore, as a chronotherapeutic approach, possible potential of the cutaneous circadian clock should be broadly conceived. In recent years, more emphasis has been placed on describing for multidisciplinary interventions of circadian and epigenetic mechanisms in transcriptional regulation of genes encoding circadian proteins (Sahar and Sassone-Corsi 2009; Masri and Sassone-Corsi 2013). Further investigation is required to define epigenetic regulation of the circadian clock. Of all the circadian mechanisms and chronotherapeutic applications discussed throughout this review, a better understanding of the cutaneous circadian system will lead to developing better strategies to treat cutaneous diseases.

Acknowledgments S. G. is supported by NIEHS (4R00ES022640) and receives additional support from WSU College of Pharmacy.

References

Akashi M, Takumi T (2005) The orphan nuclear receptor RORα regulates circadian transcription of the mammalian core-clock Bmal1. Nat Struct Mol Biol 12(5):441–448

Albrecht U (2012) Timing to perfection: the biology of central and peripheral circadian clocks. Neuron 74(2):246–260

Asher G, Schibler U (2011) Crosstalk between components of circadian and metabolic cycles in mammals. Cell Metab 13(2):125–137

Aston-Jones G, Chen S, Zhu Y, Oshinsky ML (2001) A neural circuit for circadian regulation of arousal. Nat Neurosci 4(7):732–738

Bjarnason GA, Jordan RC, Wood PA, Li Q, Lincoln DW, Sothern RB, Hrushesky RB, Ben-David Y (2001) Circadian expression of clock genes in human oral mucosa and skin: association with specific cell-cycle phases. Am J Pathol 158(5):1793–1801

Boivin DB (2000) Influence of sleep-wake and circadian rhythm disturbances in psychiatric disorders. J Psychiatry Neurosci 25(5):446–458

Bowden GT (2004) Prevention of non-melanoma skin cancer by targeting ultraviolet-B-light signalling. Nat Rev Cancer 4(1):23–35
Bunger MK, Walisser JA, Sullivan R, Manley PA, Moran SM, Kalscheur VL, Colman RJ, Bradfield CA (2005) Progressive arthropathy in mice with a targeted disruption of the Mop3/Bmal-1 locus. Genesis 41(3):122–132
Burgess HJ, Sharkey KM, Eastman CI (2002) Bright light, dark and melatonin can promote circadian adaptation in night shift workers. Sleep Med Rev 6(5):407–420
Chen ST, Choo KB, Hou MF, Yeh KT, Kuo SJ, Chang JG (2005) Deregulated expression of the PER1, PER2 and PER3 genes in breast cancers. Carcinogenesis 26(7):1241–1246
Cho K, Mabasa L, Bae S, Walters MW, Park CS (2012) Maternal high-methyl diet suppresses mammary carcinogenesis in female rat offspring. Carcinogenesis 33(5):1106–1112
Colwell CS (2011) Linking neural activity and molecular oscillations in the SCN. Nat Rev Neurosci 12(10):553–569
Dagan Y (2002) Circadian rhythm sleep disorders (CRSD). Sleep Med Rev 6(1):45–54
Davis S, Mirick DK, Stevens RG (2001) Night shift work, light at night, and risk of breast cancer. J Natl Cancer Inst 93(20):1557–1562
de Gruijl FR, van Kranen HJ, Mullenders LH (2001) UV-induced DNA damage, repair, mutations and oncogenic pathways in skin cancer. J Photochem Photobiol B 63(1):19–27
Desotelle JA, Wilking MJ, Ahmad N (2012) The circadian control of skin and cutaneous photodamage. Photochem Photobiol 88(5):1037–1047
Dibner C, Schibler U, Albrecht U (2010) The mammalian circadian timing system: organization and coordination of central and peripheral clocks. Annu Rev Physiol 72:517–549
Dickmeis T, Lahiri K, Nica G, Vallone D, Santoriello C, Neumann CJ, Hammerschmidt M, Foulkes NS (2007) Glucocorticoids play a key role in circadian cell cycle rhythms. PLoS Biol 5(4):854–864
Dubrovsky YV, Samsa WE, Kondratov RV (2010) Deficiency of circadian protein CLOCK reduces lifespan and increases age-related cataract development in mice. Aging (Albany NY) 2 (12):936–944
Fischer TW, Slominski A, Zmijewski MA, Reiter RJ, Paus R (2008) Melatonin as a major skin protectant: from free radical scavenging to DNA damage repair. Exp Dermatol 17(9):713–730
FitzGerald GA (2014) Temporal targets of drug action. Science 346(6212):921–922
Fu L, Lee CC (2003) The circadian clock: pacemaker and tumour suppressor. Nat Rev Cancer 3(5):350–361
Gaddameedhi S, Selby CP, Kaufmann WK, Smart RC, Sancar A (2011) Control of skin cancer by the circadian rhythm. Proc Natl Acad Sci 108(46):18790–18795
Gaddameedhi S, Selby CP, Kemp MG, Ye R, Sancar A (2015) The circadian clock controls sunburn apoptosis and erythema in mouse skin. J Invest Dermatol 135(4):1119–1127
Gery S, Komatsu N, Baldjyan L, Yu A, Koo D, Koeffler HP (2006) The circadian gene per1 plays an important role in cell growth and DNA damage control in human cancer cells. Mol Cell 22(3):375–382
Geyfman M, Kumar V, Liu Q, Ruiz R, Gordon W, Espitia F, Cam E, Millar SE, Smyth P, Ihler A, Takahashi JS, Andersen B (2012) Brain and muscle Arnt-like protein-1 (BMAL1) controls circadian cell proliferation and susceptibility to UVB-induced DNA damage in the epidermis. Proc Natl Acad Sci 109(29):11758–11763
Guillaumond F, Dardente H, Giguère V, Cermakian N (2005) Differential control of Bmal1 circadian transcription by REV-ERB and ROR nuclear receptors. J Biol Rhythms 20(5):391–403
Hardeland R, Coto-Montes A, Poeggeler B (2003) Circadian rhythms, oxidative stress, and antioxidative defense mechanisms Chronobiol Int 20(6):921–962
Hardman JA, Tobin DJ, Haslam IS, Farjo N, Farjo B, Al-Nuaimi Y, Grimaldi B, Paus R (2015) The peripheral clock regulates human pigmentation. J Invest Dermatol 135(4):1053–1064
Harmer SL, Panda S, Kay SA (2001) Molecular bases of circadian rhythms. Annu Rev Cell Dev Biol 17(1):215–253
Hastings M, O'Neill JS, Maywood ES (2007) Circadian clocks: regulators of endocrine and metabolic rhythms. J Endocrinol 195(2):187–198

Hecht M, Zimmer L, Loquai C, Weishaupt C, Gutzmer R, Schuster B, Gleisner S, Schulze B, Goldinger SM, Berking C, Forschner A, Clemens P, Grabenbauer G, Müller-Brenne T, Bauch J, Eich HT, Grabbe S, Schadendorf D, Schuler G, Keikavoussi P, Semrau S, Fietkau R, Distel LV, Heinzerling L (2015) Radiosensitization by BRAF inhibitor therapy—mechanism and frequency of toxicity in melanoma patients. Ann Oncol 26(6):1238–1244

Huang W, Ramsey KM, Marcheva B, Bass J (2011) Circadian rhythms, sleep, and metabolism. J Clin Invest 121(6):2133–2141

Inoue I, Shinoda Y, Ikeda M, Hayashi K, Kanazawa K, Nomura M, Matsunaga T, Haiyuan Xu, Kawai S, Awata T, Komoda T, Katayama S (2005) CLOCK/BMAL1 is involved in lipid metabolism via transactivation of the peroxisome proliferator-activated receptor (PPAR) response element. J Atheroscler Thromb 12(3):169–174

Jaenisch R, Bird A (2003) Epigenetic regulation of gene expression: how the genome integrates intrinsic and environmental signals. Nat Genet 33:245–254

Jetten AM, Ueda E (2001) The ROR nuclear orphan receptor subfamily: critical regulators of multiple biological processes. Prog Nucleic Acid Res Mol Biol 69:205–247

Jhappan C, Noonan FP, Merlino G (2003) Ultraviolet radiation and cutaneous malignant melanoma. Oncogene 22(20):3099–3112

Johnson CH, Egli M (2014) Metabolic compensation and circadian resilience in prokaryotic cyanobacteria. Annu Rev Biochem 83:221–247

Jung-Hynes B, Reiter RJ, Ahmad N (2010) Sirtuins, melatonin and circadian rhythms: building a bridge between aging and cancer. J Pineal Res 48(1):9–19

Kang HS, Angers M, Beak JY, Wu X, Gimble JM, Wada T, Xie W, Collins JB, Grissom SF, Jetten AM (2007) Gene expression profiling reveals a regulatory role for RORα and RORγ in phase I and phase II metabolism. Physiol Genomics 31(2):281–294

Kang TH, Reardon JT, Kemp M, Sancar A (2009) Circadian oscillation of nucleotide excision repair in mammalian brain. Proc Natl Acad Sci 106(8):2864–2867

King DP, Takahashi JS (2000) Molecular genetics of circadian rhythms in mammals. Annu Rev Neurosci 23(1):713–742

Kliukiene J, Tynes T, Andersen A (2001) Risk of breast cancer among Norwegian women with visual impairment. Br J Cancer 84(3):397–399

Ko CH, Takahashi JS (2006) Molecular components of the mammalian circadian clock. Hum Mol Genet 15(suppl 2):R271–R277

Lamia KA, Storch KF, Weitz CJ (2008) Physiological significance of a peripheral tissue circadian clock. Proc Natl Acad Sci 105(39):15172–15177

Laposky AD, Bass J, Kohsaka A, Turek FW (2008) Sleep and circadian rhythms: key components in the regulation of energy metabolism. FEBS Lett 582(1):142–151

Lee C, Etchegaray JP, Cagampang FR, Loudon AS, Reppert SM (2001) Posttranslational mechanisms regulate the mammalian circadian clock. Cell 107(7):855–867

Lévi F, Zidani R, Misset JL (1997) Randomised multicentre trial of chronotherapy with oxaliplatin, fluorouracil, and folinic acid in metastatic colorectal cancer. The Lancet 350(9079):681–686

Lévi F, Okyar A, Dulong S, Innominato PF, Clairambault J (2010) Circadian timing in cancer treatments. Annu Rev Pharmacol Toxicol 50:377–421

Logan RW, Sarkar DK (2012) Circadian nature of immune function. Mol Cell Endocrinol 349(1):82–90

Lowrey PL, Takahashi JS (2011) Genetics of circadian rhythms in Mammalian model organisms. Adv Genet 74:175

Manzella N, Bracci M, Strafella E, Staffolani S, Ciarapica V, Copertaro A, Rapisarda V, Ledda C, Amati M, Valentino M, Santarelli L (2015) Circadian modulation of 8-oxoguanine DNA damage repair. Sci Rep 5:13752

Marcheva B, Ramsey KM, Buhr ED, Kobayashi Y, Su H, Ko CH, Ivanova G,Omura C, Mo S, Vitaterna MH, Lopez JP, Philipson LH, Bradfield CA, Crosby SD, JeBailey L, Wang X, Takahashi JS, Bass J (2010) Disruption of the clock components CLOCK and BMAL1 leads to hypoinsulinaemia and diabetes. Nature 466(7306):627–631

Masri S, Sassone-Corsi P (2013) The circadian clock: a framework linking metabolism, epigenetics and neuronal function. Nat Rev Neurosci 14(1):69–75

Maury E, Ramsey KM, Bass J (2010) Circadian rhythms and metabolic syndrome from experimental genetics to human disease. Circ Res 106(3):447–462
Mohawk JA, Green CB, Takahashi JS (2012) Central and peripheral circadian clocks in mammals. Annu Rev Neurosci 35:445–462
Mormont MC, Levi F (2003) Cancer chronotherapy: principles, applications, and perspectives. Cancer 97(1):155–169
Morris CJ, Aeschbach D, Scheer FA (2012) Circadian system, sleep and endocrinology. Mol Cell Endocrinol 349(1):91–104
Narayanan DL, Saladi RN, Fox JL (2010) Review: ultraviolet radiation and skin cancer. Int J Dermatol 49(9):978–986
Nichols JA, Katiyar SK (2010) Skin photoprotection by natural polyphenols: anti-inflammatory, antioxidant and DNA repair mechanisms. Arch Dermatol Res 302(2):71–83
Noonan FP, Zaidi MR, Wolnicka-Glubisz A, Anver MR, Bahn J, Wielgus A, Cadet J, Douki T, Mouret S, Tucker MA, Popratiloff A, Merlino G, De Fabo EC (2012) Melanoma induction by ultraviolet A but not ultraviolet B radiation requires melanin pigment. Nat Commun 3:884
Ohdo S (2010) Chronotherapeutic strategy: rhythm monitoring, manipulation and disruption. Adv Drug Deliv Rev 62(9):859–875
Partch CL, Green CB, Takahashi JS (2014) Molecular architecture of the mammalian circadian clock. Trends Cell Biol 24(2):90–99
Petrovsky N, Harrison LC (1997) Diurnal rhythmicity of human cytokine production: a dynamic disequilibrium in T helper cell type 1/T helper cell type 2 balance? J Immunol 158(11):5163–5168
Plikus MV, Vollmers C, de la Cruz D, Chaix A, Ramos R, Panda S, Chuong CM (2013) Local circadian clock gates cell cycle progression of transient amplifying cells during regenerative hair cycling. Proc Natl Acad Sci 110(23):E2106–E2115
Premi S, Wallisch S, Mano CM, Weiner AB, Bacchiocchi A, Wakamatsu K, Bechara EJ, Halaban R, Douki T, Brash DE (2015) Chemiexcitation of melanin derivatives induces DNA photoproducts long after UV exposure. Science 347(6224):842–847
Rahman SA, Kollara A, Brown TJ, Casper RF (2008) Selectively filtering short wavelengths attenuates the disruptive effects of nocturnal light on endocrine and molecular circadian phase markers in rats. Endocrinology 149(12):6125–6135
Reiter RJ (1991) Pineal melatonin: cell biology of its synthesis and of its physiological interactions. Endocr Rev 12(2):151–180
Reppert SM, Weaver DR (2002) Coordination of circadian timing in mammals. Nature 418 (6901):935–941
Rigel DS (2008) Cutaneous ultraviolet exposure and its relationship to the development of skin cancer. J Am Acad Dermatol 58(5):S129–S132
Sack RL, Auckley D, Auger RR, Carskadon MA, Wright KP Jr, Vitiello MV, Zhdanova IV (2007) Circadian rhythm sleep disorders: part II, advanced sleep phase disorder, delayed sleep phase disorder, free-running disorder, and irregular sleep-wake rhythm: an American academy of sleep medicine review. Sleep 30(11):1484–1501
Sahar S, Sassone-Corsi P (2009) Metabolism and cancer: the circadian clock connection. Nat Rev Cancer 9(12):886–896
Sancar A (2008) The intelligent clock and the Rube Goldberg clock. Nat Struct Mol Biol 15(1):23–24
Sancar A, Lindsey-Boltz LA, Ünsal-Kaçmaz K, Linn S (2004) Molecular mechanisms of mammalian DNA repair and the DNA damage checkpoints. Annu Rev Biochem 73(1):39–85
Sancar A, Lindsey-Boltz LA, Gaddameedhi S, Selby CP, Ye R, Chiou YY, Kemp MG, Hu J, Lee JH, Ozturk N (2015) Circadian clock, cancer, and chemotherapy. Biochemistry 54(2): 110–123
Scheer FA, Hilton MF, Mantzoros CS, Shea SA (2009) Adverse metabolic and cardiovascular consequences of circadian misalignment. Proc Natl Acad Sci 106(11):4453–4458
Scheiermann C, Kunisaki Y, Frenette PS (2013) Circadian control of the immune system. Nat Rev Immunol 13(3):190–198

Schultz TF, Kay SA (2003) Circadian clocks in daily and seasonal control of development. Science 301(5631):326–328
Sharma S, Kelly TK, Jones PA (2010) Epigenetics in cancer. Carcinogenesis 31(1):27–36
Shearman LP, Sriram S, Weaver DR, Maywood ES, Chaves I, Zheng B, Kume K, Lee CC, Hastings MH, Reppert SM (2000) Interacting molecular loops in the mammalian circadian clock. Science 288(5468):1013–1019
Siegel RL, Miller KD, Jemal A (2015) Cancer statistics, 2015. CA Cancer J Clin 65(1):5–29
Simonneaux V, Ribelayga C (2003) Generation of the melatonin endocrine message in mammals: a review of the complex regulation of melatonin synthesis by norepinephrine, peptides, and other pineal transmitters. Pharmacol Rev 55(2):325–395
Sinha RP, Häder DP (2002) UV-induced DNA damage and repair: a review. Photochem Photobiol Sci 1(4):225–236
Slominski A, Wortsman J, Tobin DJ (2005) The cutaneous serotoninergic/melatoninergic system: securing a place under the sun. FASEB J 19(2):176–194
Slominski A, Zbytek B, Nikolakis G, Manna PR, Skobowiat C, Zmijewski M, Li W, Janjetovic Z, Postlethwaite A, Zouboulis CC, Tuckey RC (2013) Steroidogenesis in the skin: implications for local immune functions. J Steroid Biochem Mol Biol 137:107–123
Smedby KE, Hjalgrim H, Melbye M, Torrång A, Rostgaard K, Munksgaard L, Adami HO, Hansen M, Porwit-MacDonald A, Jensen BA, Roos G (2005) Ultraviolet radiation exposure and risk of malignant lymphomas. J Natl Cancer Inst 97(3):199–209
Smolensky MH, Peppas NA (2007) Chronobiology, drug delivery, and chronotherapeutics. Adv Drug Deliv Rev 59(9):828–851
Spörl F, Korge S, Jürchott K, Wunderskirchner M, Schellenberg K, Heins S, Spechta A, C Stollc C, Klemzb R, Maierb B, Wencka H, Schradera A, Kunzc D , Blatta T, Kramer A (2012) Krüppel-like factor 9 is a circadian transcription factor in human epidermis that controls proliferation of keratinocytes. Proc Natl Acad Sci 109(27):10903–10908
Srinivasan V, Pandi-Perumal SR, Trahkt I, Spence DW, Poeggeler B, Hardeland R, Cardinali DP (2009) Melatonin and melatonergic drugs on sleep: possible mechanisms of action. Int J Neurosci 119(6):821–846
Storch KF, Lipan O, Leykin I, Viswanathan N, Davis FC, Wong WH, Weitz CJ (2002) Extensive and divergent circadian gene expression in liver and heart. Nature 417(6884):78–83
Takahashi JS, Hong HK, Ko CH, McDearmon EL (2008) The genetics of mammalian circadian order and disorder: implications for physiology and disease. Nat Rev Genet 9(10):764–775
Tanioka M, Yamada H, Doi M, Bando H, Yamaguchi Y, Nishigori C, Okamura H (2009) Molecular clocks in mouse skin. J Invest Dermatol 129(5):1225–1231
Triqueneaux G, Thenot S, Kakizawa T, Antoch MP, Safi R, Takahashi JS, Delaunay F, Laudet V (2004) The orphan receptor Rev-erbα gene is a target of the circadian clock pacemaker. J Mol Endocrinol 33(3):585–608
Vitaterna MH, Selby CP, Todo T, Niwa H, Thompson C, Fruechte EM, Hitomi K, Thresher RJ, Ishikawa T, Miyazaki J, Takahashi JS, Sancar A (1999) Differential regulation of mammalian period genes and circadian rhythmicity by cryptochromes 1 and 2. Proc Natl Acad Sci 96(21):12114–12119
Wang Y, DiGiovanna JJ, Stern JB, Hornyak TJ, Raffeld M, Khan SG, Oh KS, Hollander MC, Dennis PA, Kraemer KH (2009) Evidence of ultraviolet type mutations in xeroderma pigmentosum melanomas. Proc Natl Acad Sci 106(15):6279–6284
Yarosh DB, Canning MT, Teicher D, Brown DA (2005) After sun reversal of DNA damage: enhancing skin repair. Mutat Res/Fundam Mol Mech Mutagen 571(1):57–64
Zhang R, Lahens NF, Ballance HI, Hughes ME, Hogenesch JB (2014) A circadian gene expression atlas in mammals: implications for biology and medicine. Proc Natl Acad Sci 111(45):16219–16224
Zheng B, Albrecht U, Kaasik K, Sage M, Lu W, Vaishnav S, Li Q, Sun ZS, Eichele G, Bradley A Lee CC (2001) Nonredundant roles of the mPer1 and mPer2 genes in the mammalian circadian clock. Cell 105(5):683–694
Zvonic S, Floyd ZE, Mynatt RL, Gimble JM (2007) Circadian rhythms and the regulation of metabolic tissue function and energy homeostasis. Obesity 15(3):539–543

Chapter 21
Psychological Stress as a Determinant of Skin Barrier Function: Immunological Pathways and Therapeutic Opportunities

Mark E. Mummert

Abstract Psychological stress is proposed to be an evolutionary adaptation to the flight or fight response. Physiological changes occur in a number of systems during psychological stress, including the immune response. Classically, acute psychological stress leads to activation of the immune response and chronic psychological stress leads to suppression of the immune response. Skin is the outer most barrier of the body and possesses both innate and adaptive immune responses. Because many dermatological diseases have an immune system component (e.g., atopic dermatitis) we will assess the impact of psychological stress on the skin immune responses herein. Psychological stress has been reported to affect both the innate and adaptive immune responses in experimental systems and in skin disease states. A number of mechanisms have been proposed to explain how psychological stress exerts its impact on the skin immune response including redistribution of the lymphocytes, modulation of immune cell functions and differential expression of cytokines. Although rare, psychtropic drugs can also cause unwanted skin pathologies. The finding that adverse reactions of psychotropic drugs are related to major histocompatability haplotype may suggest an immune mechanism of action. On the other hand, some drugs used to treat skin diseases can results in psychiatric disorders. Finally, a number of psychological methods have been used to successfully treat or reduce the symptoms of skin diseases including hypnosis, cognitive behavioral therapy, psychotherapy and biofeedback.

Keywords Psychological stress · Immune response · Skin · Psychotropic medication · Psychological methods

---

M.E. Mummert (✉)
Mental Sciences Institute, University of North Texas Health Science Center, 3500 Camp Bowie Blvd., Fort Worth, TX, USA
e-mail: mark.mummert@unthsc.edu

M.E. Mummert
Department of Dermatology, University of Texas Southwestern Medical Center, Dallas, TX, USA

G.T. Wondrak (ed.), *Skin Stress Response Pathways*,
DOI 10.1007/978-3-319-43157-4_21

21.1 Introduction

The concept that psychological stress could cause physiological responses was proposed over a century ago by Canon who hypothesized that the release of substances (e.g., adrenalin, epinephrine) by the adrenal medulla during "pain and the major emotions" (fear, rage, and asphyxia) increased cardiac vigor and increased sugar content in the blood and led to cessation of the activities of the alimentary canal (Cannon 1914). These physiological alterations, which operate to endow the organism to flee or to fight, were considered an evolutionary adaptation for survival. However, for most modern human's physiological changes induced by psychological stress, including the skin can be unwanted.

Skin is the largest sensory organ of the body. Due to its anatomic location the skin also serves as a protective barrier to the internal organs from a variety of environmental agents including: (1) microorganisms, (2) ultraviolet radiation (3) ozone, (4) mechanical damage and (5) allergens. In addition to providing a physical barrier, the skin is also an immunological organ equipped with antigen presenting cells (i.e., epidermal Langerhans cells and dermal dendritic cells) that continuously monitor their microenvironment. Exposure of skin to pro-inflammatory stimuli results in the migration of these cells to the lymph nodes where they behave as antigen presenting cells by presenting antigen to their cognate T cells.

In addition to the role of skin in performing its role as a physiological and immunological barrier to physical threats, the skin is also linked to the nervous system. In fact, the skin and nervous system are derived from a common ectodermal origin. Skin is highly innervated and reacts to psychological stimuli induced by neuroendocrine factors. The cells of the immune system are also generally equipped with receptors to react to neuroendocrine factors. Thus, the skin and the cutaneous immune system can respond to psychological factors. As a result, factors such as psychological stress can result in changes to the skin. Indeed, a number of dermatological diseases are exacerbated by psychological stress including relatively common dermatoses such as psoriasis and atopic dermatitis. The importance of psychiatric conditions with skin disease is highlighted by the finding that co-occurring psychiatric disorders in patients with skin disorders show a prevalence of around 30 % (Shenefelt 2011).

21.2 Types of Psychological Stress

Dhabhar and McEwen have proposed that psychological stress exists as a spectrum, with acute psychological stress and chronic psychological stress at the far and opposite ends of a spectrum (Dhabhar and McEwen 1997a). This model also predicts an area of resilience, which is defined by the authors as the ability of physiological systems to enable survival for extended periods of time under increasingly challenging conditions. Acute psychological stress has been defined as isolated, single stress events that last only minutes to hours while chronic psychological stress has been defined as several stress events that last multiple hours per day for a time period of several weeks or months (Dhabhar et al. 2012). Acute and chronic psychological stress generally is different in terms of their immunological outcome with acute psychological stress enhancing the immune response and chronic psychological stress suppressing the immune response.

Although the immunological outcomes of psychological stress has been viewed mostly in a negative light, the findings that acute psychological stress enhances the immune response and chronic psychological stress suppress' the immune response may have potential benefits. Evolutionarily the immune enhancing activity induced by acute psychological stress may have benefitted the organism by preparing it to sustain injury and consequent infection. Such a scenario is especially easy to appreciate in the context of predation where the prey is attacked by a predator.

Immunosuppression due to chronic psychological stress at first glance appears harder to reconcile. However, previous research has shown that larger numbers of social networks appear to lower the immune response, particularly under stress. Segerstrom has argued that ecological immunosuppression due to high energy demands (such as during chronic psychological stress) is offset by conserving energy due to social connectedness (Segerstrom 2008). Thus, in this model social connectedness is likely to outweigh the cost of changes in immunity.

21.3 Skin and the Neuroendocrine System

The central hypothalamic-pituitary-adrenal (HPA) axis is activated following stress signals including factors such as 5-hydroxytryptamine (Calogero et al. 1989; Tsagarakis et al. 1989) and inflammatory cytokines (Kariagina et al. 2004; Raber et al. 1998). Stress signals also activate the locus coeruleus of the brain stem eliciting a sympathetic nervous system response. When the HPA axis is activated, stress hormones are released including corticotropin-releasing hormone (CRH) and arginine vasopressin (Bernardini et al. 1994) from the hypothalamus which induces adrenocorticotropic hormone (ACTH) release from the anterior pituitary (Whitnall 1993). CRH also activates the noradrenergic pathways resulting in norepinephrine secretion by the peripheral sympathetic nervous system and norepinephrine and epinephrine secretion from the adrenal medulla (Tausk et al. 2008). ACTH regulates secretion of glucocorticoids including cortisol from the adrenal gland (Tsigos and Chrousos 2002) while cortisol negatively regulates CRH production in a feedback loop mechanism (Miyazaki et al. 2000). Norepinehrine, a major neurotransmitter, is released by sympathetic fibers to innervated tissues, including the skin (Kellogg 2006; Pergola et al. 1993; Zimmerman and Whitmore 1967).

Investigations have shown that human skin expresses CRH as well as CRH receptors (CRH-R). The CRH-R1α isoform is the predominant CRH receptor in skin and is expressed in all major cell populations of epidermis, dermis and sub-cutis. In addition to CRH, human skin also expresses urocortin I (Slominski et al. 2000a) and urocortin II mRNA (Slominski et al. 2004). CRH-R1 binds to urocortin I,but not to urocortin II while CRH-R2 binds to urocortin II but not urocortin I (Grammatopoulos and Chrousos 2002; Hsu and Hsueh 2001), (Slominski et al. 2000b). Finally, skin produces the precursor protein proopiomelanocortin protein (POMC) and POMC derived peptides that give rise to ACTH and other polypeptide products (Kono et al. 2001; Slominski et al. 2000b). Interestingly, human hair follicles can synthesizes cortisol, and cortisol synthesis is regulated by endogenous feedback controls (Ito et al. 2005). Thus, the skin apparently has a fully functional peripheral equivalent of the HPA axis. The peripheral skin HPA axis may coordinate or fine tune peripheral stress responses with the central HPA axis. In addition to expressing components of the HPA axis, skin also produces a number of other neuroendocrine signals including prolactin (Langan et al. 2010; Ramot et al. 2010), melatonin (Slominski et al. 2008) and catecholamines (Schutz et al. 2008; Weihe et al. 2005).

Skin is also highly innervated with sensory nerves that produce neurotrophins and neuropeptides. Psychological stress has been shown to lead to increased concentrations of cutaneous nerve growth factor (NGF) (Joachim et al. 2007). A number of biological activities are associated with NGF, including axon sprouting of peptidergic and sympathetic neurons, promoting cross-talk between neural cells, glia and immune cells and facilitating monocyte/macrophage migration through vascular endothelium (Levi-Montalcini et al. 1996). Moreover, NGF results in upregulation of SP + nerve fibers in the dermis of stressed mice. Calcitonin gene-related peptide (CGRP) is a potent vasodilator that is also upregulated in response to NGF (Joachim et al. 2007). SP and CGRP have different distributions within the skin with SP nerve fibers detected in the dermis and subcutis and CGRP nerve fibers are in the epidermis around the distal hair follicle and the arrector pili muscle (Peters et al. 2001).

21.4 Impact of Psychological Stress on Skin Immune Responses

The innate immune response consists of elements that contribute to the immediate and generic defense of the skin and immunological memory does not develop. By contrast, the adaptive immune response requires time for the development of a specific defense and can create immunological memory.

21.4.1 Innate Immune Responses to Stress

The stratum corneum is terminally differentiated epidermis that forms the outer most skin layer. The corneocytes forming the stratum corneum arise from the underlying keratinocytes. The spaces between the corneocytes contain high concentrations of non-polar lipids which contribute to the water impermeability of the stratum corneum. The stratum corneum plays a role in maintaining tissue hydration, and its disruption results in transepidermal water loss. The stratum corenum is normally sloughed off, potentially removing skin microorganisms such as potential pathogens. Lastly, the stratum corneum protects the skin from ultraviolet radiation via melanin derived from melanocytes (Marks 2004). Investigations have evaluated the impact of immobilization stress and crowding stress on the barrier function of the stratum corneum as measured by barrier recovery after its removal by tape stripping or sodium dodecyl sulfate treatment in rats. In that study, immobilization induced stress and crowding stress both significantly delayed barrier recovery for up to 7 days in both male and female mice. However, the tranquillizers diazepam and chlorpromazine resulted in an increased rate of barrier recovery suggesting that pharmacological reduction of psychological stress promoted stratum corneum formation (Denda et al. 1998).

The impact of psychological stress on barrier recovery in humans has also been studied (Garg et al. 2001). Individuals with high levels of perceived psychological stress had significantly delayed barrier recovery rates as compared with those reporting low perceived stress levels. Based on these findings these investigators concluded that stress-induced changes in epidermal function may precipitate dermatoses. Using mice and stress induced by continuous light and radio noise, Choi et al. found that impaired stratum corneum barrier function was linked to decreased synthesis of epidermal lipids (Choi et al. 2005). Treatment of psychologically stressed mice with RU-486 (a glucocorticoid receptor antagonist) or antalarmin (a CRH antagonist that blocks increased glucocorticoid production) returned stratum corneum recovery to normal rates. These results underscore the potential importance of glucocorticoids induced during psychological stress and stratum corneum homeostasis.

Anti-microbial peptides encapsulated in lamellar bodies are synthesized and secreted by skin. Aberg et al. evaluated the effect of cutaneous *Streptococcus pyogenes* infections on psychologically stressed mice (Aberg et al. 2007). Stressed mice downregulated anti-microbial peptides (cathelin-related peptide and β-defensin) and developed significantly more severe cutaneous infections as compared with non-stressed control animals. Pharmacological blockade of CRH or glucocorticoid production returned anti-microbial peptides to normal levels and reduced the infection severity. These results suggested that psychological stress is directly linked to the innate immunity conferred by anti-microbial peptides via the central or peripheral HPA axis.

Mast cells are found throughout connective tissues, including the dermis (Cowen et al. 1979; Eady et al. 1979; Graham et al. 1955). ACTH and CRH activate mast cells, and human mast cells express CRH receptors (Cao et al. 2005). Asadi et al. has shown that SP can induce the expression of functional CRH receptor-1 in human mast cells (Asadi et al. 2012). Moreover, acute psychological stress is associated with mast cell activation and the release of IL-6. The finding that serum levels of IL-6 are abrogated in mast cell deficient mice following restraint stress as compared with their wild-type control counterparts shows the importance of mast cells in the production of systemic IL-6 (Huang et al. 2002). IL-6 can cross the blood/brain barrier (Banks et al. 1994) and activate the HPA axis (Mastorakos et al. 1993) and can also induce immune reactions including lymphocyte activation (Takeda et al. 1998; Kitani et al. 1992) and increased antibody production via CD4 + T cell help (Dienz et al. 2009). Systemic effects of IL-6 include induction of fever (Kagiwada et al. 2004; Castell et al. 1989a, 1989b) and acute phase protein production (Castell et al. 1989a, 1989b). Mast cells also play a role in neurogenic inflammation. Singh et al. reported that restraint induced stress resulted in significantly enhanced degranulation of mast cells in mice as compared with their non-stressed counterparts. Pre-treatment of mice before stress with CRH antiserum, the neurotensin receptor antagonist SR48692 and capsacin to deplete sensory neurons were all found to inhibit mast cell degranulation. These results suggested a role for neurogenic inflammation in psychological stress in addition to the HPA axis (Singh et al. 1999).

21.4.2 Adaptive Immune Responses to Stress

The adaptive immune response requires the interaction of antigen presenting cells with antigen specific T cells. Activation of T cells requires their interplay with antigen presenting cells and co-stimulatory molecules on the surfaces of both cell types as well as the production of cytokines.

In classic experiments, Dhabhar and McEwen investigated the impact of acute stress on contact hypersensitivity (CHS) reactions in rats using stress induced by a 2 h confinement in a box (Dhabhar and McEwen 1999). Briefly, animals were sensitized using 2,4-dinitrofluorobenzene (DNFB), stressed on day 5 following sensitization and challenged on the pinna of the ear on day 6 and the ear swelling measured after the DNFB challenge. Acute stress significantly increased the ear swelling response in stressed rats as compared with the control animals. Elimination of glucocorticoid and epinephrine by adrenalectomy abrogated the stress-induced enhancement, highlighting the importance of these hormones for immunomodulation. Injections of corticosterone or epinephrine at low doses also enhanced stress-induced ear swelling suggesting that these hormones play a role in immunoenhancement. By contrast, high doses of corticosterone or epinephrine had the opposite effect with the ear swelling response reduced. Thus, the physiological outcome of corticostrone and epinephrine depends on their concentrations. Using a different contact sensitizing reagent (trinitrochlorobenzene) and isolation stress, Nakano also found that stress enhanced the cutaneous immune response as evaluated by ear swelling (Nakano 2007). On the other hand, stress alone did not enhance the ear swelling response of mice treated with the contact irritant, sodium dodecyl sulfate. These results showed that elements of the adaptive immune response were required for acute stress-induced immune enhancement, as irritants do not develop immunological memory.

Different strains of mice have been shown to have different skin sensitivities to psychological stressors. For example, Flint et al. reported that C57BL/6 mice had blunted ear swelling responses to restraint stress as compared with BALB/c mice (Flint and Tinkle 2001). The ear swelling responses in the stressed C57BL/6 strain could not be enhanced even after injection of corticosterone. The nature of the stressor also appears to impact the degree of the CHS response in animals. Bowers et al. compared CHS responses in mice acutely or chronically stressed by restraint, forced swim, isolation, handling and low temperature (Bowers et al. 2008). Restraint stress and forced swim stress resulted in the most dramatic increase in the CHS response.

The impact of chronic stress on skin immune responses has also been experimentally investigated. Chronic stress has been reported to lead to immunosuppression in a number of systems, including skin graft rejection (Wistar and Hildemann 1960) and in CHS responses (Hall et al. 2014; Dhabhar and McEwen 1997b). By contrast, other studies using chronic restraint-induced stress resulted in enhanced CHS responses (Bowers et al. 2008). Again, the mouse strain appears to play a role in if the psychological stress induces enhancement or suppression of the immune response.

A number of factors may account for psychological stress-induced changes in the adaptive immune response including the numbers, proportions and distributions of immune cells. For example, previous studies found that psychological stress markedly decreased the percentages of leukocytes in the blood (Hall et al. 2014; Dhabhar et al. 1994, 1995). Interestingly, administration of corticosterone to adrenalectomized mice closely mirrored the decrease in blood leukocytes observed in stressed animals (Dhabhar et al. 1995).

Psychological stress may also modulate the activities of immunological cells. For example, psychological stress has been shown to impair lymphocyte function (Bartrop et al. 1977). Psychological stress has also been shown to decrease the density of Langerhans cells in the epidermis in both mice and humans (Kleyn et al. 2008; Hosoi et al. 1998). Langerhans cells are epidermal members of the dendritic cell family of antigen-presenting cells. Conventionally, Langerhans cells have been considered pivotal for the generation of adaptive immunity; although current studies suggest their immunological activities may be considerably more complex (reviewed in (Clausen and Kel 2010)). A number of stress related molecules have been shown to impact Langerhans cells and dendritic cells. Corticosteroids have been shown to induce the apoptosis of Langerhans cells and impair their expression of co-stimulatory molecules (Hoetzenecker et al. 2004). In vitro studies have shown that epinephrine inhibits antigen presentation in epidermal cell preparations and by purified Langerhans cells (Seiffert et al. 2002). Glucocorticoids inhibit dendritic cell production of IL-12 (Panina-Bordignon et al. 1997; Elenkov et al. 1996); and IL-12 suppression may skew the TH1/TH2 balance toward TH2 and thus impact the nature of the immune response (Seiffert and Granstein 2006). Importantly, blockade of β2-AR with the antagonist ICI188, 551 impaired the migration of Langerhans cells to the lymph nodes and blunted the subsequent CHS response when mice were sensitized with the fluorescein isothiocyanate contact sensitizing reagent (Seiffert et al. 2002). By contrast, other stress related molecules appear to enhance dendritic cell functions. For example, it has been shown that noradrenaline enhanced phosphatidylinositol 3-kinase induced antigen endocytosis by dendritic cells in vitro (Yanagawa et al. 2010).

21.5 Human Skin Diseases Linked to Psychological Stress

A number of human skin diseases may be preceded or exacerbated by psychological stress including urticaria, alopecia areata, rosacea, psoriasis and atopic dermatitis (Jaffernay 2007). Despite the number of animal studies showing a correlation between psychological stress and the immune response, mechanistic studies in humans are much rarer. Perhaps the best studied human dermatopsychological disease is atopic dermatitis. Atopic dermatitis affects approximately 6 % of the population in the USA and is a chronic inflammatory disorder that is characterized by eczematous lesions and pruritus (Hanifin et al. 2007). A psychological profile that includes excitability, depression and anxiety has been linked to this disease. Although the etiologic agent(s) that causes atopic dermatitis remain to be fully identified results of sequential patch testing have suggested that it has a biphasic TH1/TH2 T cell response. The initial acute inflammation is primarily TH2 with a shift toward TH1 chronification (Grewe et al. 1998; Thepen et al. 1996).

Studies comparing atopic and nonatopic controls using the Trier Social Stress Test (TSST) have been conducted (Buske-Kirschbaum et al. 2002b). Importantly, both groups showed similar levels in serum levels of lymphocytes, monocytes, neutrophils and basophils. On the other hand, eosinophil numbers were significantly higher in patients with atopic dermatitis as compared with nonatopic controls. Moreover, concentrations of IgE were greater in patients with atopic dermatitis as compared with nonatopic controls.

In addition to higher numbers of eosinophils and increased IgE concentrations, patients with atopic dermatitis had reduced concentrations of cortisol and ACTH as compared with nonatopic controls when TSST stressed. These results suggested that atopic dermatitis patients have a blunted HPA axis. By contrast, catecholamine concentrations were significantly higher in patients with atopic dermatitis as compared with nonatopic control patients. These results suggested that atopic dermatitis patients had an overactive sympathetic adrenomedullary system (SAM) (Buske-Kirschbaum et al. 2002a). These results may provide a plausible explanation for how psychological stress enhances atopic dermatitis. Both the HPA axis and SAM inhibit TH1 activity, possibly through IL-12. Psychological stress impedes TH1 activity via the suppressed HPA axis skewing the TH1/TH2 balance to TH2 and thus, acute disease symptoms.

21.6 Cutaneous Side Effects to Psychtropic Medications

Treatment of psychiatric disorders with psychotropic drugs can result in undesirable side reactions in the skin. Although the overall incidence of skin side effects is reportedly rare (incidence of 0.1 %) (Lange-Asschenfeldt et al. 2009) some psychotropic drugs can lead to significantly higher incidences. For example, up to 17 % of patients may have cutaneous side effects to the loading dose of the mood stabilizer, carbamazepine (Chadwick et al. 1984). Clinically relevant skin side effects follow the general scheme that mood stabilizers have a greater incidence than antidepressants (39 % vs. 29 %). In turn, antidepressants have a greater incidence than neuroleptics (29 % vs. 19 %) (Lange-Asschenfeldt et al. 2009).

Risk factors associated with cutaneous side effects to psychotropic drugs include female gender (Arndt and Jick 1976), African American ethnicity (Kalow 1982), age (Hajjar et al. 2003; Ives et al. 1992) and concurrent abuse of illicit drugs (Lange-Asschenfeldt et al. 2009). Although the mechanisms underlying these propensities are somewhat speculative, immunogenetic background appears to underlie sensitivity to some drugs. Patients with the HLA-B1502 allele are 100 times more likely to develop epidermal necrolysis and those carrying the HLA-A3101 allele are 9 times more susceptible than the general population. Among the antiepileptic drugs HLA-B1502, HLA-A3101, HLA-B1508, HLA-B1511, HLA-B1518 and HLA-B1521 all have increased incidences as compared with the population as a whole (Mitkov et al. 2014).

It is interesting to note that adverse psychiatric effects to drugs used in dermatology have also been reported. Depression due to treatment with isotretinoin and IFNα is one example and psychosis due to treatment with daposone is a second example (Locala 2009).

21.7 Psychological Methods to Reduce Dermatological Diseases

The notion that skin is intertwined with the psyche, and that psychological methods can impact the skin, is not a new concept. For example, Ullman reported that under hypnosis it was possible to cause blister formation and to induce the recurrence of Herpes simplex (Ullman 1947). Moreover, hypnosis has been used to treat skin diseases. An early report showed that ichthyosis could be significantly cleared after the patient was given the hypnotic suggestion that the disease would clear (Mason 1952). Shenefelt performed a MEDLINE search that covered the years 1966–1998 using search terms related to hypnosis and skin disease (Shenefelt 2011). Results from MEDLINE showed that a wide range of dermatological disorders could be improved using hypnosis as an alternative or complementary therapy for skin disease treatment, including (1) atopic dermatitis, (2) psoriasis, (3) alopecia areata, (4) rosacea, (5) vitiligo, (6) hyperhidrosis, and (7) ichthyosis vulgaris (Shenefelt 2000).

The apparent psychophysiologic responses of many dermatoses suggests that treatment programs structured at the dermatology/psychiatry interface may be useful for patient treatment, including programs that incorporate (1) psychotherapy, (2) biofeedback, (3) hypnosis, and (4) cognitive behavioral methods (Heller et al. 2011; Shenefelt 2000, 2003).

Other psychological methods have also been found to lead to resolution of skin disease. For example, Fortune et al. has reported that patients that chose to participate in a cognitive behavioral therapy program reported less frequencies and numbers of psoriasis symptoms up to 6 months after the program ended (Fortune et al. 2004).

21.8 Conclusions

Skin is a highly innervated organ that arises from an ectodermal origin in common with the nervous system. Both the innate and adaptive immune responses of the skin respond to psychological stimuli. In fact, many skin diseases have been shown to precede or to be exacerbated by psychological stress. Perhaps the most studied human skin disease to date is atopic dermatitis, which is a TH2 disease with TH1 chronification. Psychological stress impedes TH1 activity via the suppressed HPA axis skewing the TH1/TH2 balance to TH2 and thus, acute disease symptoms. In addition to disease, psychotropic medications can affect skin, mostly by inducing exanthematous eruptions. Conversely, drugs used to treat skin diseases can also induce psychiatric comorbidity. The ability to manipulate reactions in the skin by psychological means may be one way to alleviate skin disease. The apparent psychophysiologic responses of many dermatoses suggests that treatment programs structured at the dermatology/psychiatry interface may be useful for patient treatment, including programs that incorporate (1) psychotherapy, (2) biofeedback, (3) hypnosis, and (4) cognitive behavioral methods.

References

Aberg KM, Radek KA, Choi EH, Kim DK, Demerjian M, Hupe M, Kerbleski J, Gallo RL, Ganz T, Mauro T, Feingold KR, Elias PM (2007) Psychological stress downregulates epidermal antimicrobial peptide expression and increases severity of cutaneous infections in mice. J Clin Invest 117:3339–3349

Arndt KA, Jick H (1976) Rates of cutaneous reactions to drugs. a report from the Boston Collaborative Drug Surveillance Program. JAMA 235:918–923
Asadi S, Alysandratos KD, Angelidou A, Miniati A, Sismanopoulos N, Vasiadi M, Zhang B, Kalogeromitros D, Theoharides TC (2012) Substance P (SP) induces expression of functional corticotropin-releasing hormone receptor-1 (CRHR-1) in human mast cells. J Invest Dermatol 132:324–329
Banks WA, Kastin AJ, Gutierrez EG (1994) Penetration of interleukin-6 across the murine blood-brain barrier. Neurosci Lett 179:53–56
Bartrop RW, Luckhurst E, Lazarus L, Kiloh LG, Penny R (1977) Depressed lymphocyte function after bereavement. Lancet 1:834–836
Bernardini R, Chiarenza A, Kamilaris TC, Renaud N, Lempereur L, Demitrack M, Gold PW, Chrousos GP (1994) In vivo and in vitro effects of arginine-vasopressin receptor antagonists on the hypothalamic-pituitary-adrenal axis in the rat. Neuroendocrinology 60:503–508
Bowers SL, Bilbo SD, Dhabhar FS, Nelson RJ (2008) Stressor-specific alterations in corticosterone and immune responses in mice. Brain Behav Immun 22:105–113
Buske-Kirschbaum A, Geiben A, Hollig H, Morschhauser E, Hellhammer D (2002a) Altered responsiveness of the hypothalamus-pituitary-adrenal axis and the sympathetic adrenomedullary system to stress in patients with atopic dermatitis. J Clin Endocrinol Metab 87:4245–4251
Buske-Kirschbaum A, Gierens A, Hollig H, Hellhammer DH (2002b) Stress-induced immunomodulation is altered in patients with atopic dermatitis. J Neuroimmunol 129:161–167
Calogero AE, Bernardini R, Margioris AN, Bagdy G, Gallucci WT, Munson PJ, Tamarkin L, Tomai TP, Brady L, Gold PW (1989) Effects of serotonergic agonists and antagonists on corticotropin-releasing hormone secretion by explanted rat hypothalami. Peptides 10:189–200
Cannon WB (1914) The emergency function of the adrenal medulla in pain and the major emotions. Am J Physiol 33:356–372
Cao J, Papadopoulou N, Kempuraj D, Boucher WS, Sugimoto K, Cetrulo CL, Theoharides TC (2005) Human mast cells express corticotropin-releasing hormone (CRH) receptors and CRH leads to selective secretion of vascular endothelial growth factor. J Immunol 174:7665–7675
Castell JV, Andus T, Kunz D, Heinrich PC (1989a) Interleukin-6. The major regulator of acute-phase protein synthesis in man and rat. Ann NY Acad Sci. 557, 87–99 (discussion 100-1)
Castell JV, Gomez-Lechon MJ, David M, Andus T, Geiger T, Trullenque R, Fabra R, Heinrich PC (1989b) Interleukin-6 is the major regulator of acute phase protein synthesis in adult human hepatocytes. FEBS Lett 242:237–239
Chadwick D, Shaw MD, Foy P, Rawlins MD, Turnbull DM (1984) Serum anticonvulsant concentrations and the risk of drug induced skin eruptions. J Neurol Neurosurg Psychiatry 47:642–644
Choi EH, Brown BE, Crumrine D, Chang S, Man MQ, Elias PM, Feingold KR (2005) Mechanisms by which psychologic stress alters cutaneous permeability barrier homeostasis and stratum corneum integrity. J Invest Dermatol 124:587–595
Clausen BE, Kel JM (2010) Langerhans cells: critical regulators of skin immunity? Immunol Cell Biol 88:351–360
Cowen T, Trigg P, Eady RA (1979) Distribution of mast cells in human dermis: development of a mapping technique. Br J Dermatol 100:635–640
Denda M, Tsuchiya T, Hosoi J, Koyama J (1998) Immobilization-induced and crowded environment-induced stress delay barrier recovery in murine skin. Br J Dermatol 138:780–785
Dhabhar FS, Malarkey WB, Neri E, McEwen BS (2012) Stress-induced redistribution of immune cells–from barracks to boulevards to battlefields: a tale of three hormones–Curt Richter award winner. Psychoneuroendocrinology 37:1345–1368
Dhabhar FS, McEwen BS (1997a) Acute stress enhances while chronic stress suppresses cell-mediated immunity in vivo: a potential role for leukocyte trafficking. Brain Behav Immun 11:286–306
Dhabhar FS, McEwen BS (1997b) Acute stress enhances while chronic stress suppresses cell-mediated immunity in vivo: a potential role for leukocyte trafficking. Brain Behav Immun 11:286–306

Dhabhar FS, McEwen BS (1999) Enhancing versus suppressive effects of stress hormones on skin immune function. Proc Natl Acad Sci USA 96:1059–1064

Dhabhar FS, Miller AH, McEwen BS, Spencer RL (1995) Effects of stress on immune cell distribution dynamics and hormonal mechanisms. J Immunol 154:5511–5527

Dhabhar FS, Miller AH, Stein M, McEwen BS, Spencer RL (1994) Diurnal and acute stress-induced changes in distribution of peripheral blood leukocyte subpopulations. Brain Behav Immun 8:66–79

Dienz O, Eaton SM, Bond JP, Neveu W, Moquin D, Noubade R, Briso EM, Charland C, Leonard WJ, Ciliberto G, Teuscher C, Haynes L, Rincon M (2009) The induction of antibody production by IL-6 is indirectly mediated by IL-21 produced by CD4 + T cells. J Exp Med 206:69–78

Eady RA, Cowen T, Marshall TF, Plummer V, Greaves MW (1979) Mast cell population density, blood vessel density and histamine content in normal human skin. Br J Dermatol 100:623–633

Elenkov IJ, Papanicolaou DA, Wilder RL, Chrousos GP (1996) Modulatory effects of glucocorticoids and catecholamines on human interleukin-12 and interleukin-10 production: clinical implications. Proc Assoc Am Phys 108:374–381

Flint MS, Tinkle SS (2001) C57BL/6 mice are resistant to acute restraint modulation of cutaneous hypersensitivity. Toxicol Sci 62:250–256

Fortune DG, Richards HL, Griffiths CE, Main CJ (2004) Targeting cognitive-behaviour therapy to patients' implicit model of psoriasis: results from a patient preference controlled trial. Br J Clin Psychol 43:65–82

Garg A, Chren MM, Sands LP, Matsui MS, Marenus KD, Feingold KR, Elias PM (2001) Psychological stress perturbs epidermal permeability barrier homeostasis: implications for the pathogenesis of stress-associated skin disorders. Arch Dermatol 137:53–59

Graham HT, Lowry OH, Wahl N, Priebat MK (1955) Mast cells as sources of tissue histamine. J Exp Med 102:307–318

Grammatopoulos DK, Chrousos GP (2002) Functional characteristics of CRH receptors and potential clinical applications of CRH-receptor antagonists. Trends Endocrinol Metab 13:436–444

Grewe M, Bruijnzeel-Koomen CAFM, Schöpf E, Thepen T, Langeveld-Wildschut AG, Ruzicka T, Krutmann J (1998) A role for Th1 and Th2 cells in the immunopathogenesis of atopic dermatitis. Immunol Today 19:359–361

Hajjar ER, Hanlon JT, Artz MB, Lindblad CI, Pieper CF, Sloane RJ, Ruby CM, Schmader KE (2003) Adverse drug reaction risk factors in older outpatients. Am J Geriatr Pharmacother 1:82–89

Hall JM, Witter AR, Racine RR, Berg RE, Podawiltz A, Jones H, Mummert ME (2014) Chronic psychological stress suppresses contact hypersensitivity: Potential roles of dysregulated cell trafficking and decreased IFN-gamma production. Brain Behav Immun 36:156–164

Hanifin, J.M., Reed, M.L., Eczema Prevalence and Impact Working Group (2007) A population-based survey of eczema prevalence in the United States. Dermatitis 18:82–91

Heller MM, Lee ES, Koo JY (2011) Stress as an influencing factor in psoriasis. Skin Ther Lett 16:1–4

Hoetzenecker W, Meingassner JG, Ecker R, Stingl G, Stuetz A, Elbe-Burger A (2004) Corticosteroids but not pimecrolimus affect viability, maturation and immune function of murine epidermal Langerhans cells. J Invest Dermatol 122:673–684

Hosoi J, Tsuchiya T, Denda M, Ashida Y, Takashima A, Granstein RD, Koyama J (1998) Modification of LC phenotype and suppression of contact hypersensitivity response by stress. J Cutan Med Surg 3:79–84

Hsu SY, Hsueh AJ (2001) Human stresscopin and stresscopin-related peptide are selective ligands for the type 2 corticotropin-releasing hormone receptor. Nat Med 7:605–611

Huang M, Berry J, Kandere K, Lytinas M, Karalis K, Theoharides TC (2002) Mast cell deficient W/W(v) mice lack stress-induced increase in serum IL-6 levels, as well as in peripheral CRH and vascular permeability, a model of rheumatoid arthritis. Int J Immunopathol Pharmacol 15:249–254

Ito N, Ito T, Kromminga A, Bettermann A, Takigawa M, Kees F, Straub RH, Paus R (2005) Human hair follicles display a functional equivalent of the hypothalamic-pituitary-adrenal axis and synthesize cortisol. FASEB J 19:1332–1334

Ives DG, Kuller LH, Schulz R, Traven ND, Lave JR (1992) Comparison of recruitment strategies and associated disease prevalence for health promotion in rural elderly. Prev Med 21:582–591

Jafferany M (2007) Psychodermatology: a guide to understanding common psychocutaneous disorders. Prim Care Companion J Clin Psychiatry 9:203–213

Joachim RA, Kuhlmei A, Dinh QT, Handjiski B, Fischer T, Peters EM, Klapp BF, Paus R, Arck PC (2007) Neuronal plasticity of the "brain-skin connection": stress-triggered up-regulation of neuropeptides in dorsal root ganglia and skin via nerve growth factor-dependent pathways. J Mol Med (Berl) 85:1369–1378

Kagiwada K, Chida D, Sakatani T, Asano M, Nambu A, Kakuta S, Iwakura Y (2004) Interleukin (IL)-6, but not IL-1, induction in the brain downstream of cyclooxygenase-2 is essential for the induction of febrile response against peripheral IL-1alpha. Endocrinology 145:5044–5048

Kalow W (1982) Ethnic differences in drug metabolism. Clin Pharmacokinet 7:373–400

Kariagina A, Romanenko D, Ren SG, Chesnokova V (2004) Hypothalamic-pituitary cytokine network. Endocrinology 145:104–112

Kellogg DL Jr (2006) In vivo mechanisms of cutaneous vasodilation and vasoconstriction in humans during thermoregulatory challenges. J Appl Physiol 100:1709–1718

Kitani A, Hara M, Hirose T, Harigai M, Suzuki K, Kawakami M, Kawaguchi Y, Hidaka T, Kawagoe M, Nakamura H (1992) Autostimulatory effects of IL-6 on excessive B cell differentiation in patients with systemic lupus erythematosus: analysis of IL-6 production and IL-6R expression. Clin Exp Immunol 88:75–83

Kleyn CE, Schneider L, Saraceno R, Mantovani C, Richards HL, Fortune DG, Cumberbatch M, Dearman RJ, Terenghi G, Kimber I, Griffiths CE (2008) The effects of acute social stress on epidermal Langerhans' cell frequency and expression of cutaneous neuropeptides. J Invest Dermatol 128:1273–1279

Kono M, Nagata H, Umemura S, Kawana S, Osamura RY (2001) In situ expression of corticotropin-releasing hormone (CRH) and proopiomelanocortin (POMC) genes in human skin. FASEB J 15:2297–2299

Langan EA, Foitzik-Lau K, Goffin V, Ramot Y, Paus R (2010) Prolactin: an emerging force along the cutaneous-endocrine axis. Trends Endocrinol Metab 21:569–577

Lange-Asschenfeldt C, Grohmann R, Lange-Asschenfeldt B, Engel RR, Ruther E, Cordes J (2009) Cutaneous adverse reactions to psychotropic drugs: data from a multicenter surveillance program. J Clin Psychiatry 70:1258–1265

Levi-Montalcini R, Skaper SD, Dal Toso R, Petrelli L, Leon A (1996) Nerve growth factor: from neurotrophin to neurokine. Trends Neurosci 19:514–520

Locala JA (2009) Current concepts in psychodermatology. Curr. Psychiatry Rep. 11:211–218

Marks R (2004) The stratum corneum barrier: the final frontier. J Nutr 134:2017S–2021S

Mastorakos G, Chrousos GP, Weber JS (1993) Recombinant interleukin-6 activates the hypothalamic-pituitary-adrenal axis in humans. J Clin Endocrinol Metab 77:1690–1694

Mason AA (1952) A case of congenital ichthyosiform erythrodermia of brocq treated by hypnosis. Br Med J 2:422–423

Mitkov MV, Trowbridge RM, Lockshin BN, Caplan JP (2014) Dermatological side effects of psychtropic medications. Psychosomatics 55:1–20

Miyazaki Y, Yokozeki H, Awad S, Igawa K, Minatohara K, Satoh T, Katayama I, Nishioka K (2000) Glucocorticoids augment the chemically induced production and gene expression of interleukin-1α through NF-kB and AP-1 activation in murine epidermal cells. J Invest Dermatol 115:746–752

Nakano Y (2007) Effect of chronic topical exposure to low-dose noxious chemicals and stress on skin sensitivity in mice. J Occup Health 49:431–442

Panina-Bordignon P, Mazzeo D, Lucia PD, D'Ambrosio D, Lang R, Fabbri L, Self C, Sinigaglia F (1997) $ß_2$-agonists prevent Th1 development by selective inhibition of interleukin 12. J Clin Invest 100:1513–1519

Pergola PE, Kellogg DL Jr, Johnson JM, Kosiba WA, Solomon DE (1993) Role of sympathetic nerves in the vascular effects of local temperature in human forearm skin. Am J Physiol 265: H785–H792
Peters EM, Botchkarev VA, Botchkareva NV, Tobin DJ, Paus R (2001) Hair-cycle-associated remodeling of the peptidergic innervation of murine skin, and hair growth modulation by neuropeptides. J Invest Dermatol 116:236–245
Raber J, Sorg O, Horn TF, Yu N, Koob GF, Campbell IL, Bloom FE (1998) Inflammatory cytokines: putative regulators of neuronal and neuro-endocrine function. Brain Res Rev 26:320–326
Ramot Y, Biro T, Tiede S, Toth BI, Langan EA, Sugawara K, Foitzik K, Ingber A, Goffin V, Langbein L, Paus R (2010) Prolactin–a novel neuroendocrine regulator of human keratin expression in situ. FASEB J 24:1768–1779
Schutz B, von Engelhardt J, Gordes M, Schafer MK, Eiden LE, Monyer H, Weihe E (2008) Sweat gland innervation is pioneered by sympathetic neurons expressing a cholinergic/noradrenergic co-phenotype in the mouse. Neuroscience 156:310–318
Segerstrom SC (2008) Social networks and immunosuppression during stress: Relationship conflict or energy conservation? Brain Behav Immun 22:279–284
Seiffert K, Granstein RD (2006) Neuroendocrine regulation of skin dendritic cells. Ann NY Acad Sci 1088:195–206
Seiffert K, Hosoi J, Torii H, Ozawa H, Ding W, Campton K, Wagner JA, Granstein RD (2002) Catecholamines inhibit the antigen-presenting capability of epidermal Langerhans cells. J Immunol 168:6128–6135
Shenefelt PD (2003) Biofeedback, cognitive-behavioral methods, and hypnosis in dermatology: is it all in your mind? Dermatol Ther 16:114–122
Shenefelt PD (2000) Hypnosis in dermatology. Arch Dermatol 136:393–399
Shenefelt PD (2011) Psychodermatological disorders: recognition and treatment. Int J Dermatol 50:1309–1322
Singh LK, Pang X, Alexacos N, Letourneau R, Theoharides TC (1999) Acute immobilization stress triggers skin mast cell degranulation via corticotropin releasing hormone, neurotensin, and substance P: A link to neurogenic skin disorders. Brain Behav Immun 13:225–239
Slominski A, Pisarchik A, Tobin DJ, Mazurkiewicz JE, Wortsman J (2004) Differential expression of a cutaneous corticotropin-releasing hormone system. Endocrinology 145:941–950
Slominski A, Roloff B, Curry J, Dahiya M, Szczesniewski A, Wortsman J (2000a) The skin produces urocortin. J Clin Endocrinol Metab 85:815–823
Slominski A, Szczesniewski A, Wortsman J (2000b) Liquid chromatography-mass spectrometry detection of corticotropin-releasing hormone and proopiomelanocortin-derived peptides in human skin. J Clin Endocrinol Metab 85:3582–3588
Slominski A, Tobin DJ, Zmijewski MA, Wortsman J, Paus R (2008) Melatonin in the skin: synthesis, metabolism and functions. Trends Endocrinol Metab 19:17–24
Takeda K, Kaisho T, Yoshida N, Takeda J, Kishimoto T, Akira S (1998) Stat3 activation is responsible for IL-6-dependent T cell proliferation through preventing apoptosis: generation and characterization of T cell-specific Stat3-deficient mice. J Immunol 161:4652–4660
Tausk F, Elenkov I, Moynihan J (2008) Psychoneuroimmunology. Dermatol Ther 21:22–31
Thepen T, Langeveld-Wildschut EG, Bihari IC, van Wichen DF, van Reijsen FC, Mudde GC, Bruijnzeel-Koomen CA (1996) Biphasic response against aeroallergen in atopic dermatitis showing a switch from an initial TH2 response to a TH1 response in situ: an immunocytochemical study. J Allergy Clin Immunol 97:828–837
Tsagarakis S, Navarra P, Rees LH, Besser M, Grossman A, Navara P (1989) Morphine directly modulates the release of stimulated corticotrophin-releasing factor-41 from rat hypothalamus in vitro. Endocrinology 124:2330–2335
Tsigos C, Chrousos GP (2002) Hypothalamic-pituitary-adrenal axis, neuroendocrine factors and stress. J Psychosom Res 53:865–871
Ullman M (1947) Herpes simplex and second degree burn induced under hypnosis. Am J Psych 103:828–830

Weihe E, Schutz B, Hartschuh W, Anlauf M, Schafer MK, Eiden LE (2005) Coexpression of cholinergic and noradrenergic phenotypes in human and nonhuman autonomic nervous system. J Comp Neurol 492:370–379
Whitnall MH (1993) Regulation of the hypothalamic corticotropin-releasing hormone neurosecretory system. Prog Neurobiol 40:573–629
Wistar R Jr, Hildemann WH (1960) Effect of stress on skin transplantation immunity in mice. Science 131:159–160
Yanagawa Y, Matsumoto M, Togashi H (2010) Enhanced dendritic cell antigen uptake via alpha2 adrenoceptor-mediated PI3 K activation following brief exposure to noradrenaline. J Immunol 185:5762–5768
Zimmerman BG, Whitmore L (1967) Transmitter release in skin and muscle blood vessels during sympathetic stimulation. Am J Physiol 212:1043–1054

Index

G.T. Wondrak (ed.), *Skin Stress Response Pathways*,
DOI 10.1007/978-3-319-43157-4

MIX
Papier aus verantwortungsvollen Quellen
Paper from responsible sources
FSC® C105338

If you have any concerns about our products,
you can contact us on
ProductSafety@springernature.com

In case Publisher is established outside the EU,
the EU authorized representative is:
Springer Nature Customer Service Center GmbH
Europaplatz 3, 69115 Heidelberg, Germany

Printed by Libri Plureos GmbH
in Hamburg, Germany